Crisis and Trauma

Crisis and Trauma

Developmental-Ecological Intervention

Barbara G. Collins
East Stroudsburg University

Thomas M. Collins
University of Scranton

Lahaska Press
Houghton Mifflin Company
Boston   New York

Publisher, Lahaska Press: Barry Fetterolf
Senior Editor, Lahaska Press: Mary Falcon
Editorial Assistant: Lisa Littlewood
Associate Project Editor: Shelley Dickerson
Marketing Manager: Brenda Bravener-Greville
Senior Manufacturing Coordinator: Marie Barnes

Cover image: © Noriko O. Kawamoto/Photonica

Lahaska Press, a unique collaboration between the Houghton Mifflin College Division and Lawrence Erlbaum Associates, is dedicated to publishing books and offering services for the academic and professional counseling communities. The partnership of Lahaska Press was formed in late 1999. The name "Lahaska" is a Native American Lenape word meaning "source of much writing." The small eastern Pennsylvania town of Lahaska, named by the Lenape, is the home of the Lahaska Press editorial offices.

Acknowledgments appear on page 538, which constitutes an extension of the copyright page.

Printed in the U.S.A.

Library of Congress Catalog Number: 2003103116

ISBN: 0-618-37371-3

23456789 – QUF – 08 07 06 05 04

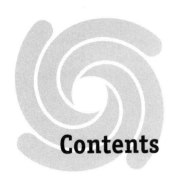

Contents

CHAPTER 8   **Substance Abuse**   240

FORD BROOKS

THOMAS M. COLLINS

CHAPTER 9   **Chronic and Terminal Illness**   280
ELIZABETH J. JACOB
THOMAS M. COLLINS

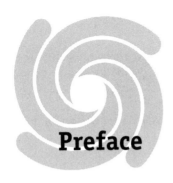

Preface

Crisis and Trauma reflects our belief that knowledge about crisis events, crisis responses, and crisis counseling is central to the competence of every human service professional, regardless of specific discipline. All individuals may experience crises in their lives, and all helping professionals will encounter individuals responding to crises—sometimes in their immediate aftermath, and sometimes months or even years later. Furthermore, the knowledge and skills that lead to competent and effective crisis counseling are applicable to many other professional roles.

Crisis represents a time of great challenge to affected individuals. The repercussions can be debilitating and long lasting, but not necessarily so. Indeed, many individuals emerge from crises with renewed appreciation of their lives and their own strength and resilience. It is the authors' belief in this later possibility that frames the orientation and approach this text presents.

This text is written at a time when societal recognition of crises and the psychological aftermath of crises is at an all-time high. We began writing *Crisis and Trauma* in the aftermath of September 11, 2001—a day that, like Pearl Harbor, will be a day of infamy and great personal, community, and societal loss and suffering. It will also be a day remembered for the heroic and altruistic behaviors of many individuals, including first responders, such as emergency personnel, police, and firefighters, as well as everyday citizens. Several of the contributors to this text were part of that effort.

AUTHORS AND CONTRIBUTORS

The primary authors and the invited contributors to this text are all experienced clinicians with many years of experience providing crisis counseling services. Our respective disciplines include mental health counseling, social work, and psychology. Many of us have also been activists involved in grassroots community organizing and creation of crisis intervention programs and services.

The authors and most of the contributors are also experienced educators and researchers. We have taught crisis intervention courses to both undergraduate and graduate students in human services, counseling, social work, and psychology. The authors of the applied crisis intervention chapters (Chapters 6 to 13) were selected because of their expertise and experience in that particular crisis arena (see author identification information).

RATIONALE

We wrote this book in large part because we were not satisfied with the other available models for working with individuals in the aftermath of crises. We strove to write a practice-oriented text that would present and apply a genuinely holistic model of crisis counseling incorporating assessment into intervention from time of immediate postimpact to resolution. We also strove to present a conceptualization that placed crisis responses on a continuum. The "continuum" concept can be utilized to accurately assess when individuals' crisis responses cross a diagnostic threshold, when responses indicate potential danger to self or others, and accordingly to accurately identify those crisis survivors requiring primarily information and connection to community resources and those requiring more intensive crisis intervention. As will be discussed in the chapter on disasters, in crisis situations involving many survivors, crisis responders must quickly triage in order to provide services according to need.

Further, contrary to the oft-stated assertion that the goal of crisis intervention is to assist individuals to return to a precrisis state, the authors' experience with crisis survivors has convinced us that individuals are changed by the experience of crisis and traumatic events. As noted, that does not mean the change is necessarily negative, though for some it may be as their struggles to adapt are compromised by poor coping skills, lack of resources, or other personal and/or environmental deficits. But many others are changed by newly found appreciation of their strength and resilience, by the development of new strategies for coping, or by a renewed sense of what is important in their lives. Ultimately, individuals must find some way to incorporate the reality of experienced crises into their ongoing personal and relational development, and they are changed if only by their recognition that such crises can and do occur. Our perspective emphasizes survivor strengths and creativity, and the crisis counselor's primary role as an empowering companion.

THEORETICAL APPROACH

As will be elaborated, this text's approach to crisis counseling assessment and intervention is based on a **developmental-ecological perspective**. This perspective draws on both developmental and systems theory to provide a holistic and integrated framework for viewing individual responses to crisis events. This perspective suggests that individuals' psychological responses (emotional, behavioral, cognitive) must be seen within the context of life-span development. Furthermore, individuals, crisis events, and recovery environments must be comprehended as situated within a particular ecology that includes personal, social, and material resources, the physical environment, the community, and the individual's unique culture. Although this comprehensive, holistic "lens" may at first glance appear overwhelming, we contend that a more reductionist approach does not yield interventions responsive to the unique complexity of each of the individuals we serve, whether our encounter is a single session or ongoing.

The assessment and intervention models that emerge from this holistic perspective also reflect an appreciation of the bio-psycho-social impact of crises. Although our assessment model does not directly name physiology as a separate domain for assessment, we speak about the physiological component of crisis response in numerous examples and references. This is a particularly salient issue discussed in the health crisis chapter and is also an essential focus in discussing posttraumatic stress symptoms and responses.

Similarly, our model does not identify spirituality as a separate assessment domain. However, we continuously acknowledge the importance of spirituality in many persons' lives and the significant role that spiritual beliefs and traditions have in affecting how individuals attribute meaning to particular crises and contemplate healing and their futures.

OVERVIEW OF TEXT

The text is organized in three parts. The first part includes the first five chapters. It introduces fundamental concepts in crisis theory and practice, and presents the authors' theoretical framework, assessment model, and intervention models. Chapter 4 introduces readers to basic counselor attributes and skills necessary for working in crisis counseling settings. Chapter 5 provides an overview of the continuum of response to crisis and covers both diagnosis and assessment of lethality.

The second part, Chapters 6 through 13, addresses a variety of unique crises, including sexual assault (Chapter 6), domestic violence (Chapter 7), substance abuse (Chapter 8), health crises (Chapter 9), crises of death (Chapter 10), child abuse and neglect (Chapter 11), school crises (Chapter 12), and disasters (Chapter 13). In each of these chapters, information regarding the dynamics and impact of that specific crisis are examined, and both single-session and ongoing crisis counseling with individuals who have experienced that type of crisis are described. Every chapter ends with an extended case example of either a single-session crisis intervention or an ongoing crisis counseling process.

Chapter 14, the final chapter in the text, discusses burnout, compassion fatigue, and vicarious traumatization. It ends with a personal reflection by the coordinator of mental health responses at "Ground Zero" in New York City following the September 11 attacks on the World Trade Center.

REAL CRISES, REAL LIVES

Each of the chapters, but particularly Chapters 6 through 14, contain numerous case vignettes and examples. Each of these vignettes is drawn from crisis counseling situations involving real individuals dealing with real crises in their lives. We carefully changed information that might identify a particular individual; however, the descriptions of situations and responses are true, and the excerpts of dialog are representative of what actually occurred.

In response to the suggestion of reviewers, we have deleted most references to individuals' culture, race, or ethnicity. Thus, unless it was specifically germane to a discussion focused on the impact of culture, the reader will not find individuals described by these characteristics. This was a conscious decision made to avoid the possible stereotyping resulting from specific racial or cultural identifiers being associated with particular crises or crises responses. However, the implications of age, gender, ability, ethnicity, and culture are discussed in varying ways throughout the text and are specifically included as one component of the ecology of individuals within our assessment and intervention models

INTENDED AUDIENCE

This book is designed as a primary text for upper-level undergraduate and graduate students in Crisis Intervention courses in a variety of disciplines, including counseling, social work, and psychology. Although we recognize that not all programs currently offer a separate course in Crisis Intervention, it is our strong hope that curriculum development will increasingly reflect the current knowledge about the role of trauma and crises in individuals' lives and the importance of preparing professionals competent to provide crisis counseling interventions. This text can usefully function as a primary and/or supplemental text in other professional preparation courses (e.g., counseling theories, counseling skills, case management, practicum, internship), and/or for specialized advanced training provided to teachers, nurses, and other education, criminal justice, and human service professionals. In addition, the book may be a reference for current helping professionals who wish to increase their knowledge about crisis and their competence as crisis counselors.

ACKNOWLEDGMENTS

The authors wish to express their appreciation to a number of individuals who have generously assisted us in this project. First we thank the East Stroudsburg University students who field-tested this text for the first time in their Fall 2002 Crisis Intervention class. Once they overcame their initial reluctance to criticize their professor's text, they offered compelling, insightful, and useful feedback, almost all of which was incorporated into the final draft. We also highlight the tremendous contribution of Tracy Moore, graduate assistant in the Counseling program at the University of Scranton, who painstakingly verified each reference used in the text.

We also express appreciation to the reviewers of this text whose detailed and constructive questions, comments, and suggestions stimulated our thinking and ultimately resulted in what we believe were important revisions and improvements. They are Amy S. Badura, Ph.D. (Creighton University), Ann C. Diver-Stamnes, Ph.D. (Humboldt State University), Noreen M. Glover, Ph.D. (Syracuse University), Douglas Guiffrida, Ph.D. (University of Rochester), Gordon Hart, Ph.D. (Temple University), Russell Lee, Ph.D. (Bemidji State Univeristy), Peter Manzi, Ph.D. (University of Rochester), and Rick A. Myer, Ph.D. (Duquesne University).

And last, we appreciate the encouragement, support, feedback, and expert editorial assistance from Barry Fetterolf, Mary Falcon, and Shelley Dickerson (Lahaska Press and Houghton Mifflin), and Nancy Benjamin (Books By Design).

DEDICATION

Finally, we dedicate this book to the two groups of individuals who are its focus: crisis survivors and crisis responders. With great respect and caring, we acknowledge the many crisis survivors we have worked with during our professional lives. It is they who have taught us about the real meaning of crisis and about the struggle to move from victim to survivor. Second, we acknowledge both the crisis counselors who on a daily basis join with crisis survivors in their struggle to rebuild their lives and the numerous first responders who at times have risked, and lost, theirs in the line of duty.

Barbara G. Collins
Thomas M. Collins

Authors and Contributors

BARBARA G. COLLINS, Ph.D., LCSW, BCD, is Professor and Chair of the Department of Sociology, Criminal Justice, and Social Work, East Stroudsburg University. She has been a community organizer and founded multiple crisis programs, including psychiatric crisis services and community programs to serve survivors of domestic violence and sexual assault. She provides consultation and training in the areas of both child and adult trauma, and has thirty years of clinical experience in community mental health and private practice, where she specializes in working with health crises, trauma survivors, and sexuality. She also presents and publishes on these topics.

THOMAS M. COLLINS, Ph.D., NCC, LPC, is Director of the Community Counseling program at the University of Scranton and Director of the collaborative Community Counseling program with Universidad Iberoamericana in Mexico City. He also co-directs a USAID TIES-ENLACES funded International Collaboration for Community Development program. Chair-Elect of the National Board for Certified Counselors, he is a licensed professional counselor and licensed psychologist, and holds a post-doctoral certificate in psychopharmacology. He has over twenty-five years of clinical experience as a therapist, supervisor, and consultant in inpatient and outpatient mental health, psychosocial oncology, child welfare, and private practice. He is active in efforts to globalize the counseling profession and to meet the mental health needs of underserved populations nationally and internationally.

CONTRIBUTORS

Ford Brooks, Ed.D., LPC, CAC, is Assistant Professor, Counselor Education, Shippensburg University. He has worked as a mental health counselor in inpatient, outpatient, and private practice settings, primarily with addicted and dually diagnosed clients. He presents and publishes on the topics of addiction, relapse, and spirituality.

LeeAnn Eschbach, Ph.D., NCC, LPC, is Director, School Counseling program, University of Scranton. She serves as a consultant to schools for special programming and supervision, and is a member of a district-wide crisis response team.

Elizabeth J. Jacob, Ph.D., NCC, LPC, is Associate Professor, Department of Counseling and Human Services, University of Scranton. Her research interests include multicultural and global/international issues, identity development of Asian Indians, and health psychology with clinical experiences in inpatient and outpatient settings. She currently co-directs a USAID TIES-ENLACES funded International Collaboration for Community Development program.

John W. Kraybill-Greggo, M.S.W., L.S.W., A.C.S.W., is the Director of the Counselor Training Center and teaches in the Department of Counseling and Human Services at the University of Scranton. Currently a Ph.D. candidate in Social Work at Rutgers University, he has provided direct and administrative services in hospice, inpatient oncology, veteran's medical care, and community-based mental health.

Marcella J. Kraybill-Greggo, M.S.W., L.S.W., currently supervises the Child Mentoring Program at Valley Youth House in Allentown, Pennsylvania, and teaches spirituality and counseling at Elizabethtown College and the University of Scranton. She has worked with bereavement issues as a certified Spiritual Director and as the Children's Program Director of a San Francisco homeless shelter.

JoAnn Packer, Psy.D., is a licensed psychologist who has maintained a private practice for over 20 years in Princeton, New Jersey, and more recently in Waitsfield, Vermont. She is a consultant to employee assistance programs and a certified Red Cross disaster responder.

Michele Ann Tavormina, M.S.W., LCSW, is a Clinical Social Worker in private practice specializing in childhood physical and sexual abuse. She provides training and consultation in the field of child maltreatment and is a Doctoral Candidate in Clinical Social Work at New York University.

Grace Telesco, Ph.D., is an assistant professor in the Department of Sociology, Criminal Justice, and Social Work at East Stroudsburg University and a retired lieutenant in the New York City Police Department. She was selected as the interagency coordinator of the mental health response at the New York Family Assistance Center following the September 11th attacks where crisis intervention and support services were provided to over 20,000 individuals. Dr. Telesco has also served as chairperson of the Behavioral Science Department at the New York Police Academy and held teaching positions at St. John's University, John Jay College of Criminal Justice, and Fordham University's Graduate School of Social Service.

Mollie Whalen, Ph.D., is professor and director of the Women's Studies program and the Women's Center at East Stroudsburg University. Author of *Counseling to End Violence Against Women*, she has been active in the battered women's movement and anti-rape movement for over fifteen years and continues to participate in the international movement to end violence against women.

CHAPTER 1

Understanding Crisis and Crisis Intervention

U.S. Attacked; Hijacked Jets Destroy Twin Towers and Hit Pentagon in Day of Terror
By N. R. KLEINFIELD *(New York Times)*
September 12, 2001

ABSTRACT—. . . scenes of horror in lower Manhattan after World Trade Center towers were rammed by two hijacked jetliners.

• • •

Terror in Littleton: The Overview
2 Students in Colorado School Said to Gun Down as Many as 23 and Kill Themselves in a Siege
By JAMES BROOKE *(New York Times)*
April 21, 1999

ABSTRACT—Armed youths identified as Eric Harris and Dylan Klebold storm into Columbine High School in Littleton, Colo., killing up to 23 students and teachers and wounding at least 20 in five-hour siege before killing themselves; at least 13 bombs are found in school; one, set with timer, explodes in school at night; three autos are found rigged with bombs, including one that explodes; bodies of gunmen and some of victims are also apparently wired with explosives; gunmen apparently targeted minorities and athletes, as well as peers who poked fun of their group in past; two other students, thought to be gunmen's friends, are being questioned.

• • •

Workers Search Quake's Wall of Dirt for Victims
By DAVID GONZALEZ *(New York Times)*
January 15, 2001

ABSTRACT—Rescuers race to save victims trapped in huge landslide set off by powerful earthquake, Santa Tecla, El Salvador; landslide smothered some 500 homes, killing scores of people; rescue officials estimate 7.6 magnitude quake, centered off El Salvador's coast, killed over 400 people nationwide, with thousands still missing.

• • •

Women Tell of Priests' Abusing Them as Girls
By SAM DILLON *(New York Times)*

DALLAS, June 14—Linda Burke said that when she was a 14-year-old growing up in Chicago, her priest began wrestling with her on the floor, roughhousing so insistently that her clothing became undone.

When she was 17, she said, another priest began to kiss and fondle her in a chapel, and later other priests used their spiritual influence to seduce her

1

into full-fledged sex. The abuse continued for years after she became an adult, she said. "I couldn't say no," said Ms. Burke, who participated here today in an encounter of women who say they have been abused by Roman Catholic clergymen.

As these news stories taken from the headlines of newspapers illustrate, a crisis can affect any one of us at any time. Whether a car accident, domestic violence, a kidnapping, mugging, rape, hurricane, earthquake, or a terrorist attack, each type of situation is potentially a crisis event in individuals' lives. Some events are so severe and threatening to one's sense of safety and security that they are physically and psychologically traumatizing.

In some situations, the impact of these crises and/or traumatic events is long lasting and life changing although crisis and crisis reactions are generally assumed to be time-limited. Many individuals faced with crisis events cope on their own, relying on the support and assistance of family, friends, or trusted individuals like clergy or family physicians. Most individuals find some means to adapt in the aftermath of a crisis. Others find that the immediate impact of the event overwhelms them and they are unable to cope even with the assistance of supportive friends and family. And still others find that the adaptations they make to cope with the immediate, acute stress and/or trauma do not work or are not healthy adaptations because in the long run they create additional difficulties.

In this brief introduction, we've used words like *crisis, trauma, crisis reaction,* and *coping*. But what exactly do these concepts mean? When is a difficult situation a crisis? What makes a situation a traumatic event? When does a person's response to a stressful situation become a crisis reaction? And how does one intervene to effectively assist individuals who are experiencing crises in their lives? As a prelude to addressing these questions, we will explore the theoretical and philosophical view of human nature that underlies our notion of crisis and crisis intervention.

CRISIS AND CRISIS THEORY

In an early book on working with people in crisis, Dixon (1979) asserted that all crisis theory is grounded in a holistic view of human nature and individual development. Drawing on various developmental theories, he described how over the course of the life span each human organism develops habitual thinking, feeling, and behavioral patterns for meeting basic needs, meeting the demands and challenges posed by the social environment, and resolving everyday problems and stresses. In general, this personal system of habitual responses enables individuals to maintain a sense of equilibrium or a "steady state." Dixon asserted that because there are always a number of conflicting internal and external stimuli with which developing human beings must contend, some degree of disequilibrium is a common aspect of human life. Despite these challenges, most of the time individuals are able to use the techniques they have developed for coping with stress and are able to engage in at least minimally successful, everyday, normal social functioning.

Crisis and Coping

Blocher (2000) discussed coping behaviors as individuals' routinized ways of garnering personal, interpersonal, and social resources in response to stressors or problems. Children develop characteristic ways of coping and those patterns are *2 major coping styles* refined and strengthened throughout their lives. Although there is tremendous variation in the characteristic coping strategies individuals develop, early writers in the field identified two major coping styles (Folkman, 1984; Lazarus & Folkman, 1984). Emotion-focused coping includes avoiding and minimizing emotions as well as expressing emotions and seeking emotional support. Problem-focused coping emphasizes the utilization of problem-solving strategies including acquisition of new skills. More recently, authors have criticized this view as an overly simplistic conception of coping behaviors and have developed more extensive typologies of characteristic coping styles. (Coping behaviors and research examining effective and ineffective coping is discussed at greater length in Chapter 2.)

① Emotion-Focused
② Problem Focused

Many individuals' characteristic coping strategies ordinarily result in effective responses to problems. Some individuals have deficits in their normal coping skills or have developed dysfunctional coping patterns. Whether or not an individual's coping strategies are functional and healthy, some experiences and some external stimuli exceed one's capacity to adapt. Strategies that have been effective may be ineffective in face of tremendous stressors. Those who have deficits in coping skills or who characteristically utilize dysfunctional coping patterns may find that their difficulties in coping are exacerbated. In such instances, when the external stimuli and/or events are of such magnitude, intensity, and/or suddenness that habitual methods for coping fail, an individual is typically considered to be in crisis.

Development of Crisis Theory

The advent of contemporary theories of crisis and crisis intervention is often traced to a tragic event that occurred in 1942: the Cocoanut Grove fire in Boston, Massachusetts. The Cocoanut Grove was a large nightclub in which 493 people perished as fire engulfed the nightclub, many trampled to death as they tried to escape. Dr. Eric Lindemann treated many of the survivors and noted that they seemed to have common emotional responses and needs. He began to theorize about what he termed "normal" grief reactions including preoccupation with lost loved ones, identification with the deceased, expressions of guilt and hostility, varying degrees of disorganization in daily routine, and varied somatic complaints (Janosick, 1984; Lindemann, 1944).

Gerald Caplan also worked with survivors in the aftermath of the Cocoanut Grove fire. That experience was a catalyst for his interest in exploring and explaining what constituted a crisis, and he is often credited with being one of the originators of contemporary crisis theory. Caplan (1961) described *crisis* as follows: "People are in a state of crisis when they face an obstacle to important life goals—an obstacle that is, for a time, insurmountable by the use of customary methods of problem-solving. A period of disorganization ensues, a period of upset, during which many abortive attempts at solution are made" (p. 18). Caplan's interest in crisis and crisis intervention eventually led to his pioneering work intervening with families in crisis at the Harvard Public Health Family Guidance Center, where he was joined by another noted figure in the development of crisis theory, Howard Parad. Especially interested in examining the impact of particular types of crises on families, Parad and Caplan identified five elements that affected families' abilities to cope with a hazardous life event and that ultimately explained what constituted a crisis for them:

1. The stressful event poses a problem which is by definition insoluble in the immediate future.
2. The problem overtaxes the psychological resources of the family, since it is beyond their traditional problem-solving methods.
3. The situation is perceived as a threat or danger to the life goals of the family members.
4. The crisis period is characterized by tension which mounts to a peak, then falls.
5. Perhaps of the greatest importance, the crisis situation awakens unresolved key problems from both the near and distant past. (Parad & Caplan, 1960, pp. 11–12)

Numerous other theorists and practitioners have since built on these ideas, attempting to delineate a clear and comprehensive definition of crisis and to identify the criteria that distinguish a crisis event and a crisis reaction from stress and stress reactions. Dixon (1979) drew a useful distinction between stress and crisis in describing stress as a process that exists over time, as, for example, the stress of working under the pressure of meeting deadlines. Stress reactions can be and often are debilitating. Many people, however, live and work under stress for years, and in most cases individuals recognize the conditions or pressures that create the sense of stress (e.g., deadlines, too many responsibilities). By contrast, a crisis event is "generally unexpected, the adverse reaction is acute, temporal in nature, and emotionally debilitating" (Dixon, 1979, p. 20).

Defining Crisis

Slaikeu (1990, p. 15) defined crisis as "a temporary state of upset and disorganization, characterized chiefly by an individual's inability to cope with a particular situation using customary methods of problem-solving, and by the potential for a radically positive or negative outcome." James and Gilliland (2001) defined crisis as "a perception or experiencing of an event or situation as an intolerable difficulty that exceeds the person's current resources and coping mechanisms" (p. 3).

What do these multiple descriptions of crisis suggest are the elements by which an event becomes a crisis and a person's response a crisis reaction? First, it is clear that in crisis situations there is *an identifiable stimulus or catalyst: an obstacle to an important goal, a life event, or a traumatic incident.* This "catalyst event" may be predictable and identified in advance, as, for example, a retirement or the death of an individual with a terminal illness, or it may be unpredictable, as, for example, a sexual assault, the diagnosis of a debilitating health condition, or a natural disaster. Notably, in either case, a specific identifiable event is the catalyst for the crisis reaction. Second, there is *the individual's perception of the stimulus or event and its impact.* What one person perceives as an unbearably traumatic event may not be as disruptive to another. How the individual sees the event and perceives its meaning in his or her life ultimately determines the sense of it as "intolerable." Third, whatever the specific catalyst event, its impact on the individual *exceeds his or her ability to cope using his or her normal adaptive capacities.* Using the words of various theorists, the event creates a temporary "state of disorganization" (Brammer, 1985, p. 94) or disequilibrium characterized by the individual's inability to resolve the disruption by "the use of customary methods of problem-solving" (Caplan, 1961, p. 18). And last, there is an assumption that the state of being in crisis, the "intolerable" period during which one is unable to cope and/or successfully problem-solve, must be *time-limited.* According to Caplan (1961), the immediate impact of a crisis usually lasts from four to six weeks depending on the nature and intensity of the crisis event and reaction. This is not to say that there are no longer-lasting effects of many crises. The period of intense disorganization or disequilibrium, however, cannot be tolerated indefinitely; thus individuals will find some means of reestablishing needed stability.

Defining Trauma and Traumatic Events

Traumatic events are a particular kind of crisis event. In general, traumatic events are so extreme, powerful, and threatening that they overwhelm an individual's sense of safety and security. Some traumatic events are short-term—single, relatively brief but extreme threats like rape, assault, or a natural disaster. Others are long-term events that occur over time and result in prolonged or repeated exposure to the extreme threat. Examples of the latter include childhood sexual abuse, domestic violence, and some technological disasters.

According to the *Diagnostic and Statistical Manual of Mental Disorders* (American Psychiatric Association, 2000), a traumatic event is one that involved "actual or threatened death or serious injury, or a threat to the physical integrity of self or others" and one in which "the person's response involved intense fear, helplessness, or horror" (pp. 218–219). Individuals may experience both acute and chronic responses following exposure to traumatic events (see Chapter 5). Although not all individuals who are exposed to traumatic events develop trauma responses, many experience crisis reactions of some intensity, and the prevalence of Acute Stress Disorder and Posttraumatic Stress Disorder (PTSD) is quite high.

Crises and Reactivated Responses

The last element to discuss regarding crisis and trauma responses was first identified by Parad and Caplan (1960) in their description of family crises. As previously noted, they asserted that crisis situations might reawaken unresolved problems and needs in individuals' lives. They described the reappearance of emotional or behavioral problems long after an initial crisis has subsided. The typical pattern is one in which the original crisis event was not fully resolved at the time, but rather pushed aside or submerged until a new stressor resonates with the old and reactivates the unresolved or "unfinished" business.

Even individuals who have adjusted to a prior crisis or traumatic event may find that exposure to a new trauma reactivates the emotions and arousal associated with the original event, complicating their current responses. For example, many victims of the Oklahoma City federal building bombing had begun to recover and move forward with their lives by September 2001. When the World Trade Center in New York City and the Pentagon were attacked, however, many experienced renewed but all too familiar responses of terror, horror, and grief.

In uncomplicated reactivation of traumatic responses, individuals who previously recovered from trauma symptoms experience a reemergence of those symptoms in response to the current trauma exposure. In complicated reactivation, individuals who were still experiencing residual posttraumatic reactions experience exacerbation of their symptoms and in some instances significantly increased impairment (Hiley-Young, 1992).

Recognition of this potential for continued risk directs attention to the idea that crisis events pose both danger and opportunity. For a crisis or trauma event to truly be resolved and integrated into individuals' lives, affected persons must either be able to return, unchanged, to their prior ways and level of functioning or they must develop new skills and may need to change their ways of thinking and believing. For example, a person may become aware of personal strengths previously unnoticed or untested. If a crisis remains unresolved, however, or if the behaviors used to cope merely institute a fragile on-the-surface stability, the individual may function in a compromised manner in order to maintain that fragile equilibrium. An increased risk for future traumatic responses may also result.

Types of Crises

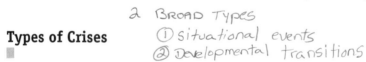

2 Broad Types
① Situational events
② Developmental transitions

Crises are typically divided into two broad types: those precipitated by *situational events,* and those related to and precipitated by *developmental transitions.* As will be discussed in later chapters, all crisis reactions, whatever the catalyst, take place during a particular developmental period in an individual's life and thus have potential developmental implications and/or impact. In defining different types of crises, however, it is helpful to recognize that in some crises the precipitating or stimulus event that causes the crisis reaction is actually embedded in normal maturational processes rather than an external event like sexual assault or the diagnosis of a life-threatening illness.

Developmental crises Individuals who have studied human experiences across the life span have noted that as human beings age they are constantly changing and growing (see Chapter 3). Various theorists have further noted that the types of changes that humans experience appear to be similar and to occur at similar times in individuals' lives. The concept of normal development essentially means that individuals change over time in predictable ways, with "normal" referring to what is typical for most people in a particular age group whether the age group is infancy, adolescence, or over the age of sixty-five.

Developmental theorists have also noted that human beings' ability to grow and change in expected ways is a product of the interaction between individual physiological needs and abilities and social expectations, demands, resources, and opportunities (Bronfenbrenner, 1979, 1989). Healthy growth, which entails the accomplishment of cognitive, emotional, and/or behavioral tasks and the successful enactment of expected social roles, is a process that can occur only within the context of a sustaining environment (Bronfenbrenner, 1979; Erikson, 1963; Piaget, 1929).

Various theories have been proposed to explain the diverse areas or domains of growth and change (e.g., cognitive, physical, socioemotional). Erikson (1963), who focused on psychosocial development, asserted that at each stage of development there is a major task or conflict to be resolved by the individual in order to move on to the next stage. For example, Erikson suggested that a major task in the development of the prepubescent child (age 6–12) is to establish "industry," or the ability to approach and succeed in new challenges such as the tasks of mastering school subjects, relating to peers and teachers, and developing problem-solving skills.

Developmental crisis refers to a situation in which an individual is overwhelmed, unable to cope, and/or unable to function adaptively in response to expected developmental role transitions. Inherent in all developmental stages are particular stressors and potential conflicts. How individuals cope depends in part on their vulnerability due to other factors (e.g., financial, personal, social support). If an individual is unable to successfully navigate those stressors and resolve those conflicts, a developmental crisis may result.

For example, a child whose developmental tasks include learning to relate to peers and teachers may experience peer conflict or conflict with teachers. This difficulty could potentially create a crisis for the individual child because the successful mastery of the peer and student roles is fundamental to the cultural expectations of adolescence and contributes to a developing sense of self and identity. Developmental crises may also emerge in midlife as some individuals experience anxiety, sadness, or fear of growing old. Individuals face potentially stressful developmental transitions as they adjust to their changing roles in retirement, adjust to aging bodies, and begin to directly confront their mortality as they see themselves and their contemporaries affected by declining health. A woman who has spent her life caring for her children may experience a crisis of identity as she sees her grown children leaving home and along with them the major purpose and meaning of her life. Certainly not everyone experiences crises as they navigate these life transitions, but for some individuals the normal developmental passages do indeed precipitate crisis responses.

[handwritten margin note: Empty Nest Syndrome]

It should be emphasized that when persons are experiencing what may be developmental crises, they may not identify their concerns as such to helping professionals. Rather, they may present with other complaints or symptoms. Thus an adolescent who is experiencing a developmental crisis may be referred to treatment because he is abusing drugs or alcohol. Or a man going through a midlife crisis may come to treatment because his wife has learned of his involvement with a younger woman and is threatening to leave him or is furious about his "adolescent" behavior. Although outsiders may smile at such behaviors, the fears and anxieties that may have precipitated these actions are often exceedingly distressing and anxiety-producing. The middle-aged man may be struggling as he faces his diminished sexual capacity, realizes that he will never be the business or athletic success that he had hoped to be, and contends with his growing sense that he is out of touch and irrelevant to his adolescent children's world. The crisis counselor must recognize the identified problem behaviors as symptoms of the individual's struggle to cope with the emotional and interpersonal crises associated with a culturally situated, developmental transition.

Situational crises   *Situational crises* are what most people imagine crises to be, and all of the events reported at the beginning of this chapter were, in fact, situational crises. The most distinguishing characteristic of a situational crisis is a clear external precipitating event. Unlike developmental crises, situational crises occur suddenly and unexpectedly, and can occur at any stage or period in an individual's life. In fact, *sudden onset,* when an event strikes without forewarning, and *unexpectedness,* when an event occurs that the individual never seriously considered as a potential risk, are two characteristics of situational crises. A third characteristic is the *emergency* nature of situational crises, which means that they are threatening in a number of potential ways (e.g., physical, emotional), necessitating immediate actions to prevent further harm (Slaikeu, 1990).

Examples of situational crises, some of which are potentially highly traumatizing, include car accidents, diagnosis of chronic or terminal illness, death of a loved one, and victimization, as in assault, hate crimes, domestic violence, rape, or childhood sexual abuse. Situational crises also include events that can affect more than one person at a single time, perhaps affecting an entire community. Natural disasters such as firestorms that destroy thousands of acres of woodlands, torching homes in their wake, hurricanes, tornadoes, floods, and human-instigated disasters such as the school shooting in Littleton, Colorado, the bombing of the federal building in Oklahoma City, and the ruthless destruction of human life caused by hijacked planes used as bombs at the World Trade Center and the Pentagon are all sudden, unpredictable emergencies that create untold suffering, taxing the abilities of individuals to cope in their aftermath. They are all clearly potential situational crisis events in many individuals' lives. Although some situational crisis events affect many people at the same time, individuals must still cope with the event according to their own unique life circumstances and personal and social resources. There are often common symptoms when traumatic events affect an entire group or community, warranting group interventions designed to enable individuals to come together in community to grieve and heal. It is also important, however, to assess the individualized impact and to intervene when necessary.

Responding to Crises and Traumatic Events: A Continuum of Response

As mentioned earlier, individuals in crisis are experiencing an inability to adapt using their customary coping strategies. They are experiencing severe upset and disorganization in functioning. Individuals who have suffered traumatic exposure may be experiencing acute physiologic and anxiety responses. Although individuals may continue to make attempts to cope, they may perceive the event to be so threatening, to pose such an insoluble difficulty, and/or to so challenge important goals or beliefs, that their efforts are ineffectual. One result is increased vulnerability. Because the normal defenses that enable individuals to function are overwhelmed, the individual is often highly suggestible and open to direction. This increased vulnerability means that whatever happens during this time period will likely have a heightened impact because the individual is significantly less defended. Thus, for example, the responses by medical personnel, police, crisis workers, and family members to a woman who has been sexually assaulted often strongly affect the victim's own inclination to either avoid or engage in self-blaming interpretations of what occurred.

Because acute crisis reactions can be so debilitating, it is generally believed that the individual cannot tolerate the disequilibrium indefinitely and thus must find some means to restore a sense of order and/or stability. As noted, however, although it is important to achieve some stability, constructive resolution of the crisis may require significantly more time. The more severe and/or the longer lasting a precipitating crisis event is, the greater the likelihood this will be true. Thus an individual who was subjected to repeated physical and/or sexual abuse over a period of years or an individual who was held captive by a kidnapper and saw other captives killed may experience distress long beyond the time when the traumatizing event(s) ends.

Many people who are experiencing the extreme emotional upset and disorganization that ensue in the wake of a crisis event may feel that they are "going crazy." As described in our earlier discussion of crisis theory, however, a primary assumption of crisis theory is that individuals in crisis are essentially responding normally to abnormal events. In other words, when individuals are faced by sudden, intensely disruptive and/or destructive situations that threaten their sense of meaning and well-being, it is normal and expected for them to react with intense emotions and to be overwhelmed and temporarily unable to adapt or cope. The symptoms experienced by persons in crisis—heart pounding, thoughts racing, inability to eat or sleep, relational problems, extreme emotionality or restricted emotion—are also not unexpected, but rather reflect the normal limits in the human capacity to immediately adapt in the face of extremely threatening circumstances.

Many people show remarkable resilience in the aftermath of crisis events. With the support of significant others, individuals are often gradually able to draw on their normal coping resources to effectively deal with both the pragmatic and subjective injuries sustained. Further, as will be examined, some individuals not only recover, but grow as the result of their enhanced sense of strength and survivorship.

Diagnosis and crisis reactions   Although acute responses to traumatic events should not be considered abnormal or indicative of either mental illness or weakness, individuals seen by crisis counselors may be experiencing a constellation of symptoms that compromise their daily functioning. In some cases, the frequency, intensity, and duration of the crisis symptoms reach a diagnostic threshold (American Psychiatric Association, 2000). Basically, the more severe a person's reactions over a sustained period of time, the more likely that person's overall functioning has been significantly affected, and thus the more likely that person's symptoms indicate a clinical syndrome.

Diagnosis has been a controversial issue in many areas of crisis work, particularly among individuals involved in the rape crisis and battered women's fields. Historically, the mental health system's response to survivors of childhood sexual abuse, sexual assault, and battering coupled disbelief with a psychiatric diagnosis that seemed to blame women for their difficulties. Many adult female trauma survivors, particularly those who suffered repeated victimization, were thought to have personality disorders, with diagnoses ranging from "masochistic" to "borderline" to "paranoid." Early responses to Vietnam veterans similarly both discounted and misdiagnosed the range of severe symptoms frequently presented. An early response by feminist crisis programs was to eschew mental health approaches completely, operating from an assumption that the only thing wrong with survivors was their victimization, and that once freed from the range of violating and controlling circumstances that harmed them, survivors would be fine. This view gradually moderated as many feminist advocates and professionals documented the negative physiological and psychological outcome of repeated exposure to violence (Herman, 1997; Walker, 1984, 1991). In truth, survivors of domestic violence and sexual assault, like Vietnam veterans and survivors of other traumatizing events, may be clinically depressed, may have become addicted to drugs or alcohol as a means of coping, or may suffer from a range of other stress reactions and symptoms.

Recently a number of crisis theorists and researchers have again challenged what they regard as a misguided emphasis on pathogenesis in the crisis literature (Stuhlmiller & Dunning, 2000; Violanti, 2000). They suggest an alternative, *salutogenic* perspective. "Instead of the assumption that stress, traumatic stress, and critical incidents cause or put people at risk to develop negative outcomes, a salutogenic perspective acknowledges the ubiquitous nature of stress and that consequences are not necessarily pathological but possibly salutary" (Stuhlmiller & Dunning, 2000, p. 34). From this perspective, crisis assessment and intervention must emphasize resistance and resilience factors in addition to illness-susceptibility factors.

This text embodies such a strength and resilience perspective. The authors also support the cautious use of diagnosis in appropriate circumstances, and contend that these ideas are not mutually exclusive. We conceptualize a continuum of crisis responses and present specific diagnoses as one way of understanding some responses to crisis and trauma. We also argue, however, against the assumption of a diagnostic perspective as a dominant paradigm for understanding crisis reactions. As Violanti (2000) reminds us: "A reliance on pathogenic intervention methods may script an individual into traumatic symptoms" by presupposing a "sick role" (p. 153).

In some instances, an appropriate diagnosis may help the crisis survivor and significant family members to understand the survivor's difficulties as a syndrome that is directly attributable to the traumatic experience. The purpose of diagnosis in such instances is not to label a person or to pathologize reactions. Rather, the diagnosis accurately conveys the manner and degree to which the capacity for normal psychological and social functioning has been compromised. The more accurate the diagnosis the more efficacious the treatment provided as interventions are targeted to the specific area of functional impairment (e.g., depression, anxiety) and at an appropriate level of intensiveness. The more disturbed the individual, the more intensive, directive, and potentially restrictive interventions must become.

Diagnosis with crisis survivors must clearly connect the presenting emotional and behavioral problems to the precipitating crisis event. In this manner crisis workers can help victims to understand what they are experiencing as crisis responses and as efforts to cope and survive, even when those responses ultimately cause distress and compromise functioning. And to reiterate a point, crisis workers' awareness of possibly debilitating crisis responses must not lead to interventions that script psychological trauma or replace a focus on an individual's strengths, resources, and positive coping techniques.

Chapter 5 examines issues of assessment with individuals whose responses to crisis events constitute a more serious impairment in functioning. It examines those diagnostic categories most commonly found among individuals who have experienced crises and/or traumatic events and also describes assessment and intervention with individuals who may be either suicidal or violent toward others.

DEVELOPMENT OF CRISIS INTERVENTION METHODS AND SERVICES

Although there were no formal mental health services at the turn of the twentieth century, the first suicide hotline was established in San Francisco in 1902 and the first suicide prevention program, the National Save a Life League, was begun in New York City in 1906. As previously described, the Cocoanut Grove fire of 1942 was the catalyst for contemporary efforts to conceptualize crisis and crisis reactions. It also raised interesting questions regarding intervention. The dominant professional thinking of that time emphasized long-term treatment provided by highly educated mental health experts as the only effective intervention for emotional and psychological problems. In the aftermath of the Cocoanut Grove fire, however, a variety of community caregivers were active in helping both individuals and the community to grieve, and follow-up showed that survivors clearly benefited from this short-term intervention. During this same general time period, crisis intervention approaches were effectively utilized to respond to World War II soldiers suffering from what was referred to at the time as "battle fatigue."

Subsequent to their experiences in the aftermath of the Cocoanut Grove fire, both Lindemann and Caplan continued their efforts to explicate the meaning of crisis and to investigate the most useful ways of intervening. Caplan (1964) emphasized the need for early intervention and observed that as a result of early intervention some individuals were able not only to reach resolution of the immediate crisis, but to actually come through the crisis functioning at a higher level than prior to the crisis. He established the Harvard Family Guidance Center, a multidisciplinary crisis research and consultation center, in 1954. Under his leadership, the center focused primarily on four types of family crises: premature birth, birth of children with congenital anomalies, birth of twins, and the impact of tuberculosis.

In 1958 the first twenty-four-hour psychiatric emergency walk-in clinic, known as the "Trouble-shooting Clinic" was established at Elmhurst City Hospital in New York. Leopold Bellak, the center's founder, was a pioneer in establishing both the theory and intervention approaches of psychiatric emergency services (Bellak & Siegel, 1983).

The 1960s yielded a host of changes both in the delivery of crisis intervention services and in the mental health system as a whole. Perhaps the most significant event during this decade was the passage of the Community Mental Health Center Act of 1963. This act mandated the establishment of community mental health centers that would provide a continuum of care including inpatient treatment, outpatient treatment, partial hospitalization, emergency services (twenty-four hours per day, seven days per week), and consultation and education services for communities. Although critics argue that the vision of every community being able to provide this broad range of services has never been realized, crisis intervention hotlines and services were identified as necessary and essential services. Also, for the most part, psychiatric emergency services were increasingly provided by community mental health centers in those communities where they were established.

In the 1990s the entire mental health system changed dramatically with the advent of managed care. Managed care proponents contended that emotional and addictive disorders could often be effectively treated with brief therapy instead of with more costly long-term psychotherapy or even more costly inpatient treatment. Although many problems have been identified with the delivery of services by managed care companies, one of the clear outcomes has been the growth of therapeutic approaches that are time-limited and problem- or solution-focused, often referred to under the umbrella term of *brief therapy*. In many instances, intensive outpatient programs and case-management programs augmented by a variety of emergency or crisis services replaced inpatient psychiatric and substance abuse treatment. Although brief therapy differs from crisis counseling in that the goals and interventions of crisis counseling are specific to assisting individuals adapt to and resolve the debilitating aftermath of exposure to crisis and/or traumatic events, both share an emphasis on time-limited efforts to enable individuals to cope with and resolve difficulties. The net effect of many of these changes has been increased emphasis on emergency crisis services supplemented by brief counseling.

As communications technology has increased our awareness of events in the world, it has also brought dramatic scenes of tragic events into our living rooms and onto our computer screens. From earthquakes in India and El Salvador, to the bombing of the Oklahoma City federal building, to the war in Bosnia, and to the terrorist attacks on the New York World Trade Center and the Pentagon, we have viewed devastation and human suffering on a much more personal and immediate level than was possible in the past. As a result, the public is keenly aware of crisis events and, correspondingly, much more aware of the psychological impact of crisis. Helping people in crisis (in the United States or abroad) has become part of our worldview, and both private organizations (e.g., the Red Cross) and government agencies (e.g., the Federal Emergency Management Agency) have increased visibility as they strive to provide services to those individuals suffering the effects of crisis events. To meet this need, numerous models of crisis assessment and crisis intervention have been developed to guide both counseling and human service professionals as well as other professionals and volunteers in the delivery of crisis intervention services.

CRISIS ASSESSMENT AND INTERVENTION: MULTIPLE MODELS

As the efficacy of crisis intervention services has been recognized, many authors and clinicians have sought to develop guidelines or models to assist those in the trenches responding to crisis situations. The complexity created by the variety of crises that individuals may face, the range of people who may encounter someone in crisis, and the growing realization that single-session crisis intervention in an emergent situation differs from longer-term crisis counseling aimed at crisis resolution has resulted in an array of differing approaches. Some authors give basic advice on what to do or not do in an emergent crisis situation that can be used by nonprofessionals and professionals alike. Other authors have developed models to be utilized in specific situations by specific types of professionals such as models of assessment and/or intervention for police officers dealing with a variety of on-the-street crises. And still others have created models that provide more sophisticated theoretically driven approaches to assessing and responding to crises in both the emergency and resolution phases of crisis intervention.

Crisis Assessment Models

Most models developed to guide crisis intervention mention, at a minimum, the importance of gauging and assessing a situation before jumping in and attempting to intervene (Hendricks & McKean, 1995; Hoff, 1995; Myer, Williams, Ottens, & Schmidt, 1992; Slaikeu, 1990). Some provide little guidance, however, and thus do little to assist crisis interventionists in knowing what or how to assess, or how to connect assessment information to their actual intervention. Myer (2001) suggested that the assessment process is often overlooked in crisis intervention although, in his view, it is the most critical aspect of crisis intervention.

At the most basic level, assessment refers to the process by which a crisis counselor comes to some understanding of the crisis event, the needs and strengths of the individual in crisis, and the deficits and strengths of the recovery environment. In most helping situations it is assumed that the understanding gained through assessment should precede and guide efforts to help clients bring about change. This is also true in crisis intervention, although in an emergency situation, assessment must be immediate and conducted simultaneously with efforts to stabilize and support the individual in crisis.

Myer (2001) recently reviewed and evaluated four current assessment models proposed for use in crisis intervention: Hoff's (1995) Vulnerability Model, Slaikeu's (1990) Multidimensional Model, Hendricks and McKean's (1995) Frontline Model, and Myer, Williams, Ottens, and Schmidt's (1992) Triage Assessment Model. Myer's assessment criteria were: user-friendly, adaptable, holistic, connected to intervention, culturally sensitive, and usable on an ongoing basis. He concluded that although each model had strengths, only the Triage Assessment Model was strong on all five of his assessment criteria. We reference Myer's (2001) evaluation of these assessment models because we find his evaluation criteria to be both reasoned and useful. We do not agree with his conclusion, however, at least in part because we differ with the assumptions he made in determining what it means for an assessment model to be user-friendly and holistic.

A basic assumption underlying the model presented in this text is the belief that a useful assessment model does not necessarily yield simplified and weighted categorizations of client functioning. Although we recommend the use of targeted assessment instruments in evaluating specific individualized aspects of a crisis client's functioning (for example, utilizing a PTSD measure or an instrument measuring the likelihood that a client will commit suicide), we believe that the primary value of a useful assessment model in crisis intervention is to develop complexity in crisis workers' perceptions and comprehension of crisis clients and the challenges they face. Correspondingly, we do not believe that assessment conclusions must lead to pre-determined intervention responses. Rather, it is the professional crisis worker's role, with knowledge of the potential range of domains affected by crisis, to individualize interventions, emphasizing the areas that are most germane for a particular individual. Although that complexity may seem messy or cumbersome, in our judgment, the goals of professional helping will not be best met by reducing those complexities to more simplified formulaic representations.

No assessment models currently proposed for use in assessing crisis reactions meet our definitions of user-friendly, adaptable across a range of crisis situations, comprehensive/holistic, connected to intervention, culturally sensitive, and usable on an ongoing basis. The Triage Assessment Model does call attention to the emotional, cognitive, and behavioral aspects of a crisis reaction, and provides useful ways of conceptualizing reactions in those areas. It fails, however, to consider the individual developmentally and does not address the degree to which both the individual in crisis and the crisis event itself are embedded in a particular ecological context. Similarly, although Slaikeu (1990) discusses the importance of utilizing a general systems framework and even presents a chart examining the systems variables that describe the crisis context, his assessment framework excludes assessment of those very variables. Hendricks and McKean's (1995) frontline model emphasizes assessment of the immediate crisis environment, however, as Myer (2001) noted, it glosses over assessment of the person and presents a very limited guide to assessment of individual areas of personal and interpersonal functioning potentially affected by crisis events.

Models of Crisis Intervention

Numerous models have also been proposed to guide those intervening with individuals in crisis (Aguilera, 1998; Greenstone & Leviton, 2002; James & Gilliland, 2001; Kanel, 2002; Roberts, 2000; Slaikeu, 1990; Wainrib & Bloch, 1998). The various models share many components. A common element of most of them is the influence of problem-solving/solution-focused approaches entailing identification of specific needs and development of specific strategies or plans to address those immediate needs. This is particularly true of those models that emphasize short-term, emergency, or single-session intervention. Some models provide very specific step-by-step problem-solving procedures designed to assist clients in a variety of emergent crisis situations (James & Gilliland, 2001; Roberts, 2000). Only one model clearly delineates the different needs and thus the different intervention processes involved in crisis counseling intended to assist clients to integrate the crisis and facilitate future growth (Slaikeu, 1990). Some of the intervention models are designed to direct helpers who are assumed to have no professional background or education as helping professionals (Greenstone & Levitan, 2002; Wainrib & Bloch, 1998), whereas others assume a crisis worker with a high level of counseling knowledge and skills (Aguilera, 1998; Kanel, 2002; Slaikeu, 1990).

Although most of the models describe the importance of establishing rapport and enabling crisis clients to feel that they are being heard and supported, attention to the helping relationship also varies across the models. The discussion on the helping relationship ranges from an emphasis on specific skills and tasks (Greenstone & Levitan, 2002; Wainrib & Bloch, 1998) to a more complex analysis of the relationship intricacies involved in effective counseling with traumatized individuals (Aguilera, 1998; Kanel, 2002; Slaikeu, 1990).

Finally, most crisis intervention models are based in crisis theory, the common practice principles derived from crisis theory including immediate intervention with limited goals, focused problem-solving, and the instilling of hope and renewed coping strategies. Crisis theory, however, is basically a perspective on crisis and crisis reactions rather than a theoretical framework directing assessment toward particular facets of psychosocial functioning or explaining why or how one might focus intervention. Crisis theory provides an essential perspective; however, the lack of a unifying theoretical perspective that provides a framework to direct crisis assessment and crisis intervention for both single-session and ongoing crisis counseling is a limitation of all current models.

In our judgment, none of the crisis intervention models reviewed completely met the criteria we find essential. A theoretically driven crisis assessment and intervention practice system that can guide crisis workers in providing both single-session crisis counseling and ongoing crisis counseling is needed. It must be holistic, attending to both the whole individual and the environment, and it must be usable across a wide range of crises. The purpose of this text is to present a practice system that meets these criteria and to illustrate its application across a range of crisis situations. The theory and model of crisis intervention presented in the following two chapters and then applied to various crises in subsequent chapters of this text is designed to prepare counselors, social workers, psychologists, and other human service professionals for the challenging and essential tasks they perform.

DISCUSSION QUESTIONS

1. Think about the events you have experienced or observed that you would label as stressful and events that you would consider crises. Given those different experiences or observations, what is the difference between a stressful event and a crisis? When does a stressful event become a crisis event?

2. Crisis has been described as an event that holds the possibility of both danger and opportunity. What does this mean? Can you identify experiences in which a crisis posed a danger? an opportunity?

EXERCISES

1. Magnet words: Write the words *stress, crisis, trauma, coping, crisis reaction,* and *crisis intervention* on the board. Divide the class into small groups. The words you have written on the board are magnet words. Ask each group to come up with words that "attach" to each of the magnet words. Words that attach to the magnet words are usually words that define, differentiate, or exemplify the magnet word.

2. Divide the class into small groups. Ask each group member to think about a crisis event that he or she has experienced either directly or indirectly. Each member should also think about what made the event feel like a crisis. Members are encouraged to share their experiences and observations with their group. Ask a member of the group to identify and list common elements that determined what constituted a crisis.

REFERENCES

Aguilera, D. C. (1998). *Crisis intervention: Theory and methodology* (8th ed.). St. Louis: Mosby.

American Psychiatric Association. (2000). *Diagnostic and statistical manual of mental disorders* (4th ed., Text Revision, DSM-IV-TR). Washington, DC: American Psychiatric Association.

Bellak, L., & Siegel, H. (1983). *Handbook of intensive brief and emergency psychotherapy*. Larchmont, NY: C.P.S., Inc.

Blocher, D. H. (2000). *Counseling: A developmental approach* (4th ed.). New York: John Wiley & Sons.

Brammer, L. M. (1985). *The helping relationship: Process and skills* (3rd ed.). Upper Saddle River, NJ: Prentice Hall.

Bronfenbrenner, U. (1979). *The ecology of human development: Experiments by nature and design*. Cambridge: Harvard University Press.

Bronfenbrenner, U. (1989). Ecological systems theory. In R. Vasta (Ed.), *Annals of child development, 6* (pp. 187–251). Greenwich, CT: JAI.

Caplan, G. (1961). *An approach to community mental health*. New York: Grune & Stratton.

Caplan, G. (1964). *Principles of preventative psychiatry*. New York: Basic Books.

Dixon, S. L. (1979). *Working with people in crisis: Theory and practice*. St. Louis: Mosby.

Erikson, E. H. (1963). *Childhood and society* (2nd ed.). New York: Norton.

Folkman, S. (1984). Personal control and stress and coping processes: A theoretical analysis. *Journal of Personality and Social Psychology, 46,* 839–852.

Greenstone, J. L., & Leviton S. C. (2002). *Elements of crisis intervention: Crises and how to respond to them*. Pacific Grove, CA: Brooks/Cole.

Hendricks, J. E., & McKean, J. B. (1995). *Crisis intervention: Contemporary issues for onsite interveners*. Springfield, IL: Charles C. Thomas Publishers.

Herman, J. (1997). *Trauma and recovery*. New York: Basic Books.

Hiley-Young, G. (1992). Trauma reactivation assessment and treatment: Integrative case examples. *Journal of Traumatic Stress, 5*(4), 545–555.

Hoff, L. A. (1995). *People in crisis: Understanding and helping* (4th ed.). Redwood City, CA: Addison-Wesley.

James, R. K., & Gilliland, B. E. (2001). *Crisis intervention strategies* (4th ed.). Belmont, CA: Wadsworth, Brooks/Cole Counseling.

Janosick, E. H. (1984). *Crisis counseling: A contemporary approach*. Monterey, CA: Wadsworth.

Kanel, K. (2002). *A guide to crisis intervention* (2nd ed.). Pacific Grove, CA: Brooks/Cole.

Lazarus, R., & Folkman, S. (1984). *Stress, appraisal, and coping*. New York: Springer.

Lindemann, E. (1944). Symptomatology and management of acute grief. *American Journal of Psychiatry, 101,* 141–148.

Meichenbaum, D. (1994). *A clinical handbook/practical therapist manual for assessing and treating adults with post-traumatic stress disorder (PTSD).* Waterloo, Ontario, Canada: Institute Press.

Myer, R. A. (2001). *Assessment for crisis intervention: A triage assessment model.* Belmont, CA: Wadsworth.

Myer, R. A., Williams, R. C., Ottens, A. J., & Schmidt, A. E. (1992). Crisis assessment: A three-dimensional model for triage. *Journal of Mental Health Counseling, 14,* 137–148.

Parad, H. J., & Caplan, G. (1960). A framework for studying families in crisis. *Social Work, 5*(3), 3–15.

Piaget, J. (1929). *The child's conception of the world.* New York: Harcourt Brace.

Roberts, A. R. (2000). *Crisis intervention handbook: Assessment, treatment and research.* New York: Oxford University Press.

Slaikeu, K. A. (1990). *Crisis intervention: A handbook for practice and research* (2nd ed.). Boston: Allyn & Bacon.

Stuhlmiller, C., & Dunning, C. (2000). Challenging the mainstream: From pathogenic to salutogenic models of posttrauma intervention. In J. Violanti, D. Paton, & C. Dunning (Eds.), *Posttraumatic stress intervention: Challenges, issues, and perspectives* (pp. 10–42). Springfield, IL: Charles C. Thomas Publisher.

Violanti, J. M. (2000). Scripting trauma: The impact of pathogenic intervention. In J. Violanti, D. Paton, & C. Dunning (Eds.), *Posttraumatic stress intervention: Challenges, issues, and perspectives* (pp. 153–165). Springfield, IL: Charles C. Thomas Publisher.

Wainrib, B. R., & Bloch, E. L. (1998). *Crisis intervention and trauma response: Theory and practice.* New York: Springer.

Walker, L. E. (1984). *The battered woman syndrome.* New York: Springer.

Walker, L. E. (1991). Post-traumatic stress disorder in women: Diagnosis and treatment of battered woman syndrome. *Psychotherapy: Theory, Research, Practice, Training, 28,* Special Issue: Psychotherapy with victims (pp. 21–29). Washington, DC: Division of Psychotherapy, American Psychological Association.

CHAPTER 2

Assessment: A Developmental-Ecological Perspective

OVERVIEW OF DEVELOPMENTAL-ECOLOGICAL PERSPECTIVE

Helping and Helping Schemas

All students in counseling, social work, psychology, psychiatric nursing, and other mental health training programs will be exposed at some point to the knowledge base associated with a developmental understanding of people, groups, and social systems, and to the various theories that assist us in conceptualizing how people change and resolve problems. What may be clear by now is that there is a seemingly endless array of theories and models. What may not be clear is how to apply those theories and models.

Your life experience and education have undoubtedly led you to conclude that no single factor can explain human behavior, and to recognize that there is more to the client than what we observe during the time we share with that person. As we work with clients, we attempt to understand them and to construct a story or working model of how they function and what factors in their environments are most critical to understanding their present difficulties. Central to this process is not only the identification of significant factors in a client's experience, but also the linking or association of those factors in the construction of meaning for that client and his or her environment. Presumably, this complex client model determines our focus, goals, and choice of intervention. In other words, we assume that assessment, or the development of understanding informed by various theories, precedes our decisions about what to do to help.

Ensuring timely and complex understanding can be difficult, however, especially in crisis intervention, because the emergent nature of the situation can yield cognitively simple responses at a time when complex understanding is necessary.

Effective crisis counseling, whether single-session or ongoing, must be based on a thought process that ensures intervention is responsive to the uniquely complex realities individuals face. Our assumption in writing this text is that complex understanding leads to successful intervention. Central to this complexity is a *developmental-ecological perspective* for understanding people and the problems they face.

Developmental Theory

The evolving shared human experience across the life span has captivated theorists and practitioners alike for many years. As described previously, theorists studying the human experience have noted that human beings appear to grow and change physically, cognitively, emotionally, and behaviorally in similar ways and in similar time sequences. Various theories of development have been proposed to try and capture the essence of those developmental changes. All development theories share some common assumptions, perhaps the most critical being that human development is a product of the interaction between individual needs and abilities and societal expectations and demands. Particularly germane to our perspective is Bronfenbrenner's (1979, 1989) ecological systems view of development, which situates development within the context of an environment and emphasizes the bidirectional nature of the interactions between developing individuals and the multilayered environments in which they are "nested."

Assumptions critical to developmental theories about the human experience include the following:

1. Growth and change are inevitable and occur at every period of life from birth through old age.
2. Development is systematic, continuous change in a valued direction.
3. Developmental changes can be most readily understood through the concepts of "stage of life" and stage-based expectations.
4. The cognitive, emotional, and behavioral changes needed at each stage (in order for the individual to continue further growth) are conceived as developmental tasks.
5. The development that takes place at each stage has a significant impact on all subsequent stages. Thus, ideally, the tasks of one stage must be achieved for healthy progression to the next stage of development.
6. An individual's biological disposition and environmental conditions interact and come together in shaping and determining ongoing development.

In essence, all developmental theories, whether explaining psychosexual, psychosocial, cognitive, or moral development, propose that at any identified stage in the life span, individuals have certain expectations to meet and they in turn need to muster personal and social resources to meet those expectations and master the developmental tasks associated with that stage. Developmental theory suggests that if they are unable to meet those expectations and accomplish those tasks, individuals will be hindered in their continued development.

Developmental theory and crisis intervention   As discussed in Chapter 1, some crises are clearly developmental in nature in that the stimulus event is directly related to developmental tasks and/or changes, for example, the "empty nest" or retirement. A developmental perspective, however, also requires us to recognize the developmental nature of all crises; even situational crises occur within the context of an individual's life span and at different times throughout one's life. Developmental crisis occurs as part of developmental transition and may exert an ongoing influence. Similarly, situational crisis occurs at specific times in a person's life and will have developmentally relevant meaning and impact. Thus, a diagnosis of cancer may have different meaning for a 32-year-old mother of two and a 76-year-old widow. And although assault is always devastating, the sexual assault of an 11-year-old child may have different meaning and impact than the sexual assault of a 25-year-old woman.

The developmental perspective provides a framework for understanding clients and for helping us to set goals on their behalf (Blocher, 2000). The following assumptions are central to this perspective:

1. Developmental intervention serves to facilitate the optimal psychological development of clients, both by enhancing higher levels of functioning and by helping to remove obstacles to further growth (Blocher, 2000).
2. Developing human beings can only be fully understood and helped within the context of their interactions with the physical, relational, and cultural environment (Blocher, 2000; Bronfenbrenner, 1979, 1989).
3. Developmental intervention facilitates a dynamic and growth-producing engagement or "fit" between the developing person and a humane and responsive environment (Blocher, 2000).

Developmental crisis intervention requires that the crisis worker be cognizant of a client's developmental functioning status. Assessment of an individual in crisis must include consideration of the cognitive and language capacities of the client as well as specific developmental meanings the crisis may have for the client. The meanings attributed to specific developmental stages and tasks are influenced by the individual's social and cultural environment. A family or culture that views being a virgin as a prerequisite for being marriageable may see a sexual assault of a young woman of marriageable age in primarily sexual terms, as terminally damaging the victim. Another young adult female may experience a sexual assault primarily as a violent and terrifying loss of control that threatens her developmentally appropriate sense of independence and self-control. Each victim has been violated, but each experiences the violation in developmentally unique ways with the tasks and conflicts of development informed by the individual's cultural context. Crisis interventionists must be attuned to the unique developmental meanings and impact of crisis events, whether those stimulus events are developmental or situational in nature.

Ecological Theory

The ecological paradigm draws on both general systems theory and the biological sciences. It utilizes the metaphor of ecology, the study of the interrelationships of living organisms and their physical and biological environments, as a perspective for understanding the interrelationships among individuals and their physical and social environments (Bronfenbrenner, 1979, 1989; Germain & Gitterman, 1996). Ecological thinking sensitizes human service professionals to interpersonal, situational, and sociocultural factors in client lives and draws attention to the nature of the transactions that occur between individuals and their environments. This perspective does not provide a specific model for intervention but is rather an "orientation to practice" or a "way of noticing" and using professional vision to encompass the client's complex reality (Meyer, 1987, p. 414). An ecological perspective of crisis calls our attention to the interrelationships among the person in crisis, the crisis event, and the environment within which the crisis occurs and within which recovery from crisis and/or mastery of specific developmental tasks must take place.

Environmental conditions and social functioning   Environmental forces, which include interpersonal relationships, community resources/conditions, and society at large, clearly have an impact on individuals and their capacity to meet their basic needs, to function adaptively, and to cope with and resolve problems and crises. Environmental forces and situational factors can affect individuals either positively or negatively. Further, the way individuals react to environmental and situational factors also differs. It is the transactions and interactions between individuals and the environment that ultimately explain individuals' differing levels of success in meeting needs, accomplishing life tasks, and coping with and resolving problems.

DuBois and Krogsrud Miley (2000) differentiated between different types of social functioning that result from the interactions between people and their social and physical environments. "Adaptive functioning" occurs when individuals are able to recognize problems and have the personal and environmental resources necessary to cope with stressors and adapt to change. Environmental resources, including informal systems like a network of friends and family and formal systems like police, hospitals, and schools, are responsive and resource-rich. In contrast, some individuals have a higher level of vulnerability. Identifiable factors, such as unemployment, drug and alcohol abuse, prejudicial or culturally incompetent social service or criminal justice institutions, make it more difficult for individuals to muster the personal, interpersonal, and institutional resources they need to address their needs and problems. And in some human systems, problems become so exacerbated that the system is immobilized. Individuals may have been previously victimized, may be addicted to drugs and/or alcohol, or may be depressed or anxious. Families may be highly chaotic, enmeshed, in conflict, or lacking in boundaries. Environments may be devoid of resources or violent and dangerous. In such situations individuals may have little or no adaptive capacity to cope with additional stressors.

Ecological theory and crisis intervention   Ecological thinking prepares a crisis counselor to view both the crisis situation and the person experiencing a crisis reaction holistically. From an ecological perspective, a crisis consists of an individual or individuals, an event or situation, and an environmental context. The person in crisis is a feeling, thinking, behaving individual who encounters the crisis event during a specific developmental stage. The individual in crisis is a member of a unique family, community, and culture. The crisis event is embedded in a particular community, school, or home. The particular community may be resource-rich or resource-poor and may include supportive or unsupportive systems that will hinder or enhance the individual's capacity to cope with and ultimately resolve the crisis situation.

Slaikeu (1990) suggested that the way an individual responds to a precipitating event and later works through the crisis experience depends not only on personal resources and coping capacities, but also on the availability and accessibility of material resources such as money, food, housing, and transportation, and social resources such as family and friends. We agree with this assessment. Additionally, we emphasize the importance of community resources. In our experience, adequate and responsive medical systems, police and criminal justice systems, and fair and flexible school systems are equally important in determining how individuals fare in efforts to cope with and resolve a crisis. Whether the crisis event is a diagnosis of cancer, natural or man-made disaster, or child abuse, individuals respond in ways that are influenced by the physical, material, social, and community resources that comprise their personal ecosystem.

Ultimately, theory and theoretical perspectives are useful to crisis counselors only to the extent that they contribute to an understanding of the dimensions of the crisis and point to procedures for intervention. In the remainder of this chapter we present a model for assessment in crisis situations based on a developmental ecological theoretical perspective. In Chapter 3 we discuss intervention, drawing on this same paradigm. As we have said, this perspective provides a holistic and complex lens through which the crisis worker can view and assess a client experiencing a crisis in his or her life. It also provides the theoretical basis for intervention models that can guide either single-session crisis counseling or ongoing crisis counseling in the aftermath of a crisis.

ASSESSING CRISIS REACTIONS: A DEVELOPMENTAL-ECOLOGICAL MODEL

Assessment is a process of coming to a complex understanding of a client system's needs and strengths. Assessment is generally thought to be the outcome of an extensive process of gathering psychosocial data about a client, and is thought to *precede* intervention. In crisis situations, however, particularly single-session interventions, assessment must be both an immediate and a continuous activity that the crisis worker engages in. In single-session crisis counseling, the assessment process begins with the crisis worker's first contact with the crisis situation or the person in crisis and continues throughout his or her involvement. In ongoing crisis counseling, the developmental-ecological model serves as a continuous lens for assessing the client's evolving status and recovery process. It also serves as a model for a formal process of gathering and assessing psychosocial data and information about precrisis functioning, resulting in the identification of a counseling focus and goals for change.

A developmental-ecological model for assessment directs our attention to both the individual and the environment, as well as the interrelationship between the two. The crisis worker seeks to assess and comprehend individual functioning, the crisis event, the client's personal ecosystem including interpersonal relationships and other social supports, and the environmental context in which the crisis event occurs. In any crisis situation, the crisis counselor must reach a quick assessment of both the client system strengths and needs. By definition, a crisis reaction entails significant disruption of normal functioning in one or more areas. Table 2.1 outlines an easy-to-remember framework for identifying what we have found to be the essential areas of person/environment functioning that must be assessed in any crisis situation.

TABLE 2.1
ABCDE ASSESSMENT MODEL

Affect	Primary feelings of client in reaction to crisis. Common responses include anxiety, anger, depression, sadness, fear, shame, confusion. May be identified or not identified by client; expressed or not expressed. Indicated verbally and nonverbally. Affective expressiveness is influenced by gender and culture.
Behavior	Client's actions/lack of action in response to crisis. Behaviors engaged in to try to cope with and resolve crisis. Possibility of dangerous or aggressive acts including suicide/homicide. Approach, avoidance, immobility (Myer, Williams, Ottens, & Schmidt, 1992).
Cognition	Thoughts, beliefs, explanations that define the meaning of the crisis and determine affective and behavioral responses. Self-image, life goals, religious and cultural beliefs. Consider developmental impact on comprehension, meaning making, verbal expression, etc. Irrational self-talk (e.g., overgeneralizing, catastrophizing, paranoia).
Development	Developmental or situational crisis. Stage of life needs/concerns/tasks affected by crisis. Assess developmental capacities in relevant areas.
Ecosystem	Culture/ethnicity of client. Presence or absence and accessibility of interpersonal, informal, and formal resources/supports. Ability and willingness to utilize supports. Perceived barriers.

Affective Responses

Understanding and responding to a crisis client's feelings has been consistently emphasized in the crisis intervention literature, with good reason. Emotions strongly influence behavior and often have a central role in a client's sense of being "out of control" or overwhelmed in the aftermath of a crisis. Although there are both gender and cultural differences in emotional expressiveness, in most cultures healthy emotional functioning is assumed to include some degree of control over the exercise of one's emotions, some ability to experience the full range of human emotions, and some ability to be attuned to and responsive to the feelings of others (Hepworth, Rooney, & Larsen, 1997). Thus individuals who are overwhelmed by their feelings or totally unable to discuss painful emotions are seen as not functioning optimally. Normal healthy emotional functioning also assumes that the affect exhibited is appropriate to the situation or circumstance. A manifestation of inappropriate affect would be extreme emotional detachment or laughing and smiling when discussing a painful or traumatic event.

Even these basic assumptions must be tempered by cultural awareness and sensitivity as the more detached or reactive emotional tendencies of individuals in some cultures might naturally lead them to different but appropriate emotional responses. Emotional expressiveness may vary when individuals switch from speaking a native language to a second language, or an individual may mask emotions because of the potential discomfort of cross-cultural communication (Lum, 1996, 1999).

The affective reactions of immediate concern to crisis interventionists typically include all of the feelings that an individual has in the aftermath of the crisis event. These include crisis clients' emotional responses to the event itself, to thoughts and efforts to make sense of what has happened (i.e., their cognitions), and to their behaviors during and after the crisis. Also of importance are emotional reactions to the responses of others, and to the circumstances and challenges crisis clients face as they try to determine the necessary steps to cope with and resolve crisis situations.

The very nature of crises and traumatic events suggests that most emotions clients experience will be negative, and further that they may not be functioning in an emotionally adaptive manner. Although the intensity of response will certainly vary among individuals, some writers have suggested that the primary negative emotions likely to be attached to crisis be symbolically described as yellow (anxiety/fear), red (anger/hostility), or black (sadness/melancholy/depressiveness) (Crow, 1977; Myer et al., 1992). Although these do seem to be common emotional responses to crises, it is also important to recognize the much wider range of emotional responses that crisis clients may experience. For some individuals a dominant emotion may be shame, for another, horror, and for a third, a sense of being alone or separate. Even when experiencing the same or similar external events such as a sexual assault, one woman may feel betrayed, another degraded, whereas a male sexual assault survivor may feel emasculated. To assume the broad range of client emotional responses can be reduced to just three types can lead to low levels of understanding and responding. Table 2.2 gives examples of a wide range of words describing feelings that can be used to more accurately distinguish

TABLE 2.2
AFFECTIVE WORD LIST: NEGATIVE EMOTIONS

Anger, Hostility

aggravated	deadly	impatient	oppressed
aggressive	discontented	inconsiderate	outraged
agitated	enraged	inhuman	resentful
angry	envious	insensitive	revengeful
arrogant	furious	intolerable	ruthless
belligerent	harsh	irritated	sadistic
callous	hateful	mad	savage
combative	heartless	malicious	unfeeling
critical	hideous	mean	vindictive
cruel	hostile	murderous	violent

Depression

abandoned	despondent	hurt	run down
alienated	discouraged	miserable	sad
alone	estranged	mistreated	tearful
battered	excluded	pathetic	terrible
crushed	grim	pitiful	unloved
defeated	hopeless	regretful	valueless
degraded	horrible	rotten	worthless
despairing	humiliated	ruined	

Distress

afflicted	dissatisfied	impaired	suspicious
anguished	distrustful	imprisoned	tormented
awkward	disturbed	lost	touchy
bewildered	doubtful	nauseated	unlovable
confused	futile	pained	unlucky
constrained	grieving	sickened	unsatisfied
disgusted	helpless	strained	unsure

Fear, Anxiety

afraid	fearful	nervous	terrified
agitated	frightened	on edge	terror-stricken
alarmed	hesitant	overwhelmed	uncomfortable
anxious	horrified	panicked	uneasy
apprehensive	insecure	scared	worried
desperate	intimidated	shaky	
dread	jumpy	tense	

Humiliation, Criticism

abused	discredited	maligned	scorned
belittled	disdained	minimized	shamed
betrayed	disgraced	mocked	slandered

TABLE 2.2 (CONTINUED)

criticized	humiliated	neglected	slighted
deprecated	ignored	put down	underestimated
diminished	libeled	ridiculed	underrated

Inadequacy

broken	exposed	incompetent	paralyzed
defective	fragile	indefensible	small
deficient	frail	ineffective	trivial
demoralized	helpless	inept	vulnerable
disabled	impotent	insecure	weak
exhausted	inadequate	insufficient	

the emotions a client is experiencing. Note that this list focuses on negative emotions, since, as we have noted, these are most common for individuals in crisis situations. Developing sensitivity to and verbal facility in identifying this wider range of feelings will enable the crisis counselor to respond to crisis clients with a much higher and more accurate level of empathic understanding. It is also important to remember that individual clients' lack of verbal proficiency in identifying feelings may be culturally defined, language-based, and/or idiosyncratic.

Crisis clients will reveal emotions in a variety of ways. Crisis counselors must therefore carefully attend to nonverbal as well as verbal clues with a goal of accurately identifying both the affective dimension and the intensity of emotional response. As Myer (2001) stated, "nervous" is not the same as "terrified," although both may be fearful responses. Clients may or may not be cognizant of and able to identify what they are feeling, particularly when they are overwhelmed. Similarly, crisis clients may or may not be able or willing to express emotions directly, and may minimize or rationalize their emotions to themselves and others as a way of avoiding the painful intensity associated with them. Observing nonverbal clues, actively listening to direct and indirect spontaneous verbal expressions, and asking probing questions directed toward understanding the emotional impact of the crisis are all common ways to facilitate the expression of painful and confusing emotions.

Behavioral Responses

Behavior, as discussed here, refers to the many actions an individual takes as he or she attempts to cope with and resolve a crisis. A crisis client's behaviors may not always appear purposeful, but they are always meaningful and always important to assess, as they are one of the most overt indicators of the individual's struggles in the aftermath of the crisis event. In assessing behavior as one component of a crisis client's functioning, it is important to notice behaviors that represent strengths and that are effective in enabling individuals to cope with problems as well as behaviors that may be problematic.

One can conceptualize behavioral problems as consisting of excesses or deficiencies. Behavioral deficiencies might include an inability or unwillingness to express feelings and thoughts or a limited ability to assert one's needs or ask for help. Behavioral excesses might include angry verbal or physical outbursts and aggressiveness, and self-destructive behaviors like excessive drinking, drug taking, or overeating. Clearly, problematic precrisis behavioral functioning, including deficits in skills, could have an impact on the crisis client's behavior in the aftermath of a crisis (Hackney & Cormier, 2000; Hepworth et al., 1997).

There have been numerous efforts to classify behavioral responses to crisis. In his early study of efforts to cope with crisis, Caplan (1964) suggested that individuals respond with either passive behaviors (e.g., aimless or repeated behaviors) or active behaviors (e.g., actively trying out new ways of problem-solving when usual ways have been unsuccessful). Koopman, Classen, and Spiegel (1996) also described active problem-focused behaviors individuals chose to directly handle traumatic stress as opposed to passive problem-solving, when the individual considered ways of taking action but seemed unable to carry them out. They also added a "passive-avoidant" category to describe the pattern of avoidance and dissociative responses whereby the individual engaged in behaviors that enabled him or her to deny the crisis. The father who refuses to talk to his wife about the death of their young child or who engages in alcohol abuse to avoid the pain of actively mourning would be an example of this last pattern.

In the Triage Assessment Model, Myer et al. (1992) classified behavioral reactions to crisis events as approach, avoidance, and immobility. A woman diagnosed with breast cancer who actively reads about alternative treatments and who joins a breast cancer support group in order to talk to and learn from other women with breast cancer is approaching the crisis and actively taking actions that enable her to cope with the cancer diagnosis. By contrast, a man diagnosed with HIV who begins to behave in a hypersexual manner or becomes obsessed with his physical appearance, bodybuilding, and exercising to excess is temporarily avoiding and denying the reality of his diagnosis. The immobilized crisis client either does nothing or engages in "self-canceling attempts" to resolve the crisis (Myer, 2001, p. 92). An example might be a woman who is abused by her fiancé and contacts a crisis hotline, but fails to follow through with agreed-upon plans and does not reveal what has happened to anyone else. Significantly, any of these clients, including those who actively approach the crisis in efforts to resolve it, can engage in behavioral patterns that are potentially detrimental.

When assessing a crisis client's behavioral functioning, it is important to remember that behavior is intimately connected to, and most often motivated by and responsive to, the individual's emotions and cognitions. An individual who perceives a threat or violation may become emotionally agitated or fearful and may react with aggressive behavior. Although behavior at times of extreme chaos or overwhelming affect may appear to be aimless and random, it nonetheless provides a clue as to the state of a client's emotions. Further, although the connection is not necessarily simple or direct, behavior is also indicative of the person's thoughts.

Behavior is clearly a primary focus of intervention, for example, when we help a client problem-solve, take specific actions, or stop particularly destructive actions. We can only understand the meaning of a client's behavior, however, when we also assess the emotions and cognitions that motivate it.

Cognitive Responses

Cognition refers to an individual's perceptions, beliefs, and judgments. As our definition of crisis suggests, the way individuals perceive and interpret the significance and meaning of events is critical to understanding how they feel and respond behaviorally. Idiosyncratic and unique perceptions and interpretations of specific events are themselves embedded in individual belief systems, values, and self-perceptions. They are also dependent on the individual's level of cognitive development and overall intellectual functioning. Thus an individual who functions at a high intellectual level and engages in complex and abstract thinking may struggle with the existential meaning of a particular crisis event. An individual who functions at a lower intellectual level and/or who engages in very concrete thinking processes may be thinking about the meaning of the crisis in a much more immediate and pragmatic way. For example, a young woman with borderline intelligence might describe how mean the man is who hurt her, whereas another woman might struggle with the fact that her perception of the world as basically fair and people as essentially good has been shattered.

Precrisis functioning is a critical determinant of how an individual will respond cognitively to a crisis event. At a minimum, healthy cognitive functioning depends on the capacity to be in touch with reality. This generally means that individuals are oriented to time, place, and person, able to reach accurate conclusions about cause-and-effect relationships, and able to distinguish their own thoughts and feelings from those of others. Individuals whose cognitive functioning is already limited or impaired would clearly experience further difficulty in coping with a crisis. Anyone, however, can experience some degree of impaired cognitive functioning in the struggle to cope cognitively with trauma and crisis events.

An individual who manifests severe cognitive impairment in response to a crisis may be incoherent, with fragmented and disconnected thoughts and speech, or may evidence a temporary lapse in reality testing as manifested in misperceptions about events or difficulty in discerning his or her feelings and thoughts from others'. A continuing pattern of such cognitive dysfunction may signify impairment requiring medication or hospitalization. Cognitive responses may also indicate the potential for suicidal or aggressive behavior. Crisis interventionists must always assess for serious cognitive impairments as well as for thoughts or ideations that could potentially lead to lethal responses to crisis (see Chapter 5).

Cognitive processes have a central role in how an individual perceives, makes sense of, and ultimately responds to a crisis emotionally, behaviorally, and interpersonally. Assessment of this area begins with understanding the crisis event as the client perceives it. This includes accurately hearing from the client's point of view both precisely what the crisis *is*, and what the meaning of the crisis is in terms of that client's belief systems, cultural meanings, and self-image. Thus, for example, in listening to a client describing an ongoing pattern of verbal and physical abuse by her husband, it would be necessary to first determine what, from the client's view, is most troubling to her. Is the crisis interpreted as, "How could someone who says he loves me do this to me?" or, alternatively, "How could I allow myself to be treated in this way?"

A number of writers have also pointed to the importance of identifying the areas or domains of a client's life that, from his or her perspective, are most affected by the crisis (Aguilera, 1998; Hoff, 1995; Myer et al., 1992). Myer (2001) identified four life dimensions that may be affected by a crisis: (1) physical safety and comfort, including food, shelter, and financial security; (2) psychological elements, including identity, self-esteem, and self-respect; (3) social relationships; and (4) moral/spiritual belief systems. He suggested that it is essential to discern the affected life dimension as the client perceives it in order to understand the significance of the crisis for that client.

The Triage Assessment Model (Myer et al., 1992) directs crisis interventionists to assign crisis clients' cognitive reactions to one of three types: (1) transgressions, the interpretation that something is currently infringing on their rights or victimizing them in some manner; (2) threats, the perception that the future is in some way compromised; or (3) loss, the sense that something has been taken away that can never be regained. This categorization is useful in sensitizing the crisis worker to the time orientation (present, future, past) as well as to general "types" of meaning that an individual may attribute to an event. It is also important, however, not to be limited by such categorizations of client responses and to recognize the diversity of meanings that a particular event may have for the individuals involved. That said, in our experience, a combined awareness of both "life dimensions" and "time orientation" can yield essential insights into the individualized meaning of a crisis. For example, a woman talking about her failing marriage may reveal the multiple ways she believes she has "lost herself" (loss/related to personal identity). A man who has learned of an abortion clinic opening in his community may speak about his unwillingness to "take the continued murder of innocent children" (transgression/related to moral belief systems). Note that in both cases the intensity of the responses could indicate the potential for lethal action.

Ultimately, the primary goal of working with crisis survivors is to help them develop adaptive ways of thinking about what has happened and its impact on them and their life. Adaptive in this sense simply means conducive to recovery and survival. In discussing crisis intervention with sexual assault survivors, Koss and Harvey (1991) identify two indicators or criteria of recovery that relate to cognition. One regards the individual's capacity to remember what has happened. "The individual has control over the remembering process and not the reverse. The individual can elect to recall or not recall events that previously intruded unbidden into awareness, taking the form of frightening dreams, troubling flashbacks, and distressing associations" (Koss & Harvey, 1991, p. 176).

The second indicator of adaptive cognition in their view would be that the individual has assigned a "tolerable meaning to the trauma and to the self as trauma survivor" (p. 177). The process of making meaning begins in the first moments of a crisis and intensifies as time passes. For any crisis client, assigning a "tolerable meaning" suggests that self-blaming cognition has been discarded and the client's self-image is of a survivor rather than merely a victim. Additionally, the survivor has named and grieved his or her losses, found a way to make sense of what happened, and has the freedom to move forward with living, perhaps with a new sense of purpose and with new concerns and motivations. For many individuals, spiritual or religious belief systems are central to the process of making meaning.

Considerable research documents that many people experience positive post-crisis changes, which are usually the result of cognitive changes as they cope with and survive a negative/traumatic event (Collins, Taylor, & Skokan, 1990; Tedeschi & Calhoun, 1995). Positive changes identified by traumatized individuals include changes in perceptions of self (e.g., the crisis made them a better person, they feel stronger), changed views of relationships (e.g., they have an increased desire to work at relationships and a stronger resolve to make decisions in their own best interest), and changed life philosophy (e.g., there are positive changes in their priorities, there is a recognition of the preciousness of life, their spiritual beliefs are strengthened) (Stuhlmiller & Dunning, 2000). Stuhlmiller and Dunning (2000) asserted that crisis interventionists must assist survivors to identify not only negative cognitive effects of trauma, but also to utilize positive-directed questions in order to "facilitate the active process of self-righting and growth" (p. 38).

In summary, cognitive reactions are the key to understanding why a crisis is a crisis for a particular individual and thus also to understanding the motive for emotional and behavioral responses. Cognitive responses are also central in the process of surviving and thriving beyond the crisis. Although cognitive responses are often more difficult to assess because they may be more difficult for the crisis worker to observe or for the client to express, they must be an essential domain of concern for the crisis worker.

Developmental Assessment

Competent developmental assessment (and intervention) evolves from the crisis interventionist's familiarity with both the basic philosophical assumptions and the concepts and theories that comprise developmental theory. This includes familiarity with the normative passages or stages postulated in various developmental theories and the direction in which these theories suggest that growth and change occurs. Optimally, change occurs in multiple functional areas including biological, cognitive, and social-emotional.

Crisis theory and developmental theories share the philosophical belief that individuals are innately motivated to grow and develop various competencies and strategies that actualize biological potential and enable mastery of environmental demands and challenges. Developmental theory suggests that as individuals confront various life transitions, both predictable milestones like beginning school or puberty and less predictable milestones like divorce, they respond by both utilizing previously developed knowledge and skills and by developing new capacities and skills. As Blocher (2000) described, many of the transitions that punctuate the course of development "result in change in assumptions about oneself and the world and thus require a corresponding change in one's behavior and relationships" (p. 27). Developmental change is seen to be continuous throughout an individual's life and to be influenced by many factors including innate biological capabilities and environments that foster mastery (Bronfenbrenner, 1979, 1989). This bio-ecological view emphasizes that human development emerges only as the result of transactions with other individuals and the environment. Social roles, social expectations, and relationship demands are thus critical dimensions of how individuals come to see themselves and how others view them.

Although it is beyond the scope of this text to teach developmental theory, a review of some basic developmental concepts that are useful in understanding a client in crisis is in order. In our experience, the two areas of developmental theory that are most useful in guiding crisis interventionists are psychosocial developmental theories that focus on the individual as a developing emotional and relational being and cognitive developmental theories that focus on the individual as a developing thinking, reasoning, and problem-solving being. In addition, it is essential that crisis workers be attuned to the impact gender and minority status have on development, for it is clear that all human growth and development occurs within the environmental and biological realities of our gender, ethnic, sexual, and cultural experiences.

Psychosocial development   Chapter 1 briefly introduced Erikson's (1963) psychosocial developmental theory. Building on the work of Erikson (1963), Havighurst (1972), and Bronfenbrenner (1979), Blocher (2000) introduced the following developmental framework: The first fifteen years of life constitute the "organization stage" of development. During this stage the individual (1) transforms into a relational individual capable of basic trust and social attachments, (2) develops an increasing sense of self as separate and able to self-regulate and handle increasingly independent tasks, (3) develops the initiative and resourcefulness that allows success in response to various learning challenges, and (4) ultimately develops a sense of stable identity. The organization stage, which focuses largely on coping with emerging physiological changes and abilities, sets the stage for the "exploration stage" (ages 16–30). During this period the individual is developmentally focused on attaining increased individual and relational maturity. This includes developing more mutual and reciprocal (as opposed to dependent) relationships and acquiring the emotional maturity to achieve, make decisions, and accept responsibility. New social roles, particularly those associated with marriage and family, require the capacity to form committed and intimate relationships.

The "realization stage" (ages 30–50) marks the end of the largely formative period of development and represents the time when individuals are most likely to achieve major life goals and values. Role expectations include successful parenting, successful careers, and the attainment of self-esteem grounded both in self-evaluation and others' recognition of one's contributions.

The stabilization stage (ages 50–65) and the examination stage (age 65 and over) both center on the "achievement of a sense of unity, stability, and harmony within one's lifestyle and between the individual and the culture" (p. 60). The midlife transitions that most often occur during the earliest part of these stages can be tumultuous as individuals review, reassess, and reorganize their priorities, recognizing that they are approaching the later years of their lives. Erikson (1963) suggested that the optimal outgrowth of the final stage is "ego integrity," or the attainment of a degree of tranquility even as individuals learn to cope with their own and loved ones' mortality, their declining physical health, and the changed social roles and living arrangements that accompany physical decline and death. Table 2.3 summarizes the major social roles and developmental tasks associated with each of these stages.

TABLE 2.3
BLOCHER'S LIFE STAGES AND DEVELOPMENTAL TASKS

Life Stages	Social Roles	Developmental Tasks
Infancy	Love-object roles, receiving and pleasing	Trust; learning to eat solid food and feed self, control elimination, manipulate objects, walk, explore immediate environment, communicate
Organization stage, early childhood (3–6 years)	Sibling, playmate, sex-appropriate roles	Autonomy; developing sense of self, sense of mutuality, realistic concepts of world, learning to be a boy or girl, manage aggression and frustration, follow verbal instructions, pay attention, become more independent
Late childhood (6–12 years)	Student, helper, big brother/big sister roles	Initiative-industry; learning to read and calculate, value self and be valued, delay gratification, control emotional reactions, deal with abstract concepts, give self to others, formulate values
Early adolescence (12–14 years)	Peer roles, sexual orientation exploration	Identity development, gender roles; belonging in various relationships, controlling impulses, being positive in work, studying, organizing time, developing relevant value hierarchy
Exploration stage, late adolescence, young adulthood (15–29 years)	Marriage roles, career roles	Intimacy and commitment, generativity; learning to commit self to goals, career, partner; be adequate parent, give unilaterally

TABLE 2.3 (CONTINUED)

Realization stage (30–50 years)	Leadership, helping, creative accomplishment roles	Ego-integrity; learning to be inner-directed, be interdependent, handle cognitive dissonance, be flexible and effective emotionally, develop creative thought processes, develop effective problem-solving techniques
Stabilization stage (50–65 years)	Leadership, helping, managing creative accomplishments, authority, prestige	Ego-integrity; learning to be aware of change, have attitude of tentativeness, develop broad intellectual curiosity, develop realistic idealism develop time perspective
Examination stage (65+ years)	Retirement roles, nonworker roles, nonauthority roles	Learning to cope with death, with retirement, affiliate with peers, cope with reduced physical vigor, cope with changed living conditions, use leisure time, care for the aging body

Adapted with permission from D. H. Blocher. (2000). *Counseling: A developmental approach* (4th ed.). New York: John Wiley & Sons.

Familiarity with these pivotal psychosocial stages is useful because whenever crisis workers encounter an individual in crisis, that individual is experiencing crisis at a specific stage in his or her life span. To be most helpful, crisis interventionists must understand the developmental factors that may influence the way an individual responds to a crisis event. These factors include significant social roles and/or developmental tasks and expectations that may be affected by the crisis and that help shape the individualized meaning of the crisis.

For example, consider a 13-year-old boy who is sexually molested, perhaps over a long period of time, by a trusted adult male. The sexual assault is the crisis event. But the meaning of that event, its impact, the victim's ability to decide what to do about it, and ultimately to process and attribute some meaning to it will be inevitably determined by the boy's developmental age and tasks. In addition to his developmental efforts to form a values-based hierarchy, he is at the formative stage of his own sexual awakening. He is also at a formative stage regarding his gender identity development. Imagine that although he was confused and frightened during the sexual molestations, he also experienced physical arousal and, perhaps, ejaculation. The confounding experience of anxiety, powerlessness, and fear coupled with sexual arousal may have a traumatizing effect on his sexual development and comfort. He may become quite confused in trying to sort out what it means about his sexuality to have been targeted by a male and to have experienced arousal during the assault. Clearly the significant developmental tasks he faces as a 13-year-old male have a tremendously important reciprocal impact on how he experiences the traumatizing event(s). His continued development may be affected if he is unable to find an acceptable way of understanding and resolving what has happened.

Or, in another example, consider a middle-aged male who loses his job when his company downsizes and twelve months later has still not found another position in his field. This man is at the developmental stage in his life when he believes he should be successful, treated with respect, and acknowledged for his contributions and importance. Although he has been doing odd jobs and has tried to keep his hopes high as he has searched for a job, he has come to believe that he will not find a similar position, given his age and the state of the economy. His wife has become the primary breadwinner, and although she tries to bolster his self-esteem, she is also increasingly critical of his growing tendency to sit at home drinking and sleeping. The crisis counselor sees him when, in a rage following an argument with his wife, he deliberately drives his car over an embankment. Although not injured seriously, he is clearly a suicide risk when he is brought to the emergency room of the local hospital. He sees himself as having lost his career as well as his position of importance within his home, and sees very little purpose in living.

In both cases, understanding psychosocial development sensitizes the crisis worker to the deeper significance of the crisis event. In each of these examples the crisis event can only be fully appreciated by understanding its developmental context and the resultant implications.

Coping behaviors   Although such life-span frameworks are useful in identifying characteristic passages through which human beings change and grow, Blocher (2000) cautioned that it is also essential to recognize the "tremendous variation in the ways people attempt to cope with or master the specific tasks and challenges that arise at each stage in the life cycle" (p. 91). He suggested that we pay equal attention to what Adler termed individual "lifestyles," or the characteristic ways individuals have learned to cope with stress or difficulties. Particularly germane to the understanding of individual lifestyles is the concept of coping behaviors.

Lazarus and Folkman (1984) defined coping as "constantly changing cognitive and behavioral efforts to manage specific external and/or internal demands that are appraised as taxing or exceeding the resources of a person" (p. 141). The concept of appraisal refers to the way the individual attributes meaning to the situation or problem, and Lazarus and Folkman delineated both primary and secondary levels of appraisal. For example, an individual may perceive a stressful event as stressful yet challenging, or conversely, as a threat that will involve damage or loss. This is referred to as a primary appraisal in that it involves what is at stake in the situation (Lazarus, 1991).

By contrast, a secondary appraisal refers to an individual's assessment regarding "which coping options are available, the likelihood that a given coping option will accomplish what it is supposed to . . ." (Lazarus & Folkman, 1984, p. 35). An appraisal of situational self-efficacy or the perception that one does or does not have the ability to do what is necessary to resolve a problem is an example of a secondary appraisal. Primary and secondary appraisals interact and affect the degree of stress an individual experiences, the type and strength of emotional reactions, and the coping approach he or she is likely to employ (Lazarus & Folkman, 1984). In this view, then, coping is an effort to manage a situation, and the way a situation is perceived is a primary determinant of both the felt need to cope and the particular coping strategies that the individual will employ. For example, an individual who perceives a situation as a threat, and also believes that he or she is unable to change the situation, is likely to experience a high level of stress. This individual is likely to cope differently than one who perceives a challenge that he or she believes can be met with either current or attainable abilities.

As noted in Chapter 1, early writers identified two major coping styles: emotion-focused coping and problem-focused coping (Folkman, 1984; Lazarus & Folkman, 1984). More recently, Cook and Heppner (1997) analyzed three separate coping measures and identified a three-factor model, including (1) problem-focused/task-oriented coping, (2) social-support/emotional expression coping, and (3) avoidance.

Blocher (2000) suggested three general coping styles that reflect the interaction between the individual and the environment: (1) minimizing and avoiding, (2) impulsive-intuitive, and (3) rational-analytic. Some individuals cope with stressful situations by physically and cognitively trying to minimize the impact of the situation or avoiding the situation altogether. Impulsive-intuitive "copers" respond to stressful situations spontaneously and without great thought, their actions based on what intuitively "feels right." By contrast, individuals who utilize more rational-analytic coping strategies tend to analyze situations and rationally determine the best course of action.

Each general coping style can be effective or ineffective depending on the situation. For example, when dealing with chronic pain, individuals who minimize attention to every ache and pain and focus instead on spending time with friends and family may find that "minimizing" helps them keep a positive perspective despite unavoidable discomfort. By comparison, an individual who is experiencing considerable physiological arousal and anxiety in response to a crisis or traumatic event (e.g., a diagnosis of cancer or a sexual assault) will not effectively cope by "just trying not to think about it." Similarly, individuals who respond to stressful situations in an unplanned and intuitive manner may usually cope successfully, but experience more difficulty coping when faced with a more complex situation.

In general, research has pointed to the efficacy of problem-solving approaches and affirmed that avoidance strategies are less successful than approaching problems with the goal of resolving them, even when the external event that precipitated the crisis (e.g., diagnosis of cancer, death of a loved one) cannot be changed (Nezu, Nezu, Friedman, Faddis, & Houts, 1998). Problem-solving approaches, however, may be insufficient in situations that arouse intense physiological and emotional responses unless the problem-solving approach includes an emotional expression and emotional support component. For example, research suggests that trying to minimize or avoid the emotional impact only serves to exacerbate the problem, as numbness and isolation replace the active pursuit of emotional expression and social support, and may increase the risk of developing PTSD (Foa & Rothbaum, 1998). (See Chapter 6, on sexual assault, and Chapter 13, on disasters, for more information.) Similarly, research on secondary stress responses among emergency and crisis personnel has documented the efficacy of "emotion-focused" and "approach" strategies rather than either "avoidance" or purely rational problem-solving (Anderson, 2000; Truman, 1997).

Crisis workers must pay attention to both the way individuals have coped with problems in the past and the way they are attempting to cope with the current crisis. Intervention can help individuals recognize and assess their coping strategies and help them develop additional coping skills, as necessary. Crisis intervention strategies also model a combined emotion-focused, problem-solving coping approach.

Cognitive development   Although we have already discussed the importance of assessing the cognitive domain, some understanding of the development of different cognitive processes can assist the crisis worker to accurately assess a client's thinking style and to intervene responsively. Contemporary cognitive development theory is rooted in the work of Jean Piaget. Piaget (1929) theorized that there is a basic human motivation to understand and cope with the world. As children attempt to make sense of their encounters with the environment, they gradually develop qualitatively different ways of thinking and understanding—what Piaget termed "basic thought processes." He developed a typology describing four basic cognitive stages: sensorimotor, preoperational, concrete, and formal.

We can benefit from Ivey's (1991) observation that these stages represent two broad types of thought patterns. The first is "concrete-focused" on the world of events, situations, and actions. Concrete thought patterns are revealed as clients speak of specific and observable details of events and specific behaviors they or others have engaged in. Abstract thought patterns, by contrast, are more concerned with ideas, thoughts, and contemplation about events. Thus an aging woman who describes feeling invisible because she has lost her youthful beauty is engaged in an abstract thought process, whereas a man who describes being angry because his wife refused his sexual advances is engaged in a more linear and concrete thought process.

Piaget saw the development from concrete to abstract thinking as a progression toward higher-order forms of cognition. Ivey (1991) cautioned that the abstract world of ideas is not necessarily more significant than the concrete world of sensory experience and action. He contended that although it is important for a counselor to be able to recognize and interact on a client's cognitive level, in accordance with the client's manner of processing information, "mismatched" interventions can also be helpful, as when a counselor helps an overly abstract client focus on more concrete specifics. At root is the counselor's ability to assess and accurately identify the client's cognitive-developmental level, which is most often revealed by the client's language and speech patterns. Further, it is helpful to bear in mind that although some individuals will present as totally concrete or totally abstract thinkers, many others will display both concrete and abstract thought patterns, perhaps in relation to specific topics.

In summary, developmental assessment requires attention to who the individual is as a developing person. This does not mean engaging in a long process of taking a social history or utilizing specific assessment devices. Rather, it means listening for and being attuned to relevant developmental issues that can inform understanding of the individual in crisis and the potential impact of the crisis. Developmental assessment includes:

1. Recognizing the developmental challenges and passages that may be affected or threatened by the crisis event.
2. Recognizing the social roles, cultural expectations, and environmental interactions that define the individual's identity, self-concept, and sense of responsibility.
3. Identifying the client's lifestyle and usual coping styles.
4. Identifying the client's characteristic thought processes.

The more these developmental ways of seeing become second nature, the more likely the crisis worker will recognize both the potential developmental implications of all crises and the inevitability that a crisis client's developmental capacities predicate his or her responses to crisis events.

Ecological Assessment

Assessment of a client's experience following a crisis must include attention to the transactions between the person and the environmental context within which the crisis occurs and the environment within which the client is embedded. A first step in assessing the environmental impact in a crisis is to determine which aspects of the environment are most salient or relevant to the particular situation and person. At a minimum, three broad areas can be identified: (1) the individual's culture and the values, traditions, and dominant belief systems of that culture; (2) the individual's social supports, including close family, friends, and others who share an ongoing involvement in that individual's life, and the nature of those relationships; and (3) the larger community within which the crisis occurs and within which the individual resides. The larger community's resources, relative safety, and supportiveness are all essential.

Joining with a client and establishing a working alliance require quick assessment and immersion in the client's worldview. This worldview is strongly influenced by the client's culture, ethnic identity, gender, and sexual orientation. Particular types of psychosocial stressors including acculturation status, prejudice and discrimination, and language barriers invariably have an impact on individual responses to crisis. Similarly, culturally diverse clients' family connectedness and relative dependence/independence with extended family vary. Family relationships are also affected by cultural values regarding gender roles, power and authority, and religion. Ecological assessment therefore begins with recognition of a crisis client's culture and degree of acculturation. Cultural competence, simply defined as the ability to work effectively with culturally diverse clients, depends on multisystem assessment (see Chapter 4).

Hepworth et al. (1997) suggested two broad foci for environmental assessments: environmental resources and social support systems. Ideal environmental resources include adequate housing and financial resources, opportunities for education and employment, and access to adequate health care, child care, and legal services including police, attorneys, and the courts.

Social systems are envisioned as concentric circles surrounding the individual, with the innermost circle being one's immediate nuclear family. (See Figure 2.1.) Moving outward, the social system circle includes extended family and close friends; more peripheral are neighbors, work associates, and members of common associations such as church and social clubs; and at the outermost edge are formal services and service providers in schools, municipal services, social services, and so on. This is a helpful way to identify and map the potential social supports that may be available to a crisis client. In formulating ecological assessments of individuals in crisis, however, it is equally necessary not only to name potential supports, but also to continually recognize the reciprocal interactions among individuals and these systems of which they are a part (Bronfenbrenner, 1979; Hepworth et al., 1997).

As has been true with each previous component, the nature of an individual's social interactions and the responsiveness of both formal and informal support systems prior to a crisis in large measure determines how an individual is able to

FIGURE 2.1
SOCIAL SUPPORT ECOSYSTEM

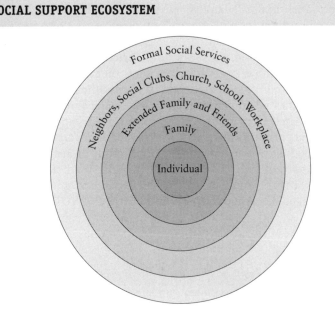

utilize those resources and potential supports during a crisis. In this regard, both the actual availability of resources and social supports and *perceived* availability and accessibility are important. An individual who perceives barriers or who fears judgment based on previous experiences, may be reluctant to reach out for assistance even if nurturing social support systems exist. Thus, for example, a gay male who is the victim of a hate crime may be hesitant to reveal what has occurred to the police or to family for fear of the reactions of these potential supporters. He may not be aware that there is a gay police detective who is respected within the local police force, or he may assume that his family would be unresponsive although he has never risked giving them the chance to understand his sexual orientation. He may, however, also be accurate in his assessment of the negative and judgmental responses he would encounter. The crisis worker must strive to both understand the crisis client's perceptions regarding potential resources and supports as well as to acquire an objective assessment of their availability and usefulness to the client. The crisis worker can present information about resources clients do not have, and can assist them to critically evaluate their a priori perceptions. The final decision as to which environmental resources and interpersonal or social supports are utilized, however, must be determined by the client.

Identifying key people in an individual's social system and the type of support they may be able to provide is key in assessing an individual's interpersonal supports. Although the use of assessment tools is rarely practical in single-session crisis intervention, when working with clients in crisis counseling, it may be helpful to utilize the Social Network Grid (Tracy & Whittaker, 1990), which can help both client and crisis worker gain an expanded awareness of the possible sources of interpersonal support in an individual's social milieu.

The last important issue of concern in ecological assessment of a crisis is assessing material resources, including the crisis client's financial condition, access to health care, housing, and transportation. A victim of domestic violence with dependent children who is financially dependent on her abuser, who does not have a car, and who cannot access counseling services without her husband's knowledge because her health insurance is in his name certainly faces many challenges if she tries to free herself from that relationship. A homeless person who experiences a brief psychotic episode is in a very different situation and has many fewer options than an individual with significant material resources at his or her disposal. It is critically important that crisis counselors understand the role of material resources in either providing options for client action or, on the contrary, in presenting additional challenges to crisis resolution.

CONCLUSION

In conclusion, any crisis assessment model should ideally alert the crisis counselor to important areas of interest or concern. The model presented here is designed to be used flexibly, continuously, and with experience and familiarity, intuitively. Our goal is not to present a specific series of questions or methods for analyzing people or situations. Rather we hope to enable crisis counselors to develop increasing complexity in comprehending crisis clients' needs and strengths. There are some very concrete assessments that must be made in any crisis situation. It is always necessary to assess the situation for possible danger and to be alert to signs of potential lethal action. Specific strategies for making such determinations are presented in Chapter 5. Beyond that crisis counselors will be most helpful to crisis clients, whether they are seen in single-session crisis counseling or in ongoing crisis counseling, when each client is seen holistically and contextually. Ultimately, assessment should lead to informed, effective intervention. That is the focus of the next chapter.

DISCUSSION QUESTIONS

1. The ABCDE assessment model is designed to guide crisis counselors in both single-session crisis intervention and ongoing crisis counseling. Discuss the differences in assessment when conducting a single-session intervention immediately following a crisis and when working with an individual in ongoing crisis counseling.

2. How does the *developmental-ecological approach* affect the perspective of a crisis counselor as he or she attempts to understand the impact of a crisis event on a given individual?

EXERCISES

1. Instruct each student to prepare for class by developing a personal "eco-map." In class, divide students into small groups and ask them to share their eco-maps with each other. Ask a group recorder or recorders to develop a list of possible sources of personal/social support as reflected in group members' eco-maps.

2. Divide the class into small groups. Write the words *Affect, Behavior, Cognition, Development, Ecosystem* on the board. Instruct each group to take each domain, and (1) identify examples of ways that domain is negatively affected by a crisis, and (2) identify examples of strengths in that domain that individuals can build upon to help them cope in the aftermath of a crisis. For example, isolation or avoidance of friends and family would be an example of a negative behavior. The belief that "I did everything I could to survive" would be an example of strength in the area of cognition. Discussion with the class as a whole can begin with the question of which list (problems or potential strengths) was easier to develop and why.

3. Ask students to identify a client, friend, or family member who has experienced a crisis. Instruct each student to interview that individual and to write a summary assessment of how he or she was affected by the crisis using the ABCDE assessment model. In class discussion following the homework assignment, consider both the process of interviewing and how useful students found the model.

REFERENCES

Aguilera, D. C. (1998). *Crisis intervention: Theory and methodology* (8th ed.). St. Louis: Mosby.

Anderson, D. G. (2000). Coping strategies and burnout among veteran child protection workers. *Child Abuse and Neglect, 24*(6), 839–848.

Blocher, D. H. (2000). *Counseling: A developmental approach* (4th ed.). New York: John Wiley & Sons.

Bronfenbrenner, U. (1979). *The ecology of human development.* Cambridge, MA: Harvard University Press.

Bronfenbrenner, U. (1989). Ecological systems theory. In R. Vasta (Ed.), *Annals of child development, 6* (pp. 187–251). Greenwich, CT: JAI.

Caplan, G. (1964). *Principles of preventive psychiatry.* New York: Basic Books.

Collins, R. L., Taylor, S. E., & Skokan, L. A. (1990). A better world or a shattered vision? Changes in perspectives following victimization. *Social Cognition, 8,* 263–285.

Cook, S. W., & Heppner, P. P. (1997). A psychometric study of three coping measures. *Educational and Psychological Measurement, 57,* 906–923.

Crow, G. A. (1977). *Crisis intervention.* New York: Association Press.

DuBois, B., & Krogsrud Miley, K. (2000). *Social work: An empowering profession* (4th ed.). Boston: Allyn & Bacon.

Erikson, E. H. (1963). *Childhood and society* (2nd ed.). New York: Norton.

Foa, E. B., & Rothbaum, B. O. (1998). *Treating the trauma of rape: Cognitive-behavioral therapy for PTSD.* New York: Guilford Press.

Folkman, S. (1984). Personal control and stress and coping processes: A theoretical analysis. *Journal of Personality and Social Psychology, 46,* 839–852.

Germain, C. B., & Gitterman, A. (1996). *The life model of social work practice* (2nd ed.). New York: Columbia University Press.

Hackney, H., & Cormier, S. (2000). *The professional counselor: A process guide to helping* (4th ed.). Boston: Allyn & Bacon.

Havighurst, R. (1972). *Developmental tasks and education.* New York: David McKay.

Hepworth, D. H., Rooney, R. H., & Larsen, J. A. (1997). *Direct social work practice: Theory and skills* (5th ed.). Pacific Grove, CA: Brooks/Cole.

Hoff, L. A. (1995). *People in crisis: Understanding and helping* (4th ed.). Redwood City, CA: Addison-Wesley.

Ivey, A. (1991). *Developmental strategies for helpers: Individual, family, and network interventions.* Pacific Grove, CA: Brooks/Cole.

Koopman, C., Classen, C., & Spiegel, D. (1996). Dissociative response in the immediate aftermath of the Oakland/Berkeley firestorm. *Journal of Traumatic Stress, 9,* 521–540.

Koss, M. P., & Harvey M. R. (1991). *The rape victim: Clinical and community interventions* (2nd ed.). Newbury Park, CA: Sage.

Lazarus, R. (1991). Progress on a cognitive-motivational-relational theory of emotion. *American Psychologist, 46,* 819–834.

Lazarus, R., & Folkman, S. (1984). *Stress, appraisal, and coping.* New York: Springer.

Lum, D. (1996). *Social work practice and people of color: A process-stage approach* (3rd ed.). Pacific Grove, CA: Brooks/Cole.

Lum, D. (1999). *Culturally competent practice: A framework for growth and action.* Pacific Grove, CA: Brooks/Cole.

Meyer, C. H. (1987). Direct practice in social work: Overview. In A. Minahan (Ed.), *Encyclopedia of social work: Vol. 1* (18th ed., pp. 409–422). Silver Spring, MD: National Association of Social Workers.

Myer, R. A. (2001). *Assessment for crisis intervention: A triage assessment model.* Belmont, CA: Wadsworth, Brooks/Cole.

Myer, R. A., Williams, R. C., Ottens, A. J., & Schmidt, A. E. (1992). Crisis assessment: A three-dimensional model for triage. *Journal of Mental Health Counseling, 14,* 137–148.

Nezu, A. M., Nezu, C. M., Friedman, S. H., Faddis, S., & Houts, P. S. (1998). *Helping cancer patients cope.* Washington, DC: American Psychological Association.

Piaget, J. (1929). The child's conception of the world. New York: Harcourt Brace.

Slaikeu, K. A. (1990). *Crisis intervention: A handbook for practice and research* (2nd ed.). Boston: Allyn & Bacon.

Stuhlmiller, C., & Dunning, C. (2000). Challenging the mainstream: From pathogenic to salutogenic models of posttrauma intervention. In J. M. Violanti, D. Paton, & C. Dunning (Eds.), *Posttraumatic stress intervention: Challenges, issues, and perspectives* (pp. 10–42). Springfield, IL: Charles C. Thomas Publisher.

Tedeschi, R. G., & Calhoun, L. G. (1995). *Trauma and transformation: Growing in the aftermath of suffering.* Thousand Oaks, CA: Sage Publications.

Tracy, E. M., & Whittaker, J. K. (1990). The social-network map: Assessing social support in clinical practice. *Families in Society, 71,* 461–470.

Truman, B. M. (1997). Secondary traumatization, counselor's trauma history, and styles of coping. *Dissertation Abstracts International: Section A: Humanities and Social Sciences, 62* (5-A), 1945.

CHAPTER 3

Crisis Intervention: A Developmental-Ecological Approach

BACKGROUND

Now that we have addressed a general theoretical and philosophical framework for envisioning crisis as well as explored important aspects of assessment, we turn in this chapter to the steps of actually helping someone experiencing a crisis reaction. As previously stated, we believe that crisis counseling in the immediate aftermath of a crisis substantively differs from intervention with someone engaged in the longer and more complex process of crisis resolution. Thus, in this text we distinguish between the goals and suggested steps of crisis counseling during the immediate post-impact phase of a crisis and the goals and strategies of ongoing crisis counseling.

As we define it, ongoing crisis counseling may be provided in the weeks and months following a crisis event or it might not be provided until months or even years later, when a person seeks counseling and his or her presenting complaints are identified as related to an unresolved crisis in the past. Slaikeu (1990) labeled single-session crisis counseling "psychological first aid" and ongoing crisis counseling "crisis therapy." He asserted that the two types of intervention differed in a number of ways including how long the crisis worker is engaged with the individual client, by whom the crisis intervention is provided, where involvement with the client occurs, and the goals and procedures of giving help (p. 102). Although we prefer to speak simply of single-session crisis counseling and ongoing crisis counseling, we concur with many of his observations.

By Whom and Where

Slaikeu (1990) contended that single-session intervention in the immediate aftermath of a crisis event was provided by a variety of "front-line caregivers" including clergy, police, medical personnel, and volunteers in various crisis service settings; not solely by mental health professionals. Although this may be the case in that any of these types of caregivers may encounter someone in crisis, this text is designed primarily for human service professionals, who we believe are the individuals most likely to function as crisis interventionists. Individuals who provide single-session crisis intervention should be proficient in utilizing beginning helping skills, knowledgeable about common crisis reactions and the dynamics of specific crises, and familiar with relevant community resources. The more complex process of assisting individuals in the long-term struggle to resolve and integrate crises in their lives requires a helping professional with even more advanced professional knowledge and skills.

Single-session crisis counseling is provided in many different community settings including hospital emergency rooms and other medical settings, schools, churches, offices, walk-in centers, and telephone hotlines. Ongoing crisis counseling is a process that may take weeks or months and is more likely to occur in more structured counseling settings such as mental health or family service centers, private therapy practices, or comprehensive crisis centers like those existing in many communities to provide assistance to survivors of domestic violence and/or sexual assault.

Goals and Processes of Intervention

Although the differences regarding the delivery of crisis intervention services are important, the more substantive distinctions between single-session crisis counseling and ongoing crisis counseling relate to their goals and counseling processes. Single-session intervention has discrete and limited goals. The primary purpose of single-session intervention is to help the individual restore some sense of control and mastery after the shattering impact of a crisis event. A crisis reaction has classically been described as a period of overwhelming emotional upset or a breakdown in coping and problem-solving, and more recently, as a violation of the individual's beliefs and images about themselves, others, and/or the world. Given this understanding of crisis, the pressing need in working with someone in the throes of a crisis reaction must be to ensure safety and promote greater stability. This entails providing emotional support as well as concrete assistance in problem-solving and linking to both informal and formal sources of ongoing support.

Ongoing crisis counseling, by contrast, has a much more ambitious goal: to treat damaging symptomatic consequences and, most important, to assist individuals to survive and thrive beyond the crisis. The goal is for individuals to rebuild those aspects of their lives that remain hostage to the crisis, whether that entails gaining greater control over one's memories and their emotional impact, finding some way to make sense of what happened, or reconnecting with significant family members and friends.

The process of resolving and integrating a crisis may in some cases result in return to a precrisis state. More often, particularly following traumatic exposure, it entails developing new ways of thinking and behaving that reflect the changed reality created by the crisis. Basic to our philosophy regarding crisis and crisis resolution is our belief that people who have experienced a significant crisis cannot simply go back to a precrisis innocence because they are inevitably changed by an intimate knowledge that crises can and do occur. This is not to suggest that crisis survivors are forever negatively affected. Rather, it is our contention that many individuals develop a greater sense of their own strength and resilience as well as a clearer understanding of what they truly value and strive for in their lives.

Although crisis counseling often contributes to growth and change rather than merely crisis stabilization, this does not mean that it is not specific in goals and processes. Ongoing crisis counseling differs from other brief therapy approaches in that it is directed toward resolution and integration of an identified crisis or traumatic event. The goals of ongoing crisis counseling thus specifically identify functional domains affected by the crisis and define what healthy adaptation or resolution of the crisis entails. It has been noted that crises represent both danger and opportunity. It is the overarching goal of all crisis counseling, both single-session and ongoing, to tilt the scale toward opportunity.

This chapter presents two models for crisis counseling—one for single-session crisis counseling and one for ongoing crisis counseling. Both are based on developmental-ecological assessment. We begin with an examination of the goals and steps of single-session crisis counseling.

SINGLE-SESSION CRISIS COUNSELING

Goals

Single-session crisis counseling can be compared to emergency room medical care in that intervention must begin immediately and must ensure that no further deterioration occurs. The overarching purpose of all single-session intervention is to help bring calm control to a potentially critical situation and to ensure that the individuals involved are more capable of taking whatever "next steps" are necessary to cope with the crisis. Single-session intervention is usually provided soon after the crisis event occurs when the individual in crisis is experiencing the most difficulty in coping with immediate needs and responses.

Three primary goals can be identified. The first, and always most immediate set of goals, is *to ensure that the client is safe and lethality is reduced.* Not every situation will include the possibility of volatility in the environment or unsafe behavior by the client or others, but it is the crisis worker's responsibility to assess that possibility and to take the directive action necessary to ensure safety. The second goal is *to ensure that the client is psychologically stable and has attained short-term mastery of him- or herself and of the situation.* This does not mean that the crisis is resolved or that the individual is no longer experiencing difficulty. What it means is that overwhelming affect has been moderated, and the individual has some idea of the next step(s) to take to gain a degree of behavioral control. Last, single-session intervention should always result in the individual's *connection with informal and formal support systems.* Single-session intervention, by definition, will not be ongoing. Thus it is vitally important for the crisis interventionist to enable persons in crisis to identify and reach out to those individuals in their network of family and friends who will be able to provide ongoing support and aid. Similarly, assisting individuals in crisis to identify formal resources they can utilize in the future and helping them to make preliminary connections with them may be the most effective step in ensuring that they utilize those resources if they need continued assistance (see Table 3.1).

TABLE 3.1
GOALS OF SINGLE-SESSION CRISIS INTERVENTION

Goals

1. Client is safe and lethality is reduced.

2. Client is psychologically stable and has attained short-term mastery of self and situation.

3. Client is connected with appropriate formal and informal supports/resources.

Components of Single-Session Crisis Intervention

As we saw in Chapter 1, most models of single-session crisis intervention have utilized a fairly straightforward problem-solving approach. Although different models have emphasized one component over another, depending on the types of situations for which they were intended, each has also included common dimensions. The six-step model presented in Table 3.2 contains familiar problem-solving components and to that extent may appear similar to other models. This model, however, is intended to bridge the gap that has too often existed between theory and practice and between assessment and intervention. It is intended to be a guide to single-session crisis intervention that can be utilized in a wide variety of crisis situations by a range of potential helpers, including hotline workers, religious leaders, caseworkers in mental health or child welfare, schoolteachers, and counselors.

Although the steps of the single-session model are presented sequentially, in any crisis situation the crisis counselor must determine the precise order in which to take these steps. Thus in a highly volatile situation, a crisis worker might be required to simultaneously assess the situation, connect with the client(s) sufficiently to begin to de-escalate, and create safety. In another situation the worker may be able to spend more time making an empathic connection with the client and gaining a more complex understanding of the client's needs and resources. Note that, as we have said before, although assessment is presented as a component of Steps 2 and 3 in the intervention process, in practice, *assessment begins at first contact and must continue throughout involvement with the person in crisis.*

TABLE 3.2
INTERVENTION MODEL: SINGLE-SESSION CRISIS INTERVENTION

Goals

1. Supportively and empathically join with client.
2. Assess and intervene immediately to:
   a. create safety in environment
   b. stabilize and de-escalate
   c. handle immediate needs
3. Explore and assess dimensions of crisis event and crisis reaction (ABCDE), encouraging ventilation.
4. Examine alternatives and develop options.
5. Assist client to mobilize personal and social resources and connect with other community resources, as needed.
6. Anticipate the future and arrange follow-up.

Step 1:
Supportively and empathically join with the client.

To be successful, any helping activity requires that the helper establish an empathic connection with the person in need. Individuals are unlikely to risk exposing their pain and suffering unless they sense that the person offering assistance truly accepts them and has the capacity at least to try to understand them. The crisis worker initially conveys acceptance through nonverbal and verbal expressions of warmth, sincere interest and concern, and respectful efforts to attend to the crisis client's comfort and privacy. Tone of voice, posture, and words all contribute to presenting a supportive and stabilizing presence.

One important way to convey interest and concern is to begin your contact with a client with a straightforward statement of your name, role, and purpose in talking to him or her. *"Hello, Mrs. Jones, my name is Mary Jane and I am a crisis counselor at Survivor's Resources. I am called to the hospital whenever there is a sexual assault reported because we know how difficult it is to know what to do, and even what to feel, in such a confusing and upsetting situation. I am available to assist you in any way that I can. . . ."* In this manner, the crisis counselor answers the inevitable but unasked question regarding who is approaching and why. Your initial introductory remarks will inform the crisis client about how you may be of assistance, begin to alleviate possible anxiety associated with a stranger's offer of help, and begin to establish a calming influence.

Perhaps the two most important relationship-building skills you bring to this interaction with the client are your capacity for empathy and authenticity. The ability to perceive and respond accurately and sensitively to the client in crisis is the elemental criterion for establishing a helping connection (see Chapter 4). Conveying authenticity or genuineness is similarly essential. When you are authentic or genuine, you relate personally and in a spontaneous manner. In a single-session intervention, although personal self-disclosure is rarely advised, self-involving statements do convey genuineness and can be used very effectively. For example, *"I want you to know I believe your decision on how to respond to him was the absolute best you could do under incredibly frightening circumstances. No one else was there to help you and you did what you were able to do at the time."* In this manner, the crisis worker conveys acceptance of the individual, respect for his or her struggle, and spontaneous and nonjudgmental support.

As the crisis worker initially assists the client to express painful and perhaps overwhelming feelings and responds empathically and supportively, the client begins to experience some lessening of anxiety. As we will see in Step 3, this opportunity to ventilate to a caring and compassionate helper can be critical in beginning to decrease the crisis client's emotional distress.

Step 2:
Intervene to create safety, stabilize, de-escalate, and handle immediate needs.

Intervene to create safety   Creating safety requires the crisis worker to assess potential dangers, both physical and psychological, and calmly and purposefully take control in a situation. In general, the more at risk the client is for harm, the more directive the crisis counselor must become. This could mean removing a person from a potentially dangerous situation, as when you direct someone to move away from an accident scene or away from electric wires that have fallen. It could also mean directing people away from a scene of mass violence to protect them from further exposure to horrific images.

It could mean ensuring the removal of anything that might cause further harm or danger in a particular situation, as when a counselor asks an individual in crisis to hand over pills he or she is threatening to swallow. Or if when working with a group of adolescent boys, one became belligerent and verbally abusive, a counselor could prevent further harm and escalation by asking a coworker to remove the other youths from the scene as the counselor calmly engages the individual in crisis. In this situation, the crisis counselor is both removing the audience and curtailing the possibility of others escalating their own behavior.

Stabilize and de-escalate   It is common for individuals in crisis to experience very high levels of agitation, anxiety, and emotionality. They may experience racing thoughts or obsessively ruminate about what has happened or will happen. This state of overwhelming affect and/or thought process cannot be maintained for long, and if allowed to continue or escalate, can lead to psychological harm, behavioral acting out, and/or emotional paralysis. A person in this condition will also be unlikely to consider his or her options rationally or to engage in problem-solving. It is thus essential that crisis workers intervene immediately to help clients moderate their responses and reestablish a sense of being in control of themselves, their thoughts, and their emotions.

The very process of feeling heard, understood, and accepted can serve to stabilize and lessen the intensity of emotional response. Similarly a calm and supportive stance by the helper can gradually serve to moderate and bring "calm control" to an otherwise potentially escalating situation.

Handle immediate needs   Immediate needs are the first concern for the victim or survivor of a crisis. In situations where an individual's physical well-being is at risk, the crisis worker must address those immediate needs first, for example, if someone has been physically injured and needs medical attention. In other instances, immediate needs are those concerns that must be addressed before other aspects of the crisis situation can be attended to. For example, most individuals who have been sexually assaulted are initially concerned with informing family members and/or their partners about what has occurred. For some individuals, fears related to the reactions of significant others may be paramount. The decision about whether to notify the police or other authorities can also be an immediate concern. Or a domestic violence survivor may need to make an immediate determination of whether it is safe for her to stay in her home, or how to leave and what to take with her if she concludes that it is not. Or an individual who cannot find a loved one following a disaster may need direction for obtaining information as it becomes available.

As individuals in crisis handle these immediate needs they begin to have an increased sense of power and control over themselves and their situation. Thus, assisting the person in crisis to identify and resolve these immediate concerns is instrumental in freeing him or her to begin to address the other dimensions of the crisis.

Step 3:
Explore and assess dimensions of crisis event and crisis reaction (ABCDE), encouraging ventilation.

The third step of single-session crisis intervention also involves several interrelated processes. For persons in crisis, this is the time when they are encouraged to talk more extensively about what has happened, to identify their most pressing needs and concerns, and to express the overwhelming emotions and recurring thoughts that are contributing to their feelings of being overwhelmed. For the crisis worker, this is the time to assist the client to talk and vent, responding supportively and empathetically to the individual's emotional needs. It is also a critical time to continue assessment, purposefully probing and listening in order to comprehend the individualized meaning and responses to what has occurred.

Exploration and ventilation   The overwhelming emotional arousal that accompanies a crisis event frequently leads to a strong urge to talk about what has happened. Talking about what has occurred is one of the primary ways an individual in crisis can release pent-up emotions and disturbing thoughts, which ultimately contributes to an increased sense of calm and control. Thus an accident victim whose car was hit head-on by a large truck that crossed the median and entered her lane might need to tell and retell the story of what she saw as the truck veered out of control, what she thought as she saw the truck heading for her and her daughter, and how the impact felt when the collision occurred. She might need to describe the smell of the air bag and the sensation of loss of feeling in her legs. In this manner she robs the incident of its psychological power and releases images and emotions that might otherwise continue to resurface in nightmares or flashbacks.

If the crisis client does not spontaneously communicate about what has happened and/or does not reveal how he or she is feeling and thinking about it, it is incumbent on the crisis worker to encourage the client to do so. For example, a crisis worker might ask the woman who was driving the car what she remembers from the crash, or what she was thinking as she waited for the ambulance to arrive. Or a crisis counselor might ask the surviving spouse of a suicide victim to share the thoughts he sees "racing through her head."

As the crisis worker explores with the client what happened, how the client feels and thinks about it, how he or she has responded so far, and who else is involved, both in the crisis situation and as potential supports, the crisis worker is simultaneously involved in the process of assessment.

Assessment   As we have stated, assessment begins at first contact with the crisis scene and/or person(s) in crisis, continues throughout involvement, and always includes an immediate consideration and determination regarding potential volatility and danger. After a situation has been evaluated as at least temporarily safe, assessment proceeds as the crisis worker observes the individual, engages him or her in exploring the situation, and actively attends to both verbal and nonverbal behaviors. The crisis worker can only fully appreciate the individual's reactions to a crisis situation when he or she sees the individual holistically (i.e., who the individual is developmentally, ecologically, and as a thinking, feeling, behaving person). The ABCDE assessment model presented in Chapter 2 can provide a continuous lens for evaluating the needs and strengths of the individual as well as his or her environmental context.

One person may respond to a frightening situation in a very emotional way, whereas another appears dazed or immobilized. The crisis worker uses reflective listening skills to attend to the verbal and nonverbal clues and responds to what is most salient for the client at that time. It is also important, however, to be attuned to what is occurring in the other functional domains. For instance, when a crisis client's behavior is assessed to be the primary issue of concern, as with a young adolescent female who has been cutting her arms with a knife, it is still necessary to assess the thoughts and feelings that her behavior may represent.

Assessment always begins with the crisis worker trying to understand both the immediate condition of the individual and the precipitating event. Comprehending a client's crisis reactions requires understanding what actually occurred, the meaning of what occurred as that unique individual perceives it, and the emotional and behavioral responses that signify the inability to cope. It also requires attention to personal and environmental strengths and resources, as these will be critical in enabling the individual to take constructive actions.

Ultimately, the crisis counselor must quickly comprehend the client and the situation while simultaneously conveying both understanding and hopeful support. An important outcome of this process is the identification of specific issues and needs that can lead to specific actions that provide at least temporary emotional relief and control.

Step 4:
Examine alternatives and develop options.

The fourth step in intervening with someone in crisis entails helping the individual to identify possible solutions to meet his or her current needs. This process is designed to enable the crisis client to engage in a rational problem-solving process, building on the identification of concerns that emerged in the earlier process of exploration. The first thing to do is determine the priority order in which to address specific needs. If immediate needs, such as whom to call for support, have already been resolved, then this step involves "what comes next?" For example, the battered woman whose immediate need was to determine whether she would be safe if she remained at home decided with the assistance of the crisis worker on the telephone that she was not safe. They agreed that she would ask her neighbor to drive her and her child to the emergency room, where the crisis worker met her. The crisis worker supportively connected with her and arranged for a student intern to attend to her child so they could talk. The crisis worker listened, empathized, and clarified as the woman ventilated and considered her situation. Now the crisis worker and her client must consider "next steps." The woman may need to consider possible legal alternatives. She must think about where to find short-term housing for herself and her child. She may have immediate financial needs.

Examining alternatives often involves a sequential process of brainstorming that begins by exploring what has been tried so far and continues with identifying other possible solutions. One of the obstacles to problem-solving in a crisis situation is that individuals may be limited in their ability to imagine a range of alternatives. Collaborative brainstorming encourages the person in crisis to identify a wider range of possibilities. (See Chapter 4 for a discussion of obstacles to problem-solving and strategies for intervening.)

The crisis worker assists the person in crisis to evaluate the pros and cons of the alternative options and to select the most acceptable ones, and the ones he or she will be most likely to follow through with. (This is usually based on an evaluation of consequences to the different alternatives.) The crisis worker often needs to structure the discussion to ensure that the individual identifies possible obstacles and is psychologically capable of carrying out the agreed-upon solutions.

This consideration of alternatives is not intended to provide solutions to long-term issues such as whether or not the individual should divorce his or her spouse or to quit his or her job. Rather, the solutions under consideration are those that address the "at the moment" needs that, once met, provide the person with the safety and stability to make later decisions. The crux of crisis intervention is re-storing equilibrium and empowering the person in crisis. Assisting individuals to identify, select, and carry through with even very short-term solutions to immedi-ate needs contributes to their renewed sense of personal control. Thus the solu-tions identified in this step of single-session crisis intervention are intended to alle-viate the immediate threats to the individual's ability to effectively cope with the crisis situation.

Step 5:
Assist the client to mobilize personal and social resources and connect with community resources, as needed.

If persons in crisis are to carry out the solutions that will enable them to begin to cope more effectively, they must draw on both their personal resources and their social support systems. When exploring the precipitating event and other factors relevant to understanding a client's reactions, the crisis worker begins to identify potential personal and social resources.

In single-session crisis intervention this means identifying both current capaci-ties for coping and precrisis levels of functioning. Thus an individual who was robbed at gunpoint and threatened with violence outside an ATM may be shaken and frightened to the point of being immobilized. If she has a network of supportive loved ones who are immediately available to provide comfort and support, how-ever, she may be able to regain at least a semblance of her precrisis emotional stabil-ity relatively quickly. She may then be able to cognitively process her fears about the assault as well as her fears about the police expectation that she identify him in court. She can draw on her precrisis strengths, including her general emotional sta-bility, her intelligence and problem-solving skills, and her loving family and friends, to assist her in handling the present crisis. As she moves forward, she may find that the experience has shaken her sense of personal safety and caused recurring fears and anxieties, and it is the crisis worker's responsibility to help her anticipate that possibility. Ensuring that this client has information about crime victim support programs and other possible forms of assistance that she may need in the future is also essential. Ultimately, however, one can expect that if the crisis worker can assist her initially to mobilize her many personal strengths and interpersonal sup-ports, the likelihood of ongoing devastating impact will be greatly reduced.

Individuals without those personal strengths or individuals who were margin-ally functional prior to a crisis may face more challenges in coping with a current crisis, but they too can be assisted to mobilize their strengths. Thus, imagine another woman—a loner and social outcast—in the same situation as the one just described. She may have difficulty experiencing the crisis worker's efforts as truly personal and supportive. Her untrusting nature may also minimize her capacity to speak honestly about herself or about what occurred. She may have few, if any, supportive friends or family. This individual, severely lacking in social supports, will be much more difficult to assist relationally. Even extremely marginal individuals, however, can be helped by single-session crisis intervention. In such cases, crisis workers need to be clear about their role and committed to providing support and compassion despite initial and, perhaps, repeated rebuffs by the individual in crisis. Also, in such cases it may be particularly important to provide the crisis client with information about other needed resources and/or to arrange follow-up services.

Crisis workers can also directly help mobilize a crisis client's social support system and enhance their ability to respond helpfully. This could mean speaking to friends or family members to help them understand their loved one's experience and to help them anticipate the needs and concerns that may develop. It may also entail preparing significant others for their own reactions, and helping them identify ways to meet their own needs so that they are capable of responding in supportive ways to the person in crisis. For example, the parents of a teenager who has been raped will have many emotional reactions to their daughter's victimization. They also undoubtedly have many beliefs, based on facts or myths, about sexual assault and its impact. The crisis worker should take the opportunity to provide them with information about rape so they are more likely to respond in ways that do not further burden or disempower the survivor. Additionally, family members may experience their own crisis responses and can benefit from crisis intervention directed to their own needs.

A growing body of literature suggests that positive changes in relationships with others often occur in the aftermath of crisis or traumatic events. Families report becoming closer as the result of their shared struggle and mutual support, and individuals commonly note an increased sense of "who their friends really are" (Calhoun & Tedeschi, 2000). Research examining people's responses to disasters has also documented the salutary effects of spontaneous sharing, social support, and a sense of community (Pennebaker & Harber, 1993). Stuhlmiller and Dunning (2000) argued that rather than reinforcing notions of illness and the need for possibly long-term treatment, crisis intervention should "convey the optimistic message that with the support of significant others, the individual has the inherent coping resources to deal with what trauma has wrought . . ." (p. 29).

Assisting crisis survivors to connect with other community resources can also be useful. This assistance may take the form of supplying information about a particular community agency or making a direct referral to a specific contact person. Referral to support groups (e.g., grief groups, rape survivor groups) can provide both emotional support and the opportunity for continued contact with agency staff, who may be able to assess ongoing needs and provide ongoing crisis counseling when warranted.

Many people in crisis have had little previous experience with the various community resources to which they now may need to turn. For example, the victim of a crime needs to understand the legal system and its major players and functions, and a family who was made homeless by a fire needs to know how to access help from the various agencies that may be able to assist with shelter resources. It is thus the crisis worker's responsibility to provide this information or be able to access it.

Chris Dunning (Stuhlmiller & Dunning, 2000), in an article challenging crisis counselors to shift their perspective from searching for signs of illness to focusing on building connections and enhancing individual and community strengths, shared a memory of a client's response in the aftermath of a tornado: "Can you restore my home, my children's baby pictures, my wedding dress? Then, what good are you?" (p. 33).

Clearly, one of the most important functions of the crisis counselor in single-session crisis counseling is serving as a liaison to natural helping networks and relevant resources. Fulfillment of this function requires a crisis worker to be familiar with regional community resources. At times it may also require the professional skills of brokering and advocating for clients.

Step 6:
Anticipate the future and arrange follow-up.

Anticipate the future   The last step of single-session crisis intervention entails two interrelated components. One component involves providing information that will prepare the crisis client for what may come next. This could mean what will happen next in specific legal or medical processes, as when a crime victim is informed that the next step will be an interview with the detective who will take his or her story in writing, or when a person with a poor medical prognosis is informed about hospice care as an alternative to staying in the hospital or going home.

It also involves helping clients anticipate what they may experience emotionally, physically, and relationally in the future. For example, experienced crisis workers know that there are usual or characteristic symptomatic responses that occur in the aftermath of significant trauma events. Physical problems with eating and sleeping, continuing emotional distress, and relational tensions are common. The crisis worker can share this information and help prepare clients for the possibility that they may experience some of those symptoms, and can help them anticipate the time and course of recovery and suggest options for ongoing assistance if their symptoms persist.

It is also useful to share information about what to anticipate in the future with significant family and friends. This information can prevent victims and their significant others from developing unrealistic expectations about quickly "getting over" the crisis, and can counteract the common tendency to negatively judge the victim if she or he appears to be "taking too long" or seems "to dwell too much" on what happened. Thus, for example, consider a young woman who calls a hotline feeling depressed, empty, and hopeless on her mother's birthday two years after her mother's sudden death. She reports that she has exhausted the patience and interest of family and friends who don't seem to understand her continued suffering. After other crisis intervention strategies have helped calm the individual and helped her plan how to spend the rest of the evening, the crisis worker can help her understand that it is normal to feel grief on days that remind one of the loved one, and can help her to anticipate similar responses in the future. With this knowledge, she may be able to plan the best way to prepare for those days so that she can allow herself to grieve, but also use that time to remember and celebrate her mother's life.

Arrange follow-up   The second component of Step 6 entails planning follow-up. The primary helper task is to arrange for follow-up contact with the crisis survivor. This last step can only be carried out with the crisis client's consent. *"I would like to be able to speak with you sometime in the next couple of days to see how you are doing and also to see if there is anything further I can do to assist you. Would it be OK with you if I called you at your mother's home sometime tomorrow afternoon?"* If the client does not give consent, the crisis worker should extend an invitation for the client to initiate further contact. *"I understand that at this time you do not want to risk a phone call that might make your family suspicious, but I want to encourage you to call me when and if you are able and let me know how you are doing and if I can be of any further assistance to you. I will be thinking about you."*

Follow-up contact with the crisis client allows the crisis worker to both assess whether the goals of single-session crisis intervention have been achieved (e.g., Is the client safe and coping more adaptively? Are interpersonal and/or community resources providing necessary support?) and to determine whether further assistance or additional referral information should be offered. Unfortunately, it is often not possible to follow up with victims of certain crisis events because, even with anticipatory preparation, many victims want to try to forget what occurred. Despite this reluctance, follow-up contact should always be offered and initiated if the client is amenable.

ONGOING CRISIS COUNSELING

Whereas the goals and activities of single-session crisis intervention are quite narrow and delimited, ongoing crisis counseling aims to assist crisis victims in the longer struggle to survive the crisis and to rebuild their lives. Whether the crisis was loss of physical or mental health, being the victim of a crime, or losing a loved one to a natural or violent catastrophe, the event often ruptures an individual's life, necessitating the process of rebuilding and redefining concepts of life and self. Koss and Harvey (1991) refer to this as a process of learning to "survive standing up" (p. 176). This is, in a nutshell, the overarching goal of crisis counseling: to help individuals to survive and thrive; to find some way of incorporating what has happened into their lives so they can move forward, continuing to live fully.

The following goals of crisis counseling are designed to contribute to that end. The domains of functioning addressed in the goals can also be utilized as assessment indicators, as each goal represents progress on a continuum of mastery and renewed stability in an essential domain of psychosocial functioning. Thus, for the crisis counselor, these objectives can serve as both indicators of the individual's needs and strengths *and* the outcomes that crisis counseling is designed to achieve.

Ongoing Crisis Counseling Goals

Ongoing crisis counseling aims to achieve five primary outcomes. The order in which they are listed is not an indicator of their priority; rather, they are easier to remember in alphabetical order. Note that each outcome relates to one of the ABCDE domains already identified in the assessment model (see Table 3.3).

TABLE 3.3
CRISIS COUNSELING GOALS

Affect stability. Individual is able to remember and speak of the crisis event with a tolerable and appropriate range of emotion or affect.

Behavioral adjustments. Negative behavioral coping strategies have been replaced by more effective/constructive patterns of behavior (e.g., client no longer depends on sleeping medicines, no longer uses drug and alcohol to cope). Threats to physical survival have been reduced or have ended.

Cognitive mastery. Individual has attributed an acceptable meaning to the crisis event and to him- or herself as a survivor. Core beliefs threatened by crisis event have been reframed.

Developmental mastery. Individual has successfully mastered developmentally appropriate life tasks and is able to continue path of normal development.

Ecosystem healthy and intact. Individual has developed or connected with interpersonal and environmental resources that enable him or her to thrive after the crisis. He or she has reestablished disconnected relationships, established new supports, or created new avenues for action (e.g., rape survivor has become active in movement opposing violence against women, surviving parent is involved with MADD, or breast cancer survivor marches in Walk for Life).

Affect stability   The first goal is affect stability, which basically means that the individual is able to remember and speak of the crisis event with a tolerable and appropriate range of emotion. A primary component of an individual's sense of being unable to cope with or to move on following a crisis is the experience of overwhelming emotion. Reminders of what has occurred may cause one to experience renewed feelings of fear, pain, or anxiety. Stability of affect suggests that the individual no longer routinely experiences such overwhelming arousal or, on the contrary, no longer needs to numb his or her emotions for fear they will explode if allowed to surface.

Behavioral adjustments   The second goal of crisis counseling is that the client makes adaptive behavioral adjustments. Behavior refers to the many actions, both adaptive and problematic, that an individual takes as he or she attempts to cope with and resolve a crisis. Successful adaptation means that the individual has developed effective or constructive patterns of behavior and eliminated negative behavioral coping strategies. This means that the individual does not engage in self-destructive activities such as excessive drug or alcohol use, or remain dependent on prescription medication to cope with disabling levels of depression or anxiety. Ultimately, the objective is for the crisis survivor to sleep, eat, work, and play in healthy ways that contribute to a sense of renewed satisfaction and happiness.

Cognitive mastery   The third goal is cognitive mastery. Because crisis events so often shatter images of safety and meaning, finding a way to make sense of what has occurred is a critical long-term task for most crisis survivors. A crisis event may challenge or threaten an individual's core beliefs about him- or herself, relationships, safety, spirituality, or trust. The individual must reexamine or reframe these beliefs in a manner that can account for or accommodate what has occurred. Ultimately, the crisis worker helps individuals to create an acceptable way to interpret and comprehend both the crisis event and themselves as survivors so they are capable of moving forward, living with a renewed sense of order, predictability, and personal understanding of the meaning of their lives.

Developmental mastery   The fourth goal is developmental mastery, which is a critical, although often overlooked, area of concern when working with survivors of crisis events. Whether the crisis is a direct result of developmental transitions and changes or an external situational event, there is a potential developmental impact because it occurs during a specific developmental period in the individual's life. Developmental mastery implies that the individual is able to accomplish or achieve developmentally appropriate tasks and is able to continue developmental growth unhampered by what has occurred. This also may include relationship or family development issues and tasks.

Ecosystem healthy and intact   The final goal of crisis counseling and the final indicator that an individual who has experienced a crisis has moved forward with his or her life is that his or her ecosystem is healthy and intact. An individual's ecosystem consists of his or her significant interpersonal social supports including close family and friends, as well as the larger community within which the individual lives including places of employment, religious worship, recreation, and other membership or affiliated associations.

Perhaps one of the most important conditions necessary for trauma survivors' recovery is their experience of belonging and meaningful connection (Herman, 1997; McFarlane & van der Kolk, 1996). Emotional attachment plays an essential role in countering the helplessness and meaningless that often surrounds the experience of trauma. Paradoxically, however, at a time when the protective role of community and connection is most necessary, many individuals withdraw from relationships or experience a failed relationship in the wake of traumatic crisis events (McFarlane & van der Kolk, 1996).

A healthy and intact ecosystem is one in which the interactions between individuals and their ecosystems contribute to their capacity to meet their needs, solve problems, grow, and develop. Thus, an indicator of recovery from a crisis and an essential goal of crisis counseling is for crisis survivors to have interpersonal and environmental sources of social support that enable them to thrive after the crisis. This means that crisis survivors have reestablished and strengthened disconnected relationships, developed new relationships and supports, and may have created new avenues for action and meaning, as when a breast cancer survivor becomes involved in planning a Walk for Life event or when a surviving parent becomes involved in Mothers Against Drunk Driving (MADD).

Ongoing Crisis Counseling Process

As Slaikeu (1990) noted, "[T]he uniqueness of crisis therapy lies not so much in its techniques, but in the fact that everything the therapist does is aimed at helping the client to deal with the impact of the crisis event on each area of the client's life" (p. 142). This is also true of the crisis counseling model presented in this text, as all strategies are directed at assisting the client to make the personal and interpersonal changes necessitated by the impact of the crisis event in his or her life. A unique aspect of this model is its theoretically grounded comprehensiveness and the effort to continuously link assessment with intervention.

Not everyone who experiences a crisis will sustain difficulties in each of the areas of psychosocial functioning. Also, although each area is described as a separate entity, the various functional domains are more likely to be dynamically interrelated, with difficulties in one area related to difficulties in others. Assessment requires that the specific areas of concern unique to each individual be identified and that those pertinent dimensions of individual and interpersonal functioning become the focus of intervention. Last, ongoing crisis counseling does not follow a linear intervention model. Table 3.4 provides a map, or schema, for recognizing *potential* areas for intervention, each based on the goals of ongoing crisis counseling.

TABLE 3.4
ONGOING CRISIS COUNSELING PROCESS

Affect stability. Assist the client in expressing and processing memories and emotions related to the crisis event.

Behavioral adjustments. Assist client in making and sustaining behavioral changes conducive to survival and ongoing optimal personal and social functioning.

Cognitive mastery. Assist client in examining and reframing core beliefs, expectations, and personal meanings (e.g., about self, others, spirituality) threatened by crisis event.

Developmental mastery. Assist client in examining impact of crisis on his/her stage of life needs/tasks and making the adjustments necessary for attaining ongoing developmental mastery.

Ecosystem healthy and intact. Assist client in examining and making needed changes in personal ecosystem (e.g., interpersonal relationships, organizational involvement, use of community resources).

All ongoing crisis counseling begins with two essential components: establishing a supportive and empowering counseling relationship and assessing crisis resolution. Both are continuous processes that the crisis worker engages in throughout the ongoing crisis counseling engagement.

Build a supportive and empowering counseling relationship   Earlier, in discussing single-session intervention, we addressed the reasons and means for making an empathic connection with a crisis survivor. Given the short-term nature of that work and the critical, immediate needs to be addressed, it is unlikely and unnecessary that a more in-depth relationship be created in that situation. If a crisis survivor is to engage in the painful and more protracted process of crisis resolution, however, the establishment of a secure and trusting therapeutic alliance is essential.

Rogers (1957, 1980) was one of the first theorists to recognize the importance of the therapeutic relationship as a necessary condition of all effective psychotherapy. From his standpoint, it is the client's *perception* of the helping professional as genuine, as emotionally responsive in an appropriate way, and as consistently warm, accepting, and concerned (showing "unconditional positive regard") that ultimately is the defining element of a meaningful relationship. Many of the helping skills taught to beginning helping professionals (e.g., attentiveness to verbal and nonverbal behaviors, empathy, paraphrasing, genuineness) are, in essence, relationship-building skills intended to assist the professional in establishing rapport and a positive working alliance. Research on drop-out rates and outcomes in therapy have generally confirmed Roger's contention, concluding that a client's positive perceptions of and reactions to the first session are strongly predictive of both continuation in treatment and positive outcomes (Garfield, 1994).

In a recent book on brief treatment, Corwin (2002) discussed the importance of establishing a working alliance, particularly with individuals who are ambivalent or resistant to therapy. She encouraged helping professionals to recognize that "resistance is motivated behavior, that it is interpersonal in nature, and that resistance can be utilized to promote understanding and change" (p. 33). This is a particularly useful insight for crisis counselors because many individuals who have experienced traumatic crises are, in fact, quite ambivalent both about trusting the helper and engaging in the process of crisis resolution. As Herman (1997) stated, disempowerment and disconnection are "core experiences" of trauma. Thus, establishing a helping relationship with survivors of trauma can be difficult because they are often ambivalent about confronting memories and feelings they may have invested considerable energy in trying to suppress. Further, survivors' presenting problems are often a product of trying to accommodate and cope with their crisis reactions, and giving up those coping strategies is frightening even when they acknowledge them to be unhealthy. And last, because many crisis survivors struggle with feelings of shame and/or self-blame, they may be particularly sensitive to criticism and rejection and thus unlikely to trust that the crisis counselor will not negatively judge them as well.

Primary components of a helping relationship include acceptance, empathy, and support. These are particularly essential when working with traumatized individuals. Corwin (2002) suggested that negative feelings such as shame, fear, or anxiety can inhibit an individual's ability and/or willingness to engage in the helping process. The helper can reduce those obstacles by providing direct support and by attempting to uncover and empathically address the individual's fears. The helper can also combat the hopelessness or helplessness that undermines motivation by "inspiring optimism." This can be facilitated both by helping the client realize that his or her reactions and feelings are normal, expected responses to extreme stress and by educating him or her about the common course of problem resolution or recovery. The helper can also employ the technique of reframing to assist the client to recognize what Corwin labeled the "healthy striving behind problematic behaviors" and the person's unrecognized or unacknowledged strengths (pp. 34–35).

Establishing an empowering connection with a survivor of a crisis or traumatic event is essential if he or she is to engage in the relationship-based, collaborative effort to explore the crisis and its impact and make the changes necessary to finally resolve it. The concept of empowerment as used here does not refer to an individual who operates solely as a separate agent. Rather, individual empowerment is viewed as emerging in a relational context and entails both the personal resources and strength to act purposefully "through a mutual, relational process" (Surrey, 1991, p. 164). See Chapter 4 for further discussion of empowerment.

As this brief review suggests, the establishment of a supportive and empowering counseling relationship is a process requiring awareness of both the processes by which the crisis counselor can reflectively and consciously join clients as an ally and collaborator and the obstacles to such an alliance. The helping relationship is unique in many respects because it is both highly intimate and inherently unequal.

It is the counselor's responsibility to use knowledge, skills, and personal authenticity to further the development of intimacy and trust, and to use the power inherent in his or her professional position to empower the crisis client in his or her own recovery process. This is particularly important when working with those who have been subjected to coercion, force, and/or authoritarian control, as the helping relationship can counteract the powerlessness endemic to the trauma experience.

Continuous assessment of crisis resolution   The assessment model presented earlier identifies essential domains of psychosocial functioning (ABCDE) that may be negatively affected by crisis events. Not everyone who becomes a candidate for crisis counseling immediately identifies a crisis event as the root of his or her difficulties. Thus all assessment processes should include inquiries to identify significant crisis events that may have precipitated current presenting problems. When a crisis event is identified, either immediately by the client or as the result of a counselor's initial assessment questioning, and that crisis event appears to be related to the current difficulties an individual is presenting, the crisis counselor must assist the client to understand the benefits of crisis counseling. The process of assessment can serve both as a means of identifying areas of need and strength and as a means of beginning to help crisis survivors recognize and name their current difficulties in terms of the need for crisis recovery or resolution. To accomplish this, the counselor should make a straightforward statement to clients followed by probing questions regarding potential difficulties of functioning in all areas.

For example, a crisis worker might say: *"When individuals experience a traumatic event, as you have, it is normal to have continuing reactions that are quite unsettling and even, perhaps, frightening because you may feel as if you're 'going off the deep end.' Some people's reactions are physical; others are emotional. Some people find that they have a hard time enjoying the things that they previously found pleasurable. What I'd like to do is try to figure out with you the kinds of reactions you are having that are causing you the most difficulty. Some of them may be things you hadn't even realized were connected to what you've been through."*

As individuals come to realize that their troublesome symptoms are not unexpected or abnormal and that you can help them work through what's happened so that they don't continue to feel so emotional, they often experience some immediate relief. Sometimes it can also be helpful to provide and explain a diagnostic label (e.g., Adjustment Disorder, Acute Stress Disorder, PTSD), as that can further assist crisis survivors to understand that their reactions are understandable, although painful, responses to abnormal events. See Chapter 5 for more information on diagnosis.

The ABCDE assessment model should serve as a guide for assessing the specific areas that indicate the crisis survivor's current levels of functioning. Implicit in each area are indicators of client difficulty as well as indicators of client strength and crisis resolution. For example, consider an individual who continues to experience a high level of guilt and self-blame following the death of her sister in an automobile accident, despite the fact that the accident was caused by another driver. Assessment might lead to the conclusion that she has been unable to assign a tolerable meaning to the event, and thus intervention, at least initially, might be focused on assisting her to reexamine her beliefs about her own power and the role of chance. Another individual may recognize intellectually that there was nothing that he could have done differently to change the outcome of a crisis, but may also suffer from recurring images of the event and overwhelming feelings of grief and depression. This person may not require intervention focused on reframing his cognitive appraisal of the crisis but rather assistance in expressing and processing painful memories and emotions. It is important to emphasize again that the crisis counselor must be attentive to all areas of psychosocial functioning and must identify both areas of strength (resolution) and areas of difficulty, always keeping in mind the interrelated, interdependent nature of the various factors.

ONGOING CRISIS COUNSELING IS A COMPLEX PROCESS

The establishment of a working alliance between client and counselor and assessment of crisis resolution are components of ongoing crisis counseling that the counselor must engage in during the initial phase of working with crisis clients. The components of crisis counseling described below, however, should not be construed as steps to follow in a linear fashion. Rather, although each is a potentially important area for intervention, the area that assumes priority will depend on the outcome of both initial and continuous assessment. Work in one area often coincides with and relates to work in another, as when emotions and cognition are explored. In reality, the idea of steps or stages to guide ongoing crisis counseling is a "convenient fiction" in that it is an attempt to "impose order and simplicity on a process that is inherently turbulent and complex" (Herman, 1997, p. 155).

It is also essential to remember that the safety of the client is the first priority. Thus if a client is engaging in unsafe behaviors or is at risk, the counselor must directly address the behavioral changes necessary to ensure the client's safety either before or while he or she is engaged in processing memories and emotions. In some instances, talking about memories and expressing emotions precedes the person's ability to try new behaviors, as is the case when a person begins to drive again after working through the anxieties associated with recurring images of an automobile collision. In other cases, behavioral changes that enable control over one's body and physical environment precede efforts to explore memories and emotions.

<u>A</u>ffect stability:
Assist the client in expressing and processing memories and emotions related to the crisis event.

The ability to remember traumatic events that have occurred with appropriate, but no longer incapacitating, emotion is a hallmark of survival following a crisis. Many individuals who have experienced major crises attempt to protect or defend themselves against overwhelming emotions and/or physiological arousal by trying not to think about or remember what happened, or by denying that there have been any lasting consequences. Unfortunately, this is rarely a successful coping approach, as ignoring images and memories of what happened and the feelings and anxieties that accompany those memories does not make them go away. More often, the images of the experience come back in the form of frightening nightmares or flashbacks or even phobic avoidance of things or places associated with the crisis event.

Thus individuals who have experienced traumatic events and who are having difficulty in the aftermath must be assisted to recall what happened in the safe and supportive environment of crisis counseling. In this way the memories gradually lose their power and the individual can tolerate them more easily. It is important that the remembering process not be a strictly intellectualized recitation of the facts of what occurred. Rather the counselor must help the individual to remember the event with all the attendant emotions. Among the most effective methods for targeting intrusive memories, heightened arousal, and anxiety responses are exposure techniques whereby counselors help trauma survivors to relive the trauma and/or confront their fears in a controlled environment in order to enhance habituation responses and correct cognitive distortions (Boudewyns & Hyer, 1990; Foa, Rothbaum, Riggs, & Murdock, 1991). Despite documented efficacy, such techniques are also quite invasive and should be utilized only by professionals with the requisite expertise. Further, full client informed consent is essential.

Foa and Rothbaum (1998) suggest that counselors help clients understand why they are being asked to engage in such a painful process by specifically explaining how recalling and speaking about what happened can gradually diminish the intense anxiety and pain associated with those images and cues. High levels of support, reassurance, and encouragement are essential to assist crisis clients as they contemplate and gradually engage in this imaginal reliving and reprocessing of the traumatic memories.

These approaches should be used only when immediate concerns regarding client safety have been addressed. Thus an individual who has been self-medicating with drugs or alcohol or an individual who expresses suicidal ideation associated with painful symptomatology should not be treated using approaches like in vivo or imaginal exposure until he or she is strong enough to handle the intensity without regression or continued self-injurious attempts to cope. (See Chapter 4 for more information on exposure techniques and Chapter 6 for information on applying these techniques with sexual assault survivors.)

Although not all crises involve trauma, painful memories are a part of most crisis responses. Traumatic events such as surviving a bomb attack or hijacking, or being subjected to ongoing abuse, or being sexually or otherwise violently assaulted are all traumatic events that may result in lingering images and memories fraught with emotion and anxieties. Other types of crises, such as learning that one's husband of many years is romantically and sexually involved with someone else, or being diagnosed with a serious illness, may not produce specific traumatic images in the same manner, but nonetheless these are experiences that may set in motion painful and disruptive crisis reactions. Remembering and talking about how one felt as one heard the word *cancer* or heard one's spouse say "I don't love you" is equally important; such recall creates the opportunity to begin the in-depth processing of the emotional responses that characterize the crisis reaction.

The expression of emotions includes both feelings tied to the images and memories of crisis events and emotions that have emerged in the aftermath of the crisis. In order for emotions to be expressed and resolved they must be accurately identified. Many clients do not know exactly what they are feeling or may be experiencing conflicting emotions (such as anger and sadness or love and hate). As we will see in Chapter 4, actively listening for cues to a client's emotional state and accurately responding with empathy is the single most useful skill crisis counselors can acquire to assist clients in this area. Crisis counselors must carefully attend to what the client says and does not say, to behavior, to verbal expressions that reveal how the client is thinking, and to direct expressions of the client's emotions. Such active listening will prepare the crisis counselor to recognize and respond to the complexity and depth of the crisis client's feelings and will provide repeated opportunities to assist the client in expressing those feelings overtly.

In many instances the crisis counselor's empathic responses will be sufficient to enable the client to emote: to cry, to express his or her confusion, to rage. In other cases, particularly with clients who are well defended and who fear the power and intensity of their feelings, the counselor's reassurances can support the client to begin to open that painful door. The counselor needs to reassure the client that his or her responses are normal and that the counselor is committed to helping the client express them in a way that will not result in loss of control.

It is the crisis counselor's responsibility to assist the crisis client to recall painful memories and to identify and express the many emotions associated with the crisis and its aftermath. As this occurs, the crisis survivor will be increasingly able to remember and endure the memories of what happened and to do so without overwhelming and disabling emotions. It will also no longer be necessary for the client to resort to denial or numbing coping strategies that contribute to the creation of other problematic physiological or behavioral symptomatology.

Behavioral adjustments:
Assist the client in making and sustaining behavioral changes conducive to survival and ongoing personal and social functioning.

Slaikeu (1990) described "behavioral change as the 'bottom line' for crisis resolution" (p. 174). What we believe he meant is that, ultimately, crises are not resolved until individuals can sleep, eat, work, and play in ways that are healthy and that contribute to renewed satisfaction and happiness. As we have noted, behavior refers to all of the actions and inaction, adaptive and maladaptive, that individuals engage in as they attempt to live their lives following a crisis event. Our charge in this domain of crisis counseling is to assist the client to eliminate negative or maladaptive behaviors and to develop or strengthen effective and constructive patterns of behavior. Crisis counselors must always be alert for indicators of self-destructive or other harmful behaviors and must be prepared to intervene in a directive fashion, when necessary. See Chapter 5 for a discussion of suicide and aggression.

Behavior is one of the most overt indicators of how an individual is functioning. A woman who is afraid to drive after a car accident and a man who refuses to be in an enclosed public space following a bomb scare are both individuals whose behavior has significantly changed following a crisis event. Similarly, a young teenage girl who begins to engage in high-risk sexual behavior after being sexually victimized and a young man who begins to behave very aggressively after being mugged are individuals whose coping behaviors are maladaptive and potentially self-injurious. The responsibility of the crisis counselor in these examples would be to assist the individuals in relinquishing or curbing those maladaptive behaviors and, equally important, in replacing them with behaviors that contributed to their well-being. This certainly is easier said than done, as the individuals may not initially identify the behaviors as maladaptive or willingly make the connection between those behaviors and other underlying reactions to a precipitating crisis. Thus, for example, the teenage girl who is behaving promiscuously may be quite defended against the interpretation that her behavior reflects a distorted self-appraisal that is a reaction to her earlier sexual victimization. Assisting crisis clients to make such associations as part of naming and ultimately changing maladaptive coping behaviors is nonetheless essential.

Other behaviors, as in the example of the woman who was afraid to drive after a car accident, are more obviously direct outcomes of a crisis event. Many individuals may actually be preoccupied with the knowledge that they must change their behaviors but at the same time resist changing them because those behaviors assist them in coping, although in a maladaptive way. In such cases, crisis counselors can employ direct behavioral techniques to assist clients to gradually approximate the behaviors they wish to initiate, and also use various other counseling interventions to help clients process and work through related thoughts and emotions (see Chapter 4).

Another potential area of behavioral change concerns the need to complete unfinished business associated with a crisis event. This might mean supporting a woman whose husband has been killed in gradually cleaning out his belongings and sorting through important papers. Or it might mean assisting a sexual abuse survivor in confronting her family about their denial of her victimization. In such instances the goal is to empower the individual to take the action that you have determined collaboratively will provide some closure and contribute to his or her ability to move on.

In addition to addressing problematic behaviors, counselors can also help crisis clients identify and initiate healthy behavioral patterns that will contribute to their overall well-being. Crisis clients often benefit from encouragement and specific advice and assistance on ways they can begin to take care of themselves. This may include improving eating or sleeping habits, or beginning an exercise regimen, or making time to read or engage in other pleasurable activities. This might also include making and carrying through with a decision to move to a new location, change a job, or return to school.

In this regard, behavior changes also serve as indicators of recovery. Other indicators include a return to precrisis activities or the development of new interests and pleasurable routines.

Cognitive mastery:
Assist the client in examining and reframing core beliefs, expectations, and personal meanings threatened by the crisis event.

As we have noted, an individual's unique perceptions and appraisal of an event are the essence of what makes a particular event a crisis for that individual. Correspondingly, the thoughts and beliefs an individual has about what occurred and its perceived impact must be of central concern in any crisis resolution process.

Crisis events may call into question expectations about the direction and course of one's life, violate beliefs about personal control, safety, trust, and spirituality, and/or shatter personalized images of self and one's relationships. During the weeks following the September 11, 2001, terrorist attacks on the World Trade Center in New York City and the Pentagon in Washington, DC, many newscasters featured conversations with religious leaders who were asked to address the question, "How could God have allowed this to happen?" Recognizing that spiritual beliefs in a fair and just God are frequently threatened and called into question when disasters resulting in great loss of life occur, broadcasters provided viewers with alternative ways of attributing meaning to what had happened. Rabbis, priests, ministers, and mullahs suggested that these acts should not be seen as *caused* by God, but could instead be understood as the result of "human beings acting on the free will that God had given them." This reframing was intended to assist religious individuals in maintaining their beliefs and thus continuing to find solace in their religious practices. Similarly, rescue workers exposed to significant physical risk, the trauma of viewing extreme horrors, and the devastating disappointment of uncovering so few survivors, were nonetheless able to perceive themselves and their fellow rescue workers as heroes and as good, caring, brave individuals who stood in stark contrast to the evildoers responsible for the devastation they encountered.

Individuals who have experienced crises or traumatic events will need to attribute a tolerable meaning to what occurred and will need to create a personal self-image that frees him or her from unrelenting shame and/or responsibility. They must also replace personal and relational myths and beliefs that keep them "stuck" with beliefs and stories that permit the restoration of self-esteem, relational connections, and hopefulness about the future. This may entail adjusting or amending previous beliefs and philosophies, defining new beliefs, and/or developing new goals and dreams.

In discussing family members' struggles to live after the losses inherent in a family member's suicide, Gutstein (1991) addresses the "ecology of personal myths," pointing to the ways in which core, and often contradictory, family fables and beliefs influence the ways individual family members come to manage and resolve the crises they face. For example, all families have a range of myths about who provides care. A given family's myths might include stories about how the loss of a crucial family member created a long-lasting vacuum in a family's functioning and stories about how extended family members took over nurturing when a parent was incapacitated.

Gutstein (1991) described the effects of a crisis on a family:

> A major crisis that eliminates or challenges a particular personal myth such as the death of a parent (i.e., "No one will ever love you as much as your mother") may lead to grief and sadness. However, a child can gradually accept the loss of the myth and replace or modify it from his/her repertoire and thus adapt to the crisis ("No one will ever love me like my mother did, but Grandma and Grandpa will always love and take care of me"). The child is able to carry on a process that I term *reconciliation* . . . an internal and external process, a compromise carried out by family members in times of crisis to alter their personal myths about the types of relationships they require and the way they and others must act to meet their needs. (p. 243)

Gutstein contended that dealing with the crisis of suicide entails not only the loss of relationship but also the disruption of basic assumptions or personal myths. In order to move on following such loss, a surviving family member must accept and mourn lost myths and ultimately modify or replace them with myths that can sustain the individual throughout life. For that to occur, the individual must be assisted to identify alternative myths, which may be competing stories from family "archives," that provide hope for future happiness.

Many beliefs about a crisis are revealed as individuals engage in the processing of memories of the event and its aftermath. It is the crisis counselor's responsibility to carefully attend to and probe for clues regarding the crisis client's thoughts about what happened and, in particular, views about him- or herself and others that have resulted. Different types of events may challenge different beliefs. An individual who was sexually assaulted may struggle with beliefs about safety, trust, power, and intimacy. A soldier returning from a tour of duty during war may struggle with beliefs about good and evil, or may be overwhelmed by an inability to justify or rationalize the behaviors he or she engaged in to revenge the deaths of friends.

A primary focus in working with crisis survivors entails examining and questioning whether the conclusions they have drawn about what happened and its impact are realistic, rational, and/or the only reasonable or possible conclusions to reach. Ultimately, if the meanings attributed to a crisis operate to maintain painful symptoms or prevent the person from future growth and adjustment, they must be considered maladaptive and should be challenged. Thus, for example, a young man who suffered massive scarring of his face after being trapped in a burning car may have concluded that his injury has rendered him sexually unattractive forever. The counselor would need to challenge this belief both as a premature conclusion and as a maladaptive belief that kept him socially isolated. Or, similarly, a counselor would need to assist a child to reexamine his belief that he is to blame for his parents' abusive behavior and their current legal difficulties.

Assisting individuals to challenge beliefs or conclusions that are self-defeating and that impair their ability to resolve crises entails the use of various cognitive therapy approaches. A fundamental tenet of cognitive therapy approaches is that an individual's thinking processes, or "inner dialogue," are the primary determinant of both emotional responses and behavior. Cognitive reframing and reality testing are useful skills in assisting clients to reexamine and replace dysfunctional beliefs (beliefs that keep the individual stuck). In working with crisis clients, this may entail assisting them to recognize the centrality of their thoughts and self-statements in affecting their feelings and behavior, and then assisting them to identify and reevaluate those beliefs and thoughts that contribute to their loss of hope regarding the future. This is often a process by which "negative personal stories are reframed as predictable responses to past situations in which [the crisis clients] were powerless." As Corwin (2002) states:

> Clients are given the opportunity to reassess the beliefs or assumptions held about their degree of personal responsibility for the event, the amount of danger or uncontrollability in their lives, their self-image as victims, their ability to cope with stressful events, and their beliefs about the reactions of others. . . . Clients are then encouraged to formulate a healing story of their past, one in which they used the resources and strengths available to them at the time in order to survive and one that offers an alternative version of what happened to them and why. (p. 21)

Ultimately, the crisis counselor must collaborate with crisis clients to identify or create beliefs and thoughts that facilitate their recovery (see Chapter 4).

In working with crisis clients it may sometimes be apparent that the client lacks information that could lead them to different conclusions about the meaning of what has occurred and their role in it. For example, consider a young woman who has a negative self-image because of the shame she feels for not stopping years of sexual abuse perpetrated by an uncle. Clearly, she could benefit from realistically reconsidering the relative size and power of a child and an adult. A counselor might encourage her to bring in a picture of herself and her uncle taken at the age when the abuse began. The stark imagery of an adult male and a prepubescent child might allow the crisis survivor to reexamine her unrealistic expectation that she, as a child, should have been able to exercise the power and control of an adult.

One of the primary purposes of psychoeducational interventions with crisis clients is to provide them with information that may lead to alternative ways of comprehending crisis events and one's role in them. Thus, for example, a counselor might give a battered woman information about power and control dynamics in relationships or provide an alcoholic with information about addiction. Information can also increase a client's perception of personal control, as, for example, when a counselor interprets a client's symptoms as outcomes of the effort to survive.

In summary, counselors must help crisis clients examine and reconsider their beliefs, expectations, and personal and family myths that have been threatened or compromised by crisis events, or that prevent them from moving forward with the process of recovery. Mutually engaging in the process of assessing the rationality and completeness of a client's beliefs and self-statements is an important part of this process. In the final analysis, the critical task is assisting clients to develop meanings, beliefs, and personal and relational myths or stories that contribute to their ongoing well-being.

Developmental mastery:
Assist clients to examine the impact of crisis on their stage-of-life needs and tasks and to make the adjustments necessary to attain ongoing developmental mastery.

This step of crisis counseling is closely tied to each of the other steps, as developmental needs and tasks are inevitably expressed and reflected in individuals' emotional states, behaviors, interpersonal relationships, and images of self and others. For example, an adolescent female who is traumatized by violence just as she is beginning to acquire a developmentally appropriate sense of independence and self-reliance may regress both emotionally and behaviorally in response to her fears and her belief that she is incapable of keeping herself safe. As part of helping her process her fears and consider whether her belief is rational, a crisis counselor might also want to assist her in thinking about her life developmentally. This could entail an honest examination and discussion about the normal, expected needs and tasks she faces, as well as her increased sense of self-doubt and vulnerability. The goal might be to help her understand the importance of continuing her normal developmental process toward self-reliance and self-efficacy, and to recognize how her thoughts and resultant behaviors are keeping her stuck.

Or consider a widow who discovers that her husband had an ongoing relationship with another woman during much of their married life. Developmentally, this woman is at the stage when much of her life is behind her and she needs to be able to look back and appraise her life with a sense of satisfaction, accomplishment, and integrity. Clearly, this discovery will challenge her images and beliefs about her marriage, her husband, and her life. The devastation she experiences is not just the result of the revealed betrayal, but the fact that it occurs *following* her husband's death, and at a time in her life when she needs to attain some closure and serenity. Awareness of the developmental impact of this crisis can prepare the crisis counselor to directly assist this client in constructing a "story" or set of explanations that can lead to such closure rather than undermining all of her previous beliefs about her marriage and her life with her husband and family.

Intervention that encompasses a developmental perspective targets those developmental tasks that may be interfered with as the result of the crisis event's impact. A 7-year-old boy whose father dies in an industrial accident must not only grieve the loss of his father, but, in order to continue healthy ongoing growth, must achieve mastery of normal developmental tasks for all children his age. For example, he must learn to read and calculate, to value his competence and initiative, to control his impulses and emotional reactions, and to establish peer relationships. Ongoing crisis counseling must attend to these developmental tasks by incorporating interventions and activities that facilitate such learning and mastery while recognizing that children who have experienced a crisis frequently regress temporarily to a previous developmental stage.

The influence of development is multidirectional. The child just described will inevitably engage in a process of grief resolution related to his father's death. This grieving process is also mediated by developmental factors. One of the most significant factors that influences the grieving process is this child's level of cognitive development. A child at the beginning of concrete operational thought is capable of understanding death only in a very logical and concrete fashion. Crisis counseling interventions must be designed to reflect this level of cognitive capacity or risk ineffective treatment.

First and foremost, assisting clients in this area requires the crisis counselor's attention to the potential development impact of any crisis event, and simultaneously to the impact of the client's development on his or her responses and coping capacities. Initially, this means watching for clues in the client's feelings, thoughts, and behaviors that reveal the ways developmental processes may have been affected. It also means designing interventions based on developmental knowledge and awareness.

The role of development is most obvious in developmental crises when it is the stage-of-life transition itself that precipitates the crisis reaction. This is the case when life transitions like the birth of a child or mandatory retirement lead to a crisis response. The developmental impact of situational crises may not be quite as obvious, but the counselor must always consider the possibility that a crisis event has had a negative impact on developmental processes. In cases such as this, the crisis counselor must intervene to address that impact and to assist the client to resolve and overcome the challenges to continued growth. This feeds directly back into the other components of the crisis counseling process: Awareness of the developmental impact of a crisis event in a client's life prepares the crisis counselor to help the client find a way of thinking/believing and a way of behaving and engaging in relationships that contributes to mastery of their current and future developmental tasks and challenges.

Ecosystem healthy and intact:
Assist clients in examining and making healthy changes in their personal ecosystem.

One of the most important factors in the resolution of crises in people's lives is their connection to other caring people. Although individuals can cry, scream, and rage alone, such solitary venting is unlikely to result in the necessary sense of closure or resolution. Rather, it is the opportunity to grieve *with others* that is most conducive to recovery. This was illustrated explicitly following the September 2001 terrorist attacks on the World Trade Center and the Pentagon. In the days following the attacks, people all over the world came together in small and large groups to pray, sing, mourn, and praise the heroes. These opportunities to come together were the way many individuals sought to process and reach an understanding of what had occurred and its impact on them, their communities, their country, and, ultimately, on their way of life. Involvement in support groups with other survivors can also provide this sense of community and ongoing connection.

Mobilization of family, friends, and community supports is often a key element in enabling individuals to cope with and, ultimately, survive crisis events. This is equally true whether the crisis event is one experienced by a single individual (e.g., a sexual assault or loss of a bodily function) or a large-scale disaster that directly affects multiple individuals and family members and indirectly affects countless additional people who are exposed through the media to dramatic details and graphic images of the event.

Some individuals have healthy, extended social support systems to meet whatever relationship and material needs they have. For others, professional support systems may be essential in order to ensure that the affected individual does not isolate him- or herself or is not financially devastated, resulting in a more serious crisis outcome. Those people who are least equipped to deal with stressors prior to a crisis due to their personal difficulties and/or social isolation are also least likely to find support and solace in connection to a community following a crisis.

Crisis counselors must engage crisis clients in conversations to examine their systems of support, and identify the perceived responsiveness and helpfulness of immediate family and friends as well as other individuals and organizations with whom the clients must interact (e.g., coworkers, employers, religious leaders). As noted in our discussion of ecological assessment, it is both the actual availability of resources and social supports and individuals' perceptions of their availability and accessibility that determine how useful and helpful those potential supports can be. Thus, intervention in this area entails assisting clients in a number of related ways. The first step is a part of ongoing assessment. It includes assisting individuals to identify the people and organizations they view as most supportive and helpful and also to examine whether they are able to ask for and use those resources. Similarly, it includes assisting individuals to identify and examine those relationships and organizational involvements they perceive as being difficult or challenging as they relate to their crisis recovery process. Second, counselors must assist individuals in identifying possible directions for change in their relationships and community involvements. And third, counselors must assist individuals to take the actions necessary to make needed changes.

Taking action to make needed changes may entail adjustments in relationship investments so that individuals spend more time and invest more energy in relationships that are mutually rewarding and sustaining, while simultaneously devoting less time and energy to relationships that are conflicted or one-sided. Alternatively, counselors may facilitate positive change by assisting individuals and their family members to change the manner in which they interact. Thus, for example, the parents of an alcoholic woman who lost custody of her children and attempted suicide can be encouraged to support their daughter without putting her under "house arrest" or constantly criticizing and blaming her as a way to try and motivate her to stay sober. And the counselor can help her accept responsibility for the fact that her parents do not trust her with their car and insist on driving her when she visits her children.

With regard to formal support systems, taking action to make needed changes may entail assisting the client to recognize, accept, and commit to ongoing, continuous use of formal resources, for example, committing to continuing participation in a Narcotics Anonymous or Alcoholic Anonymous group or an individual with persistent mental health problems continuing to live in a group home setting. Alternatively, when clients lack needed resources, such as health care or adequate housing, the crisis counselor must assist them in identifying possible resources and ultimately assist them in securing access to those formal systems of support. This could mean assisting and supporting an individual in applying for publicly subsidized housing or Supplemental Security Income or it could mean advocating for a student who needs special accommodations from his or her educational institution.

Finally, one of the important ways individuals can find a tolerable meaning in the trauma they have experienced is to become active in efforts to combat the conditions they believe contributed to their crisis. Becoming an activist who works to reform laws or to educate others, or who participates in task forces or forums, or even volunteers to provide direct services to other victims can enable individuals to create something worthwhile from their personal loss. When a young girl in New Jersey named Megan was sexually assaulted and murdered by a previously convicted sexual offender, her parents, as part of their own recovery, became actively involved in efforts to reform the law so that known sexual offenders' identities would not be kept confidential. As most readers are aware, "Megan's Law" requires communities to inform the public when a known sexual offender is released from prison and moves into their area. Similarly, most of the women who founded and continue the efforts of the advocacy group Mothers Against Drunk Drivers (MADD) were, themselves, parents who lost children as the result of accidents caused by intoxicated drivers. Many volunteers and staff members who work in sexual assault and domestic violence programs are, themselves, survivors. Many feminist rape crisis and domestic violence programs incorporate efforts to educate survivors about feminist views of violence against women and to empower survivors to become active in antirape and anti–domestic violence efforts as a crucial part of their recovery. In such instances it is the opportunity to do something meaningful with what one has learned from the personal experience of tragedy as well as the opportunity to join in community with other similarly affected individuals that appears to help people thrive after a crisis.

In summary, the goal of all crisis counseling is for the client to no longer require the assistance provided by the crisis counselor. This means that the crisis client has resolved many troublesome aspects of the crisis and has in place ongoing systems of support and access to needed resources.

DISCUSSION QUESTIONS

1. The primary purpose of single-session crisis intervention is to restore an individual's sense of control after the impact of a crisis event. The primary purpose of ongoing crisis counseling is resolution of the crisis. How do the respective goals of single-session crisis counseling and ongoing crisis counseling contribute to the achievement of these different purposes?

2. Consider the six steps of the single-session crisis intervention model. For each step, identify and discuss possible obstacles (client behaviors/characteristics, event/situation characteristics, crisis worker behaviors) that could interfere with accomplishment of these respective steps. How can crisis workers overcome these potential obstacles?

EXERCISES

Both of these exercises utilize the scenarios that follow. You can also ask students to generate their own case examples.

1. Divide the class into small groups. Explain that Step 6 of the single-session crisis intervention model entails assisting crisis clients to mobilize personal and social resources and connect with community resources. For each of the scenarios below, ask the group members to identify relevant personal, social, and community resources.

2. Divide the class into small groups. Explain that assisting a crisis client to achieve cognitive mastery in the aftermath of a crisis requires counselor sensitivity to the personal meaning of that crisis including the myths, beliefs, and/or basic assumptions that may be threatened by a crisis event. For each of the following scenarios, ask group members to identify the potential cognitive impact of the specific crisis event.

Scenarios

1. You are a residence life staff person at a small university. You are asked to come to a dorm room because a female student has just learned that her boyfriend was killed in a car crash.
2. You are employed in a domestic violence program. You are on call and have been asked to meet with a woman and her two children in the hospital emergency room. The woman and one child have been beaten by the woman's live-in companion.
3. You are a hospital crisis worker who is going to meet with a single-parent mother whose 16-year-old daughter has just been diagnosed with a rare form of bone cancer.
4. You are contacted by the director of the local Planned Parenthood agency. You are asked to provide crisis intervention for a staff of five individuals who have just learned that their medical director was killed on her way to the clinic. The police have warned the staff that the suspect is an antiabortion zealot who has not yet been apprehended.

REFERENCES

Boudewyns, P. A., & Hyer, L. (1990). Physiological response to combat memories and preliminary treatment outcome in Vietnam veteran PTSD patients treated with direct therapeutic exposure. *Behavior Therapy, 21,* 63–87.

Calhoun, L. G., & Tedeschi, R. G. (2000). Early posttraumatic intervention: Facilitating possibilities for growth. In J. M. Violanti, D. Paton, & C. Dunning (Eds.), *Posttraumatic stress intervention: Challenges, issues, and perspectives* (pp. 135–152). Springfield, IL: Charles C. Thomas Publisher.

Corwin, M. (2002). *Brief treatment in clinical social work practice.* Pacific Grove, CA: Brooks/Cole.

Foa, E. B., Rothbaum, B. O., Riggs, D., & Murdock, T. (1991). Treatment of post-traumatic stress disorder in rape victims: A comparison between cognitive-behavioral procedures and counseling. *Journal of Consulting and Clinical Psychology, 59,* 715–723.

Foa, E. B., & Rothbaum, B. O. (1998). *Treating the trauma of rape: Cognitive-behavioral therapy for PTSD.* New York: Guilford Press.

Garfield, S. L. (1994). Research on client variables in psychotherapy. In A. E. Bergin & S. L. Garfield (Eds.), *Handbook of psychotherapy and behavior change* (4th ed., pp. 190–228). New York: Wiley.

Gutstein, S. E. (1991). Adolescent suicide: The loss of reconciliation. In F. Walsh & M. McGoldrick (Eds.), *Living beyond loss: Death in the family.* New York: W. W. Norton.

Herman, J. (1997). *Trauma and recovery.* New York: Basic Books.

Koss, M. R., & Harvey, M. R. (1991). *The rape victim: Clinical and community interventions* (2nd ed.). Newbury Park, CA: Sage.

McFarlane, A. C., & van der Kolk, B. A. (1996). Trauma and its challenge to society. In B. A. van der Kolk, A. C. McFarlane, & L. Wiesaeth (Eds.), *Traumatic stress: The effects of overwhelming experience on mind, body, and society* (pp. 24–46). New York: Guilford Press.

Pennebaker, J. W., & Harber, K. (1993). A social stage model of collective coping: The Loma Prieta earthquake and the Persian Gulf War. *Journal of Social Issues, 49,* 125–145.

Rogers, C. (1957). The necessary and sufficient conditions of therapeutic personality change. *Journal of Consulting Psychology, 22,* 95–103.

Rogers, C. (1980). *A way of being.* Boston: Houghton Mifflin.

Slaikeu, K. A. (1990). *Crisis intervention: A handbook for practice and research* (2nd ed.). Boston: Allyn & Bacon.

Stuhlmiller, C., & Dunning, C. (2000). In J. M. Violanti, D. Paton, & C. Dunning (Eds.), *Posttraumatic stress intervention: Challenges, issues, and perspectives* (pp. 10–42). Springfield, IL: Charles C. Thomas Publisher.

Surrey, J. L. (1991). Relationship and empowerment. In J. Jordan, A. Kaplan, J. Miller, I. Stiver, & J. Surrey (Eds.), *Women's growth in connection: Writings from the Stone Center* (pp. 162–180). New York: Guilford Press.

CHAPTER 4

Crisis Intervention Competence

What does the concept "competence" mean in relation to the practice of crisis intervention? At its root, competence suggests that one is able to do what is necessary and suitable for the specific purpose at hand. At times, competence is measured by proof of proper qualifications or legal capacity to carry out identified roles and tasks, as in the case of licensure of helping professionals or certificates of completion of designated education, training, or examinations. We use the term *competence* primarily in the first sense. A competent crisis interventionist is one who has the ability to effectively and appropriately intervene with individuals experiencing crises in their lives.

The helping relationship is the medium through which crisis intervention is provided. The crisis worker begins a helping relationship armed with knowledge and skill and intentionally behaves in ways designed to create an atmosphere of safety and trust. This occurs through the conscious and intentional use of self.

This chapter identifies those essential qualities we have found to characterize competent crisis workers and effective crisis intervention. It also reviews the basic intervention skills most frequently employed in crisis intervention practice.

CHARACTERISTICS OF COMPETENT CRISIS COUNSELORS

As evidenced by the range of crises discussed in this text and the diversity of people served by crisis workers, the relationships formed with people in crisis may be quite varied. Reviews of the research on helping, however, suggest that there are certain core conditions or facilitative qualities demonstrated by a helping person that appear to universally enhance the likelihood that an effective helping relationship will be formed (Carkhuff, 1969; Ivey, Ivey, & Simek-Downing, 1987; Rogers, 1957, 1980). Among those qualities are self-awareness, empathy, respect, warmth, and authenticity. More recent descriptions of effective helpers have also emphasized the overarching importance of cultural self-awareness and cultural sensitivity in working with diverse peoples (Devore & Schlesinger, 1981; Sue, Arredondo, & McDavis, 1995; Sue, Ivey, & Pedersen, 1996).

Okun (1992) observed that the characteristics found to describe the effective helper are closely related to the supportive communication techniques demonstrated to enhance counseling effectiveness. Somewhat arbitrarily, in this section we describe "person-characteristics," and in the last section of this chapter we describe communication behaviors.

Self-awareness and Self-understanding

Many people are quite naïve in their self-awareness and self-knowledge, mistakenly assuming that they have no biases or prejudices and no personal preferences that affect their work with others. In reality, all individuals are a product of their unique cultural, familial, and interpersonal experiences. Thus, as Cournoyer (2000) pointed out, to be effective, professionals must have substantial and sophisticated self-understanding including awareness of how they appear to others, what issues cause anxiety, and what kinds of people or events precipitate emotional responses and/or unhelpful responses. Without such awareness and understanding, even the best-intentioned helpers may behave in ways that inadvertently diminish or undermine their effectiveness. With self-awareness, crisis workers are more likely to differentiate their own needs and feelings from those of their clients, and are more able to effectively empower clients to make determinations based on the client's perceptions and choices.

For the helping professional, the process of gaining this depth and breadth of self-awareness and self-understanding is lifelong. It is a process one continuously engages in through self-reflection and introspection, participation in personal counseling, and supervision of one's professional work. It can also be enhanced through specific structured awareness-building experiences, for example, attending a professional training on cultural awareness.

At a minimum, self-awareness must include an understanding of one's family of origin including family roles, behavioral patterns, and family influences on attitudes, beliefs, and values; gender and cultural awareness; and ongoing awareness of one's own needs and feelings. Although self-awareness is important for all helpers, it is particularly important for those providing crisis counseling because of its intensity, brevity, and the heightened vulnerability of clients experiencing a crisis reaction.

Crisis workers are confronted with situations that are volatile and that may be frightening, and are called to comfort and assist individuals who frequently are in desperate need. Some of what they see and hear may be shocking, upsetting, and/or confusing. It is essential that crisis workers be attuned to their own reactions so they can choose what and when to disclose, and also when and how to communicate calm support and understanding of clients' reactions.

Authenticity and Genuineness

Authenticity is defined as "the sharing of self by relating in a natural, sincere, spontaneous, open, and genuine manner" (Hepworth, Rooney, & Larsen, 1997, p. 120). It includes helpers' ability to be honest with themselves as well as with the individuals they seek to help.

The idea that a crisis worker should be authentic, genuine, and spontaneous may seem to contradict the previous description of the helper as someone who consciously chooses to engage in particular professional behaviors. A crisis worker's ability to be calm, thoughtful, and objective, however, does not mean that he or she is emotionally detached or too controlled. Rather, the most effective helping professional is able to relate to people personally and spontaneously. Rogers (1980) identified what he called the "appalling consequences" (p. 139) of reducing the notion of helping to simply applying specific skills. As Egan (1994) elaborated, counselor trainees must learn and use specific communication skills, but they must "use them in a fully human way" so the "skills and techniques become extensions of the helper's humanity and not just bits of helping technology" (p. 90).

This is particularly important in crisis intervention because a more detached, analytic, or professionally distanced stance would clearly fail to meet the emotional and psychological needs of the person in crisis. Herman (1997) asserted that those who provide counseling to victimized people must have a "committed moral stance" that assumes "a position of solidarity" with the client. As she described it, moral solidarity "involves an understanding of the fundamental injustice of the traumatic experience and the need for a resolution that restores some sense of justice. This affirmation expresses itself in the therapist's daily practice, in her language, and above all in her moral commitment to truth-telling without evasion or disguise" (p. 135).

Such truth telling, or authenticity, is demonstrated in a case involving a 15-year-old girl who was sadistically abused by her stepfather over a period of years. When the young woman spoke about the abuse and described the way her stepfather would "punish" her, the crisis counselor affirmed that she was, in fact, tortured. Counselors who work with children and adolescents who have been abused or molested by caregivers often find that these victims have assumed complicity and/or responsibility for what was done to them. (See Chapter 11 for more information on child abuse.) The crisis counselor's use of the word *torture* to describe the abuse acknowledged both the existence of a perpetrator and the young woman's experience of victimization rather than punishment. Similarly, a comment by a crisis worker that genuinely and spontaneously expresses sorrow about a client's experience or that affirms his or her inability to comprehend how someone could perpetrate a horrific act, affirms his or her solidarity with the survivor in an authentic manner.

Although not all crises involve victimization and trauma, it is nonetheless always important to present a personal and professional stance that conveys genuineness and honest solidarity with the crisis client. The crisis worker's ability to make a personal connection, yet still make professional decisions about when to share his or her own reactions and/or perceptions, requires a high degree of self-awareness. The more self-aware, the more likely the crisis worker is attuned to his or her reactions, and thus able to spontaneously convey genuine interest and concern, while at the same time ensuring that any self-disclosure is made for the purpose of fostering the crisis client's well-being.

Egan (1994) offered professionals the following general guidelines, which we believe are equally applicable in both single-session and ongoing crisis counseling contexts:

1. Do not overemphasize the helping role. Genuine helpers relate at deeper levels and avoid being bound by a professional role that they put on or take off at will.
2. Be spontaneous, being tactful and respectful, but avoiding artifice and studied responses.
3. Avoid defensiveness. Genuine helpers are comfortable with themselves and can encounter and examine negative criticism openly and honestly.
4. Be open and free to engage in deeper levels of sharing, as appropriate to the client's needs. This includes not having any hidden agendas (pp. 55–56).

Cultural Competence

If competence entails having the necessary knowledge and skills to behave in a manner that is effective for a given purpose, cultural competence implies a specific kind of knowledge, skill, and measure of effectiveness. The culturally competent professional is one who possesses cultural awareness and knowledge as well as the skills necessary to intervene successfully with clients from diverse cultural backgrounds (Sue & Sue, 2002). One does not develop cultural competence, however, simply by acquiring group-specific knowledge or prescriptive techniques, as this alone fails to adequately capture the multiple factors that influence a given individual or a given counseling interaction. No group of people, despite a shared sociocultural heritage, is uniform in the experience of culture. Yet all behavior, experience of the spiritual, and formation of perspectives of self and others are clearly influenced by the sociocultural environment. The presence or absence of a smile, the use of a handshake in greeting, and the notion of self are all understood within a cultural context (Pedersen, 1991).

Culture, as used here, refers to a pattern of learned beliefs, behaviors, and material objects shared by members of a given group. Cultures are complex and influence all aspects of our existence including our self-identities and worldviews. Culture is not something that belongs only to others—those we perceive as different. Rather, each of us is simultaneously individual and unique, a member of multiple cultures, thus sharing some feelings, thoughts, assumptions, and biases with others of similar cultures, and universally human. As result of one's membership in a given ethnic group, sex/gender, ability, sexuality, religion, and social class, each individual develops a particular identity, worldview, ethical/moral sense, spiritual belief, and relationship to power and oppression. Yet each individual also, in different ways, transcends these differences in the fullness of his or her individual and human existence (Fukuyama, 1990; Ho, 1995; Ibrahim, 1985; Pedersen, 1991; Speight, Myers, Cox, & Highlen, 1991).

Cultural competence begins with self-awareness. A helper's effectiveness in counseling individuals from diverse cultural backgrounds is determined both by awareness of his or her own worldview, and by understanding and appreciation of his or her clients' worldviews (Ibrahim, 1985). Cultural self-awareness includes insight into one's own cultural values, attitudes, and beliefs, as well as an understanding of how these might affect the counseling relationship. Understanding the cultural experience and worldview of clients requires a background of general knowledge about different cultural groups as well as an understanding of how cultural values and attitudes of both counselor and client affect the counseling relationship and counseling process. This includes knowledge of power structures and the impact of prejudice, oppression, and being marginalized in society, as well as knowledge of cultural duality and the bicultural experience of cultural minorities.

Cross, Bazron, Dennis, and Isaacs (1989) contended that cultural competence occurs along a continuum that ranges from cultural destructiveness to cultural proficiency. Notably, the liberal political philosophy of being unbiased—treating all people the same, regardless of ethnic and/or other cultural variables—is not valued as a competent stance. Rather, the culturally competent professional recognizes and respects cultural differences and pays attention to the "dynamics of difference"—the possibility that when people of different cultures interact with one another, one or both may misjudge the other's words and actions. "Both will bring culturally prescribed patterns of communication, etiquette and problem solving. Both may bring stereotypes with them or underlying feelings about working with someone who is 'different.' . . . Without an understanding of their cultural differences, the dynamics most likely to occur between the two are misinterpretation or misjudgment" (Research and Training Center to Improve Services for Seriously Emotionally Handicapped Children and Their Families, 1988, p. 4).

Knowledge of one's own and other cultural groups may frequently develop at the same time, for as one identifies and describes one culturally framed perspective it becomes possible to identify alternative perspectives on the same issue (Ho, 1995). For example, Hoare (1991) explored the concept of individual identity as it is understood in Western cultures and compared it to concepts of self found in non-Western cultures. In Western cultures, identity is understood and experienced as personal coherence, knowing yourself, and being an active agent in charge of your own life. By contrast, "[I[n India, the self is not a separate domain. Each person is but a small part of the entire natural, ancestral, and unknown supernatural world. . . . Indians come to their sense of being interpersonally. Disorders are those of relational difficulties in the cosmos, with nature, or in the human order" (Hoare, 1991, p. 49).

Similarly, cultures influenced by Eastern philosophy and religions such as Hinduism, Islam, and Buddhism have values and beliefs that are quite dissimilar from a traditional Western worldview. For example, according to Ho (1989), modesty in behavior, piety and deference to authority, and fatalistic acceptance of circumstances are fundamental values in Asian cultures. Such values are likely to influence help-seeking behavior, as many Asian-Americans "feel stigma and shame in talking about problems" (p. 533). The role of shame as a potential influence on seeking assistance is certainly not unique to Asian-Americans. Understanding the particular salience of "avoidance of shame" to members of this culture, however, better prepares the crisis counselor to identify with an Asian-American client's cultural influences, avoiding the possibility of acting on the basis of the counselor's own cultural beliefs about self-determination and personal power.

We do not suggest that crisis counselors memorize specific information about every possible cultural group to whom they may provide services. Yet it is clear that the more aware crisis counselors are about their own culture and the more familiar they are with the symbols and meanings of other cultures, the more likely they will accurately perceive each client's culturally mediated experience and perspective rather than impose their own perspective. Each individual's culture influences how to define family, with whom and where to seek social support, and how to explain crises or tragedies. Some culturally isolated individuals such as refugees and immigrants may have no social support system other than their immediate family. Clearly, each of these factors directly affects how one responds in times of crisis and stress (Lum, 1999).

Ultimately, cultural competence requires the ability to use one's cultural self-awareness and knowledge of diverse cultures to intervene effectively with clients from diverse ethnic or cultural origins and status. Numerous writers (Blocher, 2000; Helms & Richardson, 1997; Lum, 1996; Reynolds & Pope, 1991; Sue & Sue, 2002) have struggled to identify and describe the culturally sensitive and responsive skills believed necessary to provide effective help to diverse clients. Giordano and Giordano (1995) proposed guidelines for working with multicultural families. The following suggestions build on their ideas:

- Determine how important ethnic identification is to a crisis client, and be willing to explore the impact of that identification on perspectives related to the crisis in a validating manner.
- Be aware of and use the client's support system.
- Serve as a "culture broker," helping the individual and/or his or her family to identify and resolve value conflicts. For example, children may have adopted majority culture values that parents find unacceptable, given their own traditional cultural beliefs and practices.
- Know that there are advantages (e.g., easier establishment of rapport) and disadvantages (e.g., strong identification, projection) to being of the same ethnic background as your client.
- Don't feel that you have to know everything about every cultural group. Rather, be aware of the influence of culture, and be open to understanding your client's unique cultural perspective.
- Always try to think of differences in a way that allows for at least three possibilities. For example, remember that an individual who is Jewish may view Arab-Christian relationships differently than the Arab; or a gay Latino male may view gender differently than a heterosexual African-American male or a southern white woman.

Sue (1998) asserted that one of the fundamental attributes of multicultural competence is "scientific mindedness," wherein counselors form tentative hypotheses and test those hypotheses as they attempt to understand the meaning of their client's messages. Rather than assuming anything, the culturally effective counselor envisions possible meanings and seeks information that will lead to better conclusions. Ultimately, effective, culturally sensitive crisis intervention depends on the ability of a culturally self-aware, knowledgeable individual to listen carefully, to ask sensitive questions about the meaning of what clients reveal, and to recognize that it is each individual client who is the expert guide to his or her unique world of experience and meaning.

CHARACTERISTICS OF EFFECTIVE CRISIS INTERVENTION

Now that we have identified essential "person-characteristics" of the effective crisis counselor, in this section we focus attention on intervention. Our purpose is not to delineate specific skills (as we do later in this chapter), but rather to identify an overarching philosophy and orientation to providing assistance to individuals experiencing crises. In order to be helpful, crisis intervention must be empowering, based on an appreciation of a client's strength and resilience; and focused, always, on the individual and his or her sociocultural environment.

Empowering Crisis Intervention

> To initiate changes, you must believe that your actions are possible and that your efforts will make a difference. . . . In these circumstances, you are likely to experience empowerment. When people experience empowerment, they feel effective, conclude that they are competent, and perceive that they have power and control over the course of their lives. (DuBois & Krogsrud Miley, 2002, p. 24)

As this quotation suggests, personal empowerment entails both a sense or perception of one's own worthiness, competence, and personal control, and the availability of needed resources and the power to access and make use of them. Surrey (1987) focused on the relational context of empowerment. She defined empowerment as "the motivation, freedom, and capacity to act purposefully, with the mobilization of the energies, resources, strengths, or powers of each person through a mutual, relational process" (p. 3). Building on these notions, empowering crisis intervention requires the establishment of a helping relationship that contributes to crisis clients' enhanced power and control, with power defined as "the capacity to move or to produce change" (Miller, 1982). It is intervention that aims to increase the ability of crisis clients to make effective life decisions and to increase their ability to access and utilize needed resources and social supports.

Empowerment is thus both a means and a goal (DuBois & Krogsrud Miley, 2002). Empowerment as a means refers to the type of counseling relationship and processes that contribute to and facilitate the attainment of the goal of an empowered client. Empowerment as a goal refers to an outcome whereby individuals are capable of acting on their own behalf, believing in their own capacity to take action and having the personal and social resources to do so successfully.

Some individuals are at particular risk for disempowerment. For example, numerous writers have described the direct and indirect barriers to empowerment that many minorities experience, including underdeveloped skills and personal resources as a result of environmental obstacles, bias, stereotyping, and discrimination (Gutierrez & Lewis, 1999; Solomon, 1989). Members of stigmatized groups, such as gays and lesbians, may also experience barriers to their ability to act on their own behalf because of discriminatory attitudes and fears regarding disclosure and loss of privacy, and because of outright barriers to fair treatment. For example, following the September 11, 2001, terror attacks, many long-term domestic partners of gay and lesbian workers who were killed were denied the support and monetary compensation that was provided to married heterosexual surviving spouses. Clearly, such obstacles place added stress on already overburdened survivors.

Empowering processes aimed at increasing personal power and control are particularly relevant when working with individuals whose experiences have rendered them, at least temporarily, powerless. Each of the crises discussed in this book has that potential, and some, particularly those that involve victimization, inevitably diminish the individual's power to act. In speaking about empowering interventions with battered women, Schechter (1987) described four tasks in the empowerment process: (1) validating the woman's experiences by establishing an alliance with her and taking a stand against the violence; (2) ensuring that she is fully informed of all options and advocating for both her safety and her access to needed assistance, including shelter, welfare, and criminal justice response; (3) building on her strengths and avoiding blaming the victim; and (4) respecting her right to self-determination. These tasks are, of course, equally applicable to any victim, male or female.

Speaking about empowerment from a more general standpoint, but identifying the same basic issues, DuBois and Miley (2002) asserted that the philosophy of empowerment is translated into empowering counseling processes only when helping professionals focus on strengths, work collaboratively with their clients, and link personal and political power. Bertolino and O'Hanlon (2001) described collaborative, competency-based approaches to helping as a "third wave" in thinking about and understanding therapeutic work with individuals and families. Drawing on social constructivist thinking with its emphasis on the co-creation of both identity and meaning through social interaction, they emphasized collaboration and partnership with clients and a focus on client strengths.

Focus on strengths and competencies   Most traditional models of both assessment and counseling have primarily focused on accurately identifying what is problematic in a client's life and strategizing to change it. Thus counselors, social workers, and other helping professionals tend to notice maladaptive functioning and deficits or dysfunctions in client's families and social support systems, but may fail to notice the strengths and competencies in the client and his or her environment.

Recently, propelled in part by efforts to better serve culturally diverse clients and women, and to better recognize the creative adaptive coping capacities utilized by marginalized and oppressed individuals and communities, there has been a paradigm shift in the counseling and social work literature. This shift emphasizes the identification and assessment of strengths, competence, and resiliency, as opposed to the dominant focus on pathology (Bertolino & O'Hanlon, 2001; Cowger, 1992, 1994; Katz, 1997; Rutter, 1987; Saleebey, 1992, 1996; Stuhlmiller & Dunning, 2000).

A growing body of psychotherapy outcome research suggests that key factors predicting success include the presence of collaborative helping partnerships and approaches that emphasize client strengths and resources (Bertolino & O'Hanlon, 2001; Duncan & Miller, 2000; Stuhlmiller & Dunning, 2000). In discussing crisis interventions with individuals who have suffered traumatic events, Stuhlmiller and Dunning (2000) urged counselors to move from pathogenic to salutogenic models of posttrauma intervention. Included in such a paradigm shift is a focus on resilience and the power of "natural holding environments" that promote growth and healing.

Many years ago, Puryear (1979) emphasized the importance of identifying a crisis client's strengths as a way of helping individuals to regain control in a crisis. In some situations, identifying strengths or imagining how an individual could regain control may be quite challenging. For example, a burn victim who also lost family members and material possessions in a fire may appear to be in a hopeless situation. Or an individual diagnosed with a terminal illness may not appear to have any way to regain control of her situation. Yet even in such seemingly hopeless situations the crisis worker can search for strengths and areas in which a client can exercise personal control. The individual who is dying can exercise control by determining how he or she wishes to engage the dying process—emotionally, spiritually, and relationally.

Cowger (1992, 1994) developed a framework for "empowering practice" based on identification of strengths and deficits or obstacles in both the person and the environment. For example, he suggested that assessments of "personal factor" strengths include attention to (1) adaptive *cognition,* including views of self and the world; (2) *emotional* intelligence, as reflected in the ability to recognize, tolerate, and express one's feelings; (3) acknowledgment of problems and *motivation/* perseverance in seeking to resolve them; (4) flexible, resourceful *coping* responses; and (5) the capacity for mutual, caring, supportive relationships *(interpersonal).*

The identification of strengths and competencies is particularly important when assisting clients to take action in the aftermath of a crisis, as they need strength to take action. It is also important, however, when exploring clients' needs and challenges, as it is a way of assisting clients to see themselves and their circumstances more holistically. Recognizing the coexistence of pain and strength, vulnerability and self-protectiveness, maladaptive behaviors and successful coping enable crisis workers to validate the distress associated with unique crises situations and also facilitate individuals' adaptive coping. For example, a battered woman whose children blame her for not rescuing them from their abusive father can be helped to acknowledge her children's pain and also recognize that her decisions were made in oppressive circumstances when all options were fraught with danger.

Dual Focus on Individual and Ecological System

Our developmental-ecological perspective requires the crisis worker to attend to both the individual and the ecological systems within which the individual client lives and within which the specific crisis occurs. Systems that may be relevant to a client's situation include his or her family and primary social system as well as school, work, medical care, recreational activities, religion, neighborhood, and friendships.

Maintaining a dual focus requires that the crisis worker consistently see the crisis client in context. Years ago Barker (1978) referred to behavior settings—the environment that encloses and shapes the behavior of the human beings within it. Focused primarily on the relational and interdependent nature of behavioral and nonbehavioral components of any setting (e.g., a classroom or an office), he pioneered experimental research aimed at understanding the impact of behavior settings. Blocher (1987) suggested that counselors learn to recognize and identify relevant behavior settings: "Only when we are fully aware of the unity and coherence represented by a given behavior setting can we begin to understand and appreciate fully its impact and influence on the behavior that it encloses" (p. 182).

In fact, to comprehend every aspect of the individual's experience, the crisis counselor must recognize that experience as embedded in relationships, responsibilities and obligations, and physical and psychological locations. Similarly, the crisis counselor can only assess and utilize each potential environmental resource by considering the individual's interaction with that system.

In Chapter 3 we asserted that ecological thinking prepares a crisis counselor to view both the crisis situation and the person experiencing a crisis reaction holistically. The ecological perspective prepares us to attend to the environmental context of all human functioning and to recognize the bidirectional nature of all interactions. We reemphasize that point here, noting that this perceptual standpoint is a necessary and essential characteristic of competent crisis intervention. As Blocher (2000) noted, all human problems and difficulties arise, not from inside the individual, but "around specific interactions *between* the individual and the environment" (p. 15). Given this reality, all effective counseling must ultimately produce a better "fit" between the individual and his or her environment (Germain & Gitterman, 1996).

Competent crisis intervention *always* entails the ability to see and relate to both the individual and the environmental context of that unique individual. Further, it requires recognition of the multidirectional, interactional nature of each relationship, whether it is between two individuals (e.g., the survivor of a disaster and her spouse) or between the individual client and a system (e.g., the male sexual assault victim and the police).

CRISIS INTERVENTION SKILLS

In this section we identify and review some of the essential skills necessary for competent intervention with crisis clients. Subsequent chapters introduce additional specific assessment and prevention/intervention skills and methods particularly applicable to different crises.

For the purpose of this text, skills are defined as specific sets of behaviors engaged in by crisis interventionists that derive from knowledge about crises and about the needs and challenges facing individuals experiencing crisis reactions. They are behaviors that contribute to the accomplishment of crisis intervention/counseling goals. In other words, skills are not simply techniques or "technical tasks" that one "enacts, robot like, at the same relative time and in the same way with all clients, all problems, and all situations" (Cournoyer, 2000, p. 5). Rather, skills are both "extensions of the helper's humanity" (Egan, 1994, p. 90) and consciously chosen ways of responding to client needs in order to further the purpose of helping.

Crisis counselors must be proficient in skills that facilitate relationship development including attending and listening, client ventilation and sharing of information about the situation and personal responses, and renewed coping and survival in the aftermath of a crisis. Because crisis intervention entails assisting individuals in a wide range of domains (affective, behavioral, cognitive, developmental, ecological), the crisis worker needs a variety of ways to conceptualize and facilitate recovery and change. Goals or targets of change include (1) personal characteristics (emotions, behaviors, cognition, development), (2) interpersonal interactions, and (3) social/environmental situations, and various combinations of these (Berlin & Marsh, 1993).

Skills Associated with Relationship Development

Attending and active listening   Actively listening to what clients say both verbally and nonverbally is the essential first step of empowering crisis intervention. Unfortunately, listening with understanding to a crisis client's concerns is not as simple or easy as it sounds. Complete listening, at a minimum, includes observing, hearing, and responding to clients' nonverbal behavior, verbal messages, and the context or the ways clients are "influenced by the contexts in which they live, move, and have their being" (Egan, 1994, p. 98). For example, Kelly, a crisis client who reports in a follow-up conversation with a rape crisis worker that she is "really doing OK," may be honest in reporting her current conscious self-appraisal. Her nonverbal behavior, however, may reveal significant anxiety and/or agitation, an indication that she is not OK. Or listening to her context may reveal that it is Kelly's family that wants her to be OK.

Egan (1994) warned helpers to be aware of the "shadow side of listening to clients." He described examples of ineffective listening, including "evaluative listening," wherein the helper is judging the merits of what is being said; "filtered listening," wherein the helper filters what is heard through his or her own biases; "fact-centered" rather than person-centered listening; and, "sympathetic listening," wherein the helper's dominant response is feeling sorry for the client's pain (pp. 100–103). Each of these listening styles is particularly problematic in crisis situations, when helpers must often listen and respond quickly and actively and when both the situation and the crisis client's responses may be intense.

Attending is the behavioral complement to listening and includes both verbal and nonverbal dimensions. Attending to nonverbal behavior entails good eye contact, facial expressions that mirror and convey acceptance of the client's feelings, and body postures that reflect awareness of client needs. As is true of all skills, competent nonverbal attending requires adaptation to each individual and situation. Thus knowledge about such things as cultural differences in eye contact or sensitivity to a client's discomfort with physical closeness ultimately determines how effectively the crisis worker interacts nonverbally with a unique individual.

Attending to verbal behavior entails the use of paraphrasing or content-reflecting messages. Along with empathy, content-reflecting messages communicate the helper's comprehension of what the client is saying. More than merely parroting the exact words used by the client, an effective paraphrase identifies the key ideas and in a short response reflects the core message back to the client. It is a form of active listening that gives precise feedback leading to clarification and increased mutual understanding and facilitates further sharing by the crisis client. For example:

Crisis Client: I couldn't move, I couldn't scream, I didn't know what to do. All I did was stand and stare as the flames came closer. I simply stood there until someone, I think it was the man who was just taken in the ambulance, until he grabbed me, lifted me up, and carried me out.

Crisis Worker: *What you most remember is seeing the flames approaching you, but almost like being stuck in time. And then suddenly you were jolted into the present by the man who rescued you.*

Although it is likely that considerable emotion also surrounds this situation, the crisis worker chose, *at this time,* to actively clarify and respond to the content rather than to the feelings.

Another way to attend to verbal behavior has been described as "tracking"—verbally responding in ways that follow, accept, and encourage the client's ongoing communication. Rather than leading or directing the conversation, tracking involves staying with the client and following what he or she chooses to focus on (Minuchin, 1974).

Empathy and empathic responding Fundamentally, empathy is a way of being with a client rather than a specific skill. As Rogers (1980) declared: "It means entering the private perceptual world of the other . . . being sensitive, moment by moment, to the changing felt meanings which flow in this other person, to the fear or rage or tenderness or confusion or whatever he or she is experiencing. It means temporarily living in the other's life, moving about in it delicately without making judgments" (p. 142). Empathic crisis intervention requires that crisis workers be willing and able to momentarily suspend their own feelings and needs in order to experience the feelings of the crisis client as if those feelings were their own, but without losing their ability to maintain objectivity.

For empathy to be effective, it must be communicated both nonverbally and through the accurate and active reflection of feelings. Empathy entails selectively identifying the core emotional and content messages and selectively choosing to respond in a manner that emphasizes the client's affective responses. Thus, in responding empathically to the crisis client who was rescued from the burning building, the crisis worker might respond: *"Kelly, it sounds as though you were so terrified by the danger approaching that you literally couldn't act in response. . . . it's as if you were mesmerized by the fire."*

Empathy is not the same as sympathy, or feeling sorry for the client, nor is it projection, or assuming that one's own emotional responses are the client's. Rather, empathy requires a listener to simultaneously tune into his or her own emotional reactions and to the emotional responses of the person in crisis. Responding with empathy occurs as the listener chooses to place his or her own feelings on hold in order to experience and respond to the emotions of the other. There have been a number of research and training scales developed to measure differing levels of empathic responding (Carkhuff, 1969; Hammond, Hepworth, & Smith, 1977; Hepworth, Rooney, & Larsen, 1997). In general, lower-level responses are based in the worker's personal frame of reference and are not effective or helpful, often blocking communication. Mid-range levels are reciprocal or interchangeable empathic responses that convey understanding but do not reach beyond surface feelings. The highest levels of empathic responding are described as "reflecting each emotional nuance" and as being accurately responsive to "the full range and intensity of both surface and underlying feelings and meanings" (Hepworth, Rooney, & Larsen, 1997, p. 110).

As should be clear to the reader, attending, active listening, and empathic responding are skills that serve two primary purposes. First, they enable crisis workers to establish relationships in which clients feel heard and understood. Empathy nurtures and sustains a helping relationship, and the presence of empathy constitutes what Rogers (1957) described as one of the core conditions of helping relationships. At the same time, these skills facilitate the crisis client's sharing of his or her story.

Skills to Facilitate Exploration and Ventilation

Probing   Probing is another primary skill through which crisis workers elicit crisis clients' stories and enable them to share concerns, ideas, experiences, and feelings. Probes consist of the crisis worker's questions, requests for information, and/or clarifying and focusing responses.

The first time a crisis worker probes usually occurs when he or she requests that the client share what has happened. For example, the telephone crisis counselor might ask a caller to explain his or her situation. *"Tell me, if you can, what happened that has so upset you?"* or *"What can you tell me about what has occurred?"*

Probes are also used in the early phase and throughout crisis intervention to seek specific information necessary to assess the client's safety and identify immediate needs. Thus the crisis worker might ask a battered woman if she is safe, if someone is with her in the home, or if she has transportation to get to a shelter. Similarly, a crisis worker might ask a crisis client if he has been drinking or taking drugs, or how many pills he consumed. It is important that such closed questions be utilized only to obtain vital, specific information. Closed probes can be useful when it is important to quickly gather information necessary to assess safety, but using them too much results in clients feeling interrogated rather than helped and does little to establish an empowering and collaborative relationship.

Except for situations when very specific information is needed, open questions are a preferred means of helping crisis clients to share their experiences, feelings, and thoughts. Thus a crisis counselor might ask a suicidal client whose wife was killed in an auto accident a year earlier, *"What has kept you going since your wife's death?"* to get some insight into his coping strategies. Or in helping a crisis client begin to think about immediate options and/or alternatives, the crisis worker might ask, *"How do you think you want to handle letting your family know what has happened?"* Similarly, requests such as *"Please tell me what you're considering as possibilities"* or *"I'd like to better understand what you're feeling,"* or observations such as *"I know this situation is different, but I suspect you have ways that you usually handle stressors that you may be able to draw on"* may create an opportunity for crisis clients to ventilate and to provide more extensive insights into their reactions, ways of coping, and potential resources.

Probes can also be utilized to help crisis clients clarify or state their observations or concerns more concretely. As Egan (1994) noted, clarity means that specific experiences, specific behaviors, and specific feelings are expressed and understood. "Vagueness and ambiguity lead nowhere. It is up to the counselor to help the client move to clarity. Attending, listening, empathy, and probing are the tools counselors use to help clients achieve action-oriented clarity" (p. 140). Thus a crisis client may report "feeling like I'm going crazy." With the help of empathy and probing, the counselor can help this client to describe specifically what she means by this statement. It may be that she is overwhelmed by intrusive memories, is having panic attacks, or can't focus on her work because she keeps thinking about how angry she is. Until her statement is clarified, the work of helping cannot proceed.

Egan (1994) pointed out that skilled helpers use a judicious mix of probes and empathy to help clients express, explore, and clarify their concerns and needs. Active listening and empathic responding are clearly the skills that, combined with essential helper characteristics such as authenticity, contribute most to an effective helping alliance and helping encounter. Probes expressed as questions and requests for information have their place in assisting crisis clients to provide the specific information necessary to create safety, to talk and ventilate, and to examine alternatives and develop options. It is critically important, however, that crisis interventionists not engage clients in question-and-answer sessions.

Partializing and focusing   One of the most common manifestations of being in crisis is the individual's feeling of being overwhelmed by a number of frequently interconnected problems, needs, and concerns. The individual often doesn't know where to start to try to solve them. Thus frequently the most useful interventions are those that help clients break down interconnected problems and concerns into more manageable units. Partializing is a skill counselors use to help the crisis client explore the dimensions of the crisis event and his or her reactions. It is simply the skill of assisting the client to organize the process of examining his or her problems and to begin to take action in response to discrete concerns.

In order to use the skill of partializing, crisis workers must attempt to maintain focus and objectivity. Because crisis situations are often complex, it is easy for even the most experienced workers to find themselves overwhelmed by that complexity and intensity. Listening intently to both the whole story and parts of client stories helps maintain focus and objectivity. Consider, for example, a battered woman who is physically hurt and emotionally numb, whose children are frightened and upset, who has no money or access to money, and who is reluctant to communicate with her family because they have been unsupportive in the past. Clearly, not all of her needs can be attended to simultaneously, although her needs are intertwined. Partializing acknowledges the whole picture, but also helps her identify a way to begin to work on her problems one at a time:

Crisis Worker: *Marie, I sense that it feels as though it's just too much to deal with. You are obviously hurt—on many levels. Your children are upset. And you have no idea whom you can trust to turn to for help. I wonder if I can help you by just trying to figure out where to start. It seems to me that the first issues to address have to be medical treatment for your injuries and helping your children feel safe. What do you think?*

Once the counselor helps organize the process, the counselor and client can work collaboratively to begin to identify alternatives and actions to address immediate needs. As individual parts of the problem are identified and addressed, the client's sense of being inundated and overwhelmed gradually diminishes. As she feels less overwhelmed, she is more able to mobilize her personal strengths and engage in the process of making decisions.

Skills to Facilitate Enhanced Coping, Change, and Recovery

In order to effectively assist crisis clients attain enhanced coping and recovery, crisis workers must be competent in conceptualizing and facilitating change in a wide range of domains, including personal characteristics (e.g., affect/emotion, behavior, cognition, developmental tasks), interpersonal interactions, and social/environmental situations. Effective crisis workers must also be competent in utilizing problem-solving processes. The range of skills that can be helpful in assisting clients in crisis, particularly crisis counseling, is therefore vast, and is informed by a range of theoretical frameworks.

For ease of presentation, we divide the review of skills for facilitating enhanced coping and recovery into five broad areas that correspond with our ABCDE model: affective interventions, behavioral interventions, cognitive interventions, developmental interventions, and interventions focused on changing the social environment. Although the approaches and skills in each area clearly emanate from specific theoretical and explanatory frameworks, we focus primarily on identifying the types of specific interventions that might be useful in each area. The reader is encouraged to consult additional sources for more specific and in-depth information.

Affective interventions   Emotions are a critically important aspect of most individuals' sense of being in crisis. Thus, whether a crisis counselor strives to assist an individual who feels overwhelmed by negative emotions such as anger, sadness, fear, shame, or guilt, or to aid an individual who is numb and constricted in his or her ability to express emotions, affective interventions are always an essential aspect of effective crisis counseling. Cormier and Hackney (1993) suggested that the "primary goals of affective intervention are: a) to help the client express feelings or feeling states; b) to identify or discriminate between feelings or feeling states; c) to alter or accept feelings or feeling states; or d) in some cases, to contain feelings" (p. 147). There is a range of theoretical frameworks (e.g., person-centered, Gestalt) and skills (e.g., empathy, two-chair work, guided imagery) that the crisis interventionist can draw upon to assist him or her in accomplishing these varied goals.

We have already examined the primary role of empathy in enabling individuals to express and experience their emotions in the calm, affirming, and understanding presence of the crisis counselor. Clearly, *active listening* and responsive *empathic reflection* are both extremely helpful interventions for facilitating the expression of emotion. They are also helpful in identifying and discriminating between feelings, as the empathic responder may accurately label a feeling-state or help the client discriminate between two or more possible emotions. For example:

Crisis Worker 1: *As I listen to you talk about what happened and see your fists clench and your jaw tighten, I sense real rage.*

Crisis Worker 2: *I'm sensing so much sadness and grief. . . . Yet, I also think I'm picking up on a strong sense of resolve or determination. It's almost as though you're saying, "I'm so sad I can hardly stand up, but I'm not going to let them win."*

Focusing and *enactive exercises* can also be helpful affective interventions, particularly in helping individuals with constricted emotions. Some clients seen for crisis counseling may have coped by becoming defensively numb to their feelings and corresponding physical sensations. Bass and Davis (1988) asserted that the first step in getting in touch with one's feelings is simply to pay attention—to the sensations in one's body and to oneself as a unique person. With this in mind, a crisis counselor might encourage a client to tune into and attend to her bodily sensations. Or the counselor might ask her to pay attention to behavior that may be reflecting or masking her emotions. Or a counselor might help a crisis client who has difficulty allowing himself to feel to enact his emotions, for example, by encouraging him to scream, yell, or hit a pillow or punching bag until he begins to connect with his feelings.

Guided imagery is also a useful skill to help clients gain access to unexpressed emotions or to contain feelings that are too intense to sustain. In the first instance, a crisis counselor might ask a client to close her eyes while she describes a scene designed to evoke an emotional response. In the second case, a crisis counselor might ask a client to develop an image, or series of images, to bring to mind when the pain, fear, or anxiety became too intense. For example, Denise, an adolescent survivor of severe abuse perpetrated by her stepfather, was helped to create a scene that would take her away from the painful images, memories, and associated emotions. Once Denise imagined and described the peaceful scene, the crisis counselor rehearsed with her the process of guiding herself to the image and away from the intrusive and upsetting images and emotions.

Crisis clients can also be taught various skills for *emotional containment:* ways to calm themselves when emotions become overwhelming. Some crisis clients may be afraid that if they allow themselves to feel, they will lose control. In some situations the fear of losing control can, itself, create a sense of panic. The assistance that a crisis worker gives a crisis client in such an instance can be as simple as reminding her to breathe. It may also be helpful for crisis clients to develop a personal list of soothing and calming activities to engage in (e.g., put on a relaxation tape, do yoga, take a hot bath, pray, get on the treadmill) and people to whom they can reach out when feeling most upset (Bass & Davis, 1988). Crisis clients can be assisted to use journaling, to learn relaxation techniques, or to use art as ways of both getting in touch with and coping with difficult emotions.

Persistent anxieties, fears, and generalized arousal associated with troubling memories of traumatic events can be countered utilizing a variety of *therapeutic exposure* and *systematic desensitization techniques* such as progressive relaxation (Foa & Rothbaum, 1998; Meichenbaum, 1994). These techniques can be useful when working with crisis/trauma survivors in ongoing crisis counseling. They have been found to be particularly effective in reducing physical and emotional arousal and startle response, intrusive thoughts and images, and nightmares (the "positive" symptoms of PTSD) in trauma survivors (Meichenbaum, 1994). Direct therapy exposure, however, has not been found helpful in countering numbing or restricted affect (the "negative" symptoms of PTSD), and it is contraindicated in a variety of situations, including with individuals who have a history of psychiatric disorders (Solomon, Gerrity, & Muff, 1992) and sexual abuse survivors (Kilpatrick & Best, 1984). These interventions should not be considered unless the crisis counselor has received specialized training including information about potential hazards. In all instances, interventions designed to help clients revisit traumatic events again in order to integrate and emotionally resolve them must be collaborative, with clients well informed and in charge (Meichenbaum, 1994). See Chapter 6 for a description of exposure techniques for PTSD as possible interventions with sexual assault survivors.

One last point concerning affective interventions that is particularly relevant to those engaged in crisis counseling: Positive and/or "good" emotions can also be experienced as upsetting. For example, a woman whose husband's death prompted a crisis reaction may find that although her constant, obsessive thoughts of him are overwhelming, when she begins to think about him less, this too causes emotional distress.

Ultimately, some of the most important messages to clients are those conveying that their emotions are important. Emotions are not right or wrong or a sign of strength or weakness. They are an important aspect of our humanity, but like any aspect of functioning, they should help us adapt to living life fully and successfully.

Behavioral interventions   The behavioral aspect of crisis reactions relates to what clients do or don't do and the actions that they take or don't take as they attempt to survive in the immediate and ongoing aftermath of a crisis situation. According to Cormier and Hackney (1993), the overall goal of behavioral intervention is to "develop adaptive and supportive behaviors," which involves weakening or eliminating counterproductive behaviors and acquiring and/or strengthening desirable behaviors. Adaptive behaviors help the individual meet his or her needs, whereas maladaptive behaviors are harmful to the person's health and well-being.

In this section, we focus on three primary behavioral interventions useful in crisis counseling: the promotion of *self-management strategies, social skills training,* and *anger control*. The problematic behaviors to be targeted for change are identified first as crisis client and crisis worker engage in the collaborative process of exploring a crisis and the individual's responses. The general "exploring" skills, including probing and seeking clarification and concreteness, are the first steps in defining problem behaviors and in identifying and understanding the consequences of behavior.

Challenging skills, whereby counselors help clients to own their behavioral difficulties, to acknowledge excuses, and to commit to action (e.g., stopping behaviors that are causing difficulty, engaging in behaviors that contribute to problem management and enhanced functioning) are also essential (Egan, 1994). Used effectively, a challenge is basically an invitation to "examine behavior that seems to be self-defeating, harmful to others or both—and to change that behavior" (Egan, 1994, p. 158). Used in the spirit of empathy, challenges move individuals from identification of problematic behavioral excesses or deficiencies to action and change. Whether it is the surviving spouse who isolates him- or herself rather than confronting life alone or the abuse survivor who engages in substance abuse or self-mutilation as a form of psychic numbing, the individual must first recognize his or her behavioral pattern, acknowledge its problematic consequences, and commit to acting differently.

Self-management and *self-monitoring* interventions are among the best behavioral strategies for both facilitating specific behavioral changes and enhancing collaboration and client empowerment. Self-management emphasizes the range of ways that crisis clients can learn to change themselves rather than the interventions of the professional helper. Self-monitoring entails several discreet steps including noticing, counting, and recording specific behaviors or behavioral patterns. Through self-monitoring and self-reward, crisis clients are able to identify when and how often they are engaging in particular behaviors, and to perceive and reinforce the changes in behaviors they make successfully. Specific types of rewards that may be useful include verbal-symbolic rewards (e.g., self-praise such as "I really did that well" or "Look at me now!"), imaginal rewards (e.g., visualizing scenes that are pleasurable), and material rewards (e.g., earning points toward a desired trip or purchase) (Cormier & Hackney, 1993).

For example, a formerly battered woman could be assisted to note and record in a log each time she accepts a compliment, shares her opinion, or spends time talking to a friend rather than rushing home—all of which are behaviors that are problematically associated with her previous abusive relationship. Further, she could contract that each week she recorded at least two examples of any of the three targeted behaviors she would earn the right to purchase something frivolous for herself—also a behavior she finds difficult. Or a man who has been abusing his prescription pain medication ever since suffering injuries in a workplace accident could be assisted to note and record each time he has the desire or impulse to take a pill, but doesn't. Further, each day he refrained from using the medication, he could reward himself by buying a used CD, listening to old music being one of his favorite "positive addictions." In some instances, simply developing awareness of specific behaviors is itself sufficient impetus to produce change.

Effective coping, either in the immediate aftermath of a crisis or in long-term resolution of a crisis, requires a variety of skills. Some clients possess few skills to summon to the task and others are temporarily overwhelmed by the enormity of the stressor. In both instances, counselors can assist crisis clients to develop specific skills. Numerous researchers have demonstrated the correlation between deficiencies in problem-solving skills and ineffective coping for a broad range of populations and a wide range of problems or needs (D'Zurilla & Goldfried, 1971; Mays & Croake, 1997; Nezu & Carnevale, 1987). Hepworth, Rooney, and Larsen (1997) recommended systematic efforts to teach clients problem-solving skills in order to further the following outcomes: (1) preventing interpersonal conflicts produced by dysfunctional modes of solving problems, (2) reducing tension and anxiety by solving stress-producing problems effectively, (3) generating a wider range of options for coping, and (4) increasing confidence and self-efficacy (p. 406). We will discuss problem-solving at length in the section on cognitive interventions.

Teaching crisis clients other necessary social skills may be equally useful. Identification of specific skill limitations begins with the collaborative process of problem exploration, including exploration of strengths. Crisis clients may have limited skills including (but not limited to) assertiveness, social/relational/conversational skills, parenting skills, or anger management skills. *Social skills training* is a generalized process for teaching clients a range of particular skills or subskills. It includes a focus on cognitive and emotional aspects as well as on the specific behaviors that are targeted for development. As illustrated later in the section on anger management, an individual's thoughts and emotions are intricately related to his or her behavioral responses and thus directly impact their ability to effectively develop and utilize specific skills.

Assisting a crisis client to develop a specific skill begins with mutual recognition of a deficit in that skill and the rationale for its development. It proceeds with the identification of specific components or subskills. Modeling or role-playing, wherein the crisis counselor demonstrates the particular skill, facilitates the client's learning through observation. The modeling shows the crisis client a different way to respond in a given situation. Client role-playing of the specific skill and/or subskills follows, so the crisis client can both practice and evaluate his or her effectiveness. The last component of social skills training always entails applying the skill in real-life situations, followed by debriefing to discuss and analyze the experience.

Anger-control interventions are particularly salient when working with individuals experiencing a crisis, as anger and/or rage at what has occurred is a common response. Anger control interventions are also essential when working with individuals who are, or who have potential to be, abusive, including perpetrators of relationship violence and abusive parents.

Anger is an emotion, but it is expressed verbally and behaviorally, sometimes as violent behavior. Cognitive-behavioral theories (Beck, 1976; Ellis, 1990) suggest that angry emotional responses emerge when cognitive appraisal of a situation interprets a threat, challenge, or injustice. This cognitive perception leads to the somatic and affective response that is labeled anger, and that anger is then expressed through a particular behavior. Interventions designed to reduce or control anger and anger-related behaviors thus fall into two main categories: those that target the behavior itself and those that target the cognitive precipitating factors of the anger response, or a combination of the two. Studies that have examined the relative efficacy of these two intervention modalities have generally concluded that cognitive or combined approaches are more efficacious than behavioral interventions alone (Stordeur & Stille, 1989; Whiteman, Fanshel, & Grundy, 1987). Cognitive reframing techniques that target the beliefs, perceptions, and expectations that lead to anger are examined in the next section.

Behavioral interventions focused on anger control generally emphasize identifying both anger cues and how an individual behaves when angry. For example, does he or she behave in a mean or nasty way? become sarcastic? constantly blame others? Does the individual withdraw and let resentments fester? drink alcohol and/or get high? Teaching clients self-monitoring skills is an effective way to help them identify these and other specific anger-related behaviors that contribute to the escalation of situations and to their own anger arousal. Self-monitoring is also used to identify body cues that signal anger arousal (e.g., tenseness in arms, legs, or neck, becoming flushed or beginning to sweat, breathing faster).

Once these behaviors and physical reactions are identified, individuals can learn to identify alternative behaviors that can contribute to reduced arousal and more constructive verbal and behavioral responses. For example, counselors can encourage clients to take a time-out, acknowledging directly to themselves and others that they sense an angry buildup that they wish to avoid. The individual might then do something physical like take a walk or run to discharge the built-up tension and to give him- or herself time to calm down. Specific relaxation techniques can also be used to reduce the tension (e.g., deep breathing, progressive muscle-tensing and relaxing, imagery).

Individuals with anger control problems can also be assisted to develop interpersonal communication skills that allow them to come back to stressful or upsetting situations after tension is reduced and engage in mutually respectful dialogue. Communication skills enhance individuals' ability to communicate their thoughts and feelings assertively and constructively rather than aggressively and with contempt and disregard for another individual.

Cognitive interventions   Cognitive interventions are those intended to alter the way individuals think about and perceive themselves, others, or life situations. All cognitive approaches emanate from rational-emotive and cognitive theories that hypothesize that how one thinks is the major determinant of both behavior and emotions (Beck, 1976; Ellis, 1971, 1990; Lazarus, 1981). A basic premise of cognitive theory is that people's problematic emotions and behaviors are rooted in mistaken beliefs and errors in perceptions and thinking. The goal of any cognitive intervention, therefore, is to reduce emotional distress and maladaptive behavior by identifying and changing the relevant faulty beliefs and patterns of thought. Because misconceptions become operational through inner dialogue and self-statements, these frequently become the primary target.

According to Ellis (1971, 1990), one of the earliest cognitive theorists, it is how someone thinks that determines his or her emotional responses. He posited an intervention approach that helps clients engage in a sequential process of (1) recognizing the events that cause their troubling emotional responses, (2) identifying the belief systems that relate to those events, (3) identifying the emotional consequences that result from the event and their thoughts about it, and (4) challenging or "disputing" the problematic beliefs in order to develop more "rational" beliefs and a resultant change in emotions.

Crisis counselors can employ this cognitive strategy by first assisting crisis clients to identify both their rational and irrational beliefs about what has occurred and to recognize the emotional consequences of those beliefs. For example, a woman whose husband was killed in an automobile accident may have concluded that she is too old to ever find love again and that she is doomed to an empty and lonely old age. She may have become increasingly despondent and isolated. Helping her recognize her irrational thought pattern and its impact on her emotions and behavior is the first step. The second step in this strategy, and the real work of producing change, occurs as the counselor helps her to challenge and ultimately discard her problematic thoughts and beliefs. Finally, counselors can help clients to begin to develop an alternative belief system using a variety of tech-niques, including *rational-emotive imagery,* a strategy of helping clients imagine feeling or behaving differently. In the example above, the counselor could help the widow to imagine living a life in which she felt more energized and optimistic. As she immersed herself in that fantasy, the counselor could help her attend to the specific thoughts and words that were going through her mind that enabled her to create and experience that more positive outcome. Finally, after identifying those alternative thoughts, the counselor might ask her to practice engaging in changed self-talk (e.g., "I'm an attractive and intelligent woman" or "I have an opportu-nity to really get to know myself and develop my interests").

A related cognitive intervention is *cognitive restructuring* (Foa & Rothbaum, 1998; Meichenbaum & Fitzpatrick, 1993). Similar in outcome to other cognitive approaches, it is a strategy for helping clients become aware of self-defeating thoughts and misconceptions or faulty beliefs that result in problematic outcomes. Drawing on the work of several cognitive therapy authors, Hepworth, Rooney, and Larsen (1997) suggested the following steps for implementing this cognitive approach:

1. Help clients recognize that their beliefs, inner dialogues, and self-talk deter-mine their emotional reactions to events in their life.
2. Help clients identify the specific types of beliefs and automatic self-talk that seem to underlie their current emotional reactions and behavioral responses.
3. Help clients identify the situations in which they are most vulnerable to engag-ing in self-defeating self-talk.
4. Help clients develop and substitute self-statements that facilitate positive cop-ing emotional and behavioral responses.
5. Help clients reward themselves for enhanced coping.

Hepworth, Rooney, and Larsen cautioned that this must be a collaborative process, as clients often resist both the cognitive explanation of how and why they are experiencing difficulty and the sense of being manipulated or coerced to accept someone else's beliefs. For example, consider a man who suffered injuries in a traumatic workplace accident. He suffers from chronic pain, impaired physi-cal functioning, and high levels of anxiety and depression. He may find it difficult to accept the contention that his thought processes are an area of concern, or that his focus on his pain is actually increasing his physical and emotional discomfort. Yet the skilled application of this cognitive technique may encourage him to con-sider this premise and, through self-monitoring, to acquire information about his thinking-feeling processes.

Cognitive restructuring, or *reframing,* is a commonly used approach for assist-ing individuals with difficulty with anger control. Anger-precipitated aggressive communication and behaviors are a result of appraising a situation in a manner that leads to increasing emotional arousal rather than to constructive communi-cation. These interpretations result in self-statements that provoke a fight re-sponse, for example, *"How dare she talk to me in that way?"* or *"Stupid jerk, I'll show you what happens when you make a fool out of me"* or *"You're not going to get away with this!"* These self-statements are often grounded in an even more fundamental belief system or cognitive structure, for example, the belief that *"I have to be in control"* or *"I can't let people walk all over me."* Meichenbaum (1994) suggested that beliefs about anger including lack of emotional responsibility for becoming angry, the tendency to disparage others combined with feelings of self-righteousness and entitlement, and the belief that anger is a way to control others, particularly when one feels disrespected, "light the fuse." The outcome is situation-based self-statements that precipitate an angry emotional response.

Cognitive reframing entails assisting the individual to identify the distorted underlying belief systems, the situations that trigger responses based on those beliefs, and the self-statements that occur as those beliefs lead to interpretations and appraisals of specific situations. Individuals are then helped to develop alternative belief systems and to substitute positive self-statements for their negative, anger-producing statements.

The last area of cognitive intervention centers on how to solve problems. Skills in *problem-solving* are basic and critically important to crisis intervention. Problem-solving entails effectively engaging crisis clients in a mutual cognitive process of defining problems, developing relevant goals, identifying and utilizing appropriate resources, and ultimately planning and carrying out specific action strategies. Most crisis intervention models have utilized some variant of a basic problem-solving approach. A general problem-solving process is evident when crisis workers are instructed to identify specific problems as the result of exploration and assessment (single-session, Step 3), examine alternatives and develop options (single-session, Step 4), and assist clients to mobilize personal and social resources (single-session, Step 5). Counselors can also model and teach problem-solving thought processes to crisis clients just as they model and teach other social skills.

Problem-solving begins with the accurate identification of the specific problem(s) to focus on as the target of change. As a result of exploration and assessment, the crisis worker both reflectively captures the client's concerns and shares his or her understanding of the problem. At times, the crisis counselor identifies a problem to work on that the client has not mentioned: *"I wonder if the constant barrage of negative messages you give yourself is also part of the problem."* Or the counselor may view a problem that the client has already mentioned in a slightly different way: *"When you said you were to blame because you didn't leave, I wondered why the person who made it so difficult for you to leave was somehow off the hook. I agree that it's important to make changes at this time, and to find a way around the things that have made it difficult in the past, but it's hard for me to accept that you are to blame."* This part of the problem-solving process often entails partializing, as the counselor helps the client mentally break down numerous interrelated problems into more manageable parts.

Ultimately, one or more specific, mutually agreed upon problems are identified for work. In single-session crisis intervention, it is important to select the one or two immediate problems whose resolution will make a difference in the current crisis reality. The goals of single-session crisis intervention are delimited to short-term immediate safety and restoration of coping. Thus the problems identified for problem-solving must be problems whose resolution will contribute meaningfully to that end (Cournoyer, 2000; Egan, 1994).

The following examples illustrate the skills of two crisis workers in stating a problem as they understand it and seeking feedback from the clients.

Crisis Worker 1: *From what I understand at this point, Dan, the first problem you need to resolve now is whether you want to return home or not, and if not, where you want to go instead, even if just for the next couple of days. Is that correct?*

Crisis Worker 2: *Linda, it sounds as though the first priority is determining whether you need to be in the hospital in order to be safe. You know that you're feeling pretty suicidal, yet another part of you is also asking for help and wants to find a way through this. We're not going to solve the underlying concerns causing you to feel so much pain right now. But we do need to decide if there is a way for you to be safe at home, or if it would be better for you to have a respite and be in a safe place. What do you think about just focusing on this one question right now?*

Once the problem has been specified, the next step in problem-solving is to identify possible solutions or alternatives. The crisis client and counselor may engage in a process of brainstorming to produce a wide range of possibilities. This requires both client and counselor to expand their thinking and to be as creative as possible in identifying alternatives, even though some may initially seem to be unworkable. Thus, in the example of Linda, the second crisis client described above, the list of possibilities might include the following ideas:

1. Identify a close relative or friend whom Linda believes she can trust to know what is going on and to, in essence, "keep watch."
2. Voluntarily sign into the psychiatric unit at the hospital.
3. Ask the worker to initiate a mental-health commitment to the hospital.
4. Ask Linda to contract not to harm herself and to contact the mental health crisis line if she begins to feel like harming herself again.
5. Call her estranged husband and ask him to come home temporarily.
6. Call her parents in Florida and see if she can come down for a vacation.
7. "Suck it up" and just go back to work and "carry on."

Once this range of possibilities has been identified, the next step of the problem-solving process is to evaluate the options. Part of evaluating includes identifying the personal and social resources that the client can mobilize in order to follow through with each alternative. It is important to remember that the evaluation of options cannot occur in a vacuum. It must be based on a realistic assessment of the needs of the individual in crisis and the resources available to assist him or her. Continuing with the example above, Linda and the counselor conclude relatively quickly that options 5, 6, and 7 are not feasible. Linda will not consider options 5 and 6, and together Linda and the counselor conclude that option 7 is what Linda has been trying to do all along with little success. After reassessing Linda's current risk for harm, they also agree that commitment to the hospital is not necessary at this time *if* there are other supports in place. Ultimately, Linda and the counselor agree on a combination of options 1 and 4. Linda agrees to call her best friend and to ask her to meet her at the crisis center. She also agrees to a contract regarding the steps she will take if she experiences further thoughts of harming herself.

The last step of the problem-solving process requires taking action to implement the selected option. At times, it may be necessary to help the crisis client prepare to implement the plan. Thus, for example, a crisis client who is a runaway and who has decided he wants to contact his parents might need help rehearsing what he wants to say to them and how he will respond to his parents' possible reactions before actually calling them. Eventually, however, the crisis client carries through with the selected option. Thus, in the earlier case, Linda contacts her friend, her friend comes into the crisis center and meets with Linda and the counselor, and the two of them contract for follow-up with the counselor.

Problem-solving is an intuitive, simple process, and as Egan (1994) noted, it is widely considered to be important. Yet surprisingly few counselors are actually taught to utilize the problem-solving process and routinely utilize it in its entirety. Crisis counselors, in particular, must make problem-solving second nature, for it is the single most pragmatic approach for creating order in an otherwise overwhelming situation. It is a cognitive process that utilizes the strengths and resources of the client and a process that clients can learn and utilize in future situations.

Developmental interventions   Developmental interventions do not entail a specific type of skill, but rather reflect awareness of developmental considerations when utilizing all skills and techniques. Further, all counseling interactions are a product of the developmental capacities of both counselor and client. Skilled crisis counselors are always engaged in developmental intervention because, ideally, all interactions with crisis clients are developmentally appropriate.

We will not revisit the entire argument supporting the necessity of crisis counselors' awareness of developmental considerations. We simply reiterate that whether the focus at any given time is primarily on emotions, behavior, cognition, or environmental context including social supports, the collaboration between crisis counselor and crisis client is always influenced by developmental considerations. Additionally, the counseling relationship is always influenced by these same developmental realities. "Languaging"—the process by which individuals together create a shared understanding and experience, by necessity, reflects the development of the individuals involved (Walter & Peller, 1996). When crisis counselors fully embrace this awareness, they also recognize that all interventions are developmental interventions.

Environmental interventions   Environmental interventions are actions taken by crisis counselors to link crisis clients with necessary resources, to advance or advocate for clients' needs and interests, and to promote social justice through activism. These interventions range from client-level strategies, such as working with clients to access particular social services, to macro-level interventions that strive to bring about specific changes in social conditions. Environmental interventions grow out of awareness that clients are not always adequately served by the agencies and private and governmental programs established to serve them, and that many of the events that individuals experience as crises are embedded in a problematic social environment. For example, many of the barriers battered women face to leaving abusive homes relate to deficits in available environmental supports and resources. Further, feminists argue that it is the underlying social milieu that justifies patriarchal control that, in turn, underlies abuse. Therefore, it is societal attitudes and institutional practices that must change for battering as a social problem to be effectively addressed. In this section, we present two professional roles and accompanying strategies directed at environmental change: advocacy and social action.

Advocacy refers to the actions a crisis worker takes on behalf of an individual client *(case advocacy)* or a class of individuals, such as all breast cancer survivors in a given community *(class advocacy)*. It is a form of representing clients' needs or wishes for the purpose of producing desired change in environmental responsiveness. All competent crisis intervention, however, entails establishing an empowering and collaborative relationship with crisis clients. Advocacy must therefore contribute to the goal of client empowerment rather than the crisis counselor's need to rescue. Assisting individual clients to advocate on their own behalf and/or facilitating the development of client advocacy groups are two ways to avoid the trap of becoming a rescuer. For example, a crisis worker might assist a woman who is being treated differently by her supervisor after revealing her health status to directly challenge her supervisor and, if necessary, to speak to the director of her agency. Or a crisis worker might help organize a group of domestic violence or sexual assault survivors to engage in court monitoring.

Situations in which crisis workers, or clients and crisis workers together, might advocate include when an agency or staff person has refused or failed to provide services or benefits to which a client is entitled or when services have been delivered in a manner that dehumanizes or discriminates. Situations in which class advocacy might be indicated include when numerous people have common needs for resources that are not currently available, or when groups of people are being denied access because of discrimination or adverse procedures and/or practices. Class advocacy can occur at the local level or at the state and federal policy level.

Advocacy intervention consists of a number of specific strategies including initiating conferences with agencies or agency personnel to identify and overcome specific barriers or concerns, and appealing lower-level decisions to supervisors, administrators, review boards, or even local government overseers. In some situations, it may even mean initiating in and/or participating in legal action or providing expert testimony for a client or on behalf of a class of clients. All advocacy begins with a specific problem and demand for change.

In order to function effectively as an advocate, a crisis counselor must become comfortable with conflict and be assertive enough to raise complaints and articulate desired remedies. A counselor should assume that a target system, once presented with a documented problem, will want to collaborate to correct it. It is only if and when the assumption of collaboration proves incorrect that an advocate needs to move into a bargaining, or in some instances, conflict stance. In such cases, the operational assumption is that the target system is actively resisting making needed adjustments and/or changes (Compton & Galaway, 1994).

Because all institutional systems develop their own priorities and goals, it is essential that crisis workers always see themselves as advocating for the client's best interest, whether or not that coincides with another professional's or agency's priorities. For example, school policies that automatically expel or deny readmission to any student who has been found to have a weapon may not be in the best interest of a given student. Although the overarching goal of a no-tolerance policy is certainly one that most people can agree to, a crisis counselor might advocate that a particular student in a particular situation be given a second chance. Similarly, although prosecutors may believe that when rape victims are seen in emergency rooms the primary focus should be the collection of forensic evidence, the rape crisis advocate must insist that the primary focus should be meeting the physical and emotional needs of the individual survivor.

Social activism extends the role of the advocate to specific actions taken to raise awareness of social problems or injustices for the purpose of creating changes in attitudes as well as changes in laws and social policies. Social activists use strategies ranging from educational efforts to efforts to mobilize community members and groups to work toward common social change goals. A counselor working in a rape crisis agency might mobilize a youth drama group to teach other students about the dangers of coercive sexual behavior. Or he or she might bring together representatives from different community agencies (e.g., hospitals, police, prosecutors) involved with rape victims for the purpose of developing a more coordinated and responsive system of care. In each case, the activist role is one in which the crisis counselor goes beyond advocating for a given client's individual needs and instead works with interested others in order to reform or change social institutions that impact the well-being of an entire class of individuals (e.g., all rape survivors, all surviving parents of children killed by drunk drivers).

In order to serve as an effective advocate and activist, crisis workers must be knowledgeable about the laws, policies, programs, and standard practices of relevant social agencies and other community resources. This includes governmental and private organizations as well as various volunteer groups. The crisis worker also must be familiar with the unique needs and issues surrounding the populations they serve. The ultimate goal is always to produce a better "fit" between the needs of crisis clients and the availability and accessibility of relevant community resources and services.

DISCUSSION QUESTIONS

1. How important is the expression of emotions during a crisis? Is it possible for someone to successfully adapt to a crisis without expressing emotions? Is this a cultural issue? Does it matter?

2. Think of examples of how an individual's sex (male/female), gender (socially constructed notions of masculinity/femininity), religion, and/or ethnicity (e.g., Native American, Haitian, African American) might affect his or her responses in the following situations:

   • A child removed from the home because of serious alleged abuse
   • A man who wakes up in a psychiatric facility after a failed suicide attempt
   • A young woman who has been sexually assaulted
   • A gay couple whose home is destroyed in a hurricane

EXERCISES

1. In order to respond competently to someone in crisis, crisis counselors must know how their own experiences, dispositions, vulnerabilities, biases, and so on might affect their responses. Divide the class into small groups and ask each group to discuss what types of crises or individuals in crisis group members believe they would have the most difficulty working with and why. Students can also discuss what they can do to prepare to work effectively in such situations.

2. Divide the class into small groups. Give each group one or more of the following scenarios. Instruct group members to brainstorm the specific actions they would take to intervene. The class as a whole can then compare responses and compare their suggested actions to the steps of the single-session model.
   • You are traveling on a charter bus trip. While en route, the bus is involved in a seven-vehicle accident on a large interstate highway. Although you are uninjured except for minor bruises and cuts, many people on your bus and in surrounding vehicles have been seriously injured. The situation is chaotic and many people are dazed and/or obviously shaken.
   • You are part of a Red Cross disaster team that is called to a local industrial park in your community where there has been a chemical explosion and fire. There are numerous reported fatalities and injuries.

REFERENCES

Barker, R. (1978). *Habitats, environments, and human behavior.* San Francisco: Jossey-Bass.

Bass, E., & Davis, L. (1988). *The courage to heal: A guide for women survivors of child sexual abuse.* New York: Harper & Row.

Beck, A. T. (1976). *Cognitive therapy and the emotional disorders.* New York: International Universities Press.

Berlin, S. B., & Marsh, J. C. (1993). *Informing practice decisions.* New York: Macmillan.

Bertolino, B., & O'Hanlon, W. H. (2001). *Collaborative, competency-based counseling and therapy.* Boston: Allyn & Bacon.

Blocher, D. H. (1987). *The professional counselor.* New York: Macmillan.

Blocher, D. H. (2000). *Counseling: A developmental approach* (4th ed.). New York: John Wiley & Sons.

Carkhuff, R. R. (1969). *Helping and human relations.* New York: Holt, Rinehart, & Winston.

Compton, B. R., & Galaway, B. (1994). *Social work processes* (5th ed.). Pacific Grove, CA: Brooks/Cole.

Cormier, L. S., & Hackney, H. (1993). *The professional counselor: A process guide to helping.* Boston: Allyn & Bacon.

Cournoyer, B. (2000). *The social work skills workbook* (3rd ed.). Belmont, CA: Wadsworth.

Cowger, C. E. (1992). Assessment of client strengths. In D. Saleebey (Ed.), *The strengths perspective in social work practice* (pp. 139–147). White Plains, NY: Longman.

Cowger, C. E. (1994). Assessing client strengths: Clinical assessment for client empowerment. *Social Work, 39*(3), 262–269.

Cross, T. L., Bazron, B. J., Dennis, K. W., & Isaacs, M. R. (1989). *Towards a culturally competent system of care.* Washington, DC: CASSP Technical Assistance Center.

Devore, W., & Schlesinger, E. G. (1981). *Ethnic-sensitive social work practice.* St. Louis: C. V. Mosby.

DuBois, B., & Krogsrud Miley, K. (2002). *Social work: An empowering profession* (4th ed.). Boston: Allyn & Bacon.

Duncan, B. L., & Miller, S. D. (2000). *The heroic client: Doing client-centered, outcome-informed therapy.* San Francisco: Jossey-Bass.

D'Zurilla, T., & Goldfried, M. (1971). Problem solving and behavior modification. *Journal of Abnormal Psychology, 78,* 107–126.

Egan, G. (1994). *The skilled helper: A problem-management approach to helping* (5th ed.). Pacific Grove, CA: Brooks/Cole.

Ellis, A. E. (1971). *Rational-emotive therapy and its application to emotional education.* New York: Institute for Rational Living.

Ellis, A. E. (1990). *Rational-emotive therapy and cognitive behavior therapy.* New York: Springer.

Foa, E. B., & Rothbaum, B. O. (1998). *Treating the trauma of rape: Cognitive behavioral therapy for PTSD.* New York: Guilford Press.

Fukuyama, M. A. (1990). Taking a universal approach to multicultural counseling. *Counselor Education and Supervision, 30,* 6–17.

Germain, C., & Gitterman, A. (1996). *The life model of social work practice: Advances in theory and practice* (2nd ed.). New York: Columbia University Press.

Giordano, J., & Giordano, M. A. (1995). Ethnic dimensions in family treatment. In R. Mikesell, D. Lusterman, & S. McDaniel (Eds.), *Integrating family therapy: Handbook of family psychology and systems theory* (pp. 347–356). Washington, DC: American Psychological Association.

Gutierrez, L. M., & Lewis, E. (Eds.). (1999). *Empowering women of color.* New York: Columbia University Press.

Hammond, D., Hepworth, D., & Smith, V. (1977). *Improving therapeutic communication.* San Francisco: Jossey-Bass.

Helms, J. E., & Richardson, T. Q. (1997). How "multiculturalism" obscures race and culture as differential aspects of counseling competency. In D. B. Pope-Davis & H. L. K. Coleman (Eds.), *Multicultural counseling competencies: Assessment, education and training, and supervision* (pp. 60–79). Thousand Oaks, CA: Sage.

Hepworth, E. H., Rooney, R. H., & Larsen, J. A. (1997). *Direct social work practice: Theory and skills* (5th ed.). Pacific Grove, CA: Brooks/Cole.

Herman, J. (1997). *Trauma and recovery.* New York: Basic Books.

Ho, M. K. (1989). Social work practice with Asian Americans. In A. Morales & B. Sheafor (Eds.), *Social work: A profession of many faces* (5th ed., pp. 521–541). Boston: Allyn & Bacon.

Ho, D. Y. F. (1995). Internalized culture, culturocentrism and transcendence. *Counseling Psychologist, 23,* 4–24.

Hoare, C. H. (1991). Psychosocial identity development and cultural others. *Journal of Counseling and Development, 70,* 45–53.

Ibrahim, F. A. (1985). Effective cross-cultural counseling and psychotherapy: A framework. *The Counseling Psychologist, 13,* 625–638.

Ivey, A. E., Ivey, M. B., & Simek-Downing, L. (1987). *Counseling and psychotherapy: Integrating skills, theory and practice* (2nd ed.). Englewood Cliffs, NJ: Prentice-Hall.

Katz, M. (1997). *On playing a poor hand well: Insights from the lives of those who have overcome childhood risks and adversities.* New York: W. W. Norton.

Kilpatrick, D. G., & Best, C. L. (1984). Some cautionary remarks in treating sexual abuse victims with implosion. *Behavior Therapy, 15,* 421–423.

Lazarus, A. A. (1981). *The practice of multimodal therapy: Systematic, comprehensive, and effective psychotherapy.* New York: McGraw-Hill.

Lum, D. (1996). *Social work practice and people of color: A process-stage approach* (3rd ed.). Pacific Grove, CA: Brooks/Cole.

Lum, D. (1999). *Culturally competent practice: A framework for growth and action.* Pacific Grove, CA.: Brooks/Cole.

Mays, M., & Croake, J. W. (1997). *Treatment of depression in managed care.* New York: Brunner/Mazel.

Meichenbaum, D. (1994). *A clinical handbook/practical therapist manual for assessing and treating adults with post-traumatic stress disorder.* Waterloo, Ontario, Canada: Institute Press.

Meichenbaum, D., & Fitzpatrick, D. (1993). A constructionist narrative perspective on stress and coping: Stress inoculation applications. In L. Goldberger & S. Breznitz (Eds.), *Handbook of stress: Theoretical and clinical aspects* (2nd ed., pp. 706–723). New York: Free Press.

Miller, J. B. (1982). *Women and power: Some psychological dimensions, Work in Progress No. 1.* Wellesley, MA: Stone Center Working Papers Series.

Minuchin, S. (1974). *Families and family therapy.* Cambridge, MA: Harvard University Press.

Nezu, A. M., & Carnevale, G. J. (1987). Interpersonal problem solving and coping reactions of Vietnam veterans with post-traumatic stress disorder. *Journal of Abnormal Psychology, 96,* 155–157.

Okun, B. F. (1992). *Effective helping: Interviewing and counseling techniques* (4th ed.). Pacific Grove, CA: Brooks/Cole.

Puryear, D. A. (1979). *Helping people in crisis.* San Francisco: Jossey-Bass.

Pedersen, P. B. (1991). Multiculturalism as a generic approach to counseling. *Journal of Counseling and Development, 70,* 6–12.

Research and Training Center to Improve Services to Seriously Emotionally Handicapped Children and Their Families. (1988). Services to minority populations: What does it mean to be a culturally competent professional? *Focal Point, 2,* 3–5.

Reynolds, A. L., & Pope, R. L. (1991). The complexities of diversity: Exploring multiple oppressions. *Journal of Counseling & Development, 70,* 174–180.

Rogers, C. R. (1957). The necessary and sufficient conditions of therapeutic personality change. *Journal of Consulting Psychology, 21,* 95–103.

Rogers, C. R. (1980). *A way of being*. Boston: Houghton Mifflin.

Rutter, M. (1987). Psychosocial resilience and protective mechanisms. *American Journal of Orthopsychiatry, 57,* 316–331.

Saleebey, D. (1992). *The strengths perspective in social work practice*. White Plains, NY: Longman.

Saleebey, D. (1996). The strengths perspective in social work practice: Extension and cautions. *Social Work, 41,* 296–305.

Schechter, S. (1987). *Guidelines for mental health professionals*. Washington, DC: National Coalition Against Domestic Violence.

Solomon, B. (1989). Social work with Afro-Americans. In A. Morales & B. Sheafor (Eds.), *Social work: A profession of many faces* (5th ed., pp. 567–586). Boston: Allyn & Bacon.

Solomon, S. D., Gerrity, E. T., & Muff, A. M. (1992). Efficacy of treatments for post-traumatic stress disorder: An empirical review. *Journal of the American Medical Association, 268,* 633–638.

Speight, S. L., Myers, L. J., Cox, C. I., & Highlen, P. S. (1991). A redefinition of multicultural counseling. *Journal of Counseling and Development, 70,* 29–36.

Stordeur, R. A., & Stille, R. (1989). *Ending men's violence against their partners: One road to peace*. Newbury Park, CA: Sage.

Stuhlmiller, C., & Dunning, C. (2000). Challenging the mainstream: From pathogenic to salutogenic models of posttrauma intervention. In J. M. Violanti, D. Paton, & D. Dunning (Eds.), *Posttraumatic stress intervention: Challenges, issues, and perspectives*. Springfield, IL: Charles C. Thomas Publisher.

Sue, S. (1998). In search of cultural competence in psychotherapy and counseling. *American Psychologist, 53,* 440–448.

Sue, D. W., Arredondo, P., & McDavis, R. J. (1995). Multicultural counseling competencies and standards: A call to the profession. In J. G. Ponterotto, J. M. Casas, L. A. Suzuki, & C. M. Alexander (Eds.), *Handbook of multicultural counseling* (pp. 624–640). Thousand Oaks, CA: Sage.

Sue, D. W., Ivey, A. E., & Pedersen, P. B. (Eds.). (1996). *A theory of multicultural counseling and therapy*. Pacific Grove, CA: Brooks/Cole.

Sue, D. W., & Sue, S. (2002). *Counseling the culturally diverse: Theory and practice* (4th ed.). New York: John Wiley & Sons.

Surrey, J. L. (1987). *Work in progress: Relationship and empowerment, Work in progress series #30*. Wellesley, MA: Stone Center for Developmental Services and Studies.

Walter, J. L., & Peller, J. E. (1996). Rethinking our assumptions: Assuming anew in a postmodern world. In S. D. Miller, M. A. Hubble, & B. L. Duncan (Eds.), *Handbook of solution-focused brief therapy*. San Francisco: Jossey-Bass.

Whiteman, M., Fanshel, D., & Grundy, J. (1987). Cognitive-behavioral interventions aimed at anger of parents at risk of child abuse. *Social Work, 32*(6), 469–474.

CHAPTER 5

The Continuum
of Crisis Response:
Diagnosis and Lethality

Mary Jane is admitted to an inpatient psychiatric unit when she becomes suicidally depressed over her son's death in an automobile accident caused by a drunk driver.

• • •

John is a Gulf War veteran with a long-standing diagnosis of Posttraumatic Stress Disorder (PTSD) and a history of psychiatric hospitalization who barricades himself in a Muslim mosque with hostages after his brother is killed in the World Trade Center attack.

• • •

Vanessa has been treated for her borderline personality disorder diagnosis for many years at a community mental health clinic. Her most recent admission to an inpatient psychiatric unit occurred after she and her fiancé attempted suicide together by drug overdose. She awoke two days later to find him dead at her side.

• • •

Sally obtained a protection-from-abuse order that requires her husband, Larry, to stay at least two hundred yards away from her with no form of communication for the next six months. She is currently residing in a shelter for abused women after being released from the emergency room with multiple bruises. She informed the crisis counselor that Larry told her he would shoot her if she ever left him. He told her that he would kill her and anybody who tried to stop him and then turn the gun on himself.

Individual responses to crisis events can be conceptualized as occurring on a continuum ranging from short-term disequilibrium and disorganization in functioning to the experience of acute ongoing debilitating symptoms. Similarly, behavioral responses to high levels of arousal, anxiety, and other mood changes in the aftermath of a crisis event can range from immobility to extreme self-injurious or aggressive behavior.

This chapter examines the more severe end of the continuum of emotional response or reactions that individuals may experience in the aftermath of crisis. This includes an examination of those diagnoses that are most relevant in working with crisis survivors. The chapter also explores the potentially lethal end of the continuum of crisis responses. We specifically examine assessment and intervention with suicidal behavior and violence toward others.

Individual responses to crisis events and stressors are unique. For example, three children who grow up in the same family in which physical and sexual abuse occur on a regular basis may respond emotionally in dramatically different ways. One child may become depressed and withdraw from friends and family, whereas another child may engage in relationship violence, drug abuse, and oppositional behavior. Yet another child may experience no residual effects and live a life relatively free of early pathological influences. The uniqueness of individual responses to different types of stressors, crisis events, and traumatic events is determined by many factors, both internal and external.

Clinical disorders and lethal behavior are not assumed to co-occur, although they may. The shared significance is that they both represent the more severe end of a continuum of possible responses to crisis, necessitating more intensive and potentially more restrictive intervention. Crisis workers must accurately assess this range of potential responses and intervene appropriately when individuals are at heightened psychological or behavioral risk. In situations involving multiple crisis survivors (e.g., disasters), crisis workers must triage, immediately identifying individuals whose functioning is most compromised and target interventions accordingly.

A popularized characterization of people's emotional responses to stressors centers on the notions of "mad," "bad," "sad," and "glad." In other words, we expect children and adults to exhibit all of these emotional responses at numerous points throughout the life span. We expect children to be bad at times, for example, during the "terrible two's." Correspondingly, we expect older adults to be sad at the loss of a spouse or close friends. We expect that individuals will, in the normal course of events, exhibit each of the responses identified. Normal, in these instances, simply describes the statistical probability that the responses will occur.

There are also clear societal expectations, however, that the emotions and associated behaviors can be exhibited only so often, only so severely, and only for a limited amount of time before societal consequences emerge. At some point, a line is crossed and a determination is made that an individual is too bad, too sad, too mad, or too glad. If an individual experiences "too much" of any of these responses and they begin to interfere with daily functioning, there are diagnoses, medications, and therapeutic interventions specifically targeted to ameliorate the condition. Although this characterization may seem simplistic, the analogy is clear: There are normal affective, behavioral, and cognitive expectations of individuals in society, and there are behaviors that are considered problematic.

DIAGNOSIS

Diagnosis is a medically driven process in that specific symptoms taken together define a particular syndrome or disorder. Diagnosis has been a controversial issue in some crisis settings because of its potentially negative consequences. One such negative outcome is that the diagnosis can take on a life of its own and people may respond to the client with the diagnosis as if he or she were a disorder rather than a person with a problem who deserves dignity, respect, and compassion. Diagnosis is *not* meant to define the whole person. Furthermore, diagnoses are *not* meant to be static or unchanging.

A diagnosis is also not a final product in itself. Rather, diagnosis should lead to the prescription of strategic interventions designed to mitigate the identified condition. Failure to accurately assess the severity of a client's crisis response can have dire consequences for the client and the client's support system. The crisis intervention professional should be able to assess the client's response and determine the appropriate level and intensity of intervention.

Professional interventions occur across what has been conceptualized as a continuum of restrictiveness, or intensity, of intervention. The intensity of crisis response and concomitant level of interference in a person's life are determined by the frequency, intensity, and duration of that person's symptomatology and the resultant negative impact on functioning.

Crisis intervention thus occurs across a continuum of possible responses. Severity of emotional, behavioral, and/or cognitive impairment experienced by the individual in crisis determines the "restrictiveness," the intensity of the intervention, and the degree to which crisis counselors and other professionals become therapeutically involved in the person's life. Interventions can range from providing information on a certain topic (least restrictive) to prescription of psychotropic medication (more restrictive) to involuntary hospitalization (most restrictive).

Clearly, not all crisis responses lead to a diagnosed mental disorder. In those situations in which the diagnostic threshold is surpassed (e.g., the psychologically debilitating symptoms are sufficiently severe, frequent, and long-lasting), however, we rely on classification systems that can provide a framework for understanding the range of client responses. The *Diagnostic and Statistical Manual of Mental Disorders IV-TR* (2000), published by the American Psychiatric Association, and the *International Statistical Classification of Diseases and Related Health Problems* (ICD-9-CM2000, 2001), published by the American Medical Association in conjunction with the World Health Organization, are compatible coding systems that have been developed jointly both nationally and internationally. These systems serve as the diagnostic classification models accepted throughout the United States and most of the world. For the purposes of this chapter, we employ *DSM-IV-TR* (APA, 2000) as the diagnostic reference.

The primary disorders addressed in this chapter include Adjustment Disorders, Mood Disorders, Anxiety Disorders, and Psychotic Disorders. We have selected these disorder categories because they comprise the diagnoses most applicable to crisis survivors experiencing severe responses. This is not to say that individuals with preexisting mental disorders are immune from the experience of crisis. In fact, individuals with histories of psychiatric disturbance frequently experience multiple problems (e.g., relational, economic, vocational, physical health). Crises may be an ongoing part of life for some individuals with mental disorders, and they may serve to exacerbate the disorder and/or the severity of the problems already encountered. Similarly, an individual's preexisting emotional problems can affect responses to crisis events and thus increase or decrease the severity of reaction.

In the following discussion of specific diagnoses, we use the heuristic of a continuum to examine the progression of symptoms from those that do not merit diagnosis to those that are sufficiently severe, frequent, and long lasting to warrant diagnosis and to signal the need for more intensive crisis intervention.

ADJUSTMENT DISORDERS

According to the *DSM-IV-TR* (APA, 2000), an adjustment disorder exists when an individual experiences "marked distress" and/or "significant impairment in social or occupational functioning" in response to an "identifiable stressor" (pp. 679–683). This diagnosis makes clear that an identified stressor, whether it is divorce, unemployment, retirement, or diagnosis of chronic illness, precipitates the development of emotional (depressed mood, anxiety) or behavioral (disturbance of conduct) symptoms that then interfere with normal functioning. It is important to note that this diagnosis is appropriate only when the problematic symptoms begin within three months of the precipitating stressor (crisis).

The psychological reaction to an identifiable stressor(s) of any severity that results in the presentation of clinically significant emotional and/or behavioral symptoms is the essential feature of an Adjustment Disorder (APA, 2000, pp. 679–683). Criteria for diagnosis include:

1. Development of the emotional and/or behavioral symptoms within three months after stressor onset
2. Clinical significance, as demonstrated by one of the following:
   a. Excessive distress (more than expected for stressor exposure)
   b. Significantly impaired social or occupational (academic) functioning
3. Abatement of symptoms within six months after the stressor and/or its consequences have stopped

The catalyst that precipitates the Adjustment Disorder could be a relationship separation or divorce, being fired from one's job, or one of a number of developmental stressors such as going away to school, leaving home, failing to attain occupational goals, or retiring. As this list indicates, diagnosis may be appropriate when working with individuals experiencing either a *developmental crisis* or a *situational crisis* (the stressor) that precipitates the problematic responses. These stressors can be external events or life transitions. Adjustment Disorders are assumed to be relatively time-limited (six-month) conditions in that once the stressor and/or its consequences have ended, the diagnosis is no longer appropriate. When the stressor is ongoing (e.g., AIDS, refugee camp status), however, Adjustment Disorders may last longer. Symptoms of depression, anxiety, or disturbed conduct that persist beyond the six-month threshold automatically suggest consideration of alternative diagnoses.

The following diagram suggests a pathway for understanding the continuum of adjustment responses to a stressor:

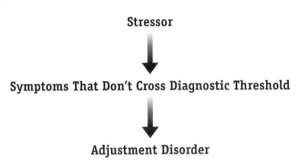

Stressor

Symptoms That Don't Cross Diagnostic Threshold

Adjustment Disorder

Adjustment Disorder subtypes include the following:

309.0 Adjustment Disorder with Depressed Mood   Prominent symptoms include depressed mood, tearfulness, or feelings of hopelessness.

309.24 Adjustment Disorder with Anxiety   Prominent symptoms include nervousness, worry, or jitteriness.

309.28 Adjustment Disorder with Mixed Anxiety and Depressed Mood   Predominant symptoms of depression and anxiety.

309.3 Adjustment Disorder with Disturbance of Conduct   Predominant presentation of disturbance in conduct in which there is violation of the rights of others or of major age-appropriate societal norms and rules.

309.4 Adjustment Disorder with Mixed Disturbance of Emotions and Conduct   Predominant presentation in which there are symptoms (depression or anxiety) and disturbance of conduct.

309.9 Adjustment Disorder, Unspecified   Reserved for maladaptive reactions that don't fit into the adjustment disorder categories above.

ANXIETY RESPONSES

Anxiety and depression are the most commonly experienced psychiatric symptoms and are endemic to crisis reactions. Clinical lore suggests that wherever you find anxiety, you find depression; and wherever you find depression, you find anxiety. Anxiety symptoms can include fear, apprehension, worry, panic, restlessness, tiredness, shakiness, muscle tension, heart palpitations, shortness of breath, dry mouth, difficulty swallowing, nausea, gastrointestinal distress, poor concentration, hypervigilance, insomnia, avoidance, and irritability. Most crisis reactions include some level of anxiety response. For purposes of diagnosis, clinical significance marks the point at which criteria observed sufficiently warrant full diagnosis. The following diagram suggests a pathway for understanding the continuum of anxiety responses to a traumatic event:

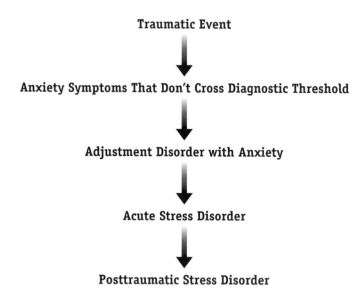

Traumatic Event

Anxiety Symptoms That Don't Cross Diagnostic Threshold

Adjustment Disorder with Anxiety

Acute Stress Disorder

Posttraumatic Stress Disorder

This pathway details the potential progression of anxiety response to a crisis or traumatic event. Initial levels of response can range from no debilitating reaction to experiencing fear, anxiety, or avoidance symptoms that don't reach diagnostic levels to experiencing a constellation of anxiety symptoms that are clearly debilitating. Some individuals who experience a level of anxiety in response to a traumatic event that does not meet Acute Stress Disorder or PTSD diagnostic criteria may fulfill the criteria for Adjustment Disorder with Anxiety.

Acute Stress Disorder and PTSD

The stress/anxiety disorders are a second general type of disorder that may be found specifically among survivors of violent crisis. As we have repeatedly emphasized, "some symptomatology following exposure to an extreme stress is ubiquitous" and thus does not require any diagnosis (APA, 2000, p. 47). If the particular constellation of symptoms persists, however, and also causes clinically significant distress or impairment in functioning, a diagnosis of Acute Stress Disorder or Posttraumatic Stress Disorder (PTSD) may be warranted.

Both Acute Stress Disorder and PTSD are diagnostically tied to exposure to a traumatic event that involved "threatened death, injury, or threat to physical integrity" (APA, 2000, p. 471). These diagnoses are therefore only applicable to individuals who have experienced such a violent or threatening crisis.

The shared criteria (APA, 2000) for both of these disorders include:

1. Exposure to an extreme traumatic stressor
2. Experience of at least three of the classic dissociative symptoms:
   a. A subjective sense of numbness, detachment, or absence of emotional responsiveness
   b. A reduction in awareness of one's surroundings
   c. Derealization (e.g., feeling that people aren't real)
   d. Depersonalization (e.g., feeling that one is watching oneself in a movie)
   e. Dissociative amnesia (e.g., difficulty recalling an important part of the trauma)
3. Experience of the traumatic event recurring through at least one of the following:
   a. Recurrent images, thoughts, dreams, illusions, flashback episodes
   b. A sense of reliving the experience
   c. Distress on exposure to reminder of the traumatic event
4. Distinct avoidance of stimuli that evoke trauma recollection (e.g., people who were involved in the event, place where the event occurred)
5. Distinct symptoms of anxiety or increased arousal (e.g., sleep difficulties, irritable mood, concentration difficulties, hypervigilance, marked startle response, motor restlessness)
6. Clinically significant distress or impairment in social, occupational, or other important functioning areas, or impairment in the person's ability to initiate or complete tasks that are necessary to secure assistance

Maxine is a 45-year-old-mother of five children who lives with her husband Dick in a rural area. Two weeks ago, the family dog began barking in the middle of the night and Maxine realized that their house was on fire. By the time Maxine and Dick got all the kids out of the smoke-filled, flame-engulfed house, they had no time to retrieve possessions and lost everything. Dick sustained second- and third-degree burns to his arms and feet in rescuing the children. The house burned to the ground before the volunteer fire department arrived. Since the fire, Maxine has become progressively more anxious and physically restless. She reports feeling as though she is watching herself in a movie and that nothing seems to feel or look the way it did before the fire. Every time she thinks about the fire she gets upset but is unable to remember the details of rescuing the children from the flames. She is sleeping, on average, two to three hours per night and wakes up repeatedly to check the children during the night. (Acute Stress Disorder)

The major difference between Acute Stress Disorder and PTSD is how long the person has experienced the anxiety response to the crisis event. Acute Stress Disorder occurs in the immediate aftermath of a crisis (within four weeks of the traumatic event), whereas PTSD cannot be diagnosed unless the problematic symptoms have persisted for more than one month. Thus if the identified constellation of symptoms occurs within one month of the stressor, a diagnosis of Acute Stress Disorder may be appropriate; however, if the symptoms persist for longer than one month or if the onset of symptoms occurs beyond the four-week time frame, a diagnosis of PTSD may be warranted.

Both Acute Stress Disorder and PTSD are complex syndromes that encompass thoughts, feelings, interactions with others, changes in self-identify and self-concept, and impaired social and occupational functioning. Whether the precipitant event is combat, sexual assault, a car accident, invasive surgery and/or loss of body parts, or experiencing an event like the World Trade Center/Pentagon disasters, trauma that exposes an individual to intense threat and horror can have a lasting and extremely troubling impact. By definition, Acute Stress Disorder and PTSD are considered only with survivors of *situational crises* as described above, as the DSM criteria require an external traumatic event in order for these diagnoses to be applicable.

DEPRESSIVE MOOD RESPONSES

Secondary to anxiety, sadness and depressed mood are common emotional reactions to crisis events. Sadness in response to a loved one's death, the diagnosis of a debilitating physical disease, or a tragedy that takes the lives of many people is to be expected. Crisis workers become concerned when sadness or depressed mood reach levels that interfere significantly with a client's life. Common symptoms of depressed mood include sustained sadness, diminished interest or pleasure in daily activities, significant weight loss or gain, insomnia or hypersomnia, psychomotor agitation or retardation, fatigue, feelings of worthlessness, inappropriate guilt, impaired cognition, and recurrent thoughts of death, suicidal ideation, and/or suicide attempts. The following diagram suggests a pathway for understanding mood responses to a crisis event that includes the full range of depressive mood responses:

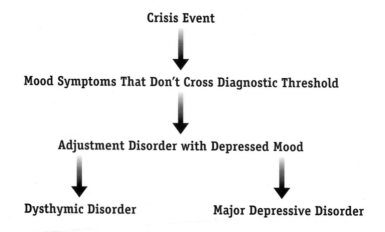

Crisis Event

↓

Mood Symptoms That Don't Cross Diagnostic Threshold

↓

Adjustment Disorder with Depressed Mood

↓   ↓

Dysthymic Disorder   **Major Depressive Disorder**

Major Depressive Disorder and Dysthymia

Of particular concern to the crisis counselor is Major Depressive Disorder (MDD) because of its close relationship to high mortality. More than 15 percent of individuals diagnosed with severe MDD eventually die by suicide, and individuals over 55 diagnosed with MDD are four times more likely to commit suicide than individuals in the general population (APA, 2000). MDD is also found among clients who experience severe pain in addition to decreased ambulatory and social functioning. Depression and medical illness are comorbid, with 20–25 percent of clients diagnosed with certain medical conditions (e.g., cancer, stroke, diabetes, myocardial infarction) having a comorbid diagnosis of MDD (APA, 2000).

DSM-IV-TR criteria for a major depressive episode include:

1. Depressed mood most of the day or nearly every day
2. Markedly diminished interest or pleasure in all or almost all activities
3. Significant weight loss or weight gain
4. Insomnia or hypersomnia
5. Psychomotor agitation or retardation
6. Fatigue or loss of energy
7. Feelings of worthlessness or excessive or inappropriate guilt
8. Diminished ability to think or concentrate, or indecisiveness
9. Recurrent thoughts of death, recurrent suicidal ideation, or suicide attempt (APA, 2000, p. 356)

The diagnostic threshold for MDD includes criteria for severity and duration of symptoms experienced in addition to the level of distress or impairment in the client's life. The client must experience at least five of the nine symptoms outlined in the list of symptoms every day or almost every day over a two-week period in order to fulfill the diagnostic criteria for this disorder.

Bertha is a 75-year-old widow who lives alone in a high-rise building for senior citizens. Her experience with major depressive episodes began twenty-eight years ago when the community she lived in for most of her life was flooded after two hurricanes in quick succession inundated the area. She lost the house she was living in, all of her possessions, and her family pets. Since that time, she has moved several times and recently obtained public housing. With each move, she lost more and more of her autonomy and slipped deeper into poverty. At the same time, her mobility has been curtailed with advancing arthritis and cardiovascular problems. She has been hospitalized psychiatrically each year for the past twenty-eight years due to major depressive episodes and concomitant social withdrawal and lack of attention to caring for herself. (Major Depressive Disorder)

Dysthymic Disorder, by contrast, is marked by depressed mood that occurs on most days, if not every day, for at least a two-year time period (one year in children or adolescents). During that time period, the person must not have been without the depressed mood or the following *DSM-IV-TR* symptoms for more than two months at a time:

1. Presence while depressed of two or more of the following:
   a. Poor appetite or overeating
   b. Insomnia or hypersomnia
   c. Low energy or fatigue

   d. Low self-esteem

   e. Poor concentration or difficulty making decisions

   f. Feelings of hopelessness (APA, 2000, p. 380)

DSM-IV-TR (APA, 2000) suggests that MDD is often a reaction to severe psychosocial stressors; these stressors are thought to play a major role in the first or second episodes but a smaller role in subsequent episodes. Dysthymic Disorder may also be a precursor to MDD: Epidemiological samples have found that each year, more than 10 percent of individuals with Dysthymic Disorder have their first major depressive episode. The seriousness of MDD and Dysthymic Disorder cannot be overstated. Left untreated, both of these disorders can lead to fatality.

PSYCHOTIC RESPONSES

Psychosis is what most people perceive of as mental illness or craziness. Psychosis actually refers to a collection of symptoms marked by bizarre content of thought, illogical thought/speech forms, perceptual disturbance, disturbed affect, lost sense of self, diminished volition, relationship withdrawal, and psychomotor abnormalities (Jongsma & Peterson, 1999). In the same way that mood or anxiety disorders can emerge in the aftermath of a traumatic stressor or crisis event, individuals can also respond psychotically to traumatic stressors. The following diagram suggests a pathway for understanding psychotic responses to a crisis event:

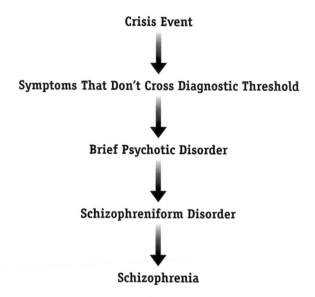

Crisis Event

↓

Symptoms That Don't Cross Diagnostic Threshold

↓

Brief Psychotic Disorder

↓

Schizophreniform Disorder

↓

Schizophrenia

   Increasing levels of psychotic responses over longer and longer periods of time can eventually lead to diagnosis of disorders with lifelong consequences. Inherent in the progression diagrammed above is the fact that mental health professionals and society at large both expect and accept that under certain circumstances individuals may have psychotic responses to crisis events. For example, individuals who survived the terrorist attacks on the World Trade Center and the Pentagon may have experienced brief periods of disorientation, bizarre thoughts, hallucinations, and disorganized speech.

A full-blown brief psychotic episode is not normal, however, and does require intensive intervention. If a person experiencing brief psychotic symptoms has a good premorbid (precrisis) level of functioning, the chance of a return to an equivalent level of functioning is good. Normal resilience in basically healthy people means that we can expect their symptoms to abate with crisis intervention, the possible use of psychotropic medications, and close observation.

Brief Psychotic Disorder

Once again, the primary determinants used to diagnose the psychotic disorders are frequency, intensity, and duration of symptoms. The diagnosis of most concern in the crisis intervention context is Brief Psychotic Disorder, especially those psychotic symptoms that develop in response to one or more events that would be severe stressors for almost anyone in a similar situation. This rare type of disordered response was once known as "brief reactive psychosis."

DSM-IV-TR criteria (APA, 2000, p. 332) for Brief Psychotic Disorder include the presence of one or more of the following symptoms over the course of an episode that is at least one day but less than one month in duration, with an eventual full return to premorbid level of functioning:

1. Delusions
2. Hallucinations
3. Disorganized speech
4. Grossly disorganized or catatonic behavior

Diagnosis is based upon the occurrence of what are referred to as "positive" psychotic symptoms (e.g., delusions, hallucinations, disorganized speech) or grossly disorganized or catatonic behavior. The onset is sudden and the symptoms last for at least one day but less than one month, with an eventual return to the premorbid level of functioning (APA, 2000).

Mary is a 26-year-old woman who worked on the fortieth floor of Tower One of the World Trade Center. On September 11, 2001, she was able to escape the building before it collapsed but not before witnessing people jumping to their deaths and seeing numerous dead or injured people. Within an hour of leaving Tower One, she began to hear voices telling her that she should have died in the building and that she would be punished for her sins. She was unable to communicate coherently to rescue workers and rambled on in chaotic sentences about punishment and the devil. She was taken to a hospital emergency room, medically cleared, and transferred to a psychiatric unit where she received antipsychotic medication.

Within two days of admission to the unit, she was able to communicate clearly and was experiencing no indications of delusions, hallucinations, or disorganized behavior. She was released to her family and given a follow-up appointment with a crisis mental health unit in her neighborhood for the same day. (Brief Psychotic Disorder)

Schizophrenia

The more severe diagnoses of Schizophreniform Disorder and Schizophrenia are based upon the duration of the psychotic symptomatology. Schizophreniform Disorder is diagnosed when the psychotic response is more than a month and less than six months in duration. Schizophrenia is diagnosed when the psychotic response lasts longer than six months with concomitant impaired social and/or occupational functioning.

The *DSM-IV-TR* criteria for Schizophrenia include:

1. Two or more of the following:
   a. Delusions
   b. Hallucinations
   c. Disorganized speech
   d. Grossly disorganized or catatonic behavior
   e. Negative symptoms (i.e., affective flattening, alogia, or avolition)
2. Social/occupational dysfunction (i.e., work, play, interpersonal relations, self-care) (APA, 2000, p. 312)

Sam is a 52-year-old man with a long history of psychiatric admissions in Veteran's Administration (VA) psychiatric units up and down the East Coast of the United States. His psychiatric troubles emerged during his second tour of combat duty in Vietnam. Sam had returned to the United States for a furlough after his first tour, and when he returned he discovered that his entire platoon had been killed. He was reassigned to another combat platoon and his overall mental status gradually deteriorated (hallucinations, delusions, disorganized speech and behavior) to the point where he was sent back to a psychiatric unit stateside. Sam's psychiatric disorder would remit with antipsychotic medications and therapy but his compliance with taking his prescribed medications and continuing treatment was poor. Within a month of being released, Sam would decompensate and be involuntarily committed to a VA psychiatric unit for observation and treatment. His first admission occurred in 1970, and his most recent admission occurred in the summer of 2002. Each time, he is admitted with psychotic symptoms parallel to those observed throughout his years of mental illness. (Schizophrenia)

Crisis counselors, in the course of their work, are exposed to the full range of emotional functioning. We have highlighted those disorders that we believe are potentially relevant to the crisis context and those for which more intensive intervention may be required. Targeted interventions to ameliorate the symptoms associated with crisis responses can be intensified through treatment of longer duration, more frequent contact, use of adjunctive psychotropic medications, and more controlled settings. Decisions to provide more restrictive intervention should not be taken lightly. The abridgement of personal freedom should always be of utmost concern, as should the risk of encouraging dependency on crisis services. Assuring a smooth transition to natural supports and community-based services is a critical component of single-session crisis intervention and ongoing crisis counseling.

DANGER TO SELF

The World Health Organization has consistently estimated that approximately one million people die from suicide each year worldwide (WHO, 2002). The global suicide rate has risen by 60 percent over the last forty-six years, with suicide attempts occurring twenty times more frequently than completed suicides. In the United States, a completed suicide occurs every eighteen minutes; an annual total of well over 30,000 deaths are due to self-inflicted injuries (CDC, 2002). Suicide ranks as the eleventh leading cause of death in the United States; the incidence of suicide among adolescents and young adults tripled from 1952 to 1995 (CDC, 2002). Given these statistics, there is little doubt that crisis workers will have occasion to counsel suicidal individuals. Rosenberg (1999) posited that suicidal behavior may be the most frequently encountered crisis situation for mental health professionals.

The need for a clear set of empirically validated guidelines for crisis counselors to intervene with suicidal individuals is obvious. We will start by attempting to dispel the common myths that have arisen in regard to suicidal behavior.

Myths of Suicide

People who talk about suicide are not going to commit suicide and just want attention.

False. Whenever a person in crisis talks about suicide, caution is in order. The crisis worker should view each mention or threat of suicide as a serious issue. Some individuals, particularly those with personality disorders, have a history of suicidal ideation and threats. These individuals require a considerable amount of energy and attention not only from family and friends but also from mental health professionals who must attempt to help them stop their self-injurious behavior. Even when a long-term client has a history of repeated suicidal threats, and lack of furtherance, the skilled professional takes all suicidal threats seriously. A cry for help is just that, and it must be answered. A crisis worker with limited knowledge of a client and limited time to intervene should *always* respond to suicidal ideation and/or intent in a consistent and well-documented fashion that places client safety and welfare first.

Suicide occurs precipitously.

Rarely. Impulsive acts of suicide are rare. The suicidal act may appear to be impulsive or even capricious, especially to surviving loved ones and friends. More than likely, however, the suicide attempt has occurred after much consideration of available options. Unfortunately the suicidal individual's thought processes can be irrational and limited by his or her coping skills or available resources. Spending a long time to consider available options does not necessarily equate with logical thought or action.

Suicidal individuals are committed to killing themselves.

Rarely. The simultaneous desire to live and to die is not incongruent for some people in the midst of great emotional upheaval. Ambivalence about wanting to live or die is overwhelming for the suicidal person. In reality, no one knows what it is like to be dead. Calling a crisis line or divulging suicidal ideation and/or plans is further evidence of an individual's ambivalence.

If a person survives a suicide attempt, there is no further danger.

False. If anything, past behavior is one of the best predictors of future behavior. Surviving a suicide attempt may lead some individuals to a new appreciation of life, but for others, the embarrassment associated with a botched suicide attempt can be emotionally painful and provide further justification for attempting suicide again. Mortensen et al. (2000) found that one of the most dangerous times for the suicidal individual was during the psychiatric hospitalization itself and in the first week following discharge.

Attempting suicide is an inherited characteristic.

Mostly false. Research identifies a family history of suicide as a risk factor for suicidal behavior (Brent, Bridge, Johnson, & Connolly, 1996; Dahlsgaard, Beck, & Brown, 1998; Mann, Waternaux, Haas, & Malone, 1999; Roy, 1992) and some types of psychiatric disorders are increasingly believed to have a biological basis rooted in genetics. At the present time, no studies have conclusively linked suicide to the human genome. There are many factors that explain suicidal behavior, and genetics is only one influence among a myriad of psychological and social influences that act singularly or in tandem with biochemistry and neuroanatomy. Would it behoove the person with a family history of suicide to be mindful of this potential? Absolutely. As with any disease or condition that has occurred in a family, people with a family history should be alert to any cues that might indicate a propensity for depression or suicidal ideation or extreme vulnerability to stress. Alertness can translate into early intervention, should the need arise.

Anyone who attempts suicide is mentally ill.

Debatable. This is a tough myth to confront because the strongest risk factors for suicide in adults are depression, alcohol abuse, cocaine use, and separation or divorce (CDC, 2002). Sanchez (2001) identified major mental illness as the strongest risk factor for suicide. The most salient risk factors for attempted suicide in youth are depression, alcohol or other drug use disorders, and aggressive or disruptive behaviors (CDC, 2002). The religious and societal injunctions against taking one's life are powerful forces; thus suicidal behavior is usually labeled as psychologically or criminally deviant (illegal).

Mental health professionals are also taught to view human behavior through a lens that utilizes suicidal ideation, intent, plans, and furtherance of threat as diagnostic indicators associated with most cases of suicide. Suicide is a complex phenomenon that results from the interplay of many complex biopsychosocial factors that cannot be oversimplified or underestimated.

If you talk about suicide with clients, you give them the idea.

False. One does not cause suicidal ideation by asking an individual if he or she is considering suicide. By contrast, ascribing words to a client's feelings and facilitating self-disclosure of suicidal ideation can be an immense relief to a client in crisis. Validation of a client's emotional state and normalization of stress-induced suicidal ideation are necessary components of intervention with suicidal clients. There is simply no alternative to the assessment of suicidal ideation/intent and targeted intervention to decrease the risk. To assess suicide risk, the crisis worker and client must talk, directly and honestly. Not to do so is irresponsible, unethical, and illegal, and makes the crisis worker culpable.

Suicide Assessment

Given the suicide mythology that exists in popular culture and the likelihood that crisis workers will encounter suicidal individuals, there is a clear need for a tool that crisis counselors can utilize to assess suicide risk. Joiner, Walker, Rudd, and Jobes (1999) proposed a seven-domain framework for suicide assessment that included "previous suicidal behavior; the nature of current suicidal symptoms; precipitant stressors; general symptomatic presentation including the presence of hopelessness; impulsivity and self-control; other predispositions, and protective factors" (p. 447). Sanchez (2001), in a similar review of various models that have been developed to understand suicide, identified common risk factors and protective factors. Risk factors were categorized as historical, personal, psychosocial-environmental, and clinical entities, whereas protective factors were seen as deterrents to committing suicide. An integration of these two frameworks in the determination of risk for suicide can assist the crisis worker in designing comprehensive interventions. To emphasize a point: The primary goal of all assessment activity is to inform treatment (Peruzzi & Bongar, 1999).

History of suicidal behavior   The practice of experienced professionals suggests that the best predictor of future behavior is past behavior. Joiner et al. (1999) viewed a prior history of suicide attempt(s) combined with current suicidal symptoms as the highest-risk combination of factors. Researchers have suggested that there are distinctive differences between suicide ideators (contemplators of suicide), single attempters, and multiple attempters (Clark & Fawcett, 1992; Rudd, Joiner, & Rajab, 1996). Logically, the crisis worker can assume that the highest risk is associated with the multiple attempter because of the type, chronicity, and severity of the psychopathology (Joiner et al., 1999). This risk in combination with any other factors discussed below always yields a moderate-to-severe-risk rating for suicide.

Current suicidal symptoms   Contemplating suicide and attempting suicide are not the same thing. Thus, thinking about suicide, planning suicide, and following through with an attempt should be viewed distinctly in suicide assessment. All suicidal symptoms are significant, but two that appear to stand out are suicidal desire or ideation and resolved plans and preparation (Joiner, Rudd, & Rajab, 1997). Not only must one want to die, one must be able to think about ending one's life. Resolved plans and preparation means that suicidal individuals must possess the competence, available means, opportunity, specific plan, preparation, duration of suicidal ideation, intensity of suicidal ideation, and conviction to attempt suicide (Joiner et al., 1999).

Suicidal desire or ideation is demarcated symptomatically by the person's expressed reason for living, death wish, ideation frequency, wish not to live, passive attempts, attempt desire, attempt expectancy, lack of attempt deterrents, and death/suicide talk (Joiner et al., 1999).

Jack is a 32-year-old married man whose wife of five years has recently died of leukemia. He reports feeling lost without her and that when he goes to bed at night, he hopes that he will die in his sleep. When he is driving, he has fleeting thoughts of driving off the road and killing himself.

Although these symptoms are clinically significant, by themselves, they don't pose severe suicidal risk. In combination with other factors, suicide risk is elevated. Any combination of risk factors should be considered a moderate-to-severe risk, as the following example illustrates:

Karl is a 42-year-old male who consistently e-mails distant family members that he no longer has a desire to live since his wife shot and killed their 12-year-old daughter with one of his hunting rifles one year ago during the Christmas holidays. She then placed the barrel of one of Karl's pistols in her mouth and shot herself. Karl lives in a rural area where his closest neighbor lives one mile away from him. He refuses any psychological intervention.

Contributing stressors   The suicide prevention literature abounds with repeated studies that have shown a link between stressful life events and suicide attempts (Brent, Perper, Moritz, & Allman, 1993; Cohen-Sandler, Berman, & King, 1982; de Wilde, Kienhorst, Diekstra, & Wolters, 1992; Marttunen, Aro, & Lonnqvist,

1993; Paykel, Prusoff, & Myers, 1975; Sanchez, 2001). Current stressors, especially interpersonal loss and relationship disruption, need to be viewed separately and in conjunction with previous suicidal behavior and/or suicidal symptoms. For single or multiple attempters, the coexistence of stressful events elevates the suicidal risk to moderate-severe levels (Joiner et al., 1999).

Historical factors Sanchez (2001) identified historical risk factors as unchangeable biological, psychosocial, mental, or medical conditions or single events that place individuals at a higher risk of suicide. One of the historical factors identified as a great risk is a person's history of major mental illness. Depressive disorders, schizophrenia, alcohol and substance abuse disorders, personality disorders, and anxiety disorders have all been associated with elevated suicide risk (Berglund, 1984; Clark & Fawcett, 1992; Duberstein & Conwell, 1997; Klatsky & Armstrong, 1993; Stoelb & Chiraboga, 1998; Tanney, 1992). Diagnostic comorbidity (two or more disorders) elevates the risk even higher (Cornelius, Salloum, Mezzich, & Cornelius, 1995). Other risk factors identified in the literature include combat-related PTSD (Kleespies, Deleppo, Gallagher, & Niles, 1999), head injury (Mann et al., 1999), childhood physical or sexual abuse (Mann et al., 1999; Yang & Clum, 1996), and a family history of suicide (Brent et al., 1996). These factors are clinically significant in and of themselves but are particularly important when found in individuals with an attempt history and significant current suicidal symptomatology. Chronicity of historical risk factors increases the concern for suicidal behavior (Sanchez, 2001).

Personal factors Personal factors encompass personality characteristics such as traits, cognitive/ attributional style, and history of emotional stability. Personal factors associated with suicidal risk include self-destructive behavior patterns (e.g., drinking and driving, combining alcohol with certain medications, binging/purging), poor impulse control, impaired judgment, low stress tolerance, poor coping skills, poor problem-solving skills, and rigid thinking/irrational beliefs (Apter, Plutchik, & van Praag, 1993; Pfeffer, Hurt, Peskin, & Siefker, 1995; Sanchez, 2001). Coexistence of these factors with any other domain identified raises the risk of a suicide attempt.

Rosalba is a 50-year-old woman with a long history of depression and psychiatric treatment who is becoming increasingly debilitated physically and emotionally by Parkinson's disease. Her first psychiatric admission occurred when she attempted suicide as a freshman in college. There have been no other suicide attempts since that time, but her entire adult life has been marked by major depressive episodes and dysthymia. She has warned her medical team that she will die before succumbing to dementia as a result of the Parkinson's disease.

Psychosocial-environmental factors Psychosocial-environmental factors include man-made and natural events that can precipitate suicidal behavior. Events influence different people in different ways. An event that overwhelms one person may be a minor event for another. Sanchez (2001) suggested categorizing psychosocial-environmental factors as acute or chronic. A death of a child would be an example of an acute factor, whereas prolonged imprisonment would be a chronic factor. Concerns related to comorbid suicidal domains remain with this group of factors.

Anthony is a 37-year-old father of two girls who has recently been sentenced to five to seven years in prison after pleading guilty to sexually molesting his younger daughter. He is fearful of how he will be treated by other inmates at the correctional facility and wonders about his emotional ability to handle so many years of isolation. His wife has begun divorce proceedings and has moved with their daughters to an undisclosed location in another part of the country. He has informed the prison guards that he will kill himself if he is singled out as a child molester by the other inmates or mistreated in any fashion.

Protective factors   Protective factors lower the risk of suicide. Sanchez (2001) reported extensive research that found that family and non-family support systems, significant relationships, a satisfying social life, and constructive use of leisure time can serve as protective factors (Fridell, Johnsson, & Traskman-Bendz, 1996; Heikkinen, Isometsa, Marttunen, & Aro, 1995; Stack, 1992). Other protective factors identified include employment (Dahlsgaard et al., 1998; Stack, 2000), religious/cultural/ethnic beliefs (Gibbs, 1997; Hovey & King, 1997; Lester, 1997; Stack, 1992), purpose for living (Jobes & Mann, 1999), suicide-related writing (Francis & Pennebaker, 1992), and involvement in psychotherapy (Dahlsgaard et al., 1998; Rudd, Joiner, & Rajab, 1995).

Thus, it appears that individuals who are embedded in their communities and have healthy coping behaviors may be at less risk of suicide because these conditions counterbalance the negative consequences of even extremely severe life events. These conditions bear particular attention when designing interventions to target these protective factors.

The existence of protective factors doesn't negate the risk of suicide but should be taken into consideration in making decisions about treatment. The lack of protective factors increases the likelihood of a suicide attempt, especially when other risk factors are present.

Rating Risk Severity

Joiner et al. (1999, pp. 447–453) proposed a continuum of suicidal behavior as a tool for rating risk severity. The continuum includes the factors just described that are predictive of level of risk:

1. *Nonexistent.* No identifiable suicidal symptoms, no past history of suicide attempts, and no or few other risk factors.

2. *Mild*. Suicidal ideation of limited intensity and duration, no resolved plans or evidence of preparation, and no or few other risk factors; a multiple attempter with no other risk factors.
3. *Moderate*. Moderate-to-severe symptoms associated with resolved plans and preparation, or no/mild symptoms associated with resolved plans and preparation, but moderate-to-severe symptoms of the suicidal desire and ideation factor and at least two other notable risk factors; a multiple attempter with any other notable finding.
4. *Severe*. Moderate-to-severe symptoms associated with resolved plans and preparation and at least one other risk factor; a multiple attempter with any two or more other notable findings.
5. *Extreme*. A multiple attempter with severe symptoms associated with resolved plans and preparation and two or more other risk factors.

Treatment Options for Suicidal Clients

Nonexistent and mild risk   For the person with a nonexistent or mild risk of suicide, recurrent evaluation and monitoring of suicide potential is indicated (Kleespies et al., 1999). The crisis worker should bear in mind the possibility that a person in either of these categories might slip over into the moderate or higher-risk category. Crisis counseling should focus on improving problem solving and adaptive coping skills, and on modulating strong emotions (Linehan, 1993; Rosenberg, 1999).

Moderate risk   The person at moderate risk of suicide should be offered recurrent evaluation for hospitalization, an increase in counseling contact, reevaluation of the treatment plan as needed, active involvement of supportive family and others, twenty-four-hour emergency availability, frequent assessment of suicide risk, consideration of medical evaluation for psychopharmacological intervention, increase in telephone contact, and use of professional consultation, as warranted (Joiner et al., 1999; Kleespies et al., 1999).

The decision to hospitalize should not be made lightly. Part of this decision rests on the availability of community services that may meet the needs of a person at moderate risk for suicide on an outpatient basis (e.g., the existence of a drop-in center at a community hospital; a short-term crisis inpatient program that can provide security for up to seventy-two hours; and/or psychopharmacological intervention). Outpatient treatment has been shown to be efficacious for clients with a mild-to-moderate suicide risk (Linehan, Armstrong, Suarez, Allmon, & Heard, 1991; Rudd et al., 1995). Clients frequently feel empowered when they realize that the crisis counselor trusts in their ability to manage their life crises without more restrictive interventions. Restrictive intervention is inevitable, however, when a client's risk increases to the severe or extreme level (Bongar, Maris, Berman, & Litman, 1998).

Severe and extreme risk   The person at severe and extreme risk of suicide should be evaluated immediately to determine whether psychiatric hospitalization is indicated. If the decision is to provide treatment services on an outpatient basis, the same services identified in the moderate risk category should be offered to the client. If hospitalization is the preferred alternative, the client may be willing to sign in voluntarily. Clients are often willing to become inpatients voluntarily (Joiner et al., 1999), but when a client refuses, a decision must be made regarding involuntary admission.

Each state has its own mental health commitment laws, which generally provide options when an individual is either a danger to self or others. The notion of danger usually implies some furtherance of threat (i.e., buying a gun, stockpiling psychotropic medication) that may or may not be known to the crisis worker and may only have been observed by the client's intimates. The individual's intimates usually have to be willing to function as the petitioner for involuntary commitment. Involuntary commitment actions taken by a mental health professional are bound to have serious repercussions for the therapeutic alliance and should be factored into post-discharge treatment strategies. Comstock (1992) considered hospitalization the treatment of choice when crisis intervention and the establishment of a treatment alliance fail, when the crisis counselor judges the person to be a risk to self or others, and when the accepted protocol for clients at imminent risk is required.

SINGLE-SESSION CRISIS COUNSELING WITH SUICIDAL INDIVIDUALS

Crisis intervention with suicidal individuals is guided by the three primary goals of single-session crisis intervention:

- Ensuring client safety, reducing lethality, and stabilizing the environment
- Assisting the client to attain immediate, short-term mastery of self and situation
- Connecting the client with appropriate formal and informal supports and resources

Step 1:
Supportively and empathically join with the client.

A crisis counselor's first responsibility is to establish a relationship with the individual in crisis in order to obtain information critical to identifying the person's focal problem and degree of suicidal risk. The counselor must establish some degree of faith and trust with the client before he or she will reveal much information. The presence of various attributes in the counselor and the use of various communication skills discussed in Chapter 4 facilitate this process.

Reaffirming depression as a normal response to perceived insurmountable problems can open the door to discussion of negative life events and possible solutions. The crisis worker gathers data from the first moments of contact with the suicidal person. Sometimes that data may save the person's life should he or she choose not to reveal identifying information in a suicidal risk situation requiring an immediate rescue.

Step 2:
Intervene to create safety, stabilize the situation, and handle the client's immediate needs.

Ensuring the person's safety while de-escalating the crisis is paramount when intervening with suicidal individuals. If the person is alone or isolated, he or she should be encouraged to stay with family or friends. With informed consent of the person in crisis, the worker may also enlist family or friends in ensuring the client's safety through periodic monitoring until the crisis subsides. Removing the means to commit suicide, such as storing weapons in a safe place outside the home or having someone else monitor potentially lethal medications, can be key activities in ensuring a suicidal person's safety.

Persuading a client to verbalize or document in writing a promise not to attempt suicide for an agreed-upon period of time can also be a useful step in preventing suicide (Jongsma & Peterson, 1999). There is a risk, however, that the promise will not be binding once the person leaves the session. By persuading a client to agree to contact a crisis service should the client have a serious urge to harm him- or herself, the crisis worker can delay a permanent solution with far-reaching impact on the client and his or her network of family and friends.

Roger, an 18-year-old high school senior, has just told his school counselor about his suicidal ideation over his realization that he may be gay. He denies having the intent or a suicide plan but he reports feeling hopeless that he or his family will ever be able to accept his homosexuality. He also refuses to allow the counselor to contact anyone. The counselor knows that there are insufficient grounds to pursue involuntary commitment and that she cannot breach confidentiality in this situation, yet she is still uncomfortable about letting Roger leave her office without some type of agreement on his part to call the school counselor or the local crisis line if he has any suicidal ideation or intent. Roger also agrees to let the school counselor contact him at home twice that evening and agrees to return to the school counselor's office first thing the next morning upon arrival at school. Roger also acknowledges in the written contract that he had no current suicidal intent or plan.

The crisis worker must then work intensively to involve the suicidal individual in close monitoring by family and friends and follow-up services to further forestall a suicide attempt. It is easier to establish a contract not to attempt suicide when the worker focuses on the client's self-professed ambivalent feelings about ending his or her life.

Step 3:
Explore and assess the dimensions of the crisis and the client's reaction to the crisis, encouraging ventilation.

Pertinent questions should include inquiries about suicidal ideation, intent/plan, lethality of plan, and access to means (Johnson, 1997). A person who is not only contemplating but intent on committing suicide is at risk, especially if he or she has access to lethal means. *Suicidal ideation* is assessed by asking directly whether the person is thinking of harming or killing him- or herself: *Do you have any thoughts about hurting yourself? Have you thought about ending your life? Have you thought about suicide as an option?*

Thoughts of suicide alone are not enough to propel a person toward a suicide attempt. A person must not only be thinking about suicide but also be intent on committing suicide. *Suicidal intent* refers to the intensity of the person's wish to die. Beck, Schuyler, and Herman (1974) developed the *Suicide Intent Scale* for potential or actual attempts, which assesses circumstances surrounding a potential or actual suicide attempt and the personal views of the suicidal person.

Circumstances of an attempt include the person's degree of isolation, timing, precautions taken against discovery, help sought during an attempt, final acts, degree of planning, suicide note, communication of intention, and purpose of the suicide act itself. These circumstances must be assessed by the crisis worker. If a person in crisis is envisioning a suicide attempt that won't be interrupted by others and has also begun to prepare privately and publicly to die with a specific purpose in mind, the intensity of that person's wish to die and thus his or her suicidal risk is quite high.

Views of the suicidal person include expectations regarding fatality risk, the choice of method, seriousness of attempt, ambivalence toward life, degree of premeditation, and ideas of reversibility. If a person in crisis is consistently envisioning a suicide in which the choice of means will ensure death with no chance of resuscitation, the intensity of that person's wish to die and thus his or her suicidal risk is quite high.

Given the significant contribution of major psychiatric disorders to the risk for suicide, an evaluation for *DSM-IV* Axis I and Axis II disorders should also be completed when time permits. Diagnostic and symptom-specific treatment recommendations (psychopharmacological and psychosocial) can help manage symptoms and mitigate the overall emotional impact on suicidal individuals (Jobes, 1995; Rudd, Joiner, Jobes, & King, 1999).

Step 4:
Identify and examine alternative actions and develop options.

Meichenbaum (1994) suggested a stance of communicating to a suicidal client that suicide is an option, but only one option. By reaffirming the suicidal person's desire to resolve pressing problems, the crisis worker can attempt to reframe suicidal ideation as a result of depression and comorbid irrational thinking. Consider the metaphor of a headache. If a person has a headache it's difficult to think clearly, given the pain's impact on concentration. Similarly, if an individual is seeing the world through a "depressed" lens, the chances of being able to think clearly are diminished.

If the suicidal person can entertain the possibility of alternatives that he or she has not considered, the crisis worker can initiate a problem-solving routine, examine alternatives, and generate options. The belief that options exist is, in itself, a sign of hope the crisis worker can nurture. The crisis worker should be fully prepared to discuss suicide as one of those options.

Expressing moral judgment will only alienate the suicidal individual. Being clear about your own religious and/or philosophical perspectives regarding suicide so that you do not impose them on clients can facilitate open communication with the suicidal person. The person in crisis has already envisioned suicide as an option but may not have really considered its advantages and disadvantages. Nor has the suicidal person been able to fully consider the advantages and disadvantages of other options. It is important to emphasize the permanence of suicide to the client in the wake of irrational thinking.

Step 5:
Help the client mobilize personal and social resources.

More than likely, the suicidal individual has exhausted the personal, social, and community resources available in his or her community. In addition to having an in-depth knowledge of social resources within a community, the crisis worker should endeavor to help the client identify potential personal resources that may be untapped or perceived to be unavailable. These resources may include family, friends, coworkers, primary care physicians, clergy, and local support groups. Reestablishing contact with external supports can play a critical role in reducing isolation and concurrently reducing dependence on professional resources after the initial suicidal phase has passed.

Step 6:
Anticipate the future and arrange follow-up contact.

Rudd et al. (1999) concluded from a review of intervention studies that intensive follow-up contact (i.e., case management, phone contact, home visits) can enhance treatment compliance for both low-risk and high-risk suicidal clients. The more personal the contact, the more compliant the suicidal person can be in successive months after a suicidal crisis. The more intensive the follow-up treatment, the more efficacious the intervention, especially for multiple attempters.

The nature of a suicidal crisis demands follow-up intervention. Suicidal ideation and intent will not be eliminated solely through brief intervention. The crisis worker thus functions as a bridge between the person in crisis and ongoing therapy. The importance of this link cannot be overstated nor can the need for the crisis worker to ensure that the person's need for services is addressed. Morgan, Jones, and Owen (1993) reported that ease of access to emergency services (e.g., twenty-four-hour availability, well-publicized access procedures), and encouragement to use crisis services resulted in reduced subsequent suicide attempts and demands for service.

DANGER TO OTHERS

Intervention with individuals who place others at risk for physical harm is a common activity of crisis workers. Crisis workers live with the threat of potential violence in their home communities, in the lives of their clients, and on the job. This threat of violence or violence itself can occur along a continuum that varies from menacing intimidation to homicide. At the extreme end of the continuum, homicide is one of the top twelve causes of death in the United States (FBI, 2000).

Homicide ranks as the second leading cause of death among males aged 15–34 years and the third leading cause of death among females in the same age range (Kramarow, Lentzer, Rooks, Weeks, & Saydah, 1999). The number of homicides in which the circumstances were unknown has almost doubled since 1976; the number of homicides resulting from arguments has declined but remains the most frequently cited circumstance (FBI, 2000). In addition, the number of homicides involving adult or juvenile gang violence has increased 500 percent since 1976.

The occurrence of nonfatal violence among youths is even more sobering. In *Youth Violence: A Report of the Surgeon General* (HHS, 2001), the authors asserted that arrest records provide only a limited picture of youth violence. The report concluded that for every youth arrested in any given year in the late 1990s, at least ten were involved in some form of violent behavior that could have seriously injured or killed another person.

At the same time, on-the-job violence experienced by mental health workers has emerged as a critical safety issue. Guy, Brown, and Poelstra (1992) reported that nearly half of all mental health clinicians would be threatened, harassed, or physically attacked during their careers, with a greater incidence of assault occurring early in one's career (Carmel & Hunter, 1991; Tardiff, 1996). Guidelines for managing the violent client have arisen in response to the experience of violence in the treatment setting (Tishler, Gordon, & Landry-Meyer, 2000). The crisis worker must protect others (the public) who are at risk for violence, protect the person who is at risk for harming another, and simultaneously safeguard his or her own safety. The crisis worker bears ethical and legal responsibility for ensuring the safety of all clients he or she encounters.

This responsibility places great expectations on the ability of the crisis worker to work effectively with the potentially violent client while attempting to protect him- or herself and others. Predicting violence is a difficult task that has challenged the mental health professions for many years (Apperson, Mulvey, & Lidz, 1993; McNeil & Binder, 1987; Skodol & Karasu, 1978). Tishler, Gordon, and Landry-Meyer (2000) concluded that although clinicians may not be able to adequately predict future violence, aggressive behavior should be viewed as a symptom of an underlying condition and therefore likely to resurface at any time. Harris and Rice (1997) found that actuarial or statistical methods of predicting violence were more reliable than clinicians' judgments about clients' aggressive behavior. The crisis worker must always be alert to signs of potential violence in the clinical context. The following risk factors derived from research and clinical practice should aid in that process.

Risk Factors for Violence

Risk factors associated with the potential for violence include a history of emotional problems (Lion, Snyder, & Merrill, 1981; Monahan, 1988; Tardiff, 1984), a history of medical illnesses associated with aggressive behavior (Pastor, 1995), a history of personality disorders, and a history of violence or impulsivity (Harris & Rice, 1997; McNeil, Binder, & Greenfield, 1988). The American Psychological Association web site provides both immediate and long-term warning signs of youth violence.

Immediate warning signs of youth violence (American Psychological Association, 2002)

- Loss of temper on a daily basis
- Frequent physical fighting
- Significant vandalism or property damage
- Increase in use of drugs or alcohol
- Increase in risk-taking behavior
- Detailed plans to commit acts of violence
- Announcing threats or plans for hurting others
- Enjoying hurting animals, and carrying a weapon

Warning signs of youth violence seen over a period of time (American Psychological Association, 2002)

- A history of violent or aggressive behavior
- Serious drug or alcohol use

- Gang membership or strong desire to be in a gang
- Access to or fascination with weapons, especially guns
- Threatening others regularly
- Trouble controlling feelings like anger
- Withdrawal from friends and usual activities
- Feeling rejected or alone,
- Having been a victim of bullying
- Poor school performance
- History of discipline problems or frequent run-ins with authority
- Feeling constantly disrespected
- Failing to acknowledge the feelings or rights of others

Mantell and Albrecht (1994) suggested a lengthy list of characteristics that might identify potentially violent employees, including

- A disgruntled attitude regarding perceived injustices in the workplace
- Social isolation, poor self-esteem
- "Cries for help of some kind"
- A fascination with military or paramilitary subjects
- Being a gun or weapon collector
- Demonstrated temper-control difficulties
- A history of threats against coworkers/supervisors
- Few, if any, healthy outlets for rage
- Excessive interest in media reports of workplace violence
- An unstable family life
- Creating fear or unrest among coworkers/supervisors
- A history of chronic labor-management disputes
- A history of numerous unresolved physical or emotional claims against the organization
- Sustained complaining about poor working conditions/unsatisfactory working environment/heightened stress
- Being a male between the ages of 30 and 40
- A migratory job history
- Drug and/or alcohol abuse
- Psychiatric impairment

Although the risk factors listed above have been identified for distinct populations, the crisis worker should be aware that the risk factors may exist in various situations. For example, a fascination with weapons or a history of run-ins with authority figures is a concern in every age group and in every possible context.

SINGLE-SESSION CRISIS COUNSELING WITH AGGRESSIVE OR VIOLENT INDIVIDUALS

Goals for crisis intervention with potentially violent or violent individuals include ensuring client safety, reducing lethality, and stabilizing the environment; assisting the client to attain immediate/short-term mastery of self and situation; and connecting the client with appropriate formal and informal supports/resources.

Step 1:
Supportively and empathically join with the client.

A true test of relationship-building skills for crisis workers is an interaction with a client who is exhibiting overt aggressive signs (e.g., noncompliance, threatening and/or loud verbalizations, impulsive body movements, hypervigilance, clenched fists). One's natural tendency is to avoid confrontation or to respond defensively when encountering threatened or actual violence. The challenge of joining with the client is best met by active listening. Verbal and nonverbal behaviors that communicate respect, patience, empathy, honesty, and understanding are essential. It is important to avoid overly friendly gestures, extended eye contact, or verbalizations that are not congruent with the crisis context.

Step 2:
Intervene to create safety, stabilize the situation, and handle the client's immediate needs.

Tishler, Gordon, and Landry-Meyer (2000) recommend three safety precautions to take in approaching a person in crisis. First, they suggest that clinicians approach the client from the front or side so as not to startle him or her, because people with violent tendencies need to keep a distance between themselves and others to feel safe. Second, they suggest that clinicians mirror a client's body language: Sit if the client is sitting; stand if the client is standing; walk alongside the client if the client is pacing. Avoid communicating physical superiority or inferiority, for example, standing over a person or walking in front of or behind him or her. Third, they advise clinicians to introduce themselves and consistently reinforce their identities as helping professionals so the client is reminded that they are trying to help.

Care should be taken in the choice of environment to interview a potentially violent individual. The best evaluation environment is one in which privacy and isolation from environmental overstimulation is balanced by visibility and quick access to help (Dubin, 1995). Depending on the available resources of the facility, closed-circuit video observation, an open door, or a staff member posted outside an office are ways to ensure the safety of the crisis counselor and the client. Crisis intervention services should always be provided in facilities that have, at a minimum, specific emergency protocols and electronic alert systems.

Counseling rooms should be free of objects that a client could use to hurt him- or herself or others (McNeil, 1998), furnished with objects that could be used as shields such as pillows (Tardiff, 1992), large enough to accommodate restraint procedures by multiple staff members, and, preferably, constructed with two exit doors (Tishler, Gordon, & Landry-Meyer, 2000). Tardiff (1991) warned that counselors should always sit close to the door in the event of a violent outbreak and the need for an immediate exit.

Stabilization and de-escalation are necessary precursors of providing crisis intervention for the potentially violent or violent individual. Crisis workers must try to communicate calmness even if they don't feel calm because the client may be hyper-alert and responsive to the worker's demeanor. A quiet and reassuring voice with moderate eye contact can help contain the client's emotional lability. It is important to be a skilled listener, to stay focused on the client's verbal and nonverbal messages, to search for commonalities or opportunities that affirm the client's perspectives (especially when the perspectives connote responsibility and rationality), and, when necessary, to communicate simple, straightforward requests.

Step 3:
Explore and assess the dimensions of the client's reaction to the crisis, encouraging ventilation.

More than likely, the aggressive/violent client has pressing immediate needs that are overwhelming his or her available coping resources. Offering the client choices, even simple ones (e.g., a glass of water, a cup of coffee, or something to eat), can suggest that the client still has some control and can contribute to calming an agitated individual. Assuring the client that you will address pressing immediate needs can be a good segue into problem solving.

The crisis worker can encourage the expression of feelings through nondirective prompts and open-ended questions. It is helpful to allow the person to vent by acknowledging his or her agitation (e.g., *"You're really angry, Bob"*). The crisis worker can facilitate appropriate ventilation by setting clear and consistent limits. For example, the crisis worker can inform the client at the outset that no one is going to get hurt and that no one will be allowed to hurt anyone else. Setting limits can help clients to understand the boundaries within which they are operating. Johnson (1997) recommended educating the client about expectations of his or her behavior and the benefits to be derived from cooperation and collaboration. The crisis worker should not respond defensively to a verbal hostility, and should watch for the point at which more rational conversation, and thus more problem solving can occur.

Discussion of ways that the client can release tension in the session can also help the client de-escalate. For example, *"Mr. Jones, I know this is very difficult for you and I'm interested in finding a way for you to get rid of the anger you've got built up. Especially here. Right now. How about if you yell into the pillow or we do some deep breathing together when you feel as if you're about to blow?"*

The crisis worker, of course, may find that for extremely agitated individuals, talking about establishing self-control is not sufficient. In those cases where verbal plans are not enough, alternatives must be available. Emergency protocols should include calling for additional help. Assuming a leadership role can assure staff and the client that you are prepared to ensure everyone's safety, including your own (Johnson, 1997).

Giving the client as many choices as possible throughout an escalating anger process can also be reassuring and empowering for the client. Offering clients a safe, quiet place gives them an opportunity to calm themselves before resuming problem solving. Different facilities have different rules and different options for physical and/or chemical restraint (medications) should the need arise. These rules and options need to be clearly articulated in emergency procedures.

There are distinct similarities between the assessment of dangerousness in suicidal, potentially violent, and homicidal clients. In fact, it is important not to underestimate the potential for a suicide attempt following nonlethal violence or a homicide but rather to plan for it as part of the crisis intervention (Hillbrand, 2001). Pertinent questions to ask the client should include questions about violent ideation, intent/plan, lethality of plan, and access to means (Johnson, 1997). A person who is not only contemplating but intent on committing violence places both him- or herself and others at risk, especially if he or she has access to lethal means.

Homicidal ideation is assessed by asking directly whether the person is thinking of harming or killing someone else and/or him- or herself: *Do you have any thoughts about hurting anyone else? How frequently do the thoughts occur? Under what circumstances? What do you do with the thoughts? Do the thoughts go away? Have you thought about ending someone else's life? Have you thought about homicide as an option? Do you have a plan? How detailed is the plan? How would you carry out the plan? Do you have the means to carry out the plan? Do you want help managing the aggressive feelings?*

Thoughts of hurting or killing someone else are not enough to propel a person toward violence. A person must not only be thinking about harming someone else but also be intent on doing so. *Intent,* in this context, refers to the intensity of the person's wish to cause harm to another. A client who has violent ideation, intent, plans, and means is a clear danger to him- or herself and others. The crisis worker is ethically and legally obligated to protect the individual(s) identified as being at risk and the crisis client. Offering the client treatment options at this point is mandatory.

If the crisis worker's assessment concludes that the individual can be maintained through closely monitored outpatient intervention, the crisis worker should make the appropriate referrals and appointments. The crisis worker should also notify the police and person(s) identified as being at risk of the potential for violence.

If the crisis worker's assessment concludes that the person is at imminent risk for harming someone else and cannot be maintained on an outpatient basis, the crisis worker should offer the client voluntary admission to a short-term, secure facility that can provide appropriate supervision and protection. Voluntary admission to an inpatient psychiatric unit may be the only recourse in some communities.

If the crisis worker's assessment concludes that the person is at imminent risk for harming someone else, cannot be maintained on an outpatient basis, is unwilling to be voluntarily admitted to a secure program, and if the grounds are met for involuntary admission, then the crisis worker should initiate commitment procedures. If the individual flees, the crisis worker should notify the police and the threatened party or parties.

Step 4:
Identify and examine alternative actions and develop options.

Clear identification of the crisis that has provoked an aggressive response and concomitant successful de-escalation can lead to an opportunity to discuss alternative responses to the crisis precipitants. Discussion of alternatives involves discussion of the consequences of proposed actions. Central to this part of the discussion is the importance of the client taking responsibility for his or her actions and making appropriate choices in the immediate future.

Step 5:
Help the client mobilize personal and social resources.

It is necessary to focus on clear, immediate steps to remedy the current crisis. Identifying alternative actions and developing options do not occur in isolation for the client or the crisis counselor. The client and the counselor should view each alternative action and corresponding set of consequences within the context of a community safety net or support system that can assist the client in maintaining a crisis resolution agenda. Engaging the client in a way that encourages relying on support from intimates is essential, as is supporting the client's efforts to make use of community services. Connecting the client with these resources is a crucial task for the crisis counselor.

Clearly, there are individuals who do not have a personal support system or, possibly, even a community resources network. In this situation the crisis counselor tries to help the client build a support system by identifying his or her needs and thoroughly canvassing the traditional and nontraditional resources currently available in a community. The client's participation in this development of options can be an empowering experience in problem solving in itself.

Step 6:
Anticipate the future and arrange follow-up contact.

Usually, the need for follow-up services with aggressive or violent clients is apparent. Johnson (1997) recommended treatment follow-up to address anger management, assertive communication, self-monitoring instruction, use of physical exercise to discharge bodily tension, and the possible need for psychopharmacological intervention. Crisis workers can anticipate continued difficulties for the client under stressful circumstances and arrange frequent contact (appointments, telephone sessions, e-mail updates, Internet chats) until the client is adequately engaged in ongoing counseling and the danger of aggression has passed.

The complexities of providing crisis intervention to those who are a danger to themselves and to others can be overwhelming initially. With explicit emergency protocols, adequate supervisory backup, and ongoing experience with suicidal/homicidal individuals, however, the crisis counselor can become very effective at preventing harm. The case study for this chapter, which involves an individual who is a danger to himself and to others, illustrates the complexities involved in responding to the potential of violence.

CASE EXAMPLE: HECTOR

Single-Session Crisis Counseling with a Potentially Violent and Suicidal Individual

Hector is a 52-year-old, married male who has called a twenty-four-hour hotline to talk with a crisis counselor at 2:00 A.M. on a Sunday morning. The call was patched through from the switchboard to an on-call worker. Hector told the switchboard operator that his wife had left him and taken the children with her.

CW: *Hi, Hector. This is Paul. I'm a crisis counselor with the county mental health program. The switchboard said you wanted to talk.*

Hector: *(Sobbing).* She left me. I came home from the pool league and she's gone. *(Some of the words are coming out quite slurred.)* The kids are gone, too. What the fuck is happening? Oh, Jesus . . .

CW: *Bring me up to speed, Hector. It sounds like a lot has happened and you're really upset. Where are you now?*

Hector: I'm downtown at a pay phone outside her mother's house. I went looking for her and I thought she might be at her mom's place. She's not there. I don't know where she is . . . I don't know where she is. *(Begins to cry again).* My children. . . . Where are my babies?

CW: *Is there anybody else with you?*

Hector: No, I'm alone. Why are you asking me all these stupid fucking questions? *(Begins to talk loudly and more animatedly.)* Don't you understand? My wife is gone and so are my kids.

CW: *I just want to make sure you're safe, Hector. That's all. Have you called the police to let them know she's missing?*

Hector: No. You can't report someone as missing until they've been gone more than twenty-four hours.

CW: *That's true, but you can at least make a report.*

Hector: No can do. They don't like me down there, trust me.

CW: *What makes you say that?*

Hector: Trust me. They know me and I know them. They've been out to the house before. My word ain't good for shit. They're all motherfuckers. Just because I wear the pants in my house and they don't, they don't think much of me.

CW: *You don't have any idea where your wife and kids might be. When did you last see her?*

Hector: Around 8:00. Before I left the house to meet my buddies at the pool league over in Pleasantville.

CW: *Did she leave you any message, or do you have any idea why she's not there?*

Hector: Yeah . . . she left me a letter. Lot of fucking good that does.

CW: *What did the letter say?*

Hector: Says she loves me but she can't live with me. Says she can't have the kids growing up in that kind of house no more with a mom and dad always fighting and the cops coming to the house. Says I got a problem with alcohol. Says she doesn't want to be hurt no more. Says she wants some time away to think things over.

CW: *Sounds like things have been pretty bad for a while now.*

Hector: We've been together since high school. Got married when I came back from Vietnam. Two kids almost out of high school. Thirty years . . . I've busted my ass to make things right for her and this is the thanks I get. I just can't fucking believe it. I just can't fucking believe she'd do this. She took my kids. *(Begins to sob again.)*

CW: *Pretty confusing time, Hector. You're feeling angry but also feeling pretty sad. How sad are you?*

Hector: What the fuck is that supposed to mean? I'm sad, Goddamn it! What do you fucking expect? *(Begins to yell but dissolves into sobs.)*

CW: *I'm concerned for your safety, Hector. This is a pretty big shock and you're feeling a lot. I just want to make sure that you get through this in one piece.*

Hector: I'm sorry. I'm so fucking sorry. Everything I fucking touch turns to shit. Everything.

CW: *You feel pretty hopeless right now because your wife left with your kids and you're not sure what's going on. It makes sense that you would be upset. When I asked how sad you were, I was trying to find out if you were so upset that you had thought about hurting yourself or your wife and kids. Have you?*

Hector: Yes. *(Begins to sob gently.)*

CW: *Who have you thought about hurting?*

Hector: Jesus, man. I would never hurt my family. . . . Only me. She doesn't really love me anymore. Why shouldn't I? I've lost her. I really fucked up this time.

CW: *Have you thought about how you would kill yourself?*

Hector: I got a gun and some bullets under the front seat of my truck. I'll just drive back into the woods and blow my fucking head off. No mess for them. Nobody has to see me go. Everyone will be better off. Including me.

CW: *Have you ever tried to kill yourself before?*

Hector: Yeah, a couple of times when I first got back from 'Nam. Right before we got married.

CW: *What was going on then?*

Hector: I was pretty fucking fried when I got out of the Army. Too much getting fucked up. Too much wacko shit in 'Nam. I was in and out of the V.A. for the first couple years. Couldn't keep my act together for shit. Tried to hang myself first time I went to the V.A. Right there on the psych unit. Right over the back of the room door but they found me before it was too late.

CW: *You said a couple of times. When else?*

Hector: One of them Korean doctors had me all fucked up on Thorazine and some other medication so I got pissed off at him one time. Got all drunked up and took my pills. All of them. Woke up two days later in the V.A. I knew then that I had to knock that shit off or I was really going to off myself. She stood by me during all that crap.

CW: *Have there been any other times?*

Hector: Naw, that's it . . . until now. I stopped drinking. Stopped smoking weed. Joined a vet's group and saw a shrink for a while. Did pretty good up until two years ago.

CW: *What happened then?*

Hector: *(Sobs heavily).* He died.

CW: *Who died, Hector?*

Hector: *(Cries steadily for a couple of minutes before regaining his ability to keep talking.)* Our son.

CW: *Your son?*

Hector: Manuel. Our 12-year-old. My boy . . . my boy. He died.

CW: *What happened?*

Hector: Cancer. He came home after a baseball game and told us his leg was sore and that he thought he had hit it with a bat. When we looked at it, there was a lump right near his right knee. We iced it but it didn't go away. We took him to see our doctor and the doctor ordered some tests. They told us he had cancer. Bone cancer. He was gone in six months. He was only 12 years old. 12 years old. Why would God do that to us . . . to me? Why?

CW: *I'm sorry your boy died, Hector. That must have been awful.*

Hector: Trust me. It still is. Things just haven't been the same since then. I picked up the bottle and I pretty much haven't stopped. I lost Manuel. I lost my job last spring. And now I've lost my wife and kids. Getting pretty near the end of the road. Wouldn't you say?

CW: *Yet you called tonight, Hector. Why'd you call?*

Hector: I don't know. Guess I was feeling sorry for myself. Misery loves company.

CW: *My bet is that you're not completely at the end of the road. There's still some belief that there might be some help or that things could get better.*

Hector: Fat fucking chance, man. Don't bullshit me.

CW: *I'm not bullshitting you. I hear that you love your wife and kids. That your heart is broken over Manuel's death. That you've dealt with some pretty mean stuff in your life and that you've stuck it out. But I also hear that you're depressed. That you know you've got a problem with booze. And that you've come too far to let it all fade away.*

Hector: Yes to most of what you've said, but I'm not sure about being able to turn it around.

CW: *Certainly sounds like what you're doing now is not working, Hector. And it hasn't been working for the past two years. You need some help and you know it. There are obviously no guarantees, but you did it before and you had a good long stretch before it all unraveled. How are you feeling right now?*

Hector: A little calmer, I guess. I still don't know where my wife and kids are.

CW: *You said your wife has stood by you until now. I suspect if you can get yourself back together there may still be hope for you and your family. I don't want you to do something that will only make it worse. Right now you need to find the strength to show yourself and your family that you're not going to continue on the same downhill track you've been on.*

Hector: I know you're right. But what the hell do I do? I'm all alone.

CW: *I can tell you're anxious to know where your wife and kids are, but how about you contract with me to let that rest for the night, and you come into the center tomorrow morning. There's a lot to sort out. Are you willing to come in to the center tomorrow? I'd like to have you talk with someone there and see if we can find some answers for you and see if you can come up with a plan to get the train back on the tracks. There's a lot to do but I think it's your best option. Are you willing to come in?*

Hector: Yeah, I guess.

CW: *Good. I'd like you to come to the center tomorrow morning at 9:00 A.M. We're at the corner of 30th and Lexington. Can I get your full name and phone number, Hector?*

Hector: Sure, why not? Martin. Hector Martin. 2013 Avenue K. 555-8832.

CW: *If anything happens between now and 9:00, Hector, give us a call. See you at 9:00.*

Hector: Thanks.

DISCUSSION QUESTION

1. Some crisis intervention professionals believe that diagnosis pathologizes individuals in crisis. Discuss the strengths and weaknesses of diagnosis in crisis intervention.

EXERCISES

1. Divide the class into groups of three in which each student will have an opportunity to participate in a role-playing activity as a suicidal individual, as a crisis counselor, and as an observer. Ask each student to invent a crisis client who has some degree of suicidal ideation, intent, and plan. The student should then play the role of that client while another student functions as the crisis counselor. After ten minutes, ask the students to stop and ask the observer to provide feedback about how well the crisis counselor was able to address the assessment (ideation/intent/plans), risk, and the development of a plan to address the client's needs. Then ask students to switch roles and engage in the same process.

2. Divide the class into groups of three in which each student will have an opportunity to participate in a role-playing activity as a potentially violent individual, as a crisis counselor, and as an observer. Ask each student to invent a crisis client who has some degree of ideation and/or intent and/or plan to harm another person. The student should then play the role of that client, while another student functions as the crisis counselor. After ten minutes, ask the students to stop and ask the observer to provide feedback about how well the crisis counselor was able to address the assessment (ideation/intent/plans), risk, and the development of a plan to address the client's needs. Then ask students to switch roles and engage in the same process.

3. Diagnosis is a controversial issue in crisis intervention. Divide the class into small work groups and assign one of the clinical chapters in this text (Chapters

6–13) to each group. Direct each group to do the following: (1) identify the pros and cons of diagnosis for the individuals in crisis in the chapter they read, and (2) report their findings to the larger class group. Process the exercise.

REFERENCES

American Medical Association. (2001). ICD-9-CM 2002: *International classification of diseases* (9th ed., Vols. 1 and 2). Chicago: Author.

American Psychiatric Association. (2000a). *Diagnostic and statistical manual of mental disorders; DSM-IV-TR* (4th ed., Text Revision). Washington, DC: Author.

American Psychiatric Association. (2000b). *Practice guidelines for the treatment of psychiatric disorders: Compendium 2000*. Washington, DC: Author.

American Psychological Association. (2002). *Warning signs of teen violence: Recognizing violence warning signs in others*. Retrieved November 10, 2002, from http://helping.apa.org/warningsigns/recognizing.html

Apperson, L. J., Mulvey, E. P., & Lidz, C. W. (1993). Short-term clinical prediction of assaultive behavior: Artifacts of research methods. *American Journal of Psychiatry, 150*, 1374–1379.

Apter, A., Plutchik, R., & van Praag, H. M. (1993). Anxiety, impulsivity, and depressed mood in relation to suicidal and violent behavior. *Acta Psychiatrica Scandinavica, 87*, 1–5.

Beck A. T., Schuyler, D., & Herman J. (1974). Development of suicidal intent scales. In T. Beck, H. Resnick, & D. Lettieri (Eds.), *The prediction of suicide* (pp. 45–55). Bowie, MD: Charles Press.

Berglund, M. (1984). Suicide in alcoholism: A prospective study of 88 suicides. The multidimensional diagnosis at first admission. *Archives of General Psychiatry, 41*, 888–891.

Bongar, B., Maris, R. W., Berman, A. L., & Litman, R. E. (1998). Outpatient standards of care and the suicidal patient. In B. Bongar, A. L. Berman, R. W. Maris, M. M.Silverman, E. A. Harris, & W. L. Packman (Eds.), *Risk management with suicidal patients* (pp. 4–33). New York: Guilford Press.

Brent, D. A., Bridge, J., Johnson, B. A., & Connolly, J. (1996). Suicidal behavior runs in families: A controlled family study of adolescent suicide victims. *Archives of General Psychiatry, 53*, 1145–1152.

Brent, D. A., Perper, J. A., Mortiz, G., & Allman, C. (1993). Psychiatric sequalae to the loss of an adolescent peer to suicide. *Journal of the American Academy of Child and Adolescent Psychiatry, 32*, 509–517.

Carmel, H., & Hunter, M. (1991). Psychiatrists injured by patient attack. *Bulletin of the American Academy of Psychiatry and the Law, 19*, 309–316.

Centers for Disease Control. (2002). Suicide in the United States. Retrieved November 12, 2002, from http://www.cdc.gov/ncipc/factsheets/suifacts.htm

Clark, D. C., & Fawcett, J. (1992). Review of empirical risk factors for evaluation of the suicidal client. In B. M. Bongar (Ed.), *Suicide: Guidelines for assessment, management, and treatment* (pp. 16–48). New York: Oxford University Press.

Cohen-Sandler, L., Berman, A. R., & King, L. A. (1982). Life stress and symptomatology: Determinants of suicidal behavior in children. *Journal of Child and Adolescent Psychiatry, 21*, 178–186.

Comstock, B. S. (1992). Decision to hospitalize and alternatives to hospitalization. In B. Bongar (Ed.), *Suicide: Guidelines for assessment, management, and treatment* (pp. 16–48). New York: Oxford University Press.

Cornelius, J. R., Salloum, I. M., Mezzich, J., & Cornelius, M. D. (1995). Disproportionate suicidality in clients with comorbid major depression and alcoholism. *American Journal of Psychiatry, 152,* 358–364.

Dahlsgaard, K. K., Beck, A. T., & Brown, G. K. (1998). Inadequate response to therapy as a predictor of suicide. *Suicide and Life-Threatening Behavior, 28,* 197–204.

de Wilde, E. J., Kienhorst, I. C., Diekstra, R. F., & Wolters, W. H. (1992). The relationship between adolescent suicidal behavior and life events in childhood and adolescence. *American Journal of Health Promotion, 149,* 45–51.

Duberstein, P., & Conwell, Y. (1997). Personality disorders and completed suicide: A methodological and conceptual review. *Clinical Psychology: Science and Practice, 4,* 359–376.

Dubin, W. R. (1995). Assaults with weapons. In B. Eichelman & A. C. Hartwig (Eds.), *Patient violence and the clinician* (pp. 53–72). Washington, DC: American Psychiatric Association.

Federal Bureau of Investigation. (2000). *FBI uniform crime report 1999.* Washington, DC: Author.

Francis, M. E., & Pennebaker, J. W. (1992). Putting stress into words: The impact of writing on physiological, absentee, and self-reported emotional well-being measures. *American Journal of Health Promotion, 6,* 280–287.

Fridell, E., Johnsson, O. A., & Traskman-Bendz, L. (1996). A 5-year follow-up study of suicide attempts. *Acta Psychiatrica Scandinavica, 93,* 151–157.

Gibbs, J. T. (1997) African American suicide: A cultural paradox. *Suicide and Life-Threatening Behavior, 27,* 68–79.

Guy, J. D., Brown, C. K., & Poelstra, P. L. (1992). Safety concerns and protective measures used by psychotherapists. *Professional Psychology: Research and Practice, 23,* 421–423.

Harris, G. T., & Rice, M. E. (1997). Risk appraisal and management of violent behavior. *Psychiatric Services, 48,* 1168–1176.

Heikkinen, M. E., Isometsa, E. T., Marttunen, M. J., & Aro, H. M. (1995). Social factors in suicide. *British Journal of Psychiatry, 167,* 747–753.

Hillbrand, M. (2001). Homicide-suicide and other forms of co-occurring aggression against self and others. *Professional Psychology: Research and Practice, 32*(6), 626–635.

Hovey, J. D., & King, C. A. (1997). Suicidality among acculturating Mexican-Americans: Current knowledge and directions for research. *Suicide and Life-Threatening Behavior, 27,* 92–103.

Jobes, D. A. (1995). The challenge and promise of clinical suicidology. *Suicide and Life-Threatening Behavior, 25,* 437–449.

Jobes, D. A., & Mann, R. E. (1999). Reasons for living versus reasons for dying: Examining the internal debate on suicide. *Suicide and Life-Threatening Behavior, 29,* 97–104.

Johnson, S. L. (1997). *Therapist's guide to clinical intervention: The 1-2-3's of treatment planning.* San Diego, CA: Academic Press.

Joiner, T. E., Rudd, M. D., & Rajab, M. H. (1997). The modified scale for suicidal ideation: Factors of suicidality and their relation to clinical and diagnostic variables. *Journal of Abnormal Psychology, 106,* 260–265.

Joiner, T. E., Walker, R. L., Rudd, M. D., & Jobes, D. A. (1999). Scientizing and routinizing the assessment of suicidality in outpatient practice. *Professional Psychology: Research and Practice, 30*(5), 447–453.

Jongsma, A. E., & Peterson, L. M. (1999). *The complete adult psychotherapy treatment Planner* (2nd ed.). New York: John Wiley & Sons, Inc.

Klatsky, A., & Armstrong, M. (1993). Alcohol use, other traits, and risk of unnatural death: A prospective study. *Alcoholism: Clinical and Experimental Research, 17,* 1156–1162.

Kleespies, P. M., Deleppo, J. D., Gallagher, P. L., & Niles, B. L. (1999). Managing suicidal emergencies: Recommendations for the practitioner. *Professional Psychology: Research and Practice, 30*(5), 454–463.

Kramarow, E., Lentzer, H., Rooks, R., Weeks, J., & Saydah, S. (1999). *Health and aging chartbook: Health United States, 1999.* Hyattsville, MD: National Center for Health Statistics.

Lester, D. (1997). The effectiveness of suicide prevention centers: A review. *Suicide and Life-Threatening Behavior, 27,* 304–311.

Linehan, M. M. (1993). *Skills training manual for treating borderline personality disorder.* New York: Guilford Press.

Linehan, M. M., Armstrong, H. E., Suarez, A., Allmon, D., & Heard, H. L. (1991). Cognitive-behavioral treatment of chronically parasuicidal borderline patients. *Archives of General Psychiatry, 48,* 1060–1064.

Lion, J. R., Snyder, W., & Merrill, G. L. (1981). Underreporting of assaults on staff in a state hospital. *Hospital and Community Psychiatry, 32,* 497–498.

Mann, J. J., Waternaux, C., Haas, G. L., & Malone, K. M. (1999) Towards a clinical model of suicidal behavior in psychiatric patients. *American Journal of Psychiatry, 156,* 181–189.

Mantell, M., & Albrecht, S. (1994). *Ticking bombs: Defusing violence in the workplace.* New York: Irwin.

Marttunen, M. J., Aro, H. M., & Lonnqvist, J. K. (1993). Adolescence and suicide: A review of psychological autopsy studies. *European Child and Adolescent Psychiatry, 2,* 10–18.

McNeil, D. E. (1998). Empirically based clinical evaluation and management of the potentially violent patient. In P. M. Kleespies (Ed.), *Emergencies in mental health practice: Evaluation and management* (pp. 95–116). New York: Guilford Press.

McNeil, D. E., & Binder, R. L. (1987). Patients who bring weapons to the psychiatric emergency room. *Journal of Clinical Psychiatry, 48,* 230–233.

McNeil, D. E., Binder, R. L., & Greenfield, T. K. (1988). Predictors of violence in civilly committed acute psychiatric patients. *American Journal of Psychiatry, 145,* 965–970.

Meichenbaum, D. (1994). *A clinical handbook/practical therapist manual for assessing and treating adults with post-traumatic stress disorder (PTSD).* Waterloo, Ontario, Canada: Institute Press.

Monahan, J. (1988). Risk assessment of violence among the mentally disordered: Generating useful knowledge. *International Journal of Law and Psychiatry, 11,* 249–257.

Morgan, H., Jones, E., & Owen, J. (1993). Secondary prevention of nonfatal deliberate self-harm: The green card study. *British Journal of Psychiatry, 163,* 111–112.

Mortensen, P. B., et al. (2000). Psychiatric illness and risk factors for suicide in Denmark. *Lancet, 355,* 9–12.

Pastor, L. H. (1995). Initial assessment and intervention strategies to reduce workplace violence. *American Family Physician, 52,* 1169–1174.

Paykel, E. S., Prusoff, B. A., & Myers, J. K. (1975). Suicide attempts and recent life events: A controlled comparison. *Archives of General Psychiatry, 31,* 327–333.

Peruzzi, N., & Bongar, B. (1999). Assessing risk for completed suicide in clients with major depression: Psychologists' views of critical factors. *Professional Psychology: Research and Practice, 30*(6), 576–580.

Pfeffer, C. R., Hurt, S. W., Peskin, J. R., & Siefker, C. A. (1995). Suicidal children grow up: Ego functions associated with suicide attempts. *Journal of the American Academy of Child and Adolescent Psychiatry, 34*, 1318–1325.

Rosenberg, J. I. (1999). An integrated training model using affective and action-based interventions. *Professional Psychology: Research and Practice, 30*(1), 83–87.

Roy, A. (1992). Genetics, biology, and suicide in the family. In R. W. Maris, A. L. Berman, J. T. Maltsberger, & R. I. Yufit (Eds.), *Assessment and prediction of suicide* (pp. 574–588). New York: Guilford Press.

Rudd, M. D., Joiner, T. E., & Rajab, M. H. (1995). Help negation after acute suicidal crisis. *Journal of Consulting and Clinical Psychology, 63*, 499–503.

Rudd, M. D., Joiner, T. E., Jobes, D. A., & King, C. A. (1999). The outpatient treatment of suicidality: An integration of science and recognition of its limitations. *Professional Psychology: Research and Practice, 30*(5), 437–446.

Sanchez, H. G. (2001). Risk factor model for suicide assessment and intervention. *Professional Psychology: Research and Practice, 32*(4), 351–358.

Skodol, A. E., & Karasu, T. B. (1978). Emergency psychiatry and the assaultive patient. *American Journal of Psychiatry, 135*, 202–205.

Stack, S. (1992). The effect of the media on suicide: The Great Depression. *Suicide and Life-Threatening Behavior, 22*, 255–267.

Stack S. (2000). Suicide: A 15-year review of the sociological literature, part II. *Suicide and Life-Threatening Behavior, 30*, 163–176.

Stoelb, M., & Chiraboga, J. (1998). A process for assessing adolescent risk for suicide. *Journal of Adolescence, 21*, 359–370.

Tanney, B. (1992). Mental disorders, psychiatric patients, and suicide. In R. Marris, A. Berman, J. Maltsberger, & R. Yufit (Eds.), *Assessment and prediction of suicide* (pp. 277–320). New York: Guilford Press.

Tardiff, K. (1984). Characteristics of assaultive patients in private hospitals. *American Journal of Psychiatry, 141*, 1232–1235.

Tardiff, K. (1991). Violence by psychiatric patients. In R. I. Simon (Ed.), *American Psychiatric Press review of clinical psychiatry and the law* (Vol. 2, pp. 175–233). Washington, DC: American Psychiatric Press.

Tardiff, K. (1992). The current state of psychiatry in the treatment of violent patients. *Archives of General Psychiatry, 49*, 493–499.

Tardiff, K. (1996). *Concise guide to assessment and management of violent patients* (2nd ed.). Washington, DC: American Psychiatric Press.

Tishler, C. L., Gordon, L. B., & Landry-Meyer, L. (2000). Managing the violent client: A guide for psychologists and other mental health professionals. *Professional Psychology: Research and Practice, 31*(1), 34–41.

U.S. Department of Health and Human Services. (2001). *Youth violence: A report of the Surgeon General.* Retrieved September 10, 2003, from http://www.mentalhealth.org/youthviolence/orderform.htm

Yang, B., & Clum, G. A. (1996). Effects of early negative life experiences on cognitive functioning and risk for suicide: A review. *Clinical Psychology Review, 16*, 177–195.

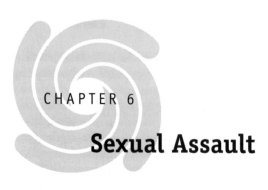

CHAPTER 6

Sexual Assault

BARBARA G. COLLINS

One Friday night during the second semester of her freshman year in college, Wendy and a couple of her friends planned to attend a fraternity party. They got together in one of the girls' rooms prior to leaving for the party and each had a shot of tequila with salt and lime "to get relaxed and in the mood." When they arrived at the party, Wendy drank a quick beer as she talked with some guys she knew from one of her classes. One of the fraternity pledges was told by a "brother" to bring another round of beers to the group, and Wendy drank her second beer. Within minutes, she began to feel dizzy and disoriented. She headed for the bathroom, realized she was only feeling worse, and made a quick decision to exit the party and head back to her dorm. She recalls stumbling and, at one point, actually falling as she walked to her dorm. She remembers entering the building, passing some other students, getting into her room, and flinging herself onto her bed. She vaguely remembers the two men from the party coming to her room "to check on her" and to get her to come back out "to party." She also remembers feeling like "a puppet" as the two men propped her up between them and walked her down the corridor and out the door with them. She passed her RA, but recollects her inability to speak and the sensation of being in a complete fog. The next thing Wendy recalled was waking up the next morning alone in a strange room, her clothes and underclothes on the floor, a foul taste in her mouth, and what she assumed to be semen coming out of her vagina. Terrified, she put on her clothes, looked around, and realized she was in one of the men's dorms. She frantically telephoned her room to reach her roommate, but there was no answer. She then called the rape crisis center.

Sexual assault directly affects hundreds of thousands of women and adolescent girls every year and indirectly affects almost all women, who are aware of their vulnerability to this personally invasive crime. Rape is the crime women fear most (Koss, 1993). Rape has been identified as a risk factor for development of a range of negative mental and physical health outcomes as well as loss of resources including unemployment, disruptions of education, reduced income, and divorce (Monnier, Resnick, Kilpatrick, & Seals, 2002). Research documents that approximately 50 percent of rape survivors develop Acute Stress Disorder and/or Post-traumatic Stress Disorder (Rothbaum, Foa, Riggs, Murdock, & Walsh, 1992).

Children, both boys and girls, are also sexually victimized, sometimes by parents, stepparents, guardians, caregivers, or other family members, and sometimes by strangers. Adolescent and adult men can also be subjected to sexual aggression and assault. In all cases, whether victims are female or male, children, adolescents, or adults, the perpetrators are most often men.

This chapter focuses on intervention with adolescent and adult victims of sexual assault. Because little is known about adult male victims, most of the information here pertains to women. It is useful to consider, however, that the available information about male victims suggests that the dynamics of sexual assault of men and the symptomatic responses of male victims are quite similar to the experiences of female victims, but they are complicated by gender-related assumptions about victimization (Goyer & Eddleman, 1984; Hutchings & Dutton, 1997; Mezey & King, 1989; Pelka, 1992). As one male rape survivor commented in describing his experience and the experience of other male victims:

> It is precisely because we have been "reduced" to the status of women that other men find us so difficult to deal with. It was obvious to me at the police station that I was held in contempt because I was a victim—feminine, hence perceived as less masculine. Had I been an accused criminal, even a rapist, chances are I would have been treated with more respect, because I would have been seen as more of a man. (Pelka, 1992, p. 40)

This male survivor's observation poignantly captures the negative view of women that too often permeates responses to both female and male victims of sexual assault. Male survivors' experiences may be further complicated by the stereotypic notion of sexual victimization as "unmanly." Sexual abuse of children is addressed in Chapter 11.

THE INCIDENCE AND PREVALENCE OF SEXUAL ASSAULT

The incidence and prevalence of sexual assault in the general population is measured in a number of ways. Official records of rapes that have been reported to local police departments are compiled and published as part of the Uniform Crime Reports (UCR) by the FBI. Because data based on official police reports dramatically understate the incidence of rape, however, crime victimization surveys are generally assumed to provide a more accurate count. The National Crime

Victimization Survey (NCVS), conducted annually by the Bureau of Justice Statistics, and several specialized surveys, like the National Violence Against Women survey, conducted collaboratively by the Department of Justice and the Centers for Disease Control and Prevention, provide a more complete picture of the extent of sexual violence in our society.

Using a definition of rape that included forced vaginal, oral, and anal sex, the NVAW survey estimated that approximately 876,100 rapes were perpetrated against adult women (age 18 and older), and 111,300 rapes were perpetrated against adult men during the twelve months preceding the survey. The survey also documented differing risks of sexual assault among minority women, with Native American and Alaskan women more likely to disclose rape and other physical assault victimization than women of other racial or ethnic groups. Calculations of lifetime experience of rape suggest that one of six U.S. women and one of thirty-three U.S. men had experienced rape or attempted rape as a child and/or as an adult (Tjaden & Thoennes, 1998).

By contrast, according to UCR data, 89,107 rapes were reported to law enforcement in the preceding twelve-month period, a 5 percent decrease in reported rapes from the previous year (FBI, 2000). Victimization data compiled by the Bureau of Justice Statistics suggested a 20 percent *increase* in rapes during the same period (Rennison, 2001).

DEFINING RAPE

The terms *rape* and *sexual assault* are used interchangeably in this chapter and refer to a broad range of types and levels of sexual victimization. Specifically, this includes any and all nonconsensual penetration, whether obtained through manipulation, pressure, coercion, force or threat of harm, or an individual's inability to give consent.

By contrast, most state statutes define rape solely in terms that require convincing evidence of nonconsensual penetration through the use of physical force, the threat of bodily harm, or the victim's inability to have given consent. Such definitions are an improvement over previous laws in that they include both vaginal and anal intercourse as well as fellatio and cunnilingus between two individuals, regardless of their sex. They do not address unwanted sexual acts that occur as the result of verbal pressures, threats, and/or false relationship promises, although some forms of sexual assault including unwanted touching and nonconsensual voyeurism are often classified as misdemeanors. Also, although all state statutes now classify marital rape as a crime, in thirty-three states exemptions from rape prosecution are still given to husbands, even when the wife is mentally or physically impaired. Bergen (1999) noted that the "existence of some spousal exemptions in the majority of states indicates that rape in marriage is still treated as a lesser crime than other forms of rape" (p. 2).

Limited legal definitions of sexual assault are problematic for a number of reasons. One problem is that official crime statistics underrepresent the amount of sexual victimization that occurs even after accounting for underreporting by victims. Second, although formal legal definitions may not include this wider range of violations, clinical data suggests that victim responses to these and other forms of sexual victimization are often quite similar to those of victims whose experiences fit more traditionally defined sexual assault (Koss & Harvey, 1991; Resnick, Kilpatrick, Dansky, Saunders, & Best, 1993). It is for this reason that most feminist definitions of rape emphasize the woman's experience of being coerced and violated rather than the specific acts committed (Brownmiller, 1975; Russell, 1984; Warshaw, 1988).

TYPES OF RAPE

Sexual assaults occur in multiple permutations. Victims can be raped by a single perpetrator, by multiple offenders, or in assaults that involve onlookers. Rapes can be perpetrated by strangers, when the offender had no previous relationship with the victim, or by offenders known to the victim, including friends, neighbors, coworkers, and family members. Two types of rape by known offenders are date rape and marital rape. In each of these types of rape, although consensual sexual activity may have occurred previously and may even be expected, rape nonetheless involves coercion, force, and lack of consent. The relationship between the victim and the offender has a major impact on prosecutors' willingness to pursue cases as well as the likelihood of conviction. The relationship between the victim and the offender may also affect friends' and family's reactions to victims.

Date Rape

Prevalence studies utilizing data based on victim surveys and self-report data from men conclude that rape by dates or romantic partners is far more extensive than reported in official statistics (Ageton, 1983; Lisak & Miller, 2002; Russell, 1991). Date rape is a particularly controversial subject, however, in part because research documents that the majority of women who self-report having experienced behaviors that *in fact* meet the legal definition of rape do not themselves identify their experience as rape. Further, the majority of these victims tell no one about the assault (Koss, 1985, 1988; Mills & Granoff, 1992; Schwartz & Leggett, 1999).

Rapes by dates, statistically, involve less violence, as measured by weapons, threats, and injury sustained, than rapes by strangers (Ellis, Atkeson, & Calhoun, 1981). More than half of date rape victims, however, perceived their offender as having used "quite a bit" of force, which involved actions such as holding the victim down or twisting her arm (Koss, 1988).

Early studies examining the relationship between assault characteristics and subsequent victim adjustment suggested that victims raped by acquaintances had more difficulty adjusting than victims of stranger rape because the former were more likely to be blamed and to blame themselves for having exercised poor judgment.

Some researchers suggested that survivors' ability to trust was shaken by the manipulative nature of the assault, and that they had more difficulty with sexual dysfunction (Burgess & Holmstrom, 1976, 1979). Later studies refined, and in some instances countered, these conclusions, finding that neither the type of assault nor the nature of the relationship between offender and victim predicted either short- or long-term reactions to rape on a variety of symptom measures, including depression, fear, anxiety, or sexual and social functioning (Frank, Turner, & Stewart, 1980; Roth, Wayland, & Woolsey, 1990). Although some studies have found a relationship between high levels of violence and poor psychological, social, and relational adjustment (Zweig, Crockett, Sayer, & Vicary, 1999), many survivors of sexually coercive date rape exhibit significant trauma symptoms and damage to sexual self-esteem (Shapiro & Chwarz, 1997).

Marital Rape

Contrary to popular belief, sexual abuse and assault of wives by their husbands are among the most common types of sexual assault (Finkelhor & Yllo, 1985; Russell, 1991). In one study, 10 percent of married or previously married women reported that their husbands "used physical force or threat to try to have sex with them" (Finkelhor & Yllo, 1985, pp. 6–7). As with date rape, marital rape is often assumed to be a situation of "He wants it; she doesn't; he goes ahead anyway," the only difference being the assumption that a husband has a right to sexual access. As Finkelhor and Yllo noted, "To most, it is a disagreement over sex that the husband wins" (p. 14).

This is not the image of rape that emerges from interviews with married women nor does it reflect the stories reported to police. Finkelhor and Yllo (1985) named and described three types of marital rape, based on their interviews with married women who reported such acts: rapes that occurred as part of a battering relationship, force-only rapes, and obsessive rape.

Battered women were the most vulnerable to marital rape and often suffered from repeated rapes. Sometimes physical beatings accompanied the sexual assaults and sometimes the sexual assaults followed physical violence and were characterized by the abusive husband as "making up." These marital rape victims were similar in many ways to other battered women in that their husband's brutality, control, and domination ruled their lives, and fear and lack of control deterred them from leaving.

Melanie's husband repeatedly abused her during their ten-year marriage. He would often accuse her of flirting or deliberately attracting the attention of other men. As he berated her for her imagined infidelities he would begin to escalate his physical attack on her, often ending with forcibly raping her as he insisted that she "show him what she wanted to do with other men."

"Force-only" rapes stand in contrast to the battered woman's story. In these rapes, husbands used only enough force to gain sexual access, and most of the rapes were prompted by the husband's desire to have sex or a particular kind of sex, and the wife's refusal. Unlike the battered woman whose rapist intended to punish, demean, and hurt, the perpetrators of force-only rapes did not routinely hit or physically harm their wives. As Finkelhor and Yllo (1985) pointed out, however, the fact that these rapes involved less brutal violence did not make them any less humiliating or upsetting for the victims.

Rebecca and her husband disagreed about the frequency of their marital sex almost from the beginning, and during the last year of their marriage these disagreements became part of a pattern of conflict and tension. Although Rebecca initially enjoyed sex with her husband, he wanted to have sex every day, was particularly insistent about oral sex, and wanted to try anal sex. Although, on occasion, she complied with his request for oral sex, most often she refused. One night he came home drunk and informed her that he was going to have sex with her. When she refused, using the weight of his body and holding her arms, he pinned her down, pulled off her pajama bottoms, and forcibly entered her.

Obsessive rapes, like force-only rapes, rarely involve the physical brutality or beatings that characterize the rapes of battered women. What distinguished these rapes was the inclusion of what Finkelhor and Yllo (1985) termed a bizarre element. In these rapes the sexual desires of the husband-rapists included more unusual sexual acts that they forced on their wives, including forced anal sex, inserting objects into her vagina, or having other people watch.

Clearly, marital rape occurs in different types of relationships and takes different forms. None of these types of rape, however, confirm the stereotype that because a woman regularly has consensual sex with her husband she cannot ever be raped by him.

Types of Rape: Differing Perpetrator Motivations

As the examples of date and marital rape exhibit, rapes appear to differ in terms of perpetrator motivation and the actions that derive from that motivation. This means that what the perpetrator does to the victim and thus her experience of the rape will also differ.

In an early examination of rape, Groth, Burgess, and Holmstrom (1977) identified three types of rape: power rape, anger rape, and sadistic rape. They argued that rapists are driven by their psychopathological need to establish power and control, to vent anger, or to gain pleasure or release through sexually sadistic violations. Feminist critiques suggested that these differing motivations usually did not reflect individual psychopathology but were, instead, an outgrowth of learned attitudes and beliefs about men, women, and sex that normalize and justify sexual coercion and violence.

Building on this early differentiation of rapists' motives, Scully and Marolla (1984, 1985) suggested that rape could be viewed as the endpoint on a continuum of sexually aggressive behaviors that reward men and victimize women. Based on interviews with convicted rapists, they concluded that men achieved different rewards (or have different motivations that are fulfilled) through their rape behavior. Some rapists express anger and/or exact revenge or punishment through raping. Such rapes tend to be violent and brutal, as individual victims are often seen to represent some collective liability for other females who are perceived as having offended the rapist. As is true with battered women who are raped by their husbands, these rapists' victims (known or strangers) are often brutalized and their lives are threatened (Groth et al., 1977; Scully & Marolla, 1985).

A second type of rape identified by Scully and Marolla (1985) were those in which the sexual assault victim was merely an easy target. In these situations, the sexual assaults occurred not because the perpetrator was intending to rape but almost as an afterthought when he realized that he was in control of a situation in which he could commit a rape. An example of this type of rape might be the sexual assault of a female clerk in a gas station that was being robbed. In this case, the woman would apparently be simply an added bonus.

In assaults termed sexual access rapes, Scully and Marolla (1985) described the motive of the rapist as simply his desire to take what was denied or perceived as inaccessible. In such rapes the purpose "was conquest, to seize what was not offered" (p. 258). In these rapes the victim is most often someone the rapist sees as being otherwise unattainable.

Other rapists were characterized as being primarily motivated by their desire to dominate and control. As one such rapist reported, "Seeing them lying there helpless gave me the confidence that I could do it. . . . In the rapes I was totally in command, she totally submissive" (quoted in Scully & Marolla, 1985, p. 259). Many of these rapists believed that women secretly desired forced sex and that the victim would, in fact, be aroused. As in what Groth et al. (1977) labeled "power rapes," the goal of the rapist was not to hurt his victim, as was the case with anger motivated rapes, but simply to dominate and control her in order to have his way.

Scully and Marolla (1985) also found that for some rapists, particularly those men who raped as part of a gang, rape represented recreation and adventure. Whether the form of gang rape was hitchhiker abduction or gang date rape, in which one perpetrator would bring a date to a predetermined location where she was then raped by multiple offenders, in each case perpetrators described it as "exciting," as an "adventure," or as one man noted, as "macho." "We felt powerful; we were in control. I wanted sex and there was peer pressure. She wasn't like a person, no personality, just domination on my part. Just to show I could do it . . . you know, macho" (p. 260).

These different types of rape and different motives and rewards of rape are clearly not mutually exclusive. A man who laces a woman's drink with a drug and then sexually assaults her is an acquaintance who apparently seeks sexual access. He also probably views the whole experience as recreation. The husband who rapes his wife may be expressing both power and control or acting out his anger or revenge.

Describing these different types of rape and varying rapist motivations does not suggest that one type of rape is worse than another. It does convey, however, that although each rape is a traumatic invasion of person, body, and spirit, each victim's experience is also unique. A woman attacked by a rapist motivated by anger will probably fear for her life, yet the knowledge that she managed to survive may assist her in her recovery. Further, because she looks like a "good victim"—beaten and brutalized—family, friends, and medical and criminal justice personnel are more likely to believe her and less likely to blame her. The victim of a power rapist who only uses as much force as necessary to conquer and dominate may not suffer the same degree of physical injury, but may blame herself or be blamed by others because she did not successfully resist the attack.

Understanding why rape occurs and the impact of rape on victims requires comprehension of the different types of rape and various motivations of rapists. Whether the perpetrator is a husband or stranger, however, and whether the woman is the victim of a gang rape, a stranger abduction, or a coercive date, rape is a degrading, sometimes violent, sexual invasion of the victim's body and of her emotional and physical integrity (Brownmiller, 1975).

From an intervention standpoint, classifying the type of rape is insignificant except as it sheds light on the functioning of the victim. Calhoun and Atkeson (1991) suggested that for purposes of intervention with rape survivors, treatment goals and methods should be largely independent of the incident itself and instead focus on each individual's responses. Such responses are impossible to predict, as individuals may experience rape trauma symptoms in response to violent, threatening assaults, but also in response to less threatening acts of sexual coercion. It is essential that crisis workers understand the various types of rapists and rapes so that they neither prejudge nor underestimate the traumatic impact of rape on victims.

DISPELLING MYTHS ABOUT RAPE

Studies of convicted rapists and research with college men who report engaging in sexually coercive and/or aggressive behavior show that these different groups of men have similar beliefs and attitudes about gender and sex that permit them to justify and rationalize their behavior (Drieschner & Lange, 1999; Hersh & Gray-Little, 1998; Malamuth, 1986; Rando, Rogers, Brittan, & Christopher, 1998; Scully & Marolla, 1984). Research also suggests that a large number of people in the general population share these beliefs, which affects their responses to victims and perpetrators (Burt, 1980, 1998; Frazier, Valtinson, & Candell, 1994; Lonsway & Fitzgerald, 1994). Burt (1980) described this constellation of beliefs about gender and sex as "rape supportive" in that they both permit and excuse men's sexually assaultive behavior and lead to a tendency to hold victims responsible for their own victimization. As Burt (1998) concluded: "Rape myths allow rapists to rape with near impunity. They teach women to blame themselves for their own victimization. They transform rape by acquaintances, friends, and intimates into no rape at all. They support the use of violence, coupled with sexuality, as a mechanism for keeping women powerless. . . . The myths make clear to her that avoiding rape is her responsibility and that she will find little sympathy for her situation should she be so careless as to allow herself to be raped" (p. 140).

Myths Regarding Men and Rape

In most rape cases, the rapist is a stranger.

It is true that most rapists who are convicted are unknown by their victims, as stranger rapists are more likely to be successfully prosecuted. The vast majority of victims, however, are raped by someone they know such as an acquaintance, family member, coworker, date, or husband.

Rapists are a small group of "sick men."

Empirical research has generally failed to find consistent patterns of psychopathology that discriminate rapists from nonrapists (Lottes, 1988). Further, researchers have found that sizable numbers of both high school and college men self-report that they have engaged in behaviors that meet the legal definition of rape and/or attempted rape (Bohmer & Parrot, 1993; Koss et al., 1987; Krahe, 1998; Rando et al., 1998).

Some psychological and personality trait differences between sexually aggressive men and non–sexually aggressive men, however, have been documented in both incarcerated and self-report populations. Sexually aggressive men have greater contempt or hostility toward women, anger/power motivations for sexual expression, higher impulsivity, lower empathy, lower femininity and hypermasculinity (Collins, 1987; Hudson & Ward, 1997; Kosson, Kelly, & White, 1997; Lisak & Ivan, 1995; Lisak & Roth, 1990; Quimette, 1997).

Rape is motivated by sexual desire.
Once aroused, a man cannot stop.

The common but false belief that rape is a crime motivated by sexual desire has been one of the most difficult to counter, at least partly because the act of rape involves sexual parts of the body. Yet, as we have noted, rapes are motivated less by sexual desire or need than they are by power and control. Rape can best be understood as sexuality in the service of power, control, and conquest. Some men experience sexual rewards through domination and conquest, just as for others sexual arousal is associated with feelings of love and intimacy. The belief that a man rapes simply because he is sexually desirous or aroused, however, is clearly a myth, as is the notion that, once aroused, he has no control over his actions.

Myths Regarding Women and Rape

Women cry rape to get revenge.

Many people, both in the past and in the present, have assumed that a woman who reported being raped was lying and that men must be protected from the possibility that a vengeful woman could "cry rape" and ruin his life. This seems to be a particularly common response to reports of acquaintance rape. Police reports contradict this assumption, however, since false reports about rape are no more common than false reports for other crimes. Further, statistics on rape incidence and reporting strongly support the conclusion that the majority of women fail to report rape. Underreporting rather than false reporting is the real problem.

A woman who does not resist (who was not beaten) has not really been raped.

The idea that a woman must prove that she resisted being raped with evidence of a physical beating or the presence of a firearm is insidious and dangerous because it implies that a woman should be able to successfully resist a man's sexually as- saultive behavior unless he uses a weapon. A woman should not have to risk fur- ther injury to her life in order to prove that she was raped. The myth that rape is merely sex compounds these beliefs because, as the distorted reasoning goes, if it's just sex and she's not "hurt," or if she had sex before, "What's the big deal?"

A woman cannot be raped by her husband.

The idea that a woman's husband cannot rape her assumes that a married woman has no right to refuse her husband sexually—that he owns her and her body. Al- though it has been a long time since marital law upheld marriage as an institution in which women and children are considered to be a man's property, state crime statutes that maintain marital exclusions in rape definitions perpetuate this idea of marriage. This myth also fails to acknowledge the violent and forcible nature of many marital rapes that occur as part of an ongoing pattern of wife battering (Finkelhor & Yllo, 1985).

She wanted it, deserved it, asked for it.
Women secretly want to be dominated and raped.

The idea that women like to be treated violently and find violence or force sexu- ally stimulating appears to be an inversion of the truth: Many men in our culture have developed a fascination with eroticized violence. Research findings suggest that sexually aggressive men are particularly likely to find sexual aggression a- ttractive and arousing, are less empathetic to victims' suffering, are more likely to have coercive and violent sexual fantasies, and are more likely to be aroused by rape stories (Collins, 1987; Drieschner & Lange, 1999; Malamuth & Donner- stein, 1982; Rice, Chaplin, Harris, & Coutts, 1994). These attitudes and person- ality traits allow sexually aggressive men to reinterpret their own and their vic- tim's behavior in order to justify their view of themselves as seductive and their victim as wanting them (Scully & Marolla, 1984).

Women provoke rape by their dress and behavior.
Nice girls don't get raped.

Numerous social-psychological studies have attempted to examine the impact of various individual characteristics on the likelihood of being raped, including a woman's character, her past sexual history, attractiveness, style of dress, the sex- ual provocativeness of her behavior, and her use of drugs or alcohol. A tacit assumption in all of these studies, closely related to the "she asked for it" myth is that victim characteristics are responsible for the perpetrator's behavior (Koss & Harvey, 1991).

Findings of a major study designed to develop a risk profile for rape using the above victim characteristics plus a range of hypothesized "vulnerability-creating early experiences" and "vulnerability enhancing situations," however, concluded that the major contributing factor to a higher risk of rape was having been sexually abused as a child. The most significant finding was that the vast majority of sexually victimized women could not be differentiated from nonvictims (Koss & Dinero, 1989).

It is true that alcohol and drug use have been implicated in many studies of sexual assault. It appears that the primary impact, however, is their effect on the man, who may be less inhibited about acting in a sexually aggressive manner when drunk or high (Koss & Gaines, 1993; Richardson & Hammock, 1991; Ullman & Brecklin, 2000). Similarly, some men apparently believe that rape is acceptable if the woman has used drugs or is drunk (Goodchilds, Zellman, Johnson, & Giarrusso, 1988; Sanday, 1990; Ullman, Karabatsos, & Koss, 1999).

The idea that women's dress, behavior, or reputation causes rape clearly serves the purpose of denying perpetrators' responsibility for their own behavior and blaming victims instead. Men may disregard women's verbal protests (Koss, 1988), may misinterpret a woman's friendly behavior as sexual (Abbey, 1991; Abbey, McAuslan, & Ross, 1998), and may justify their behavior by blaming their victims (Drieschner & Lange, 1999; Scully & Marolla, 1984). The truth about rape is that rapists want it and perpetrate it, not their victims.

Rape can happen to anyone—of any age, race, cultural background, social group, or sexual orientation. Women are raped in their own homes; in the homes of friends, acquaintances, and family members; in bars, hotels, and cars; at parties; and on the street. When a woman chooses to dress attractively, even sexily, go to a bar and have a drink, dance provocatively, party, and have fun, she is not asking for nor does she deserve to be raped. Rape occurs because of a rapist's behavior, not because of what a woman looks like or how she acts.

THE IMPACT OF RAPE

Rape Poem
by Marge Piercy

There is no difference between being raped
and being pushed down a flight of cement steps
except that the wounds also bleed inside.

There is no difference between being raped
and being run over by a truck
except that afterward men ask if you enjoyed it.

There is no difference between being raped
and being bit on the ankle by a rattlesnake
except that people ask if your skirt was short
and why you were out alone anyhow.

There is no difference between being raped
and going head first through a windshield
except that afterward you are afraid
not of cars
but half the human race.

The rapist is your boyfriend's brother.
He sits beside you in the movies eating popcorn.
Rape fattens on the fantasies of the normal male
like a maggot on garbage.

Fear of rape is a cold wind blowing
all of the time on a woman's hunched back.
Never to stroll alone on a sand road through pine woods,
never to climb a trail across a bald
without that aluminum in the mouth
when I see a man climbing towards me.

Never to open the door to a knock
without that razor just grazing the throat.
The fear of the dark side of hedges,
the back seat of the car, the empty house
rattling keys like a snake's warning.
The fear of the smiling man
in whose pocket is a knife.
The fear of the serious man
in whose fist is locked hatred.

All it takes to cast a rapist is seeing your body
as a jackhammer, as a blowtorch, as adding-machine-gun.
All it takes is hating that body
your own, your self, your muscle that softens to flab.

All it takes is to push what you hate,
what you fear onto the soft alien flesh.
To bucket out invincible as a tank
armored with treads without senses
to possess and punish in one act,
to rip up pleasure, to murder those who dare
live in the leafy flesh open to love.

Reprinted from Marge Piercy, "Rape Poem," in *Circles on the Water*
(New York: Alfred A. Knopf, 1982), 164–165.

Although individual reactions to being sexually assaulted vary considerably, for most victims rape is one of the worst experiences in their lives (Koss, 1993). Rape must always be viewed as a crisis, as a victim's life is inevitably disrupted by it, and although she may be able to integrate her rape experience into her life, it is not something that ever completely goes away or that she will ever simply "get over." Most women experience very high levels of distress in the immediate aftermath of a sexual assault. What is, perhaps, more surprising is the high likelihood of a much longer negative impact. Even years after their sexual victimization, many women survivors continue to exhibit numerous psychological effects, including depressive and anxiety disorders, drug and alcohol abuse, and Posttraumatic Stress Disorder (Atkeson, Calhoun, Resick, & Ellis, 1982; Hutchings & Dutton, 1997; Rothbaum et al., 1992; Zweig et al., 1999).

To describe in professional terms the emotional, cognitive, and physical symptoms experienced by rape survivors is to inevitably fail to capture the terror, the helplessness, and the sense of no longer owning one's own body that is the reality of the trauma of rape. Yet it is essential that crisis counselors recognize the breadth and depth of rape survivors' emotional, psychological, and behavioral reactions.

Ruch and Leon (1983) suggested viewing the long-term impact of rape and a victim's adjustment to it as a longitudinal process. Recovery is affected by the interaction of a number of variables, including the immediate effect of the assault on the victim, her coping mechanisms and preexisting life stressors, the social support she receives, and her status and experiences following the assault in other areas of her life including employment, marriage, and experience within the criminal justice system.

Koss and Harvey (1991) presented an "ecological model" of rape trauma that is compatible with the model used in this text. Assuming that any victim's postrape response is both uniquely individual and multiply determined, this model focuses on the interrelationships between characteristics of the individual victim (e.g., age, development, previous victimization history), the specific rape event that occurred (e.g., number of assailants, physical threat, and bodily injury), and the social environment within which rape recovery must occur (e.g., supportiveness, responsiveness). Research has confirmed that none of these variables taken alone determines the severity of post-rape symptomatology. For example, the severity of violence and the physical injury sustained have been found to significantly predict both Posttraumatic Stress Disorder and depression among rape survivors (Gidycz & Koss, 1990; Kilpatrick, Saunders, Amick-Mullen, Best, Veronen, & Resnick, 1989; Zweig et al., 1999). Other studies, however, have documented that it is not the characteristics of the event alone that determine the survivor's responses, but rather the *victim's perception* of the event (Creamer, Burgess, & Pattison, 1992; Girelli, Resick, Marhoefer-Dvorak, & Hutter, 1986). Thus, regardless of the actual danger she faced, if a woman feared injury and/or threat to her life, she will experience the anxiety reactions likely to emerge in the aftermath of the rape.

The Phases of Recovery

Many clinicians and researchers who have worked with victims of rape have identified typical recuperative patterns or phases of response. Burgess and Holmstrom (1974) coined the term "rape trauma syndrome" to convey the idea that most victims experience a range of common reactions that occur in a relatively predictable pattern. They described a period of acute stress and disorganization immediately following the rape and lasting from one to six months, succeeded by a longer period during which survivors gradually reorganized their lives in order to "maintain a certain equilibrium" (p. 985). Sutherland and Scherl (1970) suggested a middle phase of outward adjustment during which survivors appear to have returned to normal functioning. Notman and Nadelson (1976) described a model of rape recovery with an anticipatory or threat phase, followed by the impact phase, the posttraumatic, or recoil, phase, and finally, the posttraumatic reconstitution phase. Many researchers today investigate rape trauma syndrome primarily through the conceptual lens of PTSD. The following model builds on these ideas.

The impact and immediate aftermath   The initial responses of victims during the actual rape range from disbelief, shock, numbness, and dissociation to extreme terror and feelings of helplessness. Victims routinely describe physiological reactions such as uncontrolled trembling and heart palpitations, and some women report involuntarily vomiting or urinating.

Immediately following the assault most victims are in a state of shock, disbelief, and severe emotional distress. They may overtly react in significantly different ways. Some individuals are emotionally expressive, visibly upset, showing and verbalizing their anger, fear, and/or anxiety. Others are much more controlled, relating details about the assault without affect. These victims appear to be calm, composed, and unaffected, but are actually masking their emotions and feeling numb. Some individuals also attempt to minimize the assault and its effect on them.

Some women may experience crisis reactions that are compounded because the current crisis precipitates the recurrence of symptoms related to previous physical or mental illness and/or previous victimizations. In such instances the individual's responses to the current rape trauma are colored by her previous difficulties and/or reawakened memories. For example, an individual who was molested as a child may find that the rape reactivates unresolved feelings of powerlessness and shame that become intertwined with her responses to the current rape. Research also suggests that women who were victimized in childhood are more likely than those who were not to be victimized again, increasing the likelihood of compounding reactions (Koss & Dinero, 1989; van der Kolk, 1989).

In the immediate aftermath of the rape, victims also experience a range of physical reactions and fears. Some of these physical effects—bruising, soreness, generalized genital or anal pain, and genital or anal bleeding and/or itching—are the direct result of the assault. Physical fears regarding pregnancy and sexually transmitted diseases, including HIV infection, are common. Immediate attention to physical effects is thus extremely important.

In the days and weeks that follow a rape, most victims continue to experience a high level of emotional reactivity. Nervousness and generalized anxiety are common, as are specific fears related to being alone, meeting the attacker, experiencing further injury or threat, and fears of legal processes and the reactions of others. Many anxiety-related symptoms, including nightmares and startle responses, are likely. In the immediate aftermath of rape nearly everyone experiences intrusive and repetitive thoughts and images of what they experienced (Creamer et al., 1992; Foa & Rothbaum, 1998).

Depressive symptoms, including crying spells, sleep and eating disturbances, and fatigue are also prominent during this early recovery period (Atkeson et al., 1982). Because many rapes involve a degree of degradation, and women may have been forced to say or do things that humiliated them, they may also experience feelings of shame, self-blame, guilt, and embarrassment.

For many women, despite efforts to block the images and memories, thoughts of the assault occur repeatedly. Many women also expend considerable energy trying to figure out how they could have avoided the assault, struggling with a constant barrage of "if only I had . . ." thoughts.

Outward adjustment   As noted, Sutherland and Scherl (1970) suggested a middle phase of recovery during which victims appear to have returned to normal functioning. Also characterized as a "denial phase" (Forman, 1980), it appears to be a period during which victims attempt to forget the assault, to believe that it is an event of the past, and to get on with everyday life. Although they often resume normal activities, Forman compared this to the denial phase of grief in that it is a time of going through the motions rather than a period of actual resolution.

Trauma survivors often mobilize conscious strategies to avoid the arousal induced by memories of the trauma. If these efforts at avoidance are unsuccessful, an unconscious physiological shutting down may occur, resulting in the numbing and dissociative symptoms of the PTSD disorder.

Crisis reactivation and reorganization   For some individuals, the denial/outward adjustment phase is interrupted when images and emotional and psychological responses to the rape begin to return or can no longer be avoided. Sometimes precipitated by a particular catalyst—a smell, an image, a situation—sometimes seemingly out of nowhere, dreams and nightmares return, fears and anxieties reemerge, feelings of helplessness, vulnerability, and alienation crowd out the previous aura of normalcy. Many survivors begin to avoid friends and/or family, drop out of school, or stay home from work. They may begin to have an array of increasingly debilitating physical and psychological symptoms.

For some victims the obvious catalyst for experiencing crisis symptoms again is the beginning or continuation of criminal proceedings. Legal delays and continuances are common and can be extremely disruptive emotionally. A woman may barely have begun to return to her normal routines when another action or lack of action in the criminal process reactivates the trauma symptoms. A victim cannot successfully integrate and resolve her rape experience until criminal justice processes have ended.

When problematic symptoms recur, survivors must find a means of coping with them to restore a modicum of equilibrium. This is what Burgess and Holmstrom (1974) referred to as "reorganization." It is the phase of recovery in which the individual is forced, because of reliving the trauma incident and her reactions to it, to develop coping mechanisms to deal with those reactions. Some women develop maladaptive coping mechanisms if they suppress their memories and accompanying emotions or withdraw and isolate themselves from situations and social relationships that precipitate their responses. In such instances a woman's life may remain compromised indefinitely by the sexual assault trauma. Other women find a means to achieve long-term integration and resolution of the experience. If a woman declares her need for assistance, this is a good time for crisis counseling intervention.

For some rape survivors, the range and type of symptoms experienced and the degree of impairment of functioning that results is so severe that it meets both the symptom and duration criteria for PTSD. Studies examining the prevalence of PTSD have noted that the vast majority of rape victims experience the symptoms (although not the duration criteria) for a diagnosis of PTSD (now labeled Acute Stress Disorder) in the immediate aftermath of a sexual assault. This number gradually declines, with slightly less than 50 percent meeting the symptom criteria three to six months later. Women who did not evidence ASD/PTSD symptoms at three months post-assault showed progressive improvement over the following six-month period. For those who did evidence symptoms, however, there was no significant improvement and there was increased risk of persistent symptoms (Amir, Foa, & Cashman, 1998; Rothbaum et al., 1992).

The resolution/integration phase   The concept of resolution as applied to rape implies that the victim is no longer experiencing the debilitating symptoms of the impact and/or crisis reactivation phases. This means that she no longer struggles with recurring thoughts and nightmares nor does she expend her energy suppressing such thoughts and images lest those memories create intolerable arousal. She has overcome symptoms of anxiety, depression, and sexual dysfunction; has reconnected with others; and has developed ways of comprehending her experience that recognize her strengths and eliminate self-blaming and shame. She has become a trauma survivor.

Unfortunately, many rape victims never reach this stage of resolution; the enduring nature of symptomatic problems of fear, anxiety, hyperalertness, depression, sexual dysfunction, nightmares, and flashbacks among rape victims is well documented (Burnam, Stein, Golding, Siegel, Sorenson, Forsythe, & Telles, 1988; Calhoun, Atkeson, & Resick, 1982; Ellis et al., 1981). Large-scale studies of rape victims at varying time intervals following the sexual assault conclude that, compared to nonvictims, rape victims are significantly more likely to reveal psychological distress and to qualify for various psychiatric diagnoses including major depressive disorders, anxiety and panic disorders, alcohol abuse/dependence disorders, and Posttraumatic Stress Disorder (Hutchings & Dutton, 1997; Resick & Schnicke, 1993; Rothbaum et al., 1992; Winfield, George, Swartz, & Blazer, 1990).

SINGLE-SESSION CRISIS COUNSELING

Retrospective studies with rape victims reveal a common pattern of not seeking counseling intervention in the immediate aftermath of sexual assault. For example, one study of college student rape victims revealed that only 4 percent of them had contacted rape crisis centers (Koss, 1988), and even those who received emergency medical treatment and were offered ongoing supportive counseling were unlikely to follow through (Kilpatrick & Veronen, 1983). In fact, rape victims were less likely than other crime victims to disclose their victimization *to anyone* (Koss, Woodruff, & Koss, 1991; Mills & Granoff, 1992).

Rape victims who are seen by crisis workers in the immediate aftermath of a rape are usually seen in hospital emergency rooms, rape crisis centers, university counseling centers, or, very rarely, by private counselors. Some communities have developed collaborative sexual assault teams involving hospitals, police, prosecutors, and rape crisis centers, which have the potential to increase the likelihood that victims will receive crisis intervention services as well as pursue prosecution of perpetrators.

As we have stated, the range of victims' initial responses to rape are quite predictable, and although there are certainly compounding factors and some differences relating to ethnicity, religiosity, and related beliefs about gender and sexual violence, responses to the trauma of rape are fairly common.

The goals of crisis intervention with rape victims center on ensuring their immediate safety, both physically and emotionally, and helping them connect with other personal and social supports and resources. The goals of single-session interventions are limited, and it is not assumed that resolution of the assault will occur as the result. It is hoped that efforts to reduce a woman's emotional distress, enhance her coping, and help her connect with other sources of support and resource will prevent the emergence of maladaptive strategies for achieving equilibrium.

Because rape is extremely traumatizing, most victims are likely to be quite vulnerable and ill prepared to cope with insensitive or judgmental treatment. Thus all crisis intervention with rape victims should be nonstigmatizing and non-blaming. The crisis worker should never make a determination about whether or not the victim's experience was a legally defined rape. Rather, the role of the crisis worker is to accept what the victim says and to help her deal with her responses. It is often prudent to avoid labeling what happened as a rape or sexual assault. Intervention should include the dimensions described below, not necessarily in order; depending on the individual situation, some aspects of intervention must take precedence to others.

From first contact to termination, the crisis worker must listen carefully to comprehend the victim's sense of what happened and the manner in which she is reacting. As the single-session model presented suggests, crisis workers also must continuously assess how the individual is responding emotionally, behaviorally, and cognitively. The crisis worker must also listen for indications of how the victim's developmental level and recovery environment are affecting her responses. This is not a single step or phase of intervention, but rather a way of listening and trying to make sense of what one is hearing that occurs throughout engagement with the victim. The purpose of such continuous assessment is to guide the crisis worker to make the most appropriate interventions.

Step 1:
Supportively and empathically join with the client.

Unless a rape victim experiences the crisis worker as genuine, accepting, empathic, and supportive, she will be unlikely to reveal enough to benefit from crisis services. Rape victims have been made to feel powerless, have been degraded, humiliated, and used as objects for the gratification of their assailants. They are likely to feel scared, worried, confused, and helpless. They may also feel guilty, ashamed, soiled, and/or damaged by what has occurred.

Crisis counselors must convey their acceptance of the rape survivor and must validate her behaviors during and after the rape. Counselors can convey their acceptance through active listening, a calm and respectful demeanor, and responses that convey understanding, support, and reassurance. Counselors should acknowledge the difficulty of what a survivor has been through, her efforts to take care of herself, and her ability to survive. Counselor responses should also emphasize the perpetrator's responsibility for what occurred.

Counselor empathy also contributes to establishing a supportive relationship. The crisis worker can and should express empathy, even when the client fails to overtly identify or reveal her emotions. In cases with more controlled or inexpressive victims the crisis worker can comment on how overwhelmed/upset/distressed the individual must feel, and how understandable it is to *"not want to allow yourself to feel."* Koss and Harvey (1991) suggested that there are several helpful expressions that crisis workers should memorize for use with rape victims. They include *"I am so sorry this happened to you," "You're safe now," "No matter what you did, you did not deserve to be a victim of a crime,"* and *"I know you handled the situation right because you're alive"* (p. 166).

Step 2:
Intervene to create safety, stabilize the victim, and handle her immediate needs.

In addition to handling rape victims' overwhelming emotional needs, counselors must routinely address other immediate needs such as determining which of their significant family members and/or friends to contact for support and whether and how to attend to medical needs. In some situations, as in the case of Wendy described at the beginning of the chapter, a first-order need may be to reach a safe location and/or to attain sufficient emotional control to be able to act to seek assistance.

Seek support from significant others   It is very important that rape victims receive support and acceptance from the significant persons in their life. Unfortunately, many victims are quite fearful about disclosing what has happened for fear of how others will react, and some victims insist that they wish to tell no one. It is helpful to discuss with them both the importance of support from significant others and the victim's concerns or fears about others' expected responses. The victim may benefit from assistance in strategizing how to tell family members, and in some instances may ask you to notify someone directly.

Family members often have their own crisis reactions in hearing about their loved one's victimization, and counseling of family members may be warranted. Interventions with family members can assist them with their own responses and prepare them to support the victim. Approaches for working with family members are discussed in more detail later in this chapter.

Encourage victim to receive medical care   Counselors should strongly encourage all rape victims to receive medical care whether there are serious physical injuries or not. In some cases there are obvious physical injuries—lacerations, possible broken bones, vaginal and/or anal tissue tears—that require immediate medical attention. Even in cases without such overt injury, however, it is extremely important that victims be treated preventively for pregnancy and sexually transmitted diseases, including AIDS. When examining a victim of a possible sexual assault, hospitals are required to utilize a standardized rape evidence collection procedure. This collection of forensic evidence occurs whether or not the individual victim has decided to notify police. The evidence is kept safe—so it will be available should the individual later decide to pursue legal action.

The *idea* of a medical examination is frequently unappealing to victims, and the actual examination may feel like a revictimization. In ideal circumstances medical personnel who examine rape victims have been specially trained to handle their needs sensitively. The crisis worker can also prepare the victim by explaining the purposes and components of the examination. It is always desirable for someone to accompany the victim during the examination if she so desires. This may be a friend or family member or it may be the crisis worker or a specially trained nurse. Most important is that the individuals who interact with the victim be sensitive to her trauma and accepting of her responses.

The medical examination serves three purposes simultaneously: (1) to identify and treat physical injuries, (2) to collect forensic evidence, and (3) to prevent sexually transmitted disease and pregnancy. A gynecologist should conduct the examination and it should include the following procedures, although not necessarily in this particular order. This information is compiled from various hospital procedure manuals, victim resource guides, and the guidelines presented by the Boston Women's Health Collective in *Our Bodies, Ourselves* (1998).

1. Any serious physical injuries requiring medical attention are treated immediately. If there are no emergency physical injuries, the sexual assault examination begins.
2. A brief gynecological medical history is taken, including information about menstruation, contraceptive practices, and sexually transmitted diseases, as well as specific information about the sexual assault. This is necessary so that medical personnel are aware of any pre-assault information that might be relevant (e.g., possible pregnancy) and to guide them about what types of possible injuries and evidence to look for.
3. A physical examination of the external genitalia and internal genitals is conducted. Evidence of physical trauma including lacerations and contusions is documented and treated, if necessary. The internal examination allows the physician to view the cervix and the inside of the vagina. The doctor also performs a bimanual examination, pressing one hand on the victim's abdomen, and inserting the fingers of the other hand into the vagina.
4. Samples of pubic hair are taken both by combing the pubic area and by plucking pubic hairs from the victim. This allows identification of loose hairs that may contain the assailant's pubic hairs and plucked pubic hairs known to belong to the victim.
5. Visual observations to determine the presence of sperm are conducted and swabs are taken of the oral and rectal areas as well as other areas around the mouth, neck, breasts, and thighs, where there might be sperm.
6. Blood samples are drawn in order to determine blood type and enzyme characteristics for comparison with an identified suspect.
7. An antibiotic is routinely given for the prevention of sexually transmitted diseases (STDs). Some STDs, such as syphilis and AIDS, cannot be detected immediately, and diagnosis requires follow-up testing.
8. In most states hospital emergency room personnel are not legally required to discuss the possibility of pregnancy and the potential actions the victim may wish to consider. Thus some medical staff volunteer the following information and provide accompanying services, and others do not. If an individual victim fears pregnancy, she has several options, all of which should be explained to her so that she can make an informed choice.
   a. She can request emergency contraceptive drugs that prevent implantation of a fertilized egg in the uterus if taken correctly beginning within seventy-two hours of intercourse. There are possible side effects to the use of these drugs, which should not be taken by women with certain preexisting medical conditions. A prescribing physician should take a complete medical history and conduct a thorough examination. This treatment cannot be given to a woman who suspects she is already pregnant. A woman who suspects preexisting pregnancy should be given a pregnancy test first.
   b. She can await her next menses and, if it is late, seek an immediate menstrual extraction; in this procedure the cervix is dilated and the contents of the uterus are suctioned clean. Or she can wait longer, and if pregnancy is diagnosed, determine whether to continue the pregnancy or to have an early

first-trimester therapeutic abortion. This type of abortion most often utilizes the same method used to suction the uterus in menstrual extraction.

9. Photographs should be taken of visible injuries. Because bruises often do not show up until two to three days after a rape, victims should be encouraged to return to the hospital to be reexamined (and photographed) for bruising.

Most of the time medical personnel conduct the medical examination appropriately and collect the appropriate evidence. Hospitals with specially trained staff do a better job on many levels than hospitals without specially trained staff, and better evidence collection and treatment of survivors is likely to lead to better cases for prosecution and conviction. The growing cooperation and collaboration between the various systems serving sexual assault victims enhances the likelihood that victims will receive appropriate medical care and that forensic evidence will be collected. The remaining struggle for those who provide crisis services and serve as advocates for rape victims, however, is to ensure that the goals of the criminal justice system do not take precedence over a victim's emotional and psychological needs. The role of the crisis worker is thus to always keep the needs of the victim paramount. This means ensuring that she is informed about all medical procedures, advocating for her, if necessary, and continuously reinforcing her right to be treated with understanding and sensitivity and to make informed choices regarding her medical care.

Step 3:
Explore and assess the dimensions of the crisis and the client's reaction to the crisis, and encourage her to talk and ventilate.

Encourage the victim to talk and express emotions.

It is very helpful for the victim of a traumatic experience to be able to talk about what happened and to express his or emotions and thoughts about it. For many victims, heightened physical and emotional arousal increases the need to talk about what they have been through. With minimal encouragement from a crisis worker, many victims will thus relate with some detail the events that occurred. For more withdrawn or reticent individuals, counseling probes can serve as a catalyst (e.g., *"Where were you when it happened?" "What ran through your head when he first approached you?"*). Usually such open questions are all that is necessary to enable the individual to begin to communicate about what occurred.

The most important focus of ventilation should be the victim's feelings and emotions rather than specific details about the assault. The crisis worker can facilitate the ventilation of emotions by probing that focuses on how the victim was feeling or reacting and by responding to the victim with acceptance and empathic understanding.

As the victim tells her story to an empathic and interested listener, her experience may gradually lose some of its power. As she shares what occurred, she is no longer alone with the images and feelings and she can be assisted to challenge maladaptive thoughts about herself and her role during the assault. Ventilation, or simply getting out overwhelming thoughts and feelings, can begin the process of desensitizing the experience and decreasing attendant emotional and physiological arousal.

Assess her reaction to the crisis.

As the rape victim ventilates and tells her story, the crisis counselor listens for the purpose of comprehending her needs, strengths, and resources in all areas of functioning (ABCDE). The crisis counselor must watch, listen to, and assess her affective style, her behavioral and somatic responses, her thoughts and perceptions about what has occurred and its meaning, who she is developmentally, and what the environment surrounding her entails. When information regarding each of these components is not spontaneously forthcoming, crisis workers can facilitate attention to those areas with a simple probe. For example, *"What is going through your mind at this point?"* (cognitive probe), or *"How did your friend respond when he started pushing you out the door?"* (probe regarding situational context). The purpose of such comprehensiveness is that the crisis worker intervenes with appropriate attention to the unique needs and concerns of each individual.

Step 4:
Identify and examine alternative actions and develop options.

Rape victims have many decisions to make in the aftermath of the assault. Two of those choices are whom to tell and whether to seek medical care. Another difficult decision for most victims is whether or not to notify police or other authorities. Some hospitals notify the police of a rape automatically. The victim, however, can still determine whether or not she is willing to cooperate as a witness and report information about what occurred. The following information is compiled from various community and university police procedures for responding to sexual assault complaints.

Inform victim of police procedures for sexual assault cases.

If a victim of rape contacts the police immediately following a sexual assault, the first concern of the police dispatcher, as of the crisis worker, should be to find out whether the victim is in a safe place. If the police go to the scene of the crime they need to take action to preserve the scene and gather evidence. They need to obtain basic facts from the victim concerning what happened and the name and/or description of the assailant. The investigating officer(s) should attend to the victim's immediate emotional needs, advise the victim to seek medical treatment, accompany or transport her, if needed, and offer the services of a rape crisis worker, if one is available.

If the police are contacted after the victim is already at the hospital or at another location, the officer still needs to question the victim in order to obtain information regarding the victim herself (e.g., name, age, address, marital status, children, prior relationship with the suspect); the suspect; any witnesses who may have seen the victim and/or the perpetrator either before, during, or after the assault; and the details of the offense itself. It is helpful to inform victims about what to expect during the police interview so they are prepared to be asked for very specific information about what occurred. Some victims experience the police questioning as too invasive or assume it reflects the police officer's disbelief, blame, or judgment of her. If a victim is made aware of the necessity of such questions in order for the police to pursue her case, however, she may be somewhat less likely to experience the interview in a negative way.

Upon completion of the interview, the officer should make sure that the victim will be available the following day because a detective will need to interview her for her formal statement to the police. The officer should also be available to transport the victim home and to make arrangements to patrol the victim's neighborhood if the assault took place there. When police have obtained information about the assault and the assailant, an "all points bulletin" should be issued immediately. The investigating officer(s) then write, in their own words, the victim's account, as reported to them.

The police may or may not allow the crisis worker to be present during the police interview. Some police department procedures allow a third party to be present, whereas others, usually at the suggestion of prosecutors, do not. Police procedures must be respected. Following the interview, it is helpful to clarify with the victim what steps the police will follow and what she can expect from them next.

Provide respite.

Rape victims are likely to experience a short-term impairment in their ability to function and perform everyday responsibilities. It is thus helpful to encourage the rape survivor to consider taking a few days off from school or work or asking for assistance in caring for her children. A brief respite from meeting others' needs and expectations may be helpful; it will give her time to tend to her personal physical and emotional needs as well as to follow up with other contacts (e.g., police, medical or counseling care) if she wishes. It is important for the crisis worker to help the victim realistically evaluate her need for a brief time out without suggesting that she is now incapable of functioning. For some victims, attending to normal parenting and/or family responsibilities is in itself a means of coping and staying in connection with others.

Make a safety plan.

Because fear, helplessness, and loss of a sense of security and control are among the most common reactions following a sexual assault, it is important to consider alternatives regarding where a woman can go so she will feel safe. In some instances, such as when the crisis worker is seeing the victim in a hospital emergency room, the individual may not yet have even returned to her home. If the victim does not bring up the issue of where to go, the crisis worker should initiate a discussion concerning alternatives.

If the victim was assaulted in her home, at her place of work or school, or in her neighborhood, it is unlikely she will feel safe returning to those places until the rapist has been apprehended. In such cases it may be helpful for her to consider staying with a friend or family member either until the perpetrator is in custody or until she is able to make other arrangements that increase her sense of safety. Many victims ultimately relocate their residence, leave their job, and/or transfer to another school. Although these decisions should not be made as part of single-session crisis intervention, crisis workers must assist victims to make immediate practical arrangements to address what may be very legitimate fears, particularly if a rapist is still at large.

Step 5:
Help the victim mobilize personal and social resources.

One key component of being in crisis for some sexual assault victims is the experience of being immobilized, unable to summon their normal personal coping capacities to effective use. Rape is about power and control, thus being victimized by rape is about the experience of powerlessness. As Herman (1997) described, "Traumatic reactions occur when action is of no avail. When neither resistance nor escape is possible, the human system of self-defense becomes overwhelmed and disorganized" (p. 34). This sense of powerlessness and of the futility of action often continues beyond the period during the actual assault.

Thus in the immediate aftermath of a sexual assault, victims may experience a sense of being stuck—stuck in their emotions, immobilized in their behavior and problem solving. Finding it difficult to know how to respond, they may either do nothing or engage in "self-canceling behaviors" (Myer, 2001).

It is essential that rape victims who experience such immobility in the aftermath of an assault be helped to identify personal strengths and resources that they can draw on and specific steps that they can take. We have already discussed the process of examining alternatives. Part of enabling individuals to follow through with the options they agree to is helping them think about the tools and strengths they have within themselves and in their interpersonal networks. This includes helping victims identify the strengths already exhibited in surviving the actual assault and seeking help. It also includes helping them identify the strengths they usually draw on when faced with difficult circumstances. Even though sexual assault is uniquely traumatic, victims must draw on strengths honed in other experiences to cope.

Assisting clients to mobilize support also includes identifying those individuals in their network of family and friends on whom they can lean for support, and possibly intervening with them to enhance the likelihood that their responses will indeed be helpful. And last, this step includes connecting the rape victim with other community resources that can provide additional assistance and/or follow-up, including rape crisis centers and victim assistance programs.

Step 6:
Anticipate the future and arrange follow-up contact.

Educate the victim about symptomatic responses to rape.

Preparing victims for the types of physical and emotional reactions they may experience in the days, weeks, and months following the assault is helpful to them. It is also important to inform victims about the types of services that are available to assist them. In describing what to expect, the crisis worker's narrative should attempt to normalize the victim's reactions while simultaneously acknowledging how upsetting such reactions may be. Statements suggesting that nearly everyone experiences some physical and/or emotional problems after a rape are helpful, particularly if the crisis worker describes the kinds of symptoms that may occur. For example, Koss and Harvey (1991) suggested the following statement: *"Nearly everyone experiences some psychological problems after a rape. Particularly upsetting are nightmares or flashbacks of the experience and the feeling that you need to talk about your experience over and over again until everyone around you is fed up. These are normal psychological processes that operate after a major trauma. . . ."* (p. 174). Similarly, the crisis worker might describe the types of somatic symptoms and/or sexual difficulties that victims may experience. Each of these examples illustrates the crisis worker's responsibility to help victims anticipate distressing symptoms without pathologizing her responses.

Offer follow-up contact and referrals.

Many victims do not pursue any services following a sexual assault. It is nonetheless helpful to offer such follow-up services. The crisis worker can request permission to follow up with a phone call or can offer an appointment for a follow-up counseling session. Or the crisis worker can merely mention the availability of such follow-up services, either immediately or at a later time, should the victim desire them, and provide her with cards with names and phone numbers. In any case, the victim's decisions must be respected, and suggestions for follow-up and/or referrals must be made in a manner that empowers the victim to begin to regain some control over her life.

CRISIS INTERVENTION WITH FAMILIES AND PARTNERS

Rape is a crisis for victims and victims' families and loved ones alike. As we have noted, social support is a primary factor affecting victims' immediate and long-term adjustment to assault. Further, as van der Kolk and McFarlane (1996) noted, the personal meaning of a traumatic experience is influenced by the social context in which it occurs. The responses of significant others to victims is therefore extremely important for crisis workers who are assisting victims. Crisis intervention with partners of victims and/or other significant family members can be helpful in at least two interrelated ways: (1) it can enhance the likelihood that responses to the victim are supportive and helpful, and (2) it can facilitate family members' efforts to cope with their own crisis reactions.

Unfortunately, research suggests that families are not always as supportive and helpful as would be optimal. Family members may have the same mistaken beliefs and/or attitudes about rape found in the general public, and may thus make different assessments about what happened and the extent to which victims have been harmed. They also may have "strongly conflicting agendas to repair, create, forget, or take revenge" (McFarlane & van der Kolk, 1996, p. 27). They may respond with blame, suspicion, and/or resentment toward the victim, injuring the victim a second time, sometimes leaving deeper scars than the rape itself (Lifton, 1983; Symonds, 1982).

Responses of Male Partners and Family Members

Research suggests that men are more likely to believe myths about rape and thus are more likely to respond to the sexual aspects of the assault (Lanier, Elliott, Martin, & Kapadia, 1998; Tescavage, 1999). Although some male partners or family members may directly express anger and/or suspicion to a rape victim, it is more common for those who do not understand the nature of rape to respond by criticizing the victim for "not being careful" or wondering out loud whether she "did something" to attract or entice the perpetrator. This is particularly likely in acquaintance rape situations. Also, because some males view their female partners as belonging to them, they may see a partner who has been sexually assaulted as being in some way tainted or devalued. Although such attitudes may be very offensive to the crisis worker, it is important to respond in a manner that enables mates to work through their own feelings of fear, loss, devaluation, and shame (Benedict, 1985; Rodkin, Hunt, & Cowan, 1982; Silverman, 1978).

Fathers, brothers, and male partners may also verbalize their desire to violently punish the perpetrator on behalf of their daughter/sister/partner. As Silverman (1978) described, although such thoughts of revenge may protect the man against his own sense of helplessness and impotent rage, these threats and/or actions may additionally burden the victim with fears about what he will do and the possibility of further harm. In such cases the victim may end up calming, placating, and reassuring the men in her family, rather than having them available to support her. One study with men who were participating in a support group for male relatives of rape victims found that they, too, went through phases of crisis response (Rodkin et al., 1982). Initially, many of the men experienced the same fears and anxieties as the victim; however, their symptoms subsided much more quickly. The second phase of response was a protective stage during which the men, many of whom irrationally experienced guilt for their own failure to protect the victim, became overprotective. And last, many became impatient with the victim and her continued trauma responses and then physically and/or emotionally withdrew, leaving victims feeling abandoned and without support.

Responses of Other Family Members

Males are certainly not the only ones to believe rape mythology; some cultural and/or religious groups, especially those with very traditional beliefs about gender and women's roles, are even more likely to blame victims. For example:

Melinda revealed to her parents that she had been sexually assaulted in her older cousin's recreation room by a group of his friends. Her parents responded, questioning her about both her behavior and the truthfulness of her account. Her father, a deacon in his fundamentalist Christian church, required her to watch a video published by the church describing how "good Christian girls" make choices that prevent them from being in "compromising" situations. Her cousin was never confronted and she was never taken for counseling by her parents.

Responses such as this are quite likely to revictimize the victim. Even family members who do not adhere to such patently victim-blaming attitudes may respond to victims in ways that are not helpful, however. Family members may be overprotective and inadvertently reinforce the victim's sense of herself as helpless, thus preventing her from using her strengths as an aid in coping. Another common but unhelpful response is to try and distract the victim and to encourage her to not think about what happened. In some families the victim may be encouraged to protect other family members by not telling them about the assault. As Silverman (1978) noted, "The impact of such a stance is to deprive the woman of the opportunity to mourn the personal loss inherent in her rape experience, deny her much needed support, and communicate by inference that 'What's happened is simply too terrible to discuss,' confirming the victim's worst fears and doubts" (p. 171).

Intervening with Family Members: Ventilation and Education

Intervention with family members is designed to give them a safe and accepting place to reveal their own responses to the sexual assault. In individual sessions, which do not include the victim, crisis workers can gently and uncritically help family members unearth and share their questions and concerns as well as their often ambivalent reactions and feelings. This allows the crisis worker to empathically support family members and also provides the opportunity to educate families and partners about the actual nature of rape and its impact.

Important information to be shared with family members includes (1) explanations of rape as a crime of power and control rather than sex, (2) details about what to expect as predictable emotional and physical responses to the rape (e.g., emergence of nightmares, anxiety, fear), and (3) ideas about how to provide a supportive environment that allows the victim to release her feelings and fears yet assists her to mobilize her strengths and coping abilities. It is important to help family members understand that although there is no magical way they can make everything better, their ability to provide an emotionally supportive environment will ultimately be indispensable to the victim's recovery (Silverman, 1978).

ONGOING CRISIS COUNSELING FOR SEXUAL ASSAULT SURVIVORS

Sexual victimization frequently has a long-lasting negative impact on survivors' emotional and physical health. Although the majority of rape victims do not seek counseling assistance immediately following the sexual assault, some do, and when the negative emotional and/or relational effects become sufficiently disruptive, other survivors seek crisis counseling as well. This could be six months or six years or more after the assault occurred.

According to one study, the primary reasons for finally seeking help included persistent physical and emotional symptoms, breakups or arguments with romantic partners, withdrawal of support by family or friends, and difficulty in resuming normal sexual relations (Stewart, Hughes, Frank, Anderson, Kendall, & West, 1987). Because victims may not initially identify their sexual assault history when seeking counseling, it is generally recommended that crisis workers ask all clients (women, in particular) about experiences of violence or unwanted sexual activity as a part of routine screening and assessment.

The Counseling Relationship and Sexual Assault Survivors

When a woman presents for counseling a long time after the actual assault, she has often developed strong self-protective defenses that make it quite difficult for her to talk about what happened and to believe that she can trust the counselor not to judge her. Thus establishing a strong, trusting relationship is a prerequisite to the difficult and painful process of revisiting a previous sexual assault. Ultimately, healing from and resolving rape depend on the survivor's regaining a sense of control and power; thus the helping relationship must discourage dependency and submissiveness and enable the client to permit and sustain an intimate professional relationship.

Herman (1997) described the core experiences of any psychological trauma, including sexual assault, as disempowerment and disconnection from others. During sexual victimization one is powerless to halt the assault and/or to escape, and the victim experiences this very personal invasion alone. Frequently it is a known, perhaps trusted, individual who perpetrates the assault. Recovery thus necessitates both a renewed sense of personal power and the reestablishment of connections to others. Herman noted: "Recovery can take place only within the context of relationships, it cannot occur in isolation" (p. 133).

The helping relationship must therefore be one that restores control to the sexual assault survivor. This requires that the crisis counselor be committed to allowing and encouraging the survivor to take charge of her own life, and that the counselor restrain from advancing his or her own agenda about the correct decisions to be made. The counselor must communicate this stance both verbally and in actions that convey respect and support to the individual as she struggles to come to terms with the assault and its impact.

Preliminary and Ongoing Assessment of Rape Resolution

The primary purpose of initial assessment is to determine to what extent an individual's current difficulties are related to the sexual assault experience and aftermath and to what degree and in what ways the sexual assault remains unresolved. It is also important to comprehensively identify her current problems and needs, personal strengths, resources, and sources of support.

When a sexual assault history is identified, a number of criteria can be considered to assess whether the rape is resolved (Burgess & Holmstrom, 1979; Forman, 1980, 1983; Koss & Harvey, 1991). The criteria include (1) the individual's avoidance of or inability to talk about the assault without either "emotional glibness or overreacting" (Forman, 1983, p. 518); (2) self-blame and continued indicators of guilt; (3) negative changes in sexual functioning and/or intimate relationships; (4) presence of a variety of other symptoms that appear to have emerged or worsened following the sexual assault, including phobias and persistent fears, somatic complaints, excessive alcohol or drug abuse; and (5) elevated levels of anxiety or depression. Unresolved sexual trauma is most likely to occur when the victim has been unable to share information about the assault and receive support and assistance to work through her reactions (Burgess & Holmstrom, 1979).

The counselor must consider each of the areas identified in the developmental-ecological model of assessment presented in this text, including the individual's affective functioning, coping behaviors, cognition and ways of attributing meaning to what has occurred, developmental needs as affected by the assault, and the ecology or context of her recovery environment. Knowledge of the impact of sexual assault prepares the crisis counselor to explore and comprehend both the individual's needs and strengths. Assessment is a continuous process that evolves as ongoing crisis counseling progresses.

Goals and Processes of Ongoing Crisis Counseling with Sexual Assault Survivors

Affect stability:
Assist the survivor to express and process her memories and emotions related to the rape.

Some women may initially be reluctant to talk about a sexual assault, believing that she should no longer be reacting to it and/or that her current reactions are abnormal. Alternatively, some women may conclude that their endless thinking and talking about the rape indicates that they are not making progress in "getting over it." In both cases, the women must be reassured both that their reactions are normal and that thinking and talking about what occurred is a necessary part of the healing process.

Foa and Rothbaum (1998) theorized that in the initial period following a traumatic event, individuals engage in "emotional reprocessing," whereby they relive the event in their minds, remembering all of the details of what happened, the thoughts associated with it, and all the attendant emotions (e.g., dread, fear, horror). When the frequency and intensity of emotional reprocessing decrease over time, individuals begin to recover from the crisis. For some individuals, however, this decline does not occur, and fears, anxieties, obsessions, nightmares, and other intrusive emotional responses persist.

Some authors have suggested that when clients report continuing symptoms the crisis counselor should explain that the counseling process most useful for rape resolution is one in which she talks about her memories of the rape in a manner that comes close to her reliving it (Foa & Rothbaum, 1998; Foa, Rothbaum, Riggs, & Murdock, 1991; Koss & Harvey, 1991). The counselors should inform the client in advance that this is a painful and difficult process, but that it will return the control lost during and after the rape as she found herself powerless to control the nightmares, flashbacks, and phobias that continue to haunt her. Foa and Rothbaum (1998) suggested giving crisis clients the following rationale for engaging in this painful process:

> We are going to focus on the fears that you are experiencing, and your difficulty in coping, both of which are directly related to your assault. . . . Although most of the symptoms that you and I have talked about gradually decline with time after the trauma, some of these symptoms endure and continue to cause marked distress for many victims like yourself. . . . A major factor that prevents recovery is avoidance. . . . It is quite normal for people to want to escape or avoid memories, situations, thoughts, and feelings that are painful and distressing. However, though the strategy of avoiding painful experiences works in the short run, it actually prolongs the posttrauma reactions and prevents you from getting over your trauma related difficulties. . . . When you confront the painful experiences rather than avoiding them, you will have the opportunity to process the traumatic experience, and the pain will gradually lessen. . . . (p. 145)

It is important to empower the client to verbally agree to this process and to stop or discuss the process at any time. The counselor may also explicitly explain, particularly to a highly resistant client, that it is the counselor's responsibility to refocus the client on the work of rape resolution if the client has agreed that is the counseling goal. Some clients may need continual encouragement to stay focused on this part of the work, and may require considerable support to be able to bring up and relive their painful memories and reactions.

Roseanne is a thirty-two-year-old woman who was sexually assaulted by three men when she was fifteen years old. She told her mother and father, who blamed her because she had left the house after being told to stay at home and had gone to a place she had been warned not to go. Roseanne has seen numerous counselors previously for depression and alcohol abuse, but she has never discussed the sexual assault. When she revealed the assault to her present counselor Roseanne acknowledged that she knew she had to talk about it but was very afraid to do so. She and the counselor talked about her fears, and Roseanne decided that she wanted to go ahead and try to deal with it after all these years. Several sessions later, realizing that Roseanne's focus was always on current crises, leaving no time to work on the assault, the counselor challenged Roseanne to examine whether this was a pattern of avoidance. They contracted that the counselor would be more directive in bringing her to the topic of the assault and in supporting her in staying with the memories when they became frightening. They also discussed again the fact that Roseanne was in control and could stop or slow down at any time.

Koss and Harvey (1991) suggested that when there are high levels of anxiety surrounding verbalizing memories, techniques such as deep breathing or muscle relaxation should be taught both as a means of helping the client gain greater calm and control, and to "promote counterconditioning wherein a new set of responses can become associated with the memories" (p. 188).

Behavioral adjustments:
Assist the survivor to make and sustain necessary behavioral changes.

Efforts to process memories of a previous trauma should never proceed without attention to a client's safety. This means that if a client is suicidal or engaged in self-destructive behavior, or if she copes with her fears and anxiety through drug and/or alcohol abuse, the counselor may need to treat those behaviors first or simultaneously.

Specific targeting of problematic behaviors may be indicated. This might mean drug and alcohol treatment or counseling directed at replacing self-injurious behaviors with alternative coping strategies. In some cases, this requires treating the underlying anxiety and/or depression utilizing cognitive-behavioral strategies directly focused on symptom management.

An additional area of early behavioral change concerns countering rape-induced isolation. Although this will be discussed in greater detail later, social support clearly contributes to rape recovery, and thus early on, counselors need to assess clients' support systems and help them identify and utilize those relationships that might provide greater support during this time.

The goal is for the individual to make the behavioral changes necessary to be safe and supported as she engages in the process of rape resolution. Additional behavioral changes can be addressed as she works through specific symptomatic responses (e.g., anxiety, avoidance of sexual activity) and as she makes long-lasting changes in interpersonal relationships and possibly gets involved with other community groups.

It is also important to encourage rape survivors to engage in behaviors that contribute to their personal sense of power, confidence, and physical and mental health and well-being. This might include initiating an exercise program, identifying and engaging in pleasurable activities, or getting sufficient rest. It might also include challenging oneself to accomplish goals or to try something new, for example, going to a movie alone or going on a wilderness adventure.

Cognitive mastery:
Assist the survivor to examine and reformulate beliefs about herself and the sexual assault as well as beliefs and personal meanings that have been threatened by the assault.

The first stage of cognitive reformulation occurs when the counselor helps the client overcome cognitive avoidance and begin to process traumatic memories. As a result of the counselor's nonstigmatizing and nonblaming view of rape, at this stage the client also begins to review her own ideas about rape and victim responsibility. Many of the comments or statements we have suggested that counselors use with women in the immediate aftermath of a rape have equal value for women in ongoing crisis counseling.

Rape crisis centers often provide education about sexual assault as an essential aspect of treatment in order to introduce a way of thinking that situates what happened to the individual victim in the context of general male violence against women. If a woman can begin to perceive her victimization as one shared by many other women, it may lead to other changes in cognitions about the rape, particularly self-blaming ones. Sexual assault groups are particularly useful in challenging women's thinking about the assault, particularly self-blaming thoughts and beliefs that they could or should have prevented the assault.

Many other beliefs can be shaken by a sexual assault. Beliefs and thoughts about safety are commonly called into question, as may be beliefs about whom can be trusted. Although there are common negative cognitive effects on self-esteem, safety, trust, and personal power, the cognitive impact of a sexual assault is also unique to each person and situation.

Brenda was fourteen years old when an armed intruder broke into her family's home. After gathering the family in a central room, he demanded that Brenda's parents get him money and jewelry from another room. When they returned with the possessions he had demanded, he had already left their home, taking their daughter with them. Brenda tried to leave a trail, deliberately dropping hairpins and clothing as she was carried away; however, her parents did not locate her. After being brutally raped, sodomized, and left for dead, she managed to escape and reach a neighboring home. Although Brenda and her entire family struggled with fears regarding their safety, a particularly troubling change in beliefs for Brenda centered on her view of her father. Her image of him as strong and able to protect her was shattered by the sexual assault and his failure to rescue her.

Although irrational, this was a view that both her mother and father shared and never spoke of either.

Efforts to help Brenda and her family members included assisting them to realistically reassess their expectations for paternal omnipotence. What Brenda needed to do was to accept her father as a vulnerable human being rather than the giant he was in her childhood imagination.

Developmental mastery:
Assist the survivor to examine the impact of the sexual assault on her ongoing development.

A sexual assault occurs at a particular developmental juncture in an individual's life. Brenda, discussed above, was just fourteen years old when she was assaulted. Because the perpetrator was eventually identified as an older boy from her school, who had brothers, other relatives, and friends who also attended the same school, Brenda and her parents did not believe it was safe for her to return. Her education was disrupted, as she was forced to transfer schools and her family was eventually forced to move. Even in her new school, the very public nature of her assault made her feel that people saw and responded to her differently. Somehow, Brenda needed to be able to just be an adolescent again. She needed to be able to hang out with friends, play sports, date, and gradually explore intimate relationships. Each of these developmental needs was an appropriate and important focus of counseling intervention.

All survivors experience the impact of sexual violation in ways that resonate with their particular developmental tasks and goals. It is incumbent on the crisis counselor to be attentive to these developmentally specific impacts and to assist the survivor to work through these potential obstacles to their continued normal development.

Ecosystem healthy and intact:
Assist the survivor to make changes in her personal ecosystem in order to reestablish connection and community.

Ending isolation and reestablishing connections to others is an essential aspect of recovery. Many victims, however, are reluctant to confide in significant others, either about the initial assault or about their present difficulties. Survivors may thus feel quite alone as they attempt to confront and resolve their victimization. If this is the case, helping the survivor make changes to allow others to provide support in her struggle may be critical. In some cases, friends and family may have coped with their own reactions to her victimization by denial or suppression, or they may have become inpatient with her continuing difficulties. Intervening with them may also be helpful *if* the survivor is comfortable with that involvement.

These observations suggest that, to the extent that the survivor is willing, the counselor should encourage her to open up and reconnect with family and/or friends in the early stages of working with her. A primary purpose of devoting attention to enhancing connections with others in the early stages of recovery is to provide safety and support. The work of recovery clearly requires support and relational safe haven.

From another perspective, truly reconnecting with one's world as an empowered and healthy person is also a final step in moving forward in one's life as a sexual assault survivor. If helplessness and isolation are common outcomes of victimization and trauma, as a victim understands those effects, she gradually becomes ready to challenge herself to take greater risks and to exercise her personal sense of power, both relationally and in her everyday life. As Herman (1997) described: "In the third stage of recovery, the traumatized person recognizes that she has been a victim and understands the effects of her victimization. . . . Now she is ready to take concrete steps to increase her sense of power and control, to protect herself against future danger, and to deepen her alliances with those whom she has learned to trust" (p. 197).

Relationally, this means that the survivor is ready to begin the work of opening up and deepening her relationships with others. She is more able to be in a relationship, not as a victim, but as an empowered identity. This means that she is also more able to examine her own behaviors, not destructively, as in self-blame, but to recognize ways that her own beliefs and behaviors may have made her more vulnerable. The counselor can also help her to recognize the impact her experience has had on her partner or family members who love her, not by feeling guilty or responsible, but by acknowledging and appreciating their struggle, as well.

Sexual relationships may be a primary focus at this time as the counselor assists the survivor to reclaim her own sexual power as well as the freedom to abandon power in sexual play. Sexual experiences are often the last part of a survivor's life to be freed from intrusive memories of the assault. The crisis counselor is an important guide and support as the survivor finds ways, ideally with a committed partner, to identify and define those sexual activities that feel safe and those that do not.

For some survivors, reconnection also includes finding a way to engage in social action, thereby transforming one's own personal tragedy into a base for bringing about change. Joining together with other survivors to speak out about one's experience and to engage in educational or victim advocacy is often a way to create something meaningful despite what happened. And, by publicly acknowledging themselves as victims and survivors, some survivors both realize their connection with other survivors and join with them to address the social conditions that led to their shared victimization (Friedman, Tucker, & Neville, 2002). Such involvements also require a willingness to take risks and to master fears. Crisis counselors can help survivors envision participation, and eventually engage, in actions that are healing and empowering. Whether those actions are related to finding "a survivor mission" (Herman, 1997, p. 207), taking a self-defense course, or challenging oneself to return to school, they offer the survivor the opportunity to challenge the residue of trauma.

Termination of Crisis Counseling

It has been noted by many clinicians who work with sexual assault survivors that resolution is never truly complete (Herman, 1997; Koss & Harvey, 1991). What this means is that integration of the meaning of a survivor's experience continues to evolve. There may be times in the survivor's life when a life passage, such as the birth of a child, or some new crisis, such as being robbed or learning that one's daughter has been sexually coerced, will reignite the memories and emotions of her sexual assault. At times such as these, survivors may return to counseling, feeling upset and often blaming themselves.

For this reason, part of ending crisis counseling with a sexual assault survivor entails talking about recovery as an ongoing process that may have ups and downs. It is helpful to advise the survivor that during times of stress, or perhaps on the anniversary of the assault, she may experience a short-term return of some posttraumatic symptoms. In the course of ending counseling with the survivor, it is also always a good idea to review what has been accomplished. This includes reviewing the newly identified knowledge and skills that have enabled her to recover thus far, for she can use that knowledge and those skills when she experiences a return of her fears and sense of vulnerability.

Termination of crisis counseling with a sexual assault survivor also demands attention to the counseling relationship. Although the relationship may have become less intense as the survivor began to feel less vulnerable and more empowered, nonetheless, it was undoubtedly a relationship within which a considerable amount of personal revelation and vulnerability was expressed. Because the relationship was probably quite intense, it is essential for both the survivor and the crisis counselor to adequately prepare for termination, recognizing, that you may have become quite attached to each other. Termination of the counseling relationship must occur in a way that acknowledges that the process could not have been successful without both the client's willingness to risk trusting and the counselor's genuine caring and commitment.

CONCLUSION

Sexual assault is a crime that produces long-lasting distress for many victims. Although it was not the purpose of this chapter to discuss at length the causes of rape, it requires mentioning that rape is just one form of violence against women. It is a crime deeply embedded in society's beliefs about men and women, power and control. As such it cannot be entirely separated from the society within which it occurs. Recognizing rape as both a product of individual deviance and the acting out of dysfunctional and sexist scripts about masculinity, power and control, many individual counselors who work with sexual assault survivors also involve themselves in various social action efforts. Whether these efforts entail providing prevention workshops or advocating for victims in the criminal justice system, their overarching goal is to change the societal conditions that contribute to its prevalence. The feminist anti-rape movement and feminist rape crisis programs have had, since their inception, a primary mission of ending sexual violence. Although the provision of services to victims is essential and important work, ultimately all helpers who care about survivors must in some way engage in efforts to end this scourge (Collins & Whalen, 1989).

CASE EXAMPLE: WENDY

Single-Session Crisis Intervention

The crisis worker (CW) who answered Wendy's phone call listened as Wendy urgently described what had occurred. The crisis worker immediately determined that Wendy was quite frantic and emotionally overwhelmed. She responded in a manner intended to convey a sense of calm control and empathic understanding.

CW: *Wendy, I can hear by your voice that you are feeling pretty overwhelmed at finding yourself in this guy's room and knowing that something terrible happened to you. What I'd like you to do is take a couple of deep breaths while you listen to me. OK? One deep breath (pause); two (pause); three (pause). OK, Wendy?*

Wendy: *(Crying and hyperventilating)* Yes, yes. What should I do?

CW: *OK, breathe slowly, Wendy. Are you in danger right now?*

Wendy: No, but I don't know where they are.

CW: *Are you physically able to walk out of the dorm?*

Wendy: Yes, yes, I think I can find the stairway.

CW: *So one option is for you to do just that—to just calmly walk out the door and away from the dorm. Another option is for you to call campus police and tell them where you are, what happened, and have them come and get you.*

Wendy: No, no, I don't want to make a scene.

CW: *Wendy, it sounds to me as if something you drank knocked you out. It also sounds as though you may have been sexually assaulted, as I think you know. You have every right to have the police come and assist you.*

Wendy: *(Crying)* No, I just want to leave.

CW: *OK, Wendy. You're feeling pretty overwhelmed and upset. It's certainly up to you to decide whether to involve the police or not, but will you at least agree to come to the emergency room and get checked out? I will meet you there if you agree.*

Wendy: *(Crying)* But I don't know if I want to report this to the police . . . or to anyone.

CW: *And you don't need to make that decision right now. But Wendy, as I said before, it sounds possible to me that someone had sex with you without your consent. There may have been something in your drink that knocked you out. It's important for you to be medically examined—for your health and prevention of any other possible problems. Also, any evidence that is collected in the exam can then be available in case you do decide to take some legal action. But without that evidence you may not have that option.*

Wendy: Will you be there?

CW: *Yes, I will meet you there, and I will help you try to figure out what to do and I will support you in whatever you decide. Is there anyone who can help you get to the emergency room?*

Wendy: My roommate is not home. But I have a car. . . . Oh, no, I don't have my purse. It must be in my room, or maybe I left it at the party.

CW: *Do you have your keys? The keys to your room or to your car?*

Wendy: *(Looking)* Yes, yes, in my belt bag.

CW: *Which key, Wendy? Your room key or your car key?*

Wendy: I've got both.

CW: *OK, good. So tell me what you are going to do.*

Wendy: I'm going to walk out of the room, find the stairs down to the lobby, and walk out of the dorm.

CW: *Good. So you are going to just calmly walk. And then what?*

Wendy: I'm going to go straight to my car and drive to the hospital.

CW: *Excellent, Wendy. Be sure not to change your clothes or bathe, because any evidence of what happened is on you and your clothing. I know you're pretty sure right now that you don't want to involve the police, but as this sinks in you may change your mind, and I want to make sure you still have that choice. OK?*

Wendy: *(Sniffling, but more under control)* OK.

CW: *So, Wendy, it should take you, what, about twenty minutes to get out of there, get to your car, and drive to the hospital? And I will be waiting for you right outside the ER doors. How does that sound?*

Wendy: Good. I can do that.

CW: *Yes, I believe you can. Wendy, I'm very sorry you have to go through this, but I will help you in whatever way I can. I'll be wearing a denim jacket and blue cords and I have short dark brown hair. I will show you my identification. What kind of car are you driving so I can watch for you?*

Wendy's case is an example of single-session intervention in the immediate aftermath of a sexual assault. Although this first contact was very brief, from the moment Wendy began to speak, the crisis worker was assessing both the situation and the client's level of coping. She attempted to supportively connect with Wendy, intervened to stabilize her emotionally, and assisted her to make the immediate decisions about how to leave the men's dorm, whether to immediately call the police, and to agree to come to the emergency room. The two primary initial goals were to begin to establish a supportive relationship and to intervene to promote greater safety, both physically and emotionally. Crisis intervention with Wendy continues when she arrives at the emergency room.

The most important basis for providing assistance to a traumatized individual is the establishment of a supportive and empowering relationship. In single-session crisis intervention with a sexual assault survivor, that means that the individual in crisis feels accepted, hears that she is not being blamed or judged, and senses that the crisis worker has some understanding of what she is experiencing (empathy). Specific statements by the crisis worker that begin to create this sense of relationship include *"I am sorry this has happened to you," "I understand that you are feeling very _____," "You are understandably very _____"* Each of these statements accurately identifies and reflects what the client is feeling and at the same time directly supports her and begins to normalize her emotions, whatever they are. Statements that indicate the desire to assist are similarly instrumental in forming a supportive relationship.

At the emergency room:
After greeting Wendy, reintroducing herself, and showing identification, the crisis worker assisted Wendy in the initial emergency room intake procedure. The crisis worker and Wendy then sat down in the private room provided for them as they waited for the medical examination to begin. Before beginning, the crisis worker explained to Wendy that anything she said would be kept confidential and would be revealed only with her written permission. She then engaged Wendy in conversation again.

CW: *How are you holding up, Wendy?*

Wendy: I just want it to be over.

CW: *You'd like to be able to go back to your dorm and make what happened to you just go away.*

Wendy: *(Begins to quietly cry)* Why did they do this to me? How did it happen? I should have stopped them.

CW: *Wendy, it sounds to me as if you were not capable of stopping them. Can you recollect what happened from the time you got to the party?*

Wendy tells the story of being at the party, getting back to her dorm, and then being led out of her room by two men from the party.

CW: *So you tried to take care of yourself when you began to sense that something was wrong. You left the party and you got yourself back to your dorm. By the time the men came and got you, it sounds as if you were literally unable to resist their efforts to take you with them. We won't know for sure why you* *blacked out until the lab tests come back, but it's clear that whatever the reason, you were unable to do anything other than what you did. You were unable to stop them. Do you understand that?*

Wendy: *(Continuing to quietly sob)* Yes, I guess. But I can't remember. . . . I can't remember what they did. *(Crying harder)*

CW: *(Putting her hand on Wendy's hand) Wendy, I can hear it's terrifying to know that these two men did sexual things to you that you can't remember. It would be difficult enough to be sexually assaulted and to have images of what occurred; it may be even worse when you can only imagine.*

Wendy: *(Continuing to cry)* I'm only eighteen.

CW: *(Quietly listens for Wendy to continue)*

Wendy: I'm only a freshman. How can I ever go back to school and see them again. How can I face them?

CW: *(Realizing that medical personnel may soon arrive) Wendy, there are a lot of decisions about what you do after you leave the hospital that I want to be able to help you deal with. But I know that the nurses and doctor are probably going to be coming in shortly and I want to make sure you know what to expect. Can we stop for a bit and talk a little about what is going to happen in the medical exam?*

Wendy: OK.

The crisis worker explained the types of questions Wendy would be asked by the nurse and the reason for those questions. She also explained the medical procedures for examination of possible injuries and gathering the data necessary for the rape evidence kit, including blood work to determine both her blood alcohol level and the presence of any drugs in her system. She encouraged Wendy to answer all of the questions as honestly as she could and if she couldn't remember something to just say that. She also encouraged her to let the nurse and/or doctor know if anything was uncomfortable or painful. She then asked Wendy how she was feeling and if she had any questions. After a brief exchange, the crisis worker again asked if there was anyone whom Wendy wanted to call to come and be with her, to which Wendy again replied, "No one." The crisis worker then asked Wendy if she would like her to stay with her during the medical interview and exam or if she would prefer that she wait outside. Wendy asked the crisis worker to remain.

During the ensuing exam the crisis worker intervened to encourage the medical personnel to give Wendy as much information as possible about the exam and the purpose of specific medical procedures. She also continued to support Wendy both physically (by periodically holding her hand) and by continuing to make empathic statements. Once the exam was over the crisis worker asked the nurse if she and Wendy could briefly remain in the room to talk. She also confirmed with the nurse that the medical data would be kept safe to be used as evidence, should Wendy decide that she wants to take legal action.

During this entire time the crisis worker was actively listening and trying to comprehend information about the event and about Wendy, including her feelings, her ways of behaving, her thoughts about herself and what had occurred, her social supports, and the impact of her developmental age and lifestyle on all of the above. She was getting an image of Wendy as a relatively naïve young woman. It was revealed during the medical interview that she had not previously had sexual intercourse, and that although she had been drinking and partying with friends, she did not use drugs or routinely engage in risk-taking behavior.

Wendy's primary responses appeared to be on the withdrawal end of the continuum. Most of her thoughts appeared to be the fears and concerns of a normal peer-focused eighteen-year-old. She felt physically violated, and her newly gained sense of independence had been shattered. She was worried about others knowing what happened and concerned about her ability to return to her academic and social life at college. She refused to utilize any social supports other than the crisis worker.

The conversation resumed after the nurse left the room.

CW: *You seem to be feeling a bit calmer. Getting that exam completed helped?*

Wendy: *(Smiling wanly)* Just getting it over with.

CW: *Yes, I'm sure. What are you feeling right now?*

Wendy: I don't know. *(Pauses)* I think I'm getting angry.

CW: *(Nods head)*

Wendy: How could they do that to me? They . . . they totally manipulated me.

CW: *They certainly did that . . . and more. Wendy, it is a crime to perform sexual acts on someone without her consent. You were incapable of giving consent . . . and they may have given you something—we'll know once the blood tests come back—to guarantee that.*

Wendy: I know. I know. *(With emphasis)* That's what's making me angry. At first I was . . . sad, I guess, and scared . . . but the more I think about what happened the more I'm getting angry. They had no right to do that to me.

CW: *Wendy, please allow me to again raise the question about reporting this to someone in authority so that someone can confront these men with what they have done. What about campus police, or perhaps you could consider other campus disciplinary processes?*

Wendy: What do you mean?

CW: *Well, certainly, if you report this to the campus police there is the possibility that if there is sufficient evidence they can work with the district attorney's office to press criminal charges. That would be hard on you, but if the evidence supports what we believe happened—that you were drugged and sexually assaulted—then clearly a crime has been committed against you. The other* *option would be a campus disciplinary hearing. That wouldn't require the same degree of evidence and legal formality, but it could possibly result in the men being thrown off campus or even out of school. Either one would be difficult to go through, but . . . clearly it has to be up to you.*

Wendy: I don't know what to do. I don't want to have to see them. It all feels so . . . big.

CW: *It seems overwhelming to think about notifying the police, talking to them, and everything that follows.*

Wendy: Yes.

CW: *And it would be tough; I don't want to mislead you . . . but it will also be hard to go back to school and have to encounter these two men in classes and socially, knowing what they have done to you. My concern right now is that you shouldn't be making these tough decisions and dealing with all of this alone. I'm here and will continue to be, if you want, but how about thinking about whom you can call from your family or friends for support. (Pauses) If you had been in a car accident and were injured, whom would you call?*

Wendy: (Begins to tear up, voice quivers) My dad.

CW: *He's someone you would turn to for help?*

Wendy: *(Nods her head)* He's always there if I need him.

CW: *(Quietly) And you need him now. How about letting him know that?*

Wendy: But this is different . . . he'll be so . . . I don't know . . .

CW: *How do you think he'll react?*

Wendy: He'll be upset . . . and angry.

CW: *Angry at what?*

Wendy: At them.

CW: *And how will he be with you?*

Wendy: Worried and upset.

CW: *Worried and upset because you've been hurt?*

Wendy: Yes.

CW: *(Quietly and with emphasis) And you have been. (Pauses as she observes Wendy, who nods her head) I think you need his support as well as the support of others who care about you. How about your roommate? You said you tried to call her first.*

Wendy: Yes. I know she'll be there for me . . . and won't tell everyone if I ask her not to.

CW: *And that—not telling anyone—is important to you?*

Wendy: Not as much anymore.

CW: *So shall we call your dad and perhaps your roommate before you leave the hospital . . . before you go back? Is that what you want . . . to go back to the dorm?*

Wendy: *(Nods her head yes)*

CW: *You don't have to, you know, if you'd rather go home for a while.*

Wendy: I know. I need to decide about calling the police.

CW: *Do you want to make that decision now or wait until you call your dad and talk to him? How about we take one step at a time?*

As the session continued, the crisis worker helped Wendy call her roommate and her parents. When her roommate arrived at the hospital, Wendy decided to go back to her room with her roommate and to wait for her parents to arrive. Before Wendy left with her roommate, the crisis worker reassured her that she would continue to be available to support her and suggested that Wendy consider coming into the rape crisis center for ongoing supportive counseling.

CW: *I'm very pleased to see you feeling a little calmer and more in charge. You've been through a lot and it's not over. I know from experience that as the next few days go by and things settle down you may feel as though you can just go on and sort of pretend that this never happened. But even though that's a very normal response, I want to prepare you for the possibility that it doesn't just go away that easily. It helps to have a place and someone that you can talk to who will understand what you are going through. (Hands Wendy her card) This is our office number and address. I want to encourage you to come into the rape crisis center so that we can continue to provide you with that needed support and understanding. We offer individual counseling as well as support groups with other rape survivors, we work with family members, and we provide legal assistance and accompaniment. Please do call if I can help you in any way.*

Wendy: Thank you so much. You have helped me . . . helped me so much already. I will call.

This single-session crisis intervention with Wendy lasted approximately three and one-half hours including the time spent with medical personnel. As noted, it began on the telephone and continued in the emergency room. In this brief period the crisis worker achieved each of the goals of single-session intervention. Wendy is safe, has attained greater control over both herself and the situation, and has been informed of additional support options and resources.

Assessment began at first contact and continued throughout the crisis worker's engagement with Wendy, as did her efforts to supportively and empathically relate to Wendy. It is clear that Wendy felt accepted and affirmed. Her most pressing needs, including safety, were addressed immediately. Over the course of intervention Wendy was assisted to think about the different decisions, or alternatives, she faced, to connect or consider connecting with personal resources (parents and roommate) and social resources (hospital, police, rape crisis center), and was prepared for what to anticipate in the future. Clearly, this situation is not yet resolved for Wendy, but the work of single-session crisis intervention has been accomplished.

DISCUSSION QUESTIONS

1. Research suggests that although both men and women may believe rape myths, men are much more likely to endorse such myths. Discuss why this is so, and what might be done to effectively challenge such beliefs.

2. Feminists assert that sexual violence is a product of society rather than simply a result of individual deviance. In fact, one analyst has written about the "rape culture." Discuss how our society may perpetuate a rape culture.

EXERCISES

1. The chapter made the point that different perpetrator motives affect the way in which a sexual assault is carried out and thus the experience of victims. This exercise is designed to further sensitize class members to this point. First, divide the class into small groups. List Scully and Morolla's different perpetrator motives on the blackboard (e.g., anger/revenge, added bonus, sexual access, domination/control, recreation/adventure). Assign each group one of the types. Instruct members of each group to create a rape scenario that might typify or exemplify that type. Second, ask group members to discuss how they believe others would respond to a woman who reported being a victim of the rape scenario they created. Ask small groups to share with the class as a whole. Finally, process the exercise thoroughly.

2. *Class following Exercise 1:* Divide the class into the same groups. Ask the groups to imagine that it is a week after the rape occurred. Ask them to identify what reactions (ABCDE) they believe the victim of that rape may be experiencing. Ask small groups to share with the larger group. Process class member's thoughts and feelings.

3. *Fish-bowl role-playing activity.* Identify a student who is willing to begin a role-playing activity in which the student is the crisis counselor and the class instructor is the rape victim. The role-playing can take place in the center of a fishbowl of identified students who both serve as consultants to the crisis counselor and/or can be asked to take over that role. The remainder of the class members serve as observers, analyzing what is happening and why. The role-playing can be stopped at frequent intervals to process with the observers. At the end of the role-playing and content discussion, process class members' personal reactions.

4. Invite a police detective to come to class to demonstrate the questioning of an alleged rape victim. Have students prepare by creating a date rape scenario. The instructor or a student volunteer can role-play the victim, utilizing that

scenario. After the role-playing, process class reactions with the detective. After the detective's departure, process further with the class alone.

5. An excellent tool for sparking discussion about rape myths regarding victim responsibility is the gang rape scene from the movie *The Accused,* starring Jodie Foster. Show that scene (after preparing the class) and discuss.

REFERENCES

Abbey, A. (1991). Misperception as an antecedent of acquaintance rape: A consequence of ambiguity in communication between women and men. In A. Parrot & L. Bechhofer (Eds.), *Acquaintance rape: The hidden crime* (pp. 96–111). New York: John Wiley & Sons.

Abbey, A., McAuslan, P., & Ross, L. T. (1998). Sexual assault perpetration by college men: The role of alcohol, misperception of sexual intent, and sexual beliefs and experiences. *Journal of Social and Clinical Psychology, 17,* 167–195.

Ageton, S. S. (1983). *Sexual assault among adolescents.* Lexington, MA: D. C. Heath.

Amir, N., Foa, E. B., & Cashman, L. (1998). Predictors of posttraumatic stress disorder: A prospective study of rape and nonsexual assault victims. Symposium conducted at the meeting of the World Congress of Behavioral and Cognitive Therapies, Acapulco, Mexico.

Atkeson, B., Calhoun, K., Resick, P., & Ellis, E. (1982). Victims of rape: Repeated assessment of depressive symptoms. *Journal of Consulting and Clinical Psychology, 50,* 96–102.

Benedict, H. (1985). *Recovery: How to survive sexual assault for women, men, teenagers, their friends and families.* Garden City, NY: Doubleday.

Bergen, R. K. (1999). Marital rape. Retrieved November 15, 2002, from http://www.vaw.umn.edu/finaldocuments/Vawnet/mrape.htm

Bohmer, C., & Parrot, A. (1993). *Sexual assault on campus: The problem and the solution.* New York: Lexington Books.

Boston Women's Health Collective. (1998). *Our bodies, ourselves for the new century: A book by and for women.* New York: Simon & Schuster.

Brownmiller, S. (1975). *Against our will: Men, women, and rape.* New York: Simon & Schuster.

Burgess, A. W., & Holmstrom, L. L. (1974). Rape trauma syndrome. *American Journal of Psychiatry, 131,* 981–986.

Burgess, A. W., & Holmstrom, L. L. (1976). Coping behavior of the rape victim. *American Journal of Psychiatry, 133,* 413–418.

Burgess, A. W., & Holmstrom, L. L. (1979). Rape: Sexual disruption and recovery. *American Journal of Orthopsychiatry, 49,* 648–657.

Burnam, M. A., Stein, J. A., Golding, J. M., Siegel, J. M., Sorenson, S. B., Forsythe, A. B., & Telles, C. A. (1988). Sexual assault and mental disorders in a community population. *Journal of Consulting and Clinical Psychology, 56,* 843–850.

Burt, M. R. (1980). Cultural myths and supports for rape. *Journal of Personality and Social Psychology, 38,* 217–230.

Burt, M. R. (1998). Rape myths. In M. E. Odem & J. Clay-Warner (Eds.), *Confronting rape and sexual assault* (pp. 129–144). Wilmington, DE: Scholarly Resources Inc.

Calhoun, K. S., & Atkeson, B. M. (1991). *Treatment of rape victims: Facilitating psychosocial adjustment.* New York: Pergamon Press.

Calhoun, K. S., Atkeson, B. M., & Resick, P. A. (1982). A longitudinal examination of fear reactions in victims of rape. *Journal of Counseling Psychology, 29,* 655–661.

Collins, B. G. (1987). A discriminant analysis of the psychological characteristics, attitudes and behaviors of male readers and non-readers of soft-core pornography. *Dissertation Abstracts International, 49,* 2390.

Collins, B. G., & Whalen, M. B. (1989). Rape crisis movement: Radical or reformist? *Social Work, 34,* 61–64.

Creamer, M., Burgess, P., & Pattison, P. (1992). Reaction to trauma: A cognitive processing model. *Journal of Abnormal Psychology, 101,* 452–459.

Drieschner, K., & Lange, A. (1999). A review of cognitive factors in the etiology of rape: Theories, empirical studies, and implications. *Clinical Psychology Review, 19*(1), 57–77.

Ellis, E. M., Atkeson, B. M., & Calhoun, K. S. (1981). An assessment of long-term reaction to rape. *Journal of Abnormal Psychology, 90,* 263–266.

Federal Bureau of Investigation. (2000). *Crime in the United States, 2000.* Washington, DC: U.S. Department of Justice.

Finkelhor, D., & Yllo, K. (1985). *License to rape: Sexual abuse of wives.* New York: Holt, Rinehart & Winston.

Foa, E. B., & Rothbaum, B. O. (1998). *Treating the trauma of rape: Cognitive-behavioral therapy for PTSD.* New York: Guilford Press.

Foa, E. B., Rothbaum, B. O., Riggs, D. S., & Murdock, T. (1991). Treatment of posttraumatic stress disorder in rape victims: A comparison between cognitive-behavioral procedures and counseling. *Journal of Consulting and Clinical Psychology, 59,* 715–723.

Forman, B. D. (1980). Cognitive modification of obsessive thinking in a rape victim: A preliminary study. *Psychological Reports, 47,* 819–822.

Forman, B. D. (1983). Assessing the impact of rape and its significance in psychotherapy. *Psychotherapy: Theory, Research, and Practice, 20,* 515–519.

Frank, E., Turner, S. M., & Stewart, B. D. (1980). Initial response to rape: The impact of factors within the rape situation. *Journal of Behavioral Assessment, 2,* 39–53.

Frazier, P. A., Valtinson, G., & Candell, S. (1994). Evaluation of a coeducational interactive rape prevention program. *Journal of Counseling and Development, 73,* 153–158.

Friedman, L. N., Tucker, S. B., & Neville, P. (2002). From pain to power: Crime victims take action. In D. Shichor & S. G. Tibbetts, *Victims and victimization: Essential readings* (pp. 265–286). Prospect Heights, IL: Waveland Press.

Gidycz, C. A., & Koss, M. A. (1990). A comparison of group and individual sexual assault victims. *Psychology of Women Quarterly, 14,* 325–342.

Girelli, S. A., Resick, P. A., Marhoefer-Dvorak, S., & Hutter, C. K. (1986). Subjective distress and violence during rape: Their effects on long-term fear. *Violence and Victims, 1,* 35–45.

Goodchilds, J., Zellman, G., Johnson, P. B., & Giarrusso, R. (1988). Adolescents and their perceptions of sexual interactions. In A. W. Burgess (Ed.), *Rape and sexual assault* (Vol. 2, pp. 245–270). New York: Garland Publishing.

Goyer, P., & Eddleman, H. (1984) Same-sex rape of nonincarcerated men. *American Journal of Psychiatry, 141,* 576–579.

Groth, A. N., Burgess, A. W., & Holmstrom, L. L. (1977) Rape: Power, anger, and sexuality. *American Journal of Psychiatry, 134,* 1239–1243.

Herman, J. L. (1997). *Trauma and recovery.* New York: Basic Books.

Hersh, K., & Gray-Little, B. (1998). Psychopathic traits and attitudes associated with self-reported sexual aggression in college men. *Journal of Interpersonal Violence, 13*(4), 456–471.

Hudson, S. M., & Ward, T. (1997). Intimacy, loneliness, and attachment style in sexual offenders. *Journal of Interpersonal Violence, 12,* 323–339.

Hutchings, P., & Dutton, M. A. (1997). Symptom severity and diagnoses related to sexual assault history. *Journal of Anxiety Disorders, 11,* 607–618.

Kilpatrick, D. G., Saunders, B. E., Amick-Mullen, A., Best, C. L., Veronen, L. J., & Resnick, H. S. (1989). Victim and crime factors associated with the development of crime-related post-traumatic stress disorder. *Behavior Therapy, 20,* 199–214.

Kilpatrick, D. G., & Veronen, L. J. (1983). Treatment of rape-related problems: Crisis intervention is not enough. In L. H. Cohen, W. L. Claiborn, & G. A. Specter (Eds.), *Crisis intervention* (2nd ed., pp. 165–185). New York: Human Sciences Press.

Koss, M. P. (1985). The hidden rape victim: Personality, attitudinal, and situational characteristics. *Psychology of Women Quarterly, 9,* 193–212.

Koss, M. P. (1988). Hidden rape: Sexual aggression and victimization in a national sample of students in higher education. In A. W. Burgess (Ed.), *Rape and sexual assault* (Vol. 2, pp. 3–25). New York: Garland Publishing.

Koss, M. P. (1993). Rape: Scope, impact, interventions, and public policy responses. *American Psychologist, 48,* 1062–1069.

Koss, M. P., & Dinero, T. E. (1989). Discriminant analysis of risk factors for sexual victimization among a national sample of college women. *Journal of Consulting and Clinical Psychology, 57,* 242–250.

Koss, M. P., & Gaines, J. A. (1993). The prediction of sexual aggression by alcohol use, athletic participation, and fraternity affiliation. *Journal of Interpersonal Violence, 8*(1), 94–108.

Koss, M. P., & Harvey, M. R. (1991). *The rape victim: Clinical and community interventions* (2nd ed.). Thousand Oaks, CA: Sage.

Koss, M. P., Gidycz, C. A., & Wisniewski, N. (1987). The scope of rape: Incidence and prevalence of sexual aggression and victimization in a national sample of higher education students. *Journal of Consulting & Clinical Psychology, 55,* 162–170.

Koss, M. P., Woodruff, W. J., & Koss, P. (1991). Criminal victimization among primary care medical patients: Prevalence, incidence, and physician usage. *Behavioral Sciences and the Law, 9,* 85–96.

Kosson, D. S., Kelly, J. C., & White, J. W. (1997). Psychopathy-related traits predict self-reported sexual aggression among college men. *Journal of Interpersonal Violence, 12,* 241–254.

Krahe, B. (1998). Sexual aggression among adolescents: Prevalence and predictors in a German sample. *Psychology of Women Quarterly, 22,* 537–554.

Lanier, C. A., Elliott, N. N., Martin, D. W., & Kapadia, A. (1998). Evaluation of an intervention to change attitudes toward date rape. *Journal of American College Health, 46,* 177–180.

Lifton, R. (1983). *The broken connection: On death and the continuity of life.* New York: Basic Books.

Lisak, D., & Ivan, C. (1995). Deficits in intimacy and empathy in sexually aggressive men. *Journal of Interpersonal Violence, 10,* 296–308.

Lisak, D., & Miller, P. M. (2002). Repeat rape and multiple offending among undetected rapists. *Violence and Victims, 17,* 73–84.

Lisak, D., & Roth, S. (1990). Motives and psychodynamics of self-reported, unincarcerated rapists. *American Journal of Orthopsychiatry, 60*(2), 268–280.

Lonsway, K. A., & Fitzgerald, L. F. (1994). Rape myths: In review. *Psychology of Women Quarterly, 18,* 133–164.

Malamuth, N. M., (1986). Predictors of naturalistic sexual aggression. *Journal of Personality and Social Psychology, 50, 953–962.*

Malamuth, N. M., & Donnerstein, E. (1982). The effects of aggressive pornographic mass media stimuli. In L. Berkowitz (Ed.), *Advances in experimental social psychology (15).* New York: Academic Press.

McFarlane, A. C., & van der Kolk, B. A. (1996). Trauma and its challenge to society. In B. A. van der Kolk, A. C. McFarlane, & L. Weisaeth (Eds.), *Traumatic stress: The effects of overwhelming experience on mind, body, and society* (pp. 3–23). New York: Guilford Press.

Mezey, G., & King, M. (1989). The effects of sexual assault on men: A survey of 22 victims. *Psychological Medicine, 19, 205–209.*

Mills, C. S., & Granoff, B. J. (1992). Date and acquaintance rape among a sample of college students. *Social Work, 37, 504–509.*

Monnier, J., Resnick, H. S., Kilpatrick, D. G., & Seals, B. (2002). The relationship between distress and resource loss following rape. *Violence and Victims, 17*(1), 85–92.

Myer, R. A. (2001). *Assessment for crisis intervention: A triage assessment model.* Belmont, CA: Brooks/Cole.

Notman, M. T., & Nadelson, C. C. (1976). The rape victim: Psychodynamic considerations. *American Journal of Psychology, 133,* 408–413.

Pelka, F. (1992). Raped: A male survivor breaks his silence. *On the Issues, 22,* 8–11, 40.

Piercy, M. (1982). *Circles on the water: Selected poems of Marge Piercy.* New York: Alfred A. Knopf.

Quimette, P. C. (1997). Psychopathology and sexual aggression in nonincarcerated men. *Violence and Victims, 12,* 389–395.

Rando, R. A., Rogers, J. R., Brittan, P., and Christopher, S. (1998). Gender role conflict and college men's sexually aggressive attitudes and behavior. *Journal of Mental Health Counseling, 20,* 359–369.

Rennison, C. (2001). *Criminal victimization 2000: Changes 1999–2000 with trends 1993–2000.* Washington, DC: Bureau of Justice Statistics, U.S. Department of Justice.

Resick, P. A., & Schnicke, M. K. (1993). *Cognitive processing therapy for rape victims: A treatment manual.* Newbury Park, CA: Sage.

Resnick, H. S., Kilpatrick, D. G., Dansky, B. S., Saunders, B. E., & Best, C. L. (1993). Prevalence of civilian trauma and posttraumatic stress disorder in a representative national sample of women. *Journal of Consulting and Clinical Psychology, 61,* 984–991.

Rice, M. E., Chaplin, T. C., Harris, G. T., & Coutts, J. (1994). Empathy for the victim and sexual arousal among rapists and nonrapists. *Journal of Interpersonal Violence, 9*(4), 435–449.

Richardson, D., & Hammock, G. (1991). The role of alcohol in acquaintance rape. In A. Parrot & L. Bechhofer (Eds.), *Acquaintance rape: The hidden crime* (pp. 83–95). New York: John Wiley & Sons.

Rodkin, L., Hunt, E., & Cowan, S. (1982). A men's support group for significant others of rape victims. *Journal of Marital and Family Therapy, 8,* 91–97.

Roth, S., Wayland, K., & Woolsey, M. (1990). Victimization history and victim-assailant relationships as factors in recovery from sexual assault. *Journal of Traumatic Stress, 3*(1), 169–189.

Rothbaum, B. O., Foa, E. B., Riggs, D., Murdock, T., & Walsh, W. (1992). A prospective examination of post-traumatic stress disorder in rape victims. *Journal of Traumatic Stress, 5,* 455–475.

Ruch, L. O., & Leon, J. J. (1983). Sexual assault trauma and trauma change. *Women and Health, 8*, 5–21.

Russell, D. E. H. (1984). *Sexual exploitation: Rape, child sexual abuse, and workplace harassment.* Beverly Hills, CA: Sage.

Russell, D. E. H. (1991). Wife rape. In A. Parrot & L. Bechhofer (Eds.), *Acquaintance rape: The hidden crime* (pp. 129–139). New York: John Wiley & Sons.

Sanday, P. R. (1990). *Fraternity gang rape: Sex, brotherhood, and privilege on campus.* New York: New York University Press.

Schwartz, M. D., & Leggett, M. S. (1999). Bad dates or emotional trauma: The aftermath of campus sexual assault. *Violence Against Women, 5*, 251–271.

Scully, D., & Marolla, J. (1984). Convicted rapists' vocabulary of motive: Excuses and justifications. *Social Problems, 31*, 530–544.

Scully, D., & Marolla, J. (1985). "Riding the bull at Gilley's": Convicted rapists describe the rewards of rape. *Social Problems, 32*(3), 251–263.

Shapiro, B. L., & Chwarz, J. C. (1997). Date rape: Its relationship to trauma symptoms and sexual self-esteem. *Journal of Interpersonal Violence, 12*, 407–419.

Silverman, D. C. (1978). Sharing the crisis of rape: Counseling the mates and families of victims. *American Journal of Orthopsychiatry, 48*(1), 166–173.

Stewart, B. D., Hughes, C., Frank, E., Anderson, B., Kendall, K., & West, D. (1987). The aftermath of rape: Profiles of immediate and delayed treatment seekers. *Journal of Nervous and Mental Diseases, 175*, 90–94.

Sutherland, S., & Scherl, D. J. (1970). Patterns of response among victims of rape. *American Journal of Orthopsychiatry, 40*, 503–511.

Symonds, M. (1982) Victim's response to terror: Understanding and treatment. In F. Ochberg & D. Soskis (Eds.), *Victims of terrorism* (pp. 95–103). Boulder, CO: Westview.

Tescavage, K. (1999). Teaching women a lesson: Sexually aggressive and sexually non-aggressive men's perceptions of acquaintance and date rape. *Violence Against Women, 5*, 796–812.

Tjaden, P., & Thoennes, N. (1998). *Prevalence, incidence, and consequences of violence against women: Findings from the National Violence Against Women survey.* Washington, DC: U.S. Department of Justice.

Ullman, S. E., & Brecklin, L. R. (2000). Alcohol and adult sexual assault in a national sample of women. *Journal of Substance Abuse, 11*, 405–420.

Ullman, S. E., Karabatsos, G., & Koss, M. P. (1999). Alcohol and sexual assault in a national sample of college women. *Journal of Interpersonal Violence, 14*, 603–625.

van der Kolk, B. A. (1989). The compulsion to repeat the trauma: Re-enactment, revictimization, and masochism. *Psychiatric Clinics of North America, 12*, 389–411.

van der Kolk, B. A., & McFarlane, A. C. (1996). The black hole of trauma. In B. A. van der Kolk, A. C. McFarlane, & L. Weisaeth (Eds.), *Traumatic stress: The effects of overwhelming experience on mind, body, and society* (pp. 3–23). New York: Guilford Press.

Warshaw, R. (1988). *I never called it rape.* New York: Harper & Row.

Winfield, I., George, L. K., Swartz, M., & Blazer, D. G. (1990). Sexual assault and psychiatric disorders among a community sample of women. *American Journal of Psychiatry, 147*, 335–341.

Zweig, J. M., Crockett, L. J., Sayer, A., & Vicary, J. R. (1999). A longitudinal examination of the consequences of sexual victimization for rural young adult women. *Journal of Sex Research, 36*, 396–409.

CHAPTER 7

Battery, Control, and Power in Intimate Relationships: Designing Crisis Interventions

MOLLIE WHALEN

Francesca called the hotline, crying. "I don't know if you can help me. I'm scared. I feel awful." As Francesca's story unfolds, she reveals that her husband has never hit her, but he just treats her "so mean." When asked for examples, she describes a wide range of abusive, threatening, and controlling behaviors. Her husband has smashed all of her personal belongings; he has tortured her cats; he puts her down, calls her names, and humiliates her in front of others. He doesn't let her talk to her family or see her friends. He has a gun that he waves around when he's screaming at her. He grabs the wheel while she's driving. He forces her to have sex with him while he watches pornography. When she tries to talk to him about a divorce, he threatens to kill himself. Sometimes he threatens to kill her. Francesca is reassured that she has called the right place, and that the women's center* is there to help women who are being abused, even if they are not being physically beaten.

In 1976 two books were published: *The Battered Woman,* by Del Martin, and *Wife-beating,* by Betsy Warrior. The terms used in these titles, which underscored the gendered direction of violence in intimate relationships, have largely been replaced by the euphemism *domestic violence.* Research by scholars like Murray Straus, Richard Gelles, and Susan Steinmetz (1980) has purportedly established that men and women in intimate relationships use physical violence against one another at about the same rate. Feminist scholars and battered women's advocates (Yllo, 1993) have been quick to counter such findings by criticizing the methodology for counting incidents of hitting without assessing who initiates the violence, who is harmed more, and whether the hitting is self-defensive or retaliatory. Feminists argue that the term *domestic violence* obscures the fact that the largest proportion of battering and stringent psychological and behavioral control in intimate relationships follows the pattern of male batterer and female victim.

---

*Women's center is used in this chapter as a generic term for an organization that offers crisis intervention and short-term crisis counseling to women who are physically and emotionally abused.

It may be useful to consider two primary types of intimate relationship violence (Johnson, 1995). The type measured by the conflict scales mentioned above, which Johnson has termed "common couple violence," may be normative, and initiated and engaged in to about the same degree by both partners. The kind of violence that feminist activists in the battered women's movement discuss has sometimes been labeled "patriarchal terrorism" (Johnson, 1995; Mahoney, Williams, & West, 2001), and emanates from individual and societal acceptance of male dominance and privilege. Within this latter model, it is accepted that some men are battered, often by male partners in gay relationships; some women are batterers, usually in lesbian relationships; and, rarely, that some women use physical violence against their male partners. The latter situation, however, appears to be a very small percentage of "domestic violence" cases (less than 1 percent) and is not properly understood as arising from the same dynamics as the prototypical battering situations in heterosexual or same-sex relationships. Certainly, there is no evidence that men become entrapped in physically abusive relationships with women in the way that battered women do (Mahoney et al., 2001). Neither is there the same degree of cultural support when women batter male partners, as there is for the power and control dynamics exercised in traditional heterosexual relationships. Thus an understanding of the social and environmental conditions that support male violence against women is crucial in designing crisis counseling interventions that fit the developmental challenges women face as they cope with the possibilities and barriers to leaving violent, oppressive relationships.

It has been estimated that in as many as 25 percent of intimate relationships there will be at least one episode of physical violence during the course of the relationship (Tjaden & Thoennes, 1998). Studies that broaden the definition of violence to include verbal abuse or degradation, threatening displays of anger, and severe restrictions on a partner's personal freedom or initiative raise the estimate of relationship violence even higher. Often, unless the relationship is punctuated by overt episodes of physical violence, a woman will not consider herself to be in an abusive relationship. Verbal abuse may be labeled "just arguing." Jealous accusations or monitoring of behavior are interpreted as demonstrations of love. One incidence of violence can be explained away or excused. An ongoing pattern that affects a woman's physical health and safety or that children begin to notice is more likely to be recognized as "domestic violence." Thus, although many women may experience isolated instances of (relatively) mild physical violence, angry demands, or scolding that is degrading, and might benefit from crisis intervention at those times, most experience a longer and more severe pattern of abuse before they seek help on their own. In those cases where an abusive incident is violent enough to be brought to the attention of police or emergency room physicians, however, a crisis worker may become involved before the abuse has emerged as a pattern of the relationship.

Counseling, whether in the form of a single intervention or a longer-term crisis counseling intervention, needs to take into account the development, nature, and manifestation of abuse, broadly defined, in the course of the relationship, as part of the assessment of the victim's ecological context. In single-session crisis interventions, a crisis worker helps the woman to ensure immediate safety for herself and, perhaps, her children. But he or she also helps open a door to future interventions and assistance, should the woman return to the relationship in which she experienced violence. In crisis counseling, which may involve many sessions over several months, the crisis counselor is often working to draw connections between various kinds and degrees of violence and the overall use of power and control in the relationship. Interventions, long-term or immediate, benefit when crisis workers employ the model described here: empowering the client by validating her experience in a nonblaming and nonjudgmental manner; assessing the immediate potential for lethality (suicide or homicide) on the part of client or abuser; responsive attending to affect, cognition, and behaviors of the client; ascertaining environmental supports available to the client and helping her to access those supports; and clarifying the developmental challenges and opportunities faced by the client in her current phase of life.

DEFINING VIOLENCE IN INTIMATE RELATIONSHIPS

Research on partnership violence that uses survey methodologies strictly limits the definition of violence to discrete behavioral acts of physical assault: punching, slapping, and shoving. Although such research may provide a rough incidence count, it does little to further our understanding of the direction, severity, or chronicity of violence. Moreover, it fails to take into account the wider range of physically damaging and threatening acts that abusers typically employ, and it completely ignores the psychological abuse that often accompanies, or even supplants, direct physical violence.

In contrast to research definitions that simply measure discrete violent acts, Weis (1989) includes behavioral acts that intend, or are perceived by the victim to intend, pain, injury, or the threat of pain or injury. Ellen Pence (1987) defines battering as the ongoing abuse and coercive control of a woman by her relationship partner. Such definitions allow crisis counselors to better understand and explore the full context of abuse when confronted by a battered woman in crisis.

TYPES OF VIOLENCE AND CONTROL

Although the prototypical image of domestic violence is physical abuse resulting in bruises, abrasions, broken bones, and other internal injuries, abuse can take many other forms. For example, sexual abuse is not uncommon in abusive relationships. Rape can take the form of forced vaginal, anal, or oral intercourse, as well as penetration with an object. Sexual exploitation can include forced sexual acts with another person or persons or with animals, videotaping or photographing sexual acts or postures, or the unwanted use of pornography in sexual relations. Sexual abuse sometimes involves the control of reproduction by forcing sex without contraceptives or protection from sexually transmitted diseases (STDs), or, conversely, by inducing or insisting on abortion when pregnancy occurs.

Abusers use various means to isolate their partners, alienate them from family and friends, and control their activities and access to the outside world. Some abusers employ economic control or exploitation. For example, a woman's partner may not permit her to work outside the home, and he may control all of the household resources, perhaps giving her an "allowance" to buy food. A woman may be literally confined to the house, locked in or given no access to a car, and have no money for public transportation. Some women, even if they are allowed to use the car to drive to the supermarket or take the children to the doctor, must strictly account for their mileage and time. The abuser may paint a picture of the woman's friends and family members as evil entities who hate him, can't be trusted, or are always trying to manipulate others. He may forbid her from contacting friends or family, and monitor telephone records.

Intimidation and threats are other tactics that an abuser may use to control his partner's behavior. Yelling or screaming threats of violence, punching a fist into a wall, breaking down a door, or destroying or stealing a woman's property or clothes are all actions that may affect a woman's behavior and sense of safety, even without direct physical abuse to her body. Some abusers use threats of suicide in an attempt to prevent their partner from leaving the relationship. Others may use threats of homicide against the woman, her children, or other family members. And, indeed, those threats are too often carried out (Campbell, 1992; Greenfield et al., 1998). In the United States in 1997, for example, at least 1,217 women were killed by their partners (Fox & Zawitz, 2000). Abusers sometimes use children in the home to coerce compliance from the woman. In addition to threatening to harm children directly, abusers may threaten or actually force children to watch physical punishment or forced sex with their mother "to teach them what happens" when their mother doesn't behave.

Victims often describe emotional or verbal abuse as more harmful than physical abuse. Women sometimes feel they have more control over physical abuse, or at least they know the assault will end at some point. In addition to verbal aggression and threats, verbal abuse can include harsh criticism, denigration, belittling, and degradation about a woman's appearance, weight, intelligence, capacity as a wife or mother, or inability to "do anything right." Jealous accusations of a woman's alleged infidelity or contact with or attraction to other men are frequently used to justify abuse and control.

Even the claim of male privilege can be considered one of the many variations of emotional abuse, and it is frequently employed in addition to other forms of control. Traditional cultural messages that a woman should cater to her partner's needs, sexually satisfy him, prepare meals, maintain a clean and orderly home, nurture and protect him from the outside world, and follow his orders and demands, all work to reinforce a pattern of compliance to a man's wishes and avoidance of potential violence. It may take years for a battered woman to realize that nothing she does or fails to do will prevent the abuse from occurring.

Even when partners separate and are living apart, physical and emotional abuse can continue. In addition, a victim's home may now be subject to break-ins, burglary, or property destruction by the abuser. She may be harassed with phone calls at home or at work. She may be stalked and followed wherever she goes. Her children may be kidnapped by the abuser. A woman's sense of safety and privacy may never be secured.

PATTERNS OF VIOLENCE

Violence in intimate relationships may occur in dating relationships, marriages, cohabiting relationships, or same-sex relationships as well as after separation. Lenore Walker, a psychologist who has written seminally on battering, describes a cyclical pattern of violence that develops in many abusive relationships (Walker, 1979). Between episodes of violence there may occur a "honeymoon" phase, when the woman is relatively free from threat and the relationship seems to be going well. Eventually, tension builds up, which the woman tries to dissipate through compliance and efforts at conciliation or diffusion. Then the physical assault occurs, followed by a phase of contrition and making up. This phase may include promises that the violence will never happen again or expressions of regret that the woman behaved in such a way to bring on the abuser's anger and assault. Walker suggests that the contrition phase becomes reinforcing for both abuser and victim, so that when tension begins to build again, the assault may come sooner in order for the couple to reach the make-up phase more quickly. Over time, the contrition phase becomes shorter and shorter as the relationship endures and sometimes changes to a phase of no tension, without overt expressions of love or contrition. The periods between assaults get shorter, and the severity of the violence usually increases over time.

Other scholars have argued that the violence in many abusive relationships is sporadic rather than cyclical. Some note that the relationship stage before cohabitation or marriage may be important in understanding abusive patterns (cf. Gazmararian, Lazorick, Spitz, Ballard, Saltzman, & Marks, 1996; Kurz, 1996; Sugarman & Hotaling, 1991). Dating may be considered one stage of a relationship in which abusive behavior and controlling attitudes begin to emerge. After cohabitation or marriage begins, there is often (although not always) a honeymoon phase. Pregnancy is another relationship stage that sometimes precipitates abusive behavior. Abuse during pregnancy may include not only physical or sexual assaults, but also coerced drug or alcohol use, forced or induced abortions, or limiting a woman's access to prenatal care. The period after the birth of a child may be considered a relationship stage, as an infant demands a great deal of the woman's attention and time, taking time away from the male partner. And, finally, separation or divorce is a relationship stage that may precipitate new, additional, or more severe violence and threats.

Several scholars have written about abusive relationships using the metaphor of a spiral, in which battered women can move downward, as they become more isolated and hopeless, or upward, as they move toward decreased abuser control

(Chaplin, 1988; Kirkwood, 1993). Such metaphors emphasize the actions that women can take to change both the dynamics of abuse and her perspective on the situation.

Grassroots battered women's advocates have generally dismissed Walker's cycle of abuse theory because of her perceived victim blaming (Whalen, 1996). For example, Walker has written that "the victim becomes complicit in her own abuse" (1979, p. 69) by remaining in the relationship. Activists argue instead that women are acting in their best interests to survive (Pence, 1987).

Moreover, abuse does not always follow a particular pattern, and the victim may not be able to predict an impending assault from a stage of tension building. Some victims are awakened from sleep by being beaten. Others report that they have come to expect that physical abuse will happen under certain conditions: for example, when the abuser has been drinking, when he gets paid, when he has been viewing pornography, when she fails to prepare his dinner correctly, or when the children are noisy. Many women report that the abuse never stops and their fear never ends. The abuse just takes different forms, sometimes physical and always controlling. It is important to remember, however, even in these latter cases, that the abuser and victim also share a history of intimate, loving experiences that often confound the woman's attempts to understand the violence, as well as her efforts to leave the relationship.

DISPELLING MYTHS ABOUT DOMESTIC VIOLENCE

Myth: Women need to be disciplined periodically.

Although the notion that women need guidance, discipline, and direction may seem old-fashioned and out of date, this idea is still prevalent in many of our cultural attitudes and institutional practices. It is rooted in misogynist beliefs that women are fundamentally evil (e.g., responsible for getting man thrown out of the Garden of Eden), unclean (especially when menstruating), and potentially powerful, therefore needing to be controlled by men. Historically, cultural attitudes toward women have often equated women with children. Children, like women, are considered to be the property and responsibility of patriarchal families, their lives determined by father or husband. Children, like women, are in need of discipline, to learn to behave properly. When children, or women, talk back, get angry, or protest, they need a slap in the face to put them back in their place.

Fact: Women are independent, competent human beings, capable of making rational decisions and acting on their own behalf. Women should be protected and treated under the law in the same way men are—as citizens with rights and responsibilities.

Myth: Women who stay in abusive relationships must enjoy the abuse.

Corollary: "If I were hit just once, I'd leave." This attitude may also seem like a throwback to earlier times, but not much earlier. Only eighty years ago Freud was writing about women's masochism, a universal (for women) psychological trait that arose from girls' "knowledge" that they were castrated and must have done something terribly bad (Freud, 1925/1964). Freud contended that girls and women continue to punish themselves for their fundamental badness throughout their lives by taking some amount of pleasure from being hurt. Although Freud's theories about women's masochism are often dismissed by laypeople and contemporary psychologists alike, they still exert a powerful influence over cultural attitudes toward women. Moreover Freud's theories, although they have been modified by contemporary feminist critiques, form the basis for all contemporary psychoanalytic theory and psychoanalytic treatment modalities in psychiatry, psychology, counseling, and social work.

Related to the belief in (other) women's masochism is the conviction many women hold that if their partner ever hit them, they would immediately leave the relationship. Women who have never been abused often find it difficult to understand the conflicting emotions a woman experiences when she is physically assaulted by the man she loves, especially when he apologizes, shows contrition, and says he loves her and that it will never happen again. One assault, she believes, could have been an aberration. It may never happen again.

Fact: Women are not fundamentally masochistic by their psychological nature. One of the mantras of the battered women's movement is that "no one wants to be abused."

Fact: A persistent history of abuse, which a woman slowly comes to identify as intolerable, must be established before most women are ready to consider leaving the relationship. Before the pattern becomes apparent, women often work hard to repair the relationship after each violent incident—not because they enjoy abuse, but because they love the man and have a commitment to the relationship. Further, women fear losing "all that they have worked for"—intangibles like a good marriage, a father for their children, a home, and their possessions. In some cases, they decide to stay in the relationship because of economic concerns, concern for the welfare of their children, or because they realistically fear that the abuser will follow through on threats to kill them if they leave.

Myth: Abuse is driven by (uncontrollable) anger.

One rationale frequently offered by abusers is "She gets me so mad, I can't control myself." This rationale places the blame for the abuse squarely on the victim and suggests that anger, once unleashed, cannot be controlled and that the abuser must hit the victim.

Fact: As battered women activists have pointed out, the abuser's "uncontrollable" anger is likely elicited in other areas of his life as well (e.g., at work), yet typically does not result in assaults on bosses and coworkers. Instead, abuse occurs in intimate relationships partly because of the abuser's belief that he has the right to hit his partner and because he has the power to physically assault her without fear of physical retaliation or criminal arrest.

Some attempts at treating batterers have focused on anger management techniques, but results are largely ineffective in stopping abuse (Walker, 1980). Even if a man learns to punch a pillow or the wall instead of his partner, such displays serve to remind the woman what the abuser is capable of. That is to say, his behavior is still threatening, aimed at displaying his power and controlling her behavior, and so is still abusive by the broader definition used here.

Myth: Abuse is caused by a man's alcohol abuse.

"He only hits me when he's been drinking." "If he would stop drinking, everything would be fine." Violence in marriage has often been linked to the use and abuse of alcohol by men. Indeed, the impetus behind groups like the Women's Christian Temperance Union and the alcohol prohibition movement was the recognition that husbands were physically assaulting their wives in alarming numbers. Similar concerns have been raised about other types of substance abuse, from habitual marijuana use to cocaine or heroin addiction.

Fact: Prohibition did not stop the abuse of women. Neither did it stop alcohol use. But alcohol use or other substance abuse does not, by itself, cause violence in intimate relationships, even when it coexists with violence. When abusers make efforts to stop drinking or taking drugs, through programs like Alcoholics Anonymous (AA) or Narcotics Anonymous (NA), battering behaviors often do not stop. Moreover, most treatment programs (AA and NA, in particular) usually fail to address the male sense of entitlement with regard to "his" woman and his right to control her behaviors.

Myth: An abuser is mentally ill and can be cured through psychological treatment.

In contemporary society, people tend to believe that almost all behavior can be explained by psychological theory. Thus it can be given a diagnostic label, which suggests a particular type of treatment or cure. Therefore, if a man is abusing his partner (a misbehavior), it must be because of a psychological condition similar to a disease (with a particular diagnosis). Depending on the diagnosis, that disease or abnormality can be treated through appropriate drug therapy or counseling.

Fact: The idea that abuse is simply a product of individual aberrance is belied by the prevalence of abuse and surveys of men's attitudes toward women, and wives, in particular. The belief is widespread that when women choose to enter into relationships, they somehow belong to their partners. Moreover, the belief is widespread that a man has the right and responsibility to discipline his partner, and this belief is not limited to a small population of men who can be diagnosed with a particular disorder. Counseling programs for batterers are ineffective unless the batterer accepts responsibility for his abusive behavior (Daly, Power, & Gondolf, 2001).

Myth: Abuse can be understood as a demonstration of love.

"I wouldn't hit you if I didn't love you." "I'm jealous and suspicious of you because I love you so much." Such professions of love serve as another type of rationalization by abusers, and they often have the effect of confusing the victim.

These expressions are related to the conviction that "if I can't have you, nobody else can either," which can lead to murdering the victim.

Fact: Love, which involves mutual caring, nurturing, and the capacity to empathize, is incompatible with physical or psychological abuse and control.

Myth: Abuse is motivated by a woman's behavior.

This notion is akin to the idea that "she makes me so mad, I have to hit something." The victim's behaviors, misbehaviors, or failures to behave are viewed by the abuser, and sometimes by the victim, as the causal locus for the abuse. "She let herself get fat and ugly." "She won't keep the kids quiet." "She's always flirting with other men."

Fact: The victim is not to blame for her own abuse. No matter how she behaves, her partner could always choose not to abuse. The responsibility for abuse lies with the abuser.

Myth: Abuse is a family dynamic. The whole family must be treated.

This belief is a somewhat more sophisticated restatement of the idea that the abuser is not fully responsible for his violent behavior. Rooted in family systems theory, the hypothesis is that any dysfunction in the family can best be understood by analyzing the interacting relationships, alliances, and dynamics within the family. Thus an abuser should not seek individual treatment for his behavior, but the abuser should be treated with his partner and children, as a family unit.

Fact: Family therapy and couples counseling are usually ineffective in stopping the type of relationship violence characterized by terroristic patriarchal control (as contrasted with normative relationship violence). Indeed, a family or couples therapist might mistakenly identify male power as a strength on which to build a healthier relationship. Furthermore, traditional family therapy often fails to note a woman's intimidation by the abuser during the counseling session, as well as the endangering situation she must return to at home, especially when he is displeased with her behavior in therapy (Walker, 1980). Some feminist family therapists, while acknowledging these concerns, have suggested that with some couples and appropriate safeguards, couples or family therapy can effectively address some types of relationship violence (Lipchik, 1991; Luepnitz, 1988).

DIFFERENTIAL EXPERIENCES OF SPECIFIC GROUPS

Women and Ethnic Diversity

Although race is no longer considered a meaningful genetic or anthropological concept, institutions and people in U.S. society still commonly use race to categorize people. Moreover, perceptions of race still hold social significance for many individuals, especially those with racist attitudes. The authors of this text have chosen not to perpetuate the stereotypes that underlie the continued use of racial terminology. Thus, culturally sensitive intervention should reflect ethnic, cultural, and linguistic differences in female victims of violence. The research that employs racial variables should be viewed skeptically and critically.

Victimization studies that have used racial categorization report no significant differences in self-reported rates of intimate violence among African-American, Latina, Asian-American, and Anglo-American groups (Bachman, 1994). This finding, however, tends to reify the notion of race and further obscures the multiplicity of cultural variations within these broad categories. In general, most research employing racial or ethnic categories fails to consider or specify each of the cultural subgroups that can make up the larger racial group. Thus crisis counselors are often urged to be culturally sensitive to members of specific racial groups in a context that desensitizes them to the differences within these groups.

For example, when researchers have used the descriptor *Latina,* they may have included women from Mexico, Puerto Rico, Cuba, or other Caribbean islands, as well as countries in Central and South America, all with very different cultural ethos and different levels of acculturation. Similarly, the category Asian or Asian American may include women from cultures as diverse as China, Japan, Korea, Vietnam, and India. African Americans share a 350-year history of slavery, emancipation, and racism in the United States, but the categorization neglects the contemporary reality of many first- or second-generation Africans (with black, brown, or white skin) who have immigrated to and become citizens of the United States. There have also been secondary immigrations of black-skinned people from Caribbean island countries as diverse as Haiti, Cuba, and Jamaica, with French, Spanish, and British colonialist roots, respectively. Even the category Anglo American or European American is composed of peoples originating in multiple countries and cultures, with varying histories in the United States.

Crisis counselors of all ethnicities must be aware of this diversity when encountering the ethnic, cultural, and linguistic differences among battered women. Social class can interact with ethnic background to produce diverse experiences, attitudes, and expectations. In particular, attitudes toward women and family, including women's roles (e.g., wife and mother) and men's roles (especially husband and father), vary, based partly on cultural background.

Crisis counselors must develop sufficient cultural sensitivity to be open to hearing each woman's unique experience, and they must work to understand that experience within the ecological context of the victim's life, including her self-defined ethnic and cultural heritage. When language barriers to communication exist, counselors must also seek the translation services of an agency or trusted friend or family member of the victim. The experience of overt and covert prejudice can affect women's willingness to seek and accept help from what they perceive to be another majority white institution with mostly white counselors. Moreover, there may be pressure from some ethnic communities not to report acts that may have a negative impact on the majority's perception of that community.

Undocumented and Immigrant Women

Many of the undocumented and immigrant women in the United States suffer not only the effects of being different in America and language barriers to seeking help, but also the very real fear of deportation. Their experiences of abuse are thus compounded by the threat of being reported to or discovered by the Immigration and Naturalization Service (INS) or losing their visa if they attempt to leave the abuser. Abusers may make such threats overtly. But institutional practices that demand documentation also force battered immigrant women into untenable predicaments. Crisis counselors should be aware that in order to remain in the country, these victims might need to return to their abusers.

Lesbian Women

Although the focus of this chapter is relationship violence against women perpetrated by men, it must be acknowledged that lesbians can also be abused by their relationship partners. Indeed, the few studies available indicate that the rate of relationship violence in lesbian relationships is similar to that in heterosexual couples (Brand & Kidd, 1986; Lobel, 1986). Moreover, lesbian battering relationships feature levels of chronicity similar to heterosexual relationships and evidence not only physical abuse, but sexual and emotional abuse as well.

For reasons related to both the acknowledged homophobia of the larger society and the often-internalized homophobia of lesbian women, lesbian victims of abuse often don't seek help. When battered lesbians do seek help from battered women's programs or shelters, sometimes the relationship partner also appears for intervention, asserting that she has been abused. Thus programs are sometimes in the difficult position of having to determine which individuals will receive which services. Even when shelters do accept lesbians for temporary safeguarding, they do not knowingly accept both partners in the relationship.

Battered lesbians often suffer the same psychological effects of repeated violence as heterosexual women, including low self-esteem, powerlessness, helplessness, and hopelessness, but these effects may be compounded by internalized homophobia and self-hatred. Moreover, lesbians, unlike heterosexuals, are often concerned about being "outed" to family, friends, or coworkers. Indeed, lesbian abusers sometimes use this threat to exercise power and control in the relationship.

Crisis counselors must be sensitive to the issues particular to lesbian battering while maintaining their focus on the woman before them who is seeking help. Counselors must also be aware of the homophobia that pervades help service organizations and institutions, including some battered women's programs.

Gay Men

Battering in gay men's relationships occurs at about the same rate as battering in other types of intimate relationships (Bryant & Demian, 1990; Renzetti, 1997).

In communities where there are no services specifically for gay men, a male part-ner may call a women's center for assistance with relationship violence. Battering in relationships between gay men may raise some issues and concerns that are similar to those of battering in lesbian relationships, for example, fear of being "outed" or institutional biases against serving gays (Island & Letellier, 1991).

Blumstein and Schwartz (1983) found that in gay relationships as well as les-bian and heterosexual relationships, the partner with higher income, typically wielded more power. Because power is related to control, abuse, and violence, those with more power in a relationship are more apt to be the abusers when the relationship is characterized by violence. Kurdek (1992) found that gay men, like lesbian couples, typically experienced the most conflict around finances, affection and sex, and the sharing of household tasks.

Crisis workers, when responding to gay men or lesbians, should be cognizant of their own potential homophobia and heterosexist attitudes. Often people have negative biases toward either lesbians or gay men. Thus, crisis workers may be more open to working with gay men than they are to working with lesbians, or vice versa. Moreover, in most communities, apart from large metropolitan areas, there are no organizations to assist gay men experiencing violence in their rela-tionship. Nor can gay men avail themselves of all of the services offered by a women's center (e.g., shelter or group counseling). Crisis workers need to be aware of which services and groups are potential resources for gay men, including counselors who are accepting of them.

Rural Women

Women living in rural areas are easily subjected to the isolation tactics of abusers. For safety purposes, services for battered women are often located in towns or cities, where police protection is more readily available. Rural women may not have ready access to transportation to such services. Moreover, police response to domestic violence calls, although often delayed in urban areas, is even slower when the home is located in a rural area. Sometimes roads aren't paved or there are no street signs or house numbers to help police locate a house. Women seeking help cannot even rely upon telephone service. When toll calls are involved, an abuser can have ready access to telephone records. When the household's only telephone access is a party line, privacy and anonymity are endangered.

Although some crisis centers have developed outreach programs to assist rural women, they are usually insufficient to overcome the tactics of an abuser who is determined to keep his victim isolated from outside contact. Crisis counselors must be attuned to these issues when a rural woman does manage to make con-tact for assistance. She may not get many other chances to find out what options are available to her, and there may be no way to develop a realistic safety plan for her if she returns to the home.

Women with Physical Disabilities

Women with various physical disabilities may be dependent on their abusers for assistance with daily needs. Indeed, a physical disability may create another potential avenue for abusive and threatening behaviors. For example, an abuser might withhold essential medication; block a woman's access to particular areas of the house, such as bathrooms; or prevent access to telephones or transportation, which sometimes have special accommodations that certain people with disabilities need.

Crisis counselors, when working with women with disabilities, must strive to understand the nature of a particular disability in terms of the victim's experience and her perception of the dangers and limitations of her situation. When working with a woman with a hearing impairment, a counselor may need the services of a sign language interpreter to help with communication. Counselors must also be aware of the accessibility limits of shelters and other service providers, as these might affect the victim.

Older Women

Relationship abuse can occur within any age bracket. Women who have been in a relationship with their partner for many years may experience incidents of violence as part of an ongoing history of abuse, which they have learned to cope with. They may have developed their coping strategies at a time when battered women's services had not yet been established or when family and cultural expectations pressed women to remain in their marriages no matter how difficult they were. Sometimes an abusive pattern can begin in later years, perhaps as infirmities or illness strikes one partner. Women in such situations may be dealing with battering for the first time in their lives. Sometimes, because women tend to outlive their male partners, older women establish new relationships that become violent. In these cases, too, older women may be confronting a situation that they had never experienced or imagined.

Institutions that serve older persons and those that serve battered women sometimes compete or conflict with one another about the best, most appropriate services for abused older women. Crisis counselors should be aware of the different institutional philosophies that can affect services as they inform victims of their options. For example, federal- or state-funded programs like Area Agencies on Aging are often most concerned with housing options and financial security for older citizens. If an older woman who has been battered needs or wants to leave her home, the aging agency may have limited resources to assist her. As a result, there is often a subtle pressure on her to remain in the home with the abuser. In contrast, battered women's programs are most concerned with women's long-term safety and their need to be free from abuse. That philosophy can result in subtle pressure on a woman to leave her home and her relationship.

Religious Women

Although it is often important to attend to the religious or spiritual beliefs of a battered woman, especially in terms of how those beliefs affect her experience of violence and her devotion to the relationship, for some women religion is an especially salient and life-pervasive issue. For example, some Catholics engage in daily devotions and have strong beliefs about marriage, sex and reproduction, and women's duty. Both Protestant and Catholic religious doctrine emphasize suffering on earth as the pathway to heaven and so, implicitly or explicitly, may encourage women to put up with an abusive relationship rather than break their marriage vows. Islamic women typically show signs of their religious practice by covering the head and much of the body in a chador or other traditional dress. Islamic women come from a variety of cultural backgrounds ranging from American to African, Indian, or Asian. These cultures may impose their own variations on the religion of Islam and define different roles and appropriate behaviors for married women. Crisis counselors must strive to understand the victim's religious beliefs, as affected by her cultural heritage, especially as they affect her experience of violence, her relationship, and her attempts to seek help.

Uneducated, Unskilled Women

Uneducated or unskilled women often encounter special problems and economic hardships when attempting to leave an abusive relationship. Jobs that pay minimum wage and do not offer child care may be the only jobs available. The alternative is enrolling in the welfare system, which in recent years in most states has been severely curtailed. Although some states offer job training programs designed to help women reach self-sufficiency, the economic reality is that women who have left relationships constitute the greatest proportion of people living in poverty. Low-paying jobs simply do not allow a woman with children to survive, and women who have left their abusers cannot count on child support. Rent, utilities, child care, food, medical services, and clothing expenses typically exceed whatever income the woman is able to bring in, let alone allow for any extra amenities. Crisis counselors, although they may want to help women find ways to leave their abusive relationships, cannot ignore the economic realities of women's lives, especially those with few skills and limited or nonexistent employment experience.

BARRIERS TO LEAVING AN ABUSIVE RELATIONSHIP

Ellen Pence (1987) has developed a schema for describing the types of barriers that women may face when attempting to escape from battering relationships. This schema can help counselors organize their thinking about the explicit needs of women who contact them for help. *Personal barriers* may include feelings of shame, guilt, fear, or a sense of helplessness or hopelessness that impede decisions to leave. Other personal barriers are a lack of financial resources, family networks to rely upon, or job skills. *Relationship barriers* are those that deny a victim access to money, transportation, jobs, and, of course, the physical abuse itself, including the abuser's threats of continued harm or death if she leaves. *Institutional barriers* may include immigration policies, welfare policies, various forms of discrimination (e.g., by sex, ethnicity, or sexual orientation), or simply a lack of services in some areas. For example, the National Coalition Against Domestic Violence (NCADV, 1994) estimates that for every woman accepted into a shelter, three are turned away because of lack of space. *Cultural barriers* may include language differences, religious beliefs, and beliefs about marriage, the family, and women's roles.

THE IMPACT OF ABUSIVE RELATIONSHIPS

Some advocates and activists working in the battered women's movement have been unwilling to examine the long-term negative psychological effects of living in a violent relationship. Believing that this kind of psychological analysis has all too often led to diagnostic thinking and, ultimately, blamed the victim, they have chosen instead to emphasize the strengths developed and displayed by the woman as she works to survive the abuse (Bowker, 1993). As Pence (1987) asserts, a battered woman is always working *in her best interest,* as identified by her at the time, in her ecological situation.

Most feminist counselors and social workers place a similar emphasis on identifying client strengths, although not to the exclusion of understanding the psychological impact of being battered, both physically and emotionally. This impact can sometimes impede women's ability to act in their own best interest. Crisis counselors can assist by attending to the emotional state of the victim, while helping her reframe her sense of her personal strengths and her beliefs, as well as her options for leaving and living independently.

The focus on a victim's psychological state should emphasize the notion that her mental health problems and behaviors, like depression, psychosis, alcohol or drug abuse, do not cause the violence in intimate relationships. If a man is abusive to his partner, he would be so even if the woman had no emotional "problems" or behavioral "deficiencies." Rather, such problems may be the result of being battered over time. Abuse can lead to depression, thoughts of suicide, or attempts to escape through drug or alcohol use. Relationship violence may build on earlier instances of abuse that a victim might have experienced as a child, compounding its psychological effects.

Long-term effects of abuse often include low self-esteem and a sense of helplessness. Constantly being told that one is incompetent, ugly, incapable, or stupid by the person one loves or once loved deteriorates even the strongest self-identity. Helplessness and hopelessness may develop as the victim attempts to control or avoid the violence through her behavior toward the abuser, and fails at those attempts time after time. She develops a sense that nothing she does, or can do, will prevent the abuse. Often self-blaming thoughts emerge, with resulting feelings of guilt.

Lenore Walker (1991) has described a "battered woman syndrome" that she analyzes as a specific case of Posttraumatic Stress Disorder (PTSD). Symptoms of this syndrome include intrusive memories or flashbacks of abuse, ongoing fear that borders on terror, anxiety and sleep disturbances, and hypervigilance, which may result from long-term abuse. Although some activists in the battered women's movement have rejected the battered woman syndrome and PTSD labels because of their diagnostic flavor, these labels may help crisis workers understand the complex debilitating outcome of repeated violence and respond appropriately to the individual before them. Moreover, these diagnoses have sometimes been used in defense of women who assault or kill their abusers. Even if a woman appears to those outside the situation not to be in immediate danger of abuse, she may feel threatened and feel that she is in imminent danger. Thus an attempt to kill her abuser may be legally interpreted as an action of self-defense (Browne, 1987; Walker, 1993). Victims of relationship abuse often believe, sometimes rightly, that they will never be free of abuse until the batterer is dead. Crisis counselors should always be attuned to such beliefs in order to assess the potential for homicidal behavior in clients. Additionally, when a battered woman's feelings of despair turn to thoughts of suicide as the only means of escape, counselors need to be able to assess and respond to that crisis.

Victims are typically only able to acknowledge abuse after a pattern or history of abuse has been established, not after a single incident, no matter how severe. In cases of emotional abuse, without overt violence, acknowledgement may come even more slowly. Even when one incident is identified as abusive or violent, victims usually do not want to give up on the relationship at that point. Over the course of an abusive relationship, however, victims often seek help. Sometimes a victim may seek help by encouraging the batterer, during his stage of contrition, to seek counseling or to go to AA. Some women are willing to confide in a clergyman or a close friend. The responses they receive from such disclosures can affect their willingness to seek additional help.

Some women tell their family about the abuse. Parents or siblings may want to rescue the victim or retaliate in some way. Some women's parents merely advise them to put up with the abuse: "You've made your bed; now lie in it." "Your father beat me too, and I never left." "There's no way you can come back home." "What about your children?" "How will you support yourself?" "I told you that guy was no good."

Help is sometimes forced on victims, even when they don't ask for it. When the police respond to a domestic disturbance complaint, they may refer the victim to a battered women's program. Some states now have mandatory arrest policies for domestic violence calls. Even in those states, however, police are often reluctant to arrest a man for what may appear to them to be a "minor" incident, especially if the woman asks them not to arrest him. Yet police may still provide the woman with information about shelters or crisis programs.

When injuries are severe enough to send a woman to the hospital or family physician, health care workers may make referrals or call in a crisis worker to talk with the victim. Such responses at least let victims know that services exist to help women in similar situations, even if they do not fully understand the kinds of help available. When a victim is willing to talk with a crisis worker, the crisis worker can provide more specific information. The crisis worker then has the opportunity to demonstrate her willingness to listen, her acceptance of the woman, her belief in the victim's experience, and her hope that the woman will make safety plans, seek shelter, and eventually make a decision about whether to leave or stay in the relationship.

Crisis counselors also should be aware of the potential feelings and thoughts that a woman may have in the immediate aftermath of a single incident of violence. Whether the incident is the woman's first experience with relationship violence or is the latest in a series, each incident is a crisis and therefore presents unique opportunities for intervention. Denial or minimization of the abuse often occurs. Feelings of shame that impede full disclosure are often present. Self-blame, for bringing on the violence, may underlie communications about the assault. A woman's belief that she can help her abuser change his behavior is not uncommon. Feelings of love for her partner often exist concurrently with anger, shame, or guilt.

CRISIS INTERVENTION WITH BATTERED WOMEN

Opportunities for crisis intervention most frequently occur in conjunction with or subsequent to a single incident of violence, which may or may not yet be apparent to a victim as part of an ongoing pattern of abuse. A woman who is being psychologically or emotionally abused, but not physically battered, is much less likely to voluntarily seek out or be immediately referred for crisis intervention, as distinct from crisis counseling. Emotional abuse, however, is almost inevitably part of the context in which overt physical violence occurs, and must also be attended to.

Because physical violence is usually prominent in crisis intervention calls, crisis workers, when called to meet with a victim in person, need to contend with and respond to at least some amount of physical harm to the victim. Observing the physical bruising, broken bones, abrasions and lacerations, missing teeth, and swollen features that victims often suffer can raise complex feelings in the crisis worker, which must be dealt with in a manner that does not adversely affect the woman or the crisis intervention. It is best to expect pronounced, visible physical damage and to be prepared not to wince or cringe. It helps to stay focused on one's role as an accepting helper, not readily shocked, ready to hear and empathize with the victim's feelings and cognitive state.

Crisis Hotline/Telephone Contact: Special Concerns

Not all crisis calls involve a request to meet with the victim, although it is probably best to do so, if possible. Direct calls to a hotline from a victim may come while the woman is at home, sometimes while she is still in danger. When a woman manages to place a call to a crisis worker while the abuse is still occurring and/or when the abuser is still in the home, the crisis worker's first obligation is to try to ascertain whether the woman is safe and ensure her immediate safety from further harm.

If the abuser has not been identified as a male or a husband, or if the woman has not used the pronoun *he,* crisis workers should be careful not to assume the sex of the abuser. Because the majority of calls will come from a woman who is being abused by a man, however, most of the suggested counselor responses here are couched in gendered terms. *"Is he in the room with you now?" "Are you in danger now?" "Have you called the police?"* If the abuser is in the room with the woman, this fact may limit the kinds of responses and the amount of information the woman is able to provide, and the crisis worker must be sensitive to asking for responses that might further endanger the woman.

A woman may call a crisis worker in the hope that the telephone call will diffuse the violence, without necessitating a call to the police. She may even want the crisis worker to talk with the abuser to "calm him down." In such situations, as a crisis worker you need to respond that your job is to talk with *her,* to help *her* get to safety as soon as possible, and that if she is unable to talk openly now, although you will try to stay on the line with her, she should call again as soon as she can talk safely. If a crisis worker is actually put on the phone with an abuser, the abuser will probably attempt to justify his behavior and to further threaten the victim. Anything the crisis worker does or says to the abuser may serve to escalate the violence, so it is best to try to maintain direct contact with the victim.

In such situations, when the abuser is still in the home, and the crisis worker hears from the victim that abuse is still imminent, the crisis worker should offer to contact the police. *"Have you called the police?" "May I call them for you?"* The crisis worker should communicate not only her concern for the woman's immediate safety, but the fact that she would like to meet with her in person. If the woman refuses the offer to contact police, the crisis worker might ask, *"Where do you live?"* or *"May I have your phone number in case we are disconnected?"* Police can sometimes locate addresses from telephone numbers, using a reverse directory.

If a crisis worker's call is suddenly disconnected, and she believes the woman is still in danger, the crisis worker could contact the police and report the abuse, just as she might do if she heard neighbors fighting physically. Crisis workers, however, must also be mindful of a victim's right to confidentiality in crisis intervention, and police contact must be weighed along with an assessment of imminent danger and the client's wishes, which may be in conflict. A counselor's "duty to warn" may carry a heavier burden of legal and ethical obligation than that of a crisis volunteer, but the crisis volunteer has an obligation as well.

Perhaps the worst-case scenario is when a call is terminated before a crisis worker has sufficient information to assess the danger or to get help for the woman by reporting the abuse. Such situations, in which one is powerless to take any helpful action, may be extremely stressful and troubling for the crisis worker. The best one can hope for in such situations is that the crisis worker was able to offer sufficient empathy and concern to the caller that she is willing to call again if she has the opportunity. Such situations emphasize how critical it is to establish, through vocal intonation and caring responses, an immediate emotional connection with the caller.

SINGLE-SESSION CRISIS COUNSELING

Because many battered women's organizations have policies against crisis workers going directly to a victim's home, in most cases in-person contact with an abused woman occurs in a hospital emergency room, a police station, a church facility, or even a place like a diner. If a call comes directly from a victim, and she is able to get away, the crisis worker should try to meet her somewhere in a public space. A hospital emergency room is often the safest place, and certainly a place where injuries can be tended. Often, private counseling space is made available in hospitals for victims and crisis workers, so that a counseling connection can be more easily established and confidentiality ensured.

A crisis intervention contact, made in an atmosphere of safety, has three primary goals in addition to establishing a caring, empathic, helpful counseling connection. First, the immediate and short-term safety of the woman, and her children, if any, must be ensured. Second, the woman must attain short-term mastery of the crisis situation she confronts. Third, the woman must be helped to connect with familial, social, and community supports that are available. Perhaps most important, the crisis worker needs to open the door for continued contact or for future contacts, either with the crisis worker herself or with the organization she represents, for example, a battered women's shelter.

These are goals to keep in mind as the crisis worker also works to communicate acceptance for the woman's experience, a willingness to hear and believe, and an empowering expectation that the woman will survive and be able to change her situation. As the counseling connection is established, the crisis worker is also continuously assessing the woman's emotional, cognitive, and behavioral state, while attending to her developmental level and opportunities, and the supports available from her ecosystem. The crisis worker engages in such assessment *with* the client, rather than at a distance, and assists by offering gentle reframing, when appropriate.

Step 1:
Supportively and empathically join with the client.

Crisis intervention with battered women is often frustrating work for counselors because they may not see the full impact of their intervention or any concrete beneficial results for the victim. The woman may return home to the abuser and may not seek intervention, counseling, or follow-up for an extended period of time. If the woman does contact someone for help in the future, it may not be the original crisis counselor. Crisis intervention workers can help diffuse this frustration in the way they frame their work.

One of the primary components of crisis intervention with battered women should be establishing a sufficient counseling and empathic connection to ensure that a woman feels validated, believed, and understood. If she is able to come away from even a brief contact with some of those feelings, she is much more likely to call for assistance in the future, when the abuse occurs again, as it almost inevitably will. The crisis worker must begin to build that empathic connection from the first contact by telephone, and, if she has the opportunity to meet with the woman, will be able to further the counseling connection.

Although concern and planning for the woman's immediate safety is a practical priority, the building of the counseling connection should be the crisis worker's first concern, because it is likely to have the most beneficial long-term results. The importance of this aspect of intervention should encourage crisis counselors not to rush into problem-solving mode or overwhelm a woman with options. Building and conveying an empathic, respectful connection takes some time and must not be neglected. The counselor's listening and responding skills are crucial in this regard. Although the counselor may never know the ultimate outcome for the woman she is working with during a crisis, she needs to know that she did her best to open the door for further intervention and help-seeking. And counselors can further encourage a woman with explicit statements such as, "No *matter what you decide tonight, you can always call again.*"

Step 2:
Intervene to create safety, stabilize the situation, and handle the client's immediate needs.

The crisis worker must help the woman assess her immediate safety and that of her children by considering such factors as whether the abuser has been arrested, whether it is safe to return home, whether there are friends or family members she can stay with, or whether shelter space is available. If the abuser is still at home, and she wants to return home, does she believe the violence is over for now and that it is safe to be in the home? What about the children? Are they with her or at home with him? Many battered women assure crisis workers that their children are not in danger from the abuser, that he never hits the kids, that he's a good father. Although the crisis worker needs to hear and, to some extent, accept this assessment, it is also an opportunity to offer information about the effects on children of seeing violence in the home and seeing their mother beaten. The crisis worker can offer counseling for the children, especially when programs have trained children's advocates on staff.

When victims are experiencing overt traumatic stress reactions to an incident of physical violence, they may have difficulty thinking clearly about their immediate safety and the safety of their children. They may be initially unable to make any decisions about where to go or how to be safe, so they reject all options offered. The crisis worker then needs to help the woman stabilize her thoughts and emotions by stepping back and taking time to encourage her to tell her story and talk about how she understands her experience and how she interprets the abuse.

Even in seemingly obvious cases where physical violence has occurred, the victim may not label her experience as abuse or violence because she interprets it as "a fight," perhaps because she initiated the hitting or fought back. She may blame herself to such an extent that she accepts the entire responsibility for being beaten and is unable to understand that the responsibility for the violence lies with the abuser. Crisis counselors may need to repeat the message several times: *"No one deserves to be abused." "Nothing you did or failed to do caused his violence. He beat you and that is not OK."* (It is also against the law.)

Step 3:
Explore and assess the dimensions of the crisis and the client's reaction to the crisis.

This third step involves several interrelated steps that the crisis worker must attend to in tandem, rather than sequentially. The following discussion employs the ABCDE framework to assess and attend to the battered woman's affective, cognitive, and behavioral states, as well as her developmental issues and ecological situation.

Affect

As with intervention in all crisis situations, the counselor must attend to and assess the victim's immediate affective state. As previously noted, battered women may have difficulty fully acknowledging the extent to which violence and control affects their lives, due to feelings of shame or self-blame. Counselors can help women identify such feelings by directly asking them how it feels to talk about what happened with the counselor. References to "feeling embarrassed" are clues to shameful feelings. Comments like "it's my fault" reveal self-blame and, often, feelings of guilt. Helping victims to expand upon such feelings can help them name and clarify those feelings, while demonstrating your willingness to hear and accept.

Feelings of fear are common in battered women. Fear about the extent of one's injuries, fear of the batterer and the possibility of more violence, and fear for the safety of one's children may all be present. More practical fears, like losing one's job or what might happen to one's partner if he is incarcerated, might be better labeled concerns that a counselor can help the woman think through and come up with solutions for. But all of the fears and concerns that the victim is confronting can be temporarily incapacitating and impede decision making. Crisis counselors must listen for the specific fears expressed by the victim and help explore them one by one. A counselor should never reject a woman's fear that the batterer might kill her, because this fear might be a realistic assessment, based on threats that he has made and her intimate knowledge of what he is capable of. It is not comforting to respond that only a small percentage of abusers actually follow through on threats to kill. It is better to help the woman assess the potential for lethality and his access to a means for killing her. This kind of response communicates the counselor's belief in the woman's experience, while introducing the basis for discussing what she can do to ensure her immediate safety.

Crisis intervention counselors may sometimes hear women express angry feelings, as well. Although battered women are often too battered emotionally to consciously experience anger toward the abuser, those feelings may underlie some of the other feelings they express. Angry feelings can be seen as a source of potential strength for the woman, and should be noticed and given empathic support. Sometimes a woman, while denying her angry feelings about what has been done to her, may allow herself to be angry about what the violence is doing to the children.

Counselors should also attend to the feelings of love the woman may express for the abuser. Although counselors might prefer to hear about her negative feelings toward the abuser, it is important to recognize that there are likely to be experiences of loving times within the relationship history. Women may want to talk about the love they feel for their partner, as they attempt to understand why he abuses the person he purportedly loves. As crisis counselors listen to these expressions of love, they can also help women begin to reframe their thoughts about what counts as love by talking about trust, respect, mutual concern, and caretaking.

In attending to the victim's emotional state, crisis counselors also need to assess signs of depressive feelings that might lead to suicidal thinking. Counselors need to listen for feelings of helplessness and hopelessness as well as explicit ideation that the woman wishes she could go to sleep forever or that the only way out is to kill herself. Crisis counselors must gently probe for how far such thoughts have gone in terms of developing an actual plan.

Behavior

There is seldom a clear line of demarcation between assessing emotions, cognition, and behavior, thus, as we have noted, these areas are assessed synchronously and interactively. The emotions a victim is experiencing affects (and reflects) how she is thinking about the situation and, further, which behaviors she is likely to pursue. Thoughts and expressed emotional states are the clues the crisis counselor must use to assess the potential for certain behavior, especially behaviors like suicide or homicide.

But other behavioral possibilities must also be assessed and addressed. For example, a victim may habitually use alcohol or drugs to cope with her situation. Also, it is well documented that victims of incest or other early childhood sexual abuse are well represented among those who self-mutilate. Crisis counselors should ask the woman about how she usually deals with stress and pain, or what works to help ease the pain. Responses can provide clues about self-endangering behaviors, as well as strengths that the woman possesses, which she may call upon in this situation.

Cognition

Often a victim minimizes the extent of the abuse she has experienced during the course of a relationship or denies that she is a battered woman or a domestic violence victim. These cognitive defense mechanisms can serve an important function in terms of allowing the woman to survive and remain in the relationship day-to-day. But denial and minimization can also mean that she has yet to accept and name her experiences as abuse. A crisis intervention counselor can help by naming the violence as abuse and connecting the physical abuse to other forms of psychological control in the relationship. Timing is critical in this regard, and the counselor must find ways to offer this information without directly contradicting the woman's description of her experience.

Crisis counselors must also assess the woman's immediate capacity for decision-making and help to break down what seems to be an overwhelming task into manageable chunks. It is not necessary for a woman to decide on every step she will take in her life from this point on, but she may be thinking about all of the problems she will confront should she decide to leave the relationship. Housing, employment, children, divorce, loneliness, and safety concerns may all be impinging on her at once. Crisis counselors can help by identifying what she needs to decide upon immediately and what she can talk about and consider the next day. This tactic not only helps the woman manage immediate decisions, but also helps establish a connection for continued counseling contact and assistance.

Crisis counselors should be aware of the possibility that the victim will experience "flooding," or vivid imagery of the events that have taken place. These images can be overwhelming because they come unbidden and are largely out of the woman's control. In effect, they cause the victim to relive her experience of being beaten. Counselors should try to recognize when flooding may be occurring, offer support and empathy, name the experience, and reassure the victim that it will pass. When the imagery or reliving experience is dissipating, counselors can help by encouraging relaxation, deep breathing, and, perhaps, suggesting that the victim think about a safe place or time or event to substitute for the thoughts and feelings of terror. This may help the woman regain a sense of cognitive control.

Thoughts of suicide or homicide must be given special attention. Crisis intervention counselors must attend to and help the woman verbalize such thoughts, if present, in order to assess the likelihood that she might actually carry out a suicide or kill her abuser. Women may realistically feel that the only way to be safe from the abuser is to kill him. Crisis counselors must help the woman see that other options are available and, perhaps, remind her of the consequences to her and her children should she attempt to kill the abuser. Incarceration would serve neither her best interests nor her children's.

If the counselor determines that thoughts of suicide or homicide are likely to lead to attempts to carry out these acts, immediate action must be taken. In the case of suicide, it may be necessary to refer a woman to the mental health system or hospital emergency room to petition for temporary commitment for treatment. In the case of homicide threats, it may be necessary to call the police. The counselor should be very cautious about warning potential targets of homicide when the target is an abuser who has recently beaten his partner, for in warning that individual, one is also endangering the woman.

Development

Attention to developmental level and developmental opportunities is sometimes overlooked in crisis situations, but it behooves the crisis counselor to at least consider some developmental issues. Age is one factor that relates to developmental opportunities, although it is often less influential than life events for a particular individual. The counselor might explore the relationship stage in terms of the length of the relationship, whether there are biological or adopted children or stepchildren of the couple in the home, the children's ages, whether there have been previous attempts at separation or divorce, or whether either partner has had affairs. It is helpful to ask about the history of abuse in the current relationship and perhaps to touch upon prior experiences of abuse as a child or in other relationships. Another avenue for exploration might be the woman's job history or career efforts, as well as educational background.

In considering some of these issues, the crisis intervention counselor is trying to get as complete and holistic a picture of the woman, her current life, her history, and her future possibilities as is possible in a relatively brief, perhaps one-time, encounter. This picture can help guide the crisis intervention, but should not be used to foreclose possible avenues for further growth. Just because a woman has a prior history of abuse does not mean that she is doomed to experience violent relationships, even though she may feel that way.

Ecosystem

Crisis intervention counselors must be knowledgeable about the kinds of social and support services that are available in the community, the financial costs of such services, and the institutional barriers that make accessing some services more difficult for battered women. Counselors can then conduct options counseling from an informed base. Counselors, however, should also assess the personal supports that may be available from friends, family members, church pastors or organizations, or service providers that the woman is already connected to. It may be important to urge the woman to reach out to these people and support systems, because often she is used to keeping the abuse a secret; or she may expect or have already received an unsupportive response from them.

Crisis counselors can offer to serve as a liaison between the woman and the potential resource person or to accompany her to talk with someone. Often a victim's central concern is an economic one: "How will I pay rent, feed my children, get medical care, or pay for an attorney?" Crisis counselors may need to help women learn what financial help is available from public agencies or nonprofit groups, as well as help her explore the possibility of financial assistance from her personal support system. If a woman has access to a joint checking or savings account, she should know that she can legally withdraw money from the account.

Additional issues to consider   Crisis intervention counselors may sometimes have to attend to the crisis needs of children who accompany their mother to the hospital or an interview. If another crisis counselor or volunteer is available, it would be beneficial to call her in to assist. The crisis worker who is helping the children must be attuned to their special needs. Depending on the age of the children and their understanding of what has occurred, children may experience the same range of emotions that the victim herself does: fear, anger, shame, guilt, depression. These emotions, of course, are colored by the children's concerns about their mother's well-being, their own safety, access to their home, pets, or belongings, or, perhaps, concern for their father. Crisis intervention with children follows principles similar to those for working with adults, but adult counselors must be mindful of their tendency to infantilize, talk down to children, or "protect" them from the violent experience they have been affected by. It is important to ask respectful questions and respond seriously to their questions as well as to the emotional content behind a child's response.

Sometimes, crisis intervention counselors may also need to respond to the concerns of family members other than children. For example, a mother, father, or sibling may accompany the victim to the hospital or to an interview. In addition to feeling concern about the victim and her children, some family members can feel quite angry. They may want to urge that the abuser be arrested, or they may want to take matters into their own hands and aggressively go after the abuser. Crisis intervention with family members is necessary in such cases. If the crisis worker can call in another counselor or volunteer to work with the family, she can continue to focus on the victim and her needs. Trying to manage the often conflicting emotions, needs, and concerns of the victim and her family members can be counterproductive and, more important, can infringe on the victim's ability to explore her options and arrive at decisions that are best for her.

It is a good idea to take instant photographs of all visible injuries the victim has sustained. Some hospital emergency rooms take photographs as part of their protocol for working with domestic violence patients; or the police may request permission to take photographs to document the extent of the victim's injuries. In some communities this task is left to the battered women's program and the crisis worker. Although it may interrupt the flow of establishing the counseling connection, the crisis worker can explain the importance of documenting the victim's injuries in case she decides to pursue legal options. The crisis worker should always be sure to get the woman's informed consent before taking photographs, letting her know how they will be safeguarded, who will have access to them, and how they might be used.

Step 4:
Identify and examine alternative actions and develop options.

As the crisis worker explores the crisis event and client reactions, she is also developing alternative actions that the client can consider in order to ensure her safety. This step entails focusing on the possible actions and resources that the client has identified, as well as discussing legal and community services that she might consider using. The crisis worker should let a battered woman know about protection orders and how they function in her specific community. She needs to explore where the victim and her children will stay for the night and in the immediate future: whether they will return home, stay with family or friends, or accept a brief stay in a shelter.

It is helpful to explore a range of options for each of these issues, so that the client can empower herself by making the decisions she believes will work best for her. It is also important, however, not to overwhelm the client with too many choices. Careful listening and attention to the woman's ideas and concerns must be balanced with providing information about community services that she might not be aware of.

Crisis counselors may need to emphasize that the abuse is not likely to stop. If it happened once, it is likely to happen again. If the client returns home without any intervention, she may be putting herself and her children in danger. She may fear that if she doesn't return home, the abuser will become angry again, or even angrier, so that ultimately she and her children will be in even more danger. These kinds of fears may be the result of a realistic assessment of her specific situation. The crisis worker needs to help the client explore and weigh other possible options, while respecting her decision to return home now or in the near future.

Emergency protection orders   One option for establishing safety is an emergency protection order, enforced by police, that forces the abuser out of the home and orders him to keep away from the woman, her children, and the home until a court hearing is held. The hearing is held to determine if the order will be made permanent for a specified period of time, usually six months to one year. Such orders may not be sufficient to actually keep the man away, but he can be subject to arrest if he violates the order. Crisis workers must be familiar with how such protection orders are issued and enforced (or not enforced) in their specific localities, in order to help the victim understand the practical realities of this legal avenue and the real protection she can expect (or not expect).

If the woman believes a temporary protection order will suffice, she should know what to expect from the legal system should she decide not to follow up with the court hearing to issue a permanent order. In some communities, for example, police are less apt to respond in a timely manner to domestic disturbance calls from a woman who has failed to follow through in the court system. In a few communities, the protection-from-abuse hearing is held even when the woman decides not to appear or request a permanent order, and the order may be issued anyway, sometimes with the provision that the abuser seek counseling.

Safe housing/shelter   Another avenue for creating a short-term safe environment is to locate safe housing for the woman and her children. Sometimes family or friends can provide a temporary safe haven for the victim and her children. When such support is available, the crisis worker and client should consider the risk and possible responses if the abuser should come to the safe haven and engage in threatening behavior toward her, the children, or the supporter. Even if the woman believes that the abuser is not likely to come to the home of a safe haven provider, she should consider how to handle harassing phone calls, surveillance, or stalking by the abuser. Such actions are all intended to intimidate her into coming home. Women in these situations sometimes decide to return home simply to end the harassing behavior, and because they do not want to feel responsible for inflicting their relationship problems on friends or family. Crisis counselors should inform women that protection orders may still be available through the court if the abusive behavior persists and that, in the long run, returning home is not likely to end the physical abuse or the attempts at psychological control.

When a shelter for battered women is available and has space, the crisis counselor may offer this as an option for immediate safety. Usually, shelters also take in young children along with the battered woman, so she does not need to leave her children behind or find other options for them. Many shelters do have policies that prohibit admitting young male adolescents, however. In such cases, the crisis counselor may need to help the woman consider other options for her teenage sons. Shelters often require residents to sign agreements that include rules for living at the shelter. If the crisis counselor works directly for the shelter program, she should take time to review those rules and help the woman assess whether she might have problems following the rules. If the crisis counselor does not work directly for the shelter program and is making a referral to the program for emergency shelter, she still needs to be aware of shelter restrictions that might affect the woman, so they can be addressed before the referral is made. The woman should definitely be informed if there are specified limits on shelter stays and that she will get help making plans for what to do after leaving the shelter.

Step 5:
Help the client mobilize personal and social resources.

Once the battered woman has explored alternatives and decided upon actions to take, the crisis worker can help her make the phone calls and contacts that will connect her to the support systems that have been identified. The crisis worker should encourage the woman to make calls to family members or friends whom she has identified as supportive, to the extent that she feels able.

Sometimes, the woman may ask the crisis worker to initiate the call to help lay the groundwork for her contact. In such cases, the crisis worker should be mindful of not taking over for the battered woman. Even if the woman says she can't make the contact herself and she wants the crisis worker to speak for her, the ultimate outcome of taking over for the woman is disempowerment. The crisis worker might serve as the contact initiator in calls to the police, a district magistrate, or the battered woman's shelter, however, because such formal systems sometimes view the counselor as having more credibility and authority than the victim and so may be more responsive to offering appropriate services.

Step 6:
Anticipate the future and arrange follow-up contact.

In order to help a woman who has been a victim of relationship violence anticipate the future, the crisis worker should look for opportunities to gently inform the woman that, should she return to the relationship, the violence is likely to occur again and may escalate over time. The intent of this message is not to threaten or frighten the woman, but rather to let her know that abuse, once it starts, is likely to continue or occur again, even when the abuser is contrite, remorseful, or agrees to counseling. The crisis worker should also communicate acceptance of the woman's decision, whether she decides to leave or stay in the relationship. She should also encourage her to call again, just to talk about her situation and concerns, but especially if violence recurs.

An additional aspect of anticipating future violent behavior is helping the victim understand the impact of intimate relationship violence on her children as well as herself. The woman may be able to articulate her own sense of worthlessness, hopelessness, helplessness, or despair, yet not understand how both the violence and her affective state affect the children. Children who grow up in violent homes learn to expect violence in relationships. Although children often experience fear, anger, and a sense of responsibility for causing the abuse, they also may internalize a normative acceptance of such behavior. Men who become abusers have often grown up in abusive homes; women who are abused have sometimes witnessed violence in the relationships of their parents or stepparents.

Victims of relationship violence, as well as their children, may turn to substance use as a means of coping with or escaping the violence. As counselors know, adolescence is a particularly vulnerable time for acting-out behaviors that can endanger children. A crisis worker should supportively provide this information to the victim, to the extent possible given the time frame of a single session, to communicate her concern and empathy for the victim. When communicated effectively, information about potential effects and outcomes may eventually help a woman along the road toward "getting free" (NiCarthy, 1982) from relationship violence.

Develop a safety plan   One of the things that a crisis worker always needs to address, especially with women who intend to return home to abusers, is the development of a safety plan in the event of further violence, immediately or in the future. If the abuser becomes violent again, what can the woman do to ensure her own safety and that of her children? Does she have access to a telephone to call a hotline or the police? Are there times during the day when she might be able to make or receive a telephone call for a telephone counseling session? Are there neighbors, friends, or family members that she can contact for assistance? Can she hide some money away to call a cab, get a bus ticket, or use as a rental deposit? What kind of help might she expect from local child protective services, legal services, battered women's programs, or rental assistance programs? Are there attorneys she can contact for advice about divorce, separation, or child support? Can she get away from the home to come for counseling at the battered women's program?

Often women want to know what kind of help is available for their partners, to help the abusers stop being violent. Few communities have programs for batterers or counselors who specialize in this area. Even when such programs are available, their success is usually limited, because batterers typically refuse to take responsibility for their abusive behavior (Gondolf, 1997).

When a crisis counselor informs a woman about what services are available for batterers, she should also caution her that such counseling is often not successful in stopping abuse. Further, if the physical abuse appears to abate with the help of counseling, other manifestations of abuse and control may appear. Slowly, the crisis counselor should encourage the woman to consider the emotional abuse and psychological control that she is experiencing as well. So, developing a safety plan might include referring a batterer for counseling and at the same time helping the woman make connections between the physical and emotional violence she is experiencing.

Arrange for follow-up contact   Before ending a crisis intervention session with a woman, the crisis worker should always raise the question of follow-up. The crisis worker should always give the woman a card or a telephone number and encourage her to call again, but, if possible, she should determine a specific time when the woman might be able to contact her the next day or the following week. Establishing a specific time or day to call encourages the continuance of the counseling connection. It communicates caring about how the woman is doing and a willingness to talk and share additional ideas. If the woman is reluctant or feels unable to call, the crisis worker might ask if she could call the woman and when the best time would be. If the victim is going to a battered woman's shelter, follow-up is ensured with the program but a crisis worker might also want to work out a personal follow-up contact.

Along with arranging for follow-up contact, it may be helpful to provide the woman with a written list of referrals for assistance, with addresses, telephone numbers, and, if possible, the name of a person she can ask to speak with. If the woman feels that she cannot safely take the list with her, the crisis worker can encourage her to call again when she needs the information.

Sometimes a crisis worker may give a victim a kind of "assignment" as a way of continuing to engage her in struggling with her situation. For example, a worker may ask a woman to write an autobiography, keep a diary that analyzes her partner's efforts to control her behavior, or develop a written safety plan in the event of future violence. The crisis worker can indicate her willingness to review and talk with the woman about those "assignments" should the woman want to contact her.

If the crisis worker is successful in establishing an empathic counseling connection, she will have accomplished an important objective in anticipating and planning for the future. She will have opened a door for future contact in the event that violence occurs again, which is likely. The victim will have felt sufficiently heard, understood, and responded to that even if she returns to the violent relationship, she will be willing to contact the hotline, shelter, or battered women's program again.

The crisis worker's final communication to a woman, at the end of a single-session intervention, should always include the message that no matter what she decides to do, this night or in the future, she is always welcome to call again. This message provides an open door, and also communicates the idea that if violence occurred once in the relationship, the woman should anticipate that it is likely to happen again. In anticipating the possibility of future violence, the crisis worker should also have started the process of connecting physical violence to other forms of emotional abuse and control in the relationship, as well as the impact of these behaviors on children. Crisis workers can encourage women to contact them again when they are ready to further explore these issues and seek additional help.

ONGOING CRISIS COUNSELING WITH BATTERED WOMEN

Thus far we have been considering the counseling aspects and critical concerns for a single-session crisis intervention following a traumatic event like a physical beating. Many of the same counseling aspects and concerns are also important when a woman continues in counseling or requests longer-term crisis counseling for events that have happened in the past. Without reiterating all of the central issues, in this section we consider some of the unique aspects of crisis counseling with formerly battered women, or with women who may still be living in an abusive, although somewhat tolerable, relationship.

Crisis counseling that is precipitated by a history of living in a battering or abusive relationship is not uncommon. Sometimes a woman may still be living in an abusive relationship and might seek strength and guidance for leaving. Perhaps more often, a woman has left the abusive relationship and is living in relative safety. Women in such situations may seek crisis counseling for assistance in getting on with their lives.

Developmental issues become much more prominent in these cases. For example, women may realize the extent to which their lives have been derailed by the cycle of abuse and may be seeking job or career advice. They may be considering educational opportunities. Women may be grappling with loneliness, with living without a partner; they may want to find ways to seek out a new partner; or they may already have met someone and may be fearful of "making the same mistake twice." Women may be encountering difficulties raising children, perhaps because of the children's reactions to living in a violent home.

Some women come for crisis counseling because they are still experiencing symptoms associated with PTSD: anxiety, depression, sleeplessness, or flashbacks. Almost all formerly battered women need to address unresolved issues of loss. Clients may not initially be explicit about their history of abuse when seeking counseling, but as counselors explore a client's history of intimate relationships, whether dating, cohabiting, or marital, they should also probe for experiences of control, abuse, and violence by former partners.

Crisis counseling goals and processes with battered women or formerly battered women can be usefully conceptualized within the ABCDE framework. That is, the woman who has been a victim of intimate relationship violence will be assisted through counseling to *affect* stability, make appropriate *behavioral* adjustments, achieve *cognitive* mastery, recognize and take advantage of *developmental* opportunities, and establish and maintain healthy relationships and social and community contacts in her *ecosystem*. As is true in any counseling effort, the counselor must initially focus on establishing a relationship with the prospective client and beginning to assess her needs and strengths.

Establishing a Supportive and Empowering Counseling Relationship

In crisis counseling with formerly battered women, as with women who have been victims of sexual assault or abuse, the importance of employing an empowerment model for counseling is paramount. Because personal power has often been stripped from women who have been victimized by violence, the counseling relationship should restore power to the client. Practically, an empowering counseling relationship means that the client is seen as a fully participating partner in her own treatment. She defines her problems, establishes the pace and timing of counseling, and determines when to terminate counseling. The crisis counselor serves as an experienced consultant in helping the woman make these decisions.

Earlier definitions of feminist empowerment counseling focused on equalizing the power dynamics between counselor and client, which sometimes led to a blurring of boundaries and roles. But experience has demonstrated that a counseling relationship cannot and ought not to entail an *equal* relationship between counselor and client. The client is seeking help from a counselor with expertise in guiding people to examine their lives and offering options for future direction. The client decides whether or not to accept this assistance and what will work best for her. Together, client and counselor come to an agreement about the counseling contract, whether written or verbal. This kind of discussion and agreement about counseling establishes the basis for further empowering the client as she begins to explore and discuss her situation, feelings, and thoughts.

Preliminary and Ongoing Assessment of Crisis Resolution

The crisis counselor begins with the problem statement presented by the client. When the client explicitly presents her history of abuse as part of the problem statement, the counselor can include this background as part of their common understanding of what to examine. When a client presents a somewhat more vague complaint, like "I'm so unhappy" or "I'm feeling depressed," the counselor explores the roots of those feelings. When a client reveals a history of partner violence, abuse, and control, the crisis counselor works with the woman to incorporate these experiences into the problem definition. The counselor may need to point out some of the ways that such experiences can continue to have an impact on people's lives.

Crisis resolution is often impeded in battered women or formerly battered women because friends, family, and many grassroots counselors prefer to focus on the women's concrete needs for financial assistance, housing, employment, and child care, as well as the benefits of leaving an abusive relationship. Unfortunately, then, the emotional losses a woman might experience are denied expression and exploration (Turner & Shapiro, 1986).

As we have said, assessment is a continuous process that begins with the initial statements regarding needs and problems and extends throughout the counseling intervention. Assessment issues discussed as part of Step 3 of single-session intervention continue to be important considerations for the counselor engaged in ongoing crisis work.

Goals and Processes of Ongoing Crisis Counseling with Battered Women

Affect stability:
Assist the survivor to express and process her memories and emotions related to the abusive relationship.

After a beginning, trusting relationship has begun to form, ongoing crisis counseling always proceeds by encouraging the expression of memories and emotions surrounding the abuse and the relationship. This is often an excruciatingly painful process because the goal is not just a recitation of factual experiences, but an exploration of the meanings and emotions surrounding those experiences. Battered women have frequently survived by numbing themselves to the horror of what is occurring. Healing, however, requires a reconnection with the emotional truth of the abuse and its lasting impact. This might include grappling with the reality of seeing pet animals injured as a form of punishment, remembering sexual abuses perpetrated to demonstrate her husband's control, or struggling to accept her own failure to protect a child.

This process should include an extended exploration of feelings of loss: loss of the idealized relationship, role loss, loss of emotional security or a sense of belonging, as well as loss of the actual relationship and partner (Turner & Shapiro, 1986). Grief frameworks that help clients explore both the positive and negative effects and impacts of these losses, as well as anger that usually accompanies loss, can help move women toward resolution.

Many battered women have been subjected to a wide range of verbal abuse, denigrating their intelligence, their attractiveness, their parenting, their desirability, and their overall worth and value. In response to such painful assertions by someone who presumably knows them better than anyone else, coupled with emotional control and physical violence, many abused women become depressed and anxious. Low self-esteem, depression, and various anxiety disorders are thus common among battered women, particularly those who have been in long-term and/or emotionally controlling abusive relationships (Aguilar & Nightengale, 1994; Orava, McLeod, & Sharpe, 1996). Studies of victims have documented rates of 75 to 80 percent for depression (Dutton, 1993; Goodman, Koss, & Russo, 1993). Rates of phobias, anxiety, PTSD, dysthymia, and panic disorder have also been found to be significantly higher among samples of battered women living both in shelters and in the community compared to the normative population (Gleason, 1993).

Given the likelihood of clinical levels of depression and/or anxiety disorders (e.g., PTSD), it is essential that crisis counselors working with battered women assess and focus interventions on ameliorating these distressing symptoms. Stability of mood may be achieved in the short term through appropriate evaluation and prescription of antidepressant and/or antianxiety medications. In the long term, survivors' moods will change as they successfully process and resolve the emotional and physical arousal surrounding their vivid memories, as their view of themselves changes, and as the internalized messages about their worth are replaced by new experiences and relationships.

Behavioral adjustments:
Assist the survivor to make and sustain necessary behavioral changes.

Many battered women have developed behavioral coping strategies that have helped numb them to the reality of their abusive relationship. For some women, coping efforts have included the use of various substances, including drugs and alcohol. Often this reliance on drugs or alcohol is interpreted (by the woman and perhaps by others as well) as evidence that she is "bad" or "sick." Interventions must focus on assisting battered women to recognize the connection between the abusive relationship and their substance abuse. They must also focus on replacing these ultimately self-destructive coping behaviors with behaviors that will contribute to self-respect and freedom from harm.

The counselor assists the woman in defining her current needs, desires, and limits by exploring her thinking, feelings, and attempts to make changes in her life. Over time, the counselor and client decide together on the behavioral changes she might initiate to help her obtain her stated goals. This may include learning new coping skills (e.g., relaxation, yoga, journaling), developing new parenting behaviors, or facing the challenge of going back to school, applying for a job, or pursuing a new career.

Cognitive mastery:
Assist survivors to examine and reformulate beliefs about herself, the abuse, and the abuser.

Faulty cognitions about self are among the most difficult and important to counter and replace with more realistic self-appraisals. Just as many lay persons question why abused women stay in abusive relationships, many battered women question and blame themselves—for their failure to leave and/or for their failure to stop the batterer's abuse of others. Considering the common tendency to blame abused women for their own abuse, it is extremely important that crisis counselors understand the realities of living with violence and oppression, and the negative choices many abused women have encountered. When a woman perceives her options to be losing everything or hoping that her relationship might improve if only she could "be better," it is not surprising that she chooses to "try to be better." Similarly, if she fears losing her children or being unable to support them, it is not surprising that she tries to do what is necessary to maintain the relationship, particularly if she believes all of the negative things he says about her.

Some activists have described the "web" of control that is exerted over a battered woman as she internalizes her batterer's views of her, his behavior, and their life together. It is often only by beginning to develop an alternative vision of reality that she is able to begin to pull herself free of that "web" and to begin to move toward freedom. Given this fact, crisis counselors must pay particular attention to challenging the views abused women may have of themselves and their situation through their batterer's eyes. Education about power and control dynamics is often a part of this, as is assisting survivors to reconsider the basis for their negative self-appraisals.

The crisis counselor also assists survivors to examine faulty thinking and core beliefs that might impede the attainment of goals. A skilled counselor can help clients revisit assumptions about people and values they hold dear and to understand how they might reframe these assumptions to enhance their current life situations. This may include exploring cultural and/or spiritual beliefs that constrain the woman's attempts to move on.

Developmental mastery: Assist the survivor to examine the impact of abuse on her ongoing development.

As the abuse survivor and the crisis counselor work together, gradually a developmental picture of the individual woman emerges: where she has come from, what developmental opportunities are available to her, and, especially, where she wants to go in the future. Developmental considerations include economic goals such as getting more education or a better job or considering a career path; social goals such as establishing friendships, connecting to the community, or maintaining extended family relationships; and personal goals such as establishing healthy intimate relationships, defining her sexual desires, being a good parent, or becoming the person she wants to be. The latter goal incorporates rebuilding self-esteem and increasing self-efficacy, which may come about as a result of taking steps along the economic and social paths of development.

Ecosystem healthy and intact: Assist the survivor to make changes in her personal ecosystem in order to reestablish connection and community.

People want to be in a relationship. Some battered women may feel lonely and desperate to establish an intimate, loving, romantic, and/or sexual relationship. Others may shy away from such relationships because of their previous negative experiences. Almost all formerly battered women will be wary of getting into relationships characterized by abuse and control. The crisis counselor may need to educate a client about healthy relationships, while exploring the woman's hopes, dreams, and fears for her desired intimate relationship. It can be helpful to brainstorm about potential ways to meet people who could become prospective partners.

Whether or not a woman is actively hoping for or seeking an intimate loving relationship, it is important for her to assess and, perhaps, expand her network of close friendships. What is her history of best friend or close friend relationships? In what ways were those relationships satisfying or unsatisfying? What is she looking for from friendships now, in her current life? How might she meet people who share her interests and who could become friends?

In the course of these discussions, it is also important to consider connections to family members. Strong, healthy ties to family members can be valuable sources of support and validation. Many women feel estranged from different members of their families, however, whether parents, children, or siblings. Counselors need to assess the strength of a woman's relationships with various family members, understand the problems in some of those relationships, and help the woman decide whether she wants to reconnect, with whom, and how best to go about achieving closer relationships.

Crisis counselors sometimes ignore the developmental path that involves establishing connections to a community, as we tend to focus on individual development and personal growth in the psychological realm. It is important to understand the value to the individual of becoming a participant in the broader community, a citizen of the world. For example, many formerly battered women have experienced personal growth by volunteering in local battered women's programs. Women who engage in such activities not only feel good about helping others, but they often experience a sisterhood among women—a sense of connection to a group of people, an organization, or a social movement that helps build an identity of self-efficacy and personal power, and the feeling, "What I do matters."

Of course, becoming a battered woman's advocate is not the only kind of community participation that can benefit a woman. A woman's interests might lie elsewhere. For example, working in electoral politics, helping to create a cleaner environment, or coaching children's athletic teams are all activities that can enhance an individual's sense of contributing to the larger world.

Termination of Crisis Counseling

The crisis counseling intervention terminates as the woman is able to start taking steps along her self-defined developmental paths. Termination is a process that typically leaves the door open for future contact; the crisis counselor expresses interest in the client's successes as well as her continuing struggles and adversities, and conveys trust that the client is able to proceed on her own.

COMPARISON OF SINGLE SESSIONS AND ONGOING COUNSELING

Single-session crisis intervention and crisis counseling with individuals whose experiences include a history of abuse and violence share many important features. The time frame for each type of intervention, however, determines the issues and decisions that must be attended to immediately and those that can be explored more fully over time. In single-session intervention, the crisis worker must ensure the woman's immediate safety, assess the risk for lethality, review the legal and community resources available to her, and open the door for further contact. In ongoing crisis counseling, the crisis worker can often take a slower approach to a deeper exploration of a woman's past, the ways in which the history of abuse continues to constrain her, and her hopes and dreams for the future, empowering the woman to take advantage of the opportunities that are available to her. Both types of intervention focus on establishing an empowering counseling relationship, allowing the expression of events, feelings, and thoughts. Both assess client functioning and potential in the realms of thinking, feeling, and behavior.

Both incorporate a developmental understanding in considering the client's life. Both work to assess and build on the client's social connections and ecosystem.

CASE EXAMPLE: MANDY

Single-Session Crisis Intervention

Beep-beep. The crisis worker's cell phone sounded at 10:48, just as she was get-ting ready to go to bed. Heart pounding, she called the hotline answering service. Would this be something she could handle with a phone call, or would she need to go out and meet a victim somewhere? Would it be a call about a sexual assault or a battered woman? Although trained and prepared to respond to a range of crisis situations, whenever the beeper went off, the crisis worker was always plagued with self-doubt about her ability to help.

The answering service informed her that the hospital emergency room nurse had called with a referral for a domestic violence victim who had been physically assaulted by her husband. The victim was in the ER and had agreed to talk with a crisis volunteer from the local rape and domestic violence program. "I'll be there in five minutes."

The crisis worker began to think about the possible scenarios as she got ready to drive to the ER. How bad was the assault? Would the woman be kept in the hospital? Where was the husband? Had he been arrested? Were there any children who would need attention? At least there was room in the shelter tonight, if that should be needed. As the crisis worker began to consider these issues, her pound-ing heart slowed. She reminded herself about how she wanted to approach and present herself to the victim.

As the nurse led her back to an examination room, she reported that the patient had apparently been beaten with fists and had sustained contusions to the ab-domen and face. There was considerable edema to the face and she had lost a tooth, but there were no broken bones or internal injuries. The doctor was await-ing the results of a CT scan to rule out a concussion, but they expected her to be discharged in a little while. "Her name is Amanda Cummings. She's twenty-five. You'll have a few minutes alone with her until the CT scan comes back." The nurse whispered, "I heard her husband is a police officer."

The bright lights of the examination room revealed a woman sitting up, slouched over on the examination table. She didn't look up when the crisis worker entered the room, shutting the door behind her.

CW: *(in a soft, calm voice) Hello. Amanda Cummings? My name is Doreen. I'm from the women's center. I was told you were willing to see a crisis worker. (A nod from the woman on the table.) What may I call you?*

Client: Mandy *(not looking up).*

CW: *I want to let you know, Mandy, that anything you tell me is confidential. I'm not required to report our conversation to the doctors or the police. I just need* *to be sure that you are safe and not in further danger tonight.* [*The CW introduces the promise of confidentiality, within the limits of ensuring the client's safety.*]

Mandy: Huh. My old man *is* the police. [*Mandy responds to a piece of the communication that refers to contact and communication with the police.*]

CW: *The man who beat you, your husband?* [*Responding to what Mandy has indicated is a concern.*]

Mandy: Yep.

CW: *Can you tell me what happened?* [*Supporting Mandy in talking about the events, to hear how she presents the issues and what is of most concern; to allow her to ventilate.*]

Mandy: I don't even know. He got up pissed, around 7:00. He had to go into work for the night shift. I had his dinner ready for him. The kids were in bed. He started yelling about having chicken again, and complaining about the noise the kids made while he was trying to sleep, and why wasn't his uniform laid out. I snapped back at him about getting his own damn uniform, and he whacked me across the face. Man, I thought he broke something, it hurt so bad. My mouth was bleeding, and I was crying. That seemed to get him even more mad. He started punching me in the stomach. I couldn't even yell. Then he slugged me again in the face. I tried to get out of the house, but he grabbed me and cuffed me to the table. I think I passed out. Next thing I know I'm in an ambulance on the way to the hospital. [*The CW notes that although Mandy referred to her children in telling her story, she has not asked about where they are now.*]

CW: *You've been through a lot tonight, physically and emotionally. Are you able to look at me?* (Mandy looks up.) *Your face is pretty swollen and bruised. Are you in a lot of pain?* [*The CW demonstrates that she is able to look at and see Mandy, the person. She recognizes that Mandy may be sensitive and perhaps ashamed of how she looks after the beating. She demonstrates a willingness to talk about her physical appearance and injuries.*]

Mandy: I guess it's not as bad as it looks. [*Perhaps indicating that she is not experiencing physical pain.*]

CW: *What about the pain we can't see?* [*CW follows up by asking about painful feelings.*]

Mandy: (starting to cry) I can't believe he'd do this to me. I love him so much. He's a good husband and father. [*Expressions of disbelief and of love for her husband.*]

CW: *Has this happened before, Mandy?* [*Picking up on her disbelief and helping Mandy examine previous incidents of abuse or violence, which may not have been labeled by Mandy as abusive.*]

Mandy: Nothing this bad. [*Something has happened before, but perhaps not a beating this severe.*]

CW: *Tell me. [In an encouraging voice, rather than demanding.]*

Mandy: Well, he gets angry easy. Especially when he's tired and has to go to work. And I don't always do the right thing or say the right thing. With two kids, I can't always keep the house perfect or cook the best dinner. And I guess I don't look my best sometimes. *[Mandy does not deny that he has been violent, but is looking to her behaviors as an explanation for his anger.]*

CW: *Has he hit you before, Mandy? [Hearing the self-blame, but focusing for now on the extent of previous violence and how Mandy thinks about it.]*

Mandy: No, not really. He's slapped me a couple of times, but he usually gives me a hug right away. *[Not labeling his previous actions as hitting, but acknowledging that she's been slapped. CW notes that Mandy may be minimizing the previous violence; alternatively, she may not have conceptualized a slap as violent.]*

CW: *It must be pretty scary when he gets angry. It sounds like you kind of blame yourself sometimes, for getting him angry. [Reflecting back the self-blame heard earlier and acknowledging the feelings of fear.]*

Mandy: Well, yeah. . . . I mean, he says it's my fault, and sometimes I think it is. But I was never really scared of him before. *[Crying harder now.]*

CW: *What he did to you, Mandy, is not your fault. No one deserves to get beaten or slapped or abused for any reason. And it sounds like you do your best to take care of him, the kids, and your house. [Repeating the message that no one deserves abuse; naming the abuse, and including beatings and slaps; affirming her attempts to fulfill what she sees as her responsibilities.]*

CW: *What's your biggest concern right now, for tonight, Mandy?*

Mandy: I'm afraid to go home. I don't know what's going to happen when he gets home.

CW: *Do you know where he is now? Do you know if he was arrested?*

Mandy: I doubt it—he's a cop. I assume he just went to work.

CW: *Maybe we should try to find out for sure. If someone called the police to your home, they are supposed to make an arrest if you were harmed, and you clearly were. Maybe we can call the station and see if he's working tonight.*

Mandy: I don't want to talk to him.

CW: *You wouldn't have to. Just identify yourself and ask if your husband is on duty tonight. If the answer is no, you can ask if they know where he is. If the answer is yes, just say thanks and hang up. If he has been arrested, I can probably find out how long they're going to keep him. It's usually until the next weekday, when a judge can hear the case and decide whether or not to issue a protective order. Do you know what that is, a PFA?*

Mandy: No, not really.

CW: *It's a court order that says he has to stay away from you and the children for a period of time; sometimes it's for six months; sometimes it's for a year.*

Mandy: But he's my husband.

CW: *Yes, but he's broken the law . . . and he's hurt you pretty severely. We need to be sure that you are safe, that he's not going to hurt you again.*

Mandy: What if I don't want one, a PFA?

CW: *Most of the time, it won't be issued unless you do want it. Let's look at what you might be able to do to stay safe, if you decide not to request a PFA. Mandy, do you know where your children are now?*

Mandy: They told me in the ambulance that they had gone to my neighbor's house. She's sort of a friend—Liz Jenkins. I guess I should call and check.

CW: *That's probably a good first step. Are you comfortable having them stay there for the night?*

Mandy: What about if Jack comes home?

CW: *Do you think he'd go get them? Would they be safe with him?*

Mandy: *(crying again)* He's never hurt the kids. But they belong with me.

CW: *OK, so we might have to find a way to get the kids to you.*

The CW has switched into a problem-solving mode, as she senses Mandy is able to do so. She has provided information about the PFA process and introduced the idea that her husband may have been arrested. She has offered to help Mandy find out where he is. She has inquired about the children and ascertained that Mandy was told they were safe with a neighbor. Mandy wants the children with her, although it has not yet been decided where she will go for tonight and the immediate future.

At that moment the nurse comes in to announce that the CT scan was normal and that the doctor is ready to release the patient. The CW asks if photographs were taken of the injuries, and is told that there were and that they will be kept with her chart. The nurse says that Mandy may get dressed now. The CW asks if there is a counseling room with a phone that they can use for a while. The nurse says that there is a free room, down the hall.

CW: *Do you need any help getting dressed, Mandy? You must be pretty sore.*

Mandy: Why'd they take pictures?

CW: *It's part of the hospital protocol. Your records and the pictures can be subpoenaed if you need them to support your testimony in court. Are you concerned about the photos?*

Mandy: I'm so embarrassed. I wish they weren't there. I wish it hadn't happened.

CW: *(Silent for a bit, allowing them both to feel Mandy's shame. Then, softly) You didn't cause this to happen, Mandy. It's not your shame.*

Mandy: I know, but I married him. Everyone thinks it's so great, being married to a cop. I don't want to tell anyone.

CW: *Why don't you get dressed now, Mandy? I'll wait outside for you and we'll go down the hall to talk some more.*

Mandy gets dressed and comes out. CW shows her the counseling room, and they sit down, closing the door.

CW: *What gets in the way when you think of telling someone what happened? Who would you tell?*

Mandy: My mom. She just won't believe it.

CW: *Seems like she'd have to believe it if she saw you, saw how you were beaten. Are you afraid she'll blame you?*

Mandy: Yeah, 'cause she always warned us not to take guff from any man, like she did from her first husband. And I try not to take his guff. But when I talk back, look what happens.

CW: *It sounds as though no matter what you do, you're afraid your mother will be disappointed in you.*

Mandy: I guess I could tell my sister.

CW: *She might be able to help you?*

Mandy: She's been through this . . . maybe not as bad. She lives over in the next town.

CW: *Is that a place you might be able to stay for a while, with your kids?*

Mandy: Maybe. We get on each other's nerves after a while.

CW: *Why don't we make that call now to your neighbor, to check on the kids. If things are OK there, just let her know that you may want to pick up the kids later, before Jack gets back.*

Mandy places the call and Liz apparently picks up the phone.

"Hi, Liz? It's Mandy."

"Yeah, I'm OK. Well, I don't look so good, but nothing's broken. My head's OK."

"I'm sorry you had to see all that, but I sure appreciate your taking the kids. Are they OK?"

"Sleeping now, huh?"

"Oh, yeah? They actually arrested him? Ohmigod! Oh man, is he going to be hot."

"Really? The hospital's 'sposed to call the cops before I'm released? They need to talk to me? Am I in trouble?"

"OK. OK. Look, I'm going to find out what's going on. I may come to get the kids tonight or tomorrow. I'll talk to you later."

Mandy: They arrested him. And the cops want to talk to me. They're all his buddies. I can just imagine.

CW: *If they arrested him, Mandy, they're doing their job. And you're right, they may not be happy about it. But the reason the police need to talk to you tonight is to let you know about the arrest, when he will be released, and to* *ask you if you want a PFA hearing. That will be your decision, no matter what his buddies want you to do.*

Mandy: I don't want him in jail. I just need to be away from him for a while, 'til he calms down.

CW: *Do you think he would voluntarily stay away? Would he have a place to go?*

Mandy: No, probably not.

CW: *Maybe we should make that call to your sister. But you should also know that we do have a shelter where you and the kids could stay for awhile.*

Mandy: A shelter?

CW: *It's a house, owned by the women's center. Women who are battered can stay in one of the bedrooms with their children. They live together, cook, and take care of the house, sometimes share their experiences, and help each other along the path to getting free from abuse.*

CW introduces the idea of temporary shelter with other battered women and the women-helping-women model. She also suggests that there is a path to getting free and implies that Mandy has taken the first step.

Mandy: Do the cops know where it is?

CW: *Yes, unofficially they do. Sometimes we need to call them for protection. But we wouldn't allow your husband to come there or contact you there. I think you'd be safe. But maybe you want to check with your sister first?*

Mandy: I think I want to call her. But the shelter sounds like a good idea to me.

CW: *OK. The shelter might offer a little more protection than your sister's house. And it can give you some time to meet with our counselors and figure out what you want to do from here.*

Mandy: Won't I see you again?

CW: *Yes, if you like we can talk again. I certainly would like to help you think through this situation a bit more. We can talk about all your options. But we can also talk about your hopes and dreams for your life.*

Mandy: Huh, my dream's turned into a nightmare.

CW: *Yeah, I bet it feels that way.*

Mandy: How do we get to the shelter? I need to get my kids . . . and some things from the house.

CW: *Let's see if we can talk to the police about that, since they may have been called about your release. They can go with us while you get some clothes and pick up the kids. If you have a checkbook or savings book, it might be a good idea to get that while you're there. Then I'll drive you all to the shelter. We'll have to go over some paperwork there, and I'll want to review the rules with you.*

Mandy: The rules?

CW: *Well, we don't want you to ever give out the address of the shelter to anyone. And we don't allow drugs or alcohol there. They're mostly rules that help protect the safety of everyone in the house.*

Mandy: Thank you so much for all your help.

As the CW checks with the nurse about the police notification and to arrange an escort to go with Mandy to her home, she reviews the pieces of the intervention that she has touched on and those that are still to be addressed at some point. She has started to establish a counseling connection with Mandy, as evidenced by Mandy's thanking her and wanting to continue talking with her during her shelter stay. The stay at the shelter will ensure at least some immediate follow-up to this night's crisis. She has helped Mandy develop a plan to ensure her safety and that of her children, tonight and over the next several weeks, if necessary. Affectively, Mandy is in touch with her feelings of vulnerability, shame, fear, and guilt.

Conclusion

The crisis worker has done a good job of attending to and empathizing with Mandy's feelings, while beginning to lay the groundwork for challenging her self-blaming thoughts. Mandy still expresses feelings of love for her husband, even though she fears him. She is only dimly aware of some of her anger toward him. The crisis worker knows that if Mandy is ever going to consider leaving this relationship, she must capitalize on that anger and legitimize it as a source of strength. Cognitively, Mandy is just beginning the process of defining her relationship as an abusive one. The crisis worker will want to talk with Mandy about her mother's history of abuse, as well as the history of Mandy's relationship. The crisis worker has suggested that there is a path that leads toward freedom from violence.

With the crisis worker's help, Mandy has been able to make the decisions she needed to make tonight. The crisis worker has seen no indications of suicidality or homicidality on Mandy's part. In terms of her ecosystem, Mandy may have some family support from her sister, whom she plans to call. Her mother may be another source of support, as well. The legal system options are complicated by the fact that her husband is a police officer, and enforcement of a protection order may be attenuated by his coworkers' sympathy for him. Mandy has not talked about her own employment, and the crisis worker has not explicitly asked about it yet. The crisis worker understands that Mandy is at a developmental stage in which she is attempting to be a good wife and mother to her young children. This crisis poses an opportunity for Mandy to examine that definition of herself and to consider other possibilities.

The crisis worker has indicated an interest not only in solving the immediate problem, but talking with Mandy about her hopes and dreams for her life. What level of education has she attained, or might she hope for? What kinds of interests, hobbies, or skills does she have? What kind of work has she done, or what might she like to do? What does she hope for her children? If Mandy decides to return to the relationship, the crisis worker hopes she will do so from a position of greater strength, a firmer sense of her desires, needs, and goals. She hopes, too, that Mandy will know she can call the women's center again, should she ever need to.

DISCUSSION QUESTIONS

1. People who have never experienced an abusive relationship often have difficulty understanding why someone would remain in such a relationship. They tend to *underestimate* the impact of a particular situation on another's behavior and to *overestimate* the impact of the person's individual personality. To increase your ability to empathize with crisis clients' experiences, develop a list of contextual or situational circumstances that might lead a woman to remain in an abusive relationship after one incident of violence that resulted in her hospitalization.

2. Develop a list of contextual or situational circumstances that might lead a woman to continue in an abusive relationship despite several years of abuse.

3. In what ways do these lists differ? In what ways are they similar?

EXERCISES

1. Violence against women can take many forms. Some forms, especially those resulting in physical injury, are readily labeled violent or abusive. Others seem almost innocuous and are often ignored. Even these "milder" forms of violence, however, have a cumulative negative effect on a woman's self-worth. Consider a continuum of violence that runs from unasked-for compliments, to catcalls and whistling, to unasked-for touching, to language that infantilizes, to deprecating media images, to sexual harassment, sexual assault, domestic violence, and murder. Consider a time when you experienced a form of violence (based on your sex, gender role, ethnicity, or sexuality). Did you label the experience as violent at the time? Focus on your feelings at the time and your feelings about the experience now. Would you prefer to live in a world where these kinds of experiences happened only rarely? What would need to change in order for that to happen?

2. Imagine that a woman says to you, "He says he's so sorry that this happened and it will never happen again. He loves me so much and doesn't want me to leave. I believe him and I don't want to lose him." Develop several supportive responses that accept the woman's view of the situation, yet challenge her to think beyond her perspective.

3. Imagine that a woman from Ghana tells you, "You don't understand. In my country, men always beat their wives. It's expected." How would you communicate sensitivity to her cultural background, while helping her find ways to be safe from further violence?

REFERENCES

Aguilar, R. J., & Nightengale, N. N. (1994). The impact of specific battering experiences on the self-esteem of abused women. *Journal of Family Violence, 9*(1), 35–45.

Bachman, R. (1994). *Violence against women: A national crime victimization survey report.* Washington, DC: United States Department of Justice.

Blumstein, P., & Schwartz, P. (1983). *American couples: Money, work, sex.* New York: William Morrow.

Bowker, L. (1993). A battered woman's problems are social, not psychological. In R. J. Gelles & D. Loseke (Eds.), *Current controversies on family violence* (pp. 47–62). Newbury Park, CA: Sage.

Brand, P., & Kidd, A. (1986). Frequency of physical aggression in heterosexual and female homosexual dyads. *Psychological Reports, 59,* 1307–1313.

Browne, A. (1987). *When battered women kill.* New York: Free Press.

Bryant, S., & Demian, R. (Eds.). (1990). *Partners: Newsletter for gay and lesbian couples.* Seattle, WA: Partners.

Campbell, J. (1992). "If I can't have you, no one can": Power and control in homicide of female partners. In J. Radford & D. Russell (Eds.), *Femicide: The politics of woman killing* (pp. 99–113). New York: Twayne.

Chaplin, J. (1988). *Feminist counseling in action.* London: Sage.

Daly, J., Power, T., & Gondolf, E. (2001). Predictors of batterer program attendance. *Journal of Interpersonal Violence, 16,* 971–992.

Dutton, M. A. (1993). Understanding women's responses to domestic violence: A redefinition of battered woman syndrome. *Hofstra Law Review, 21,* 1191–1242.

Fox, J., & Zawitz, M. (2000). *Homicide trends in the United States* (NCJ 179767). Washington, DC: Bureau of Justice Statistics.

Freud, S. (1964). Some psychological consequences of the anatomical distinction between the sexes. In J. Strachey (Ed. and Trans.), *Standard edition of the complete psychological works of Sigmund Freud, Vol. 19* (pp. 243–258). London: Hogarth Press. (Original work published 1925).

Gazmararian, J., Lazorick, S., Spitz, A., Ballard, T., Saltzman, L., & Marks, L. (1996). Prevalence of violence against pregnant women. *Journal of the American Medical Association, 275,* 1915–1920.

Gleason, W. J. (1993). Mental disorders in battered women: An empirical study. *Violence and Victims, 8,* 53–68.

Gondolf, E. (1997). Batterer programs: What we know and need to know. *Journal of Interpersonal Violence, 12,* 83–98.

Goodman, L. A., Koss, M. P., & Russo, N. F. (1993). Violence against women: Physical and mental health effects: Part I. Research findings. *Applied and Preventative Psychology, 2,* 79–89.

Greenfield, L., Rand, M., Crave, D., Klaus, P., Ringel, C., Warchol, G., Maston, C., & Fox, J. (1998). *Violence by intimates: Analysis of data on crimes by current or former spouses, boyfriends, and girlfriends.* Washington, DC: United States Department of Justice.

Island, D., & Letellier, P. (1991). *Men who beat the men who love them: Battered gay men and domestic violence.* New York: Harrington Park.

Johnson, M. (1995). Patriarchal terrorism and common couple violence: Two forms of violence against women. *Journal of Marriage and the Family, 57,* 283–294.

Kirkwood, C. (1993). *Leaving abusive partners.* London: Sage.

Kurdek, L. (1992). Conflict in gay and lesbian cohabiting couples. Paper presented at the meeting of the American Psychological Association, Washington, DC.

Kurz, D. (1996). Separation, divorce, and woman abuse. *Violence Against Women, 2*(1), 63–81.

Lipchik, E. (1991). Spouse abuse: Challenging the party line. *Networker,* May/June, 59–63.

Lobel, K. (Ed.). (1986). *Naming the violence: Speaking out about lesbian battering.* Seattle, WA: Seal Press.

Luepnitz, D. (1988). *The family interpreted.* New York: Basic Books.

Mahoney, P., Williams, L., & West, C. (2001). Violence against women by intimate relationship partners. In C. Renzetti, J. Edleson, & R. Bergen (Eds.), *Sourcebook on violence against women* (pp. 143–178). Thousand Oaks, CA: Sage.

National Coalition Against Domestic Violence. (1994). Program and discussion papers from the Sixth National Conference and Membership Meeting held in Saint Paul, MN, July 29–August 3, 1994.

NiCarthy, G. (1982). *Getting free: You can end abuse and take back your life.* Seattle, WA: Seal Press.

Orava, T. A., McLeod, P. J., & Sharpe, D. (1996). Perceptions of control, depressive symptomatology, and self-esteem of women in transition from abusive relationships. *Journal of Family Violence, 11,* 167–186.

Pence, E. (1987). *In our best interest: A process for personal and social change.* Duluth, MN: Minnesota Program Development.

Renzetti, C. (1997). Violence and abuse among same sex couples. In A. Cardarelli (Ed.), *Violence between intimate partners: Patterns, causes, and effects* (pp. 79–89). Boston: Allyn & Bacon.

Straus, M., Gelles, R., & Steinmetz, S. (1980). *Behind closed doors: Violence in the American family.* Garden City, NJ: Anchor.

Sugarman, D., & Hotaling, G. (1991). Dating violence: A review of contextual and risk factors. In B. Levy (Ed.), *Dating violence: Young women in danger.* Seattle, WA: Seal Press.

Tjaden, P., & Thoennes, N. (1998). *Prevalence, incidence, and consequences of violence against women: Findings from the National Violence Against Women Survey* (NCJ 172837). Washington, DC: United States Department of Justice.

Turner, S., & Shapiro, C. (1986, September–October). Battered women: Mourning the death of a relationship. *Social Work,* 372–376.

Walker, L. (1979). *The battered woman.* New York: Harper & Row.

Walker, L. (1980). Battered women. In A. Brodsky & R. Hare-Mustin (Eds.), *Women and psychotherapy: An assessment of research and practice* (pp. 339–363). New York: Guilford Press.

Walker, L. (1991). Post-traumatic stress disorder in women: Diagnosis and treatment of battered woman syndrome. *Psychotherapy: Theory, research, practice, training, 28,* Special Issue: Psychotherapy with victims (pp. 21–29). Washington, DC: Division of Psychotherapy, American Psychological Association.

Walker, L. (1993). Legal self-defense for battered women. In M. Hansen & M. Harway (Eds.), *Battering and family therapy: A feminist perspective* (pp. 200–216). Thousand Oaks, CA: Sage.

Weis, J. (1989). Family violence research methodology and design. In L. Ohlin & M. Tonry (Eds.), *Family violence* (pp. 117–162). Chicago: University of Chicago Press.

Whalen, M. (1996). *Counseling to end violence against women: A subversive model.* Newbury Park, CA: Sage.

Yllo, K. (1993). Through a feminist lens: Gender, power and violence. In R. J. Gelles & D. Loseke (Eds.), *Current controversies on family violence* (pp. 47–62). Newbury Park, CA: Sage.

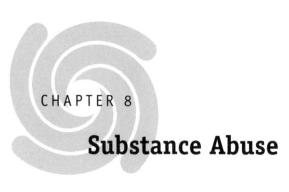

CHAPTER 8

Substance Abuse

FORD BROOKS
THOMAS M. COLLINS

Rose is a thirty-four-year-old woman who was discharged from an inpatient alcohol and drug treatment program five months ago. She has been attending group therapy three times a week and individual counseling once a month. She has also been involved in Alcoholics Anonymous meetings at least twice a week and maintaining contact with her sponsor.

The precipitating event leading to Rose's inpatient admission five months ago was significant physical withdrawal resulting from her discontinuation of alcohol, loss of her employment due to drinking, and related marital difficulties. It was Rose's third hospital admission for addiction and, when released, she was referred to a relapse prevention program.

Prior to her relapse, she had been sober for four years. She attended Alcoholics Anonymous meetings on a regular basis and was involved in outpatient treatment during the first year of her sobriety. She regained employment, but continues to experience marital conflict and tensions. Her husband is also in recovery.

Recently Rose has become increasingly more emotional and reports having unsettling nightmares about herself as a child once or twice a week. She remains abstinent but reports that she has an intense desire to drink. In the past she has repeatedly relapsed, in what appears to be an effort to medicate the emotions that seem to take over whenever she thinks about her past.

On this particular day Rose called her counselor in a panic asking for an emergency appointment. She arrived looking disheveled and tired, but sober. She reported that she couldn't sleep because every time she fell asleep she had the same nightmares. As she talked about the nightmares in response to her counselor's gentle probing, she began to cry uncontrollably. Although she was able to verbalize some of the pain associated with the images of her childhood abuse, by the end of the session Rose was again ambivalent about maintaining abstinence. She angrily asked, "Why would I want to stay sober if I have to deal with these painful memories each time I stop drinking? It pays off in some strange way to continue drinking and not face it at all."

Rose is at a crisis point in her recovery. Traumatic events from her youth are beginning to resurface, complicating her addiction recovery and creating a current crisis warranting crisis counseling.

• • •

Johnny is a twenty-five-year-old gay male who was arrested for possession of cocaine. Johnny pleaded no contest and was referred for assessment and recommendation for treatment by the court. Johnny's mother paid his bail and brought him directly from jail to the counselor's office. Johnny insisted that his cocaine use was not a problem, and he was very angry at the legal system and at the counselor because he did not believe he needed to be in treatment. His problem, as he saw it, was that he was unlucky to get caught carrying. The crisis counselor will see Johnny for the three court-mandated assessment sessions and will try to enlist his willingness to follow through with treatment.

• • •

Julie is an eighteen-year-old first-year student at a large university. She contacted the emergency services unit of the university counseling center one week after a three-day hospital admission for depression, her out-of-control eating disorder, and amphetamine abuse. Julie presented as gaunt and depressed. Upon discharge from the hospital, Julie began taking her amphetamines almost immediately, but she was scared and recognized that she could not continue this pattern or she would die. When she left the hospital she was referred for individual counseling; she went to her initial session but felt she wasn't going to make it to her next appointment. Her eating disorder was still a problem, she was continuing to abuse amphetamines, and she was extremely depressed. It was apparent to both Julie and the crisis worker that she needed medically monitored inpatient care to specifically address her addiction to amphetamines and her eating disorder.

A major barrier was that her insurance would not pay for inpatient care and Julie's father was primarily focused on his daughter "pulling herself together" and getting back to school before "she blew the entire semester."

In this case, the crisis was brought about by the combination of Julie's addiction, eating disorder, and depression. Although she saw the need for intensive treatment, her father's denial of the seriousness of his daughter's addiction and related problems emerged as a key issue needing to be addressed in order to obtain familial and financial support.

Chemical abuse and dependency are pervasive and chronic problems in our society. According to data collected by the U.S. Department of Health and Human Services (2001a), in the year 2000 there were an estimated 14 million illicit drug users in the United States, and marijuana was the most commonly abused illicit drug. Of the 5.7 million users of illicit drugs other than marijuana, 3.8 million were using prescription drugs, including pain relievers, tranquilizers, stimulants, and sedatives, for nonmedical reasons. According to the same study, 46.6 percent of Americans over age twelve reported that they currently drink alcohol, and 5.6 percent reporting "heavy drinking," defined as five drinks at a time on multiple occasions over the course of each month. More than 12 percent of women reported using alcohol while pregnant. Although not everyone who uses illicit drugs or drinks alcohol is addicted, the ubiquitous drug and alcohol use in this society must be recognized as a factor contributing to the problem of substance abuse and addiction.

The Institute of Medicine (1990) estimated that approximately 5.5 million individuals in the United States are in need of treatment for drug use disorders, and an additional 13 million individuals need treatment for alcohol use disorders. Of those, two-thirds are men and approximately one-third have more than one substance use disorder. The lifetime risk for developing dependence on alcohol is 15 percent in the general population, with the overall rate of current alcohol dependence approaching 5 percent (American Psychiatric Association, 2000).

Crisis is synonymous with a substance-abusing lifestyle. Some of the most commonly identified life crises associated with substance abuse include overdose, attempted suicide, loss of domicile, disappearance from domicile, loss of employment, losses in close personal relationships, medical emergencies, and legal crises (Newman & Wright, 1994; Ramsay & Newman, 2000).

CHARACTERISTICS OF ADDICTION

Since 1956, the American Medical Association (AMA) has described alcoholism as a disease characterized by *primary, progressive, chronic, potentially fatal,* and *symptomatic* aspects (Royce, 1989). These aspects also describe the nature of addiction to both licit and illicit drugs.

The *primary* nature of addiction means that although there may be other significant issues in an individual's life, the addiction needs to be treated as a primary or central concern. For example, a client who presents with issues of marital discord, financial problems, and Monday morning jitters due to "stress" may be treated for each separately. A helping professional not trained in addiction symptomatology may focus on bringing in the partner, or referring the client for financial counseling or to a psychiatrist for a medication evaluation; however, the addiction may be the underlying issue. When counselors evaluate and assess crises associated with substance use, it is necessary to keep in mind the primary nature of addiction. Treatment must address the symptoms and associated crises, but if the counselor does not treat the illness as one of the primary foci, the client may continue to drink or drug as the counseling focus is directed toward secondary and tertiary problems.

The second aspect is *progression.* Addiction is an illness that progresses and becomes worse as the individual continues use of the substance (Royce, 1989). For example, a client who has been sober for five years who starts drinking again will not start drinking in the same way he or she did five years earlier. Rather, disease progression suggests that within a short period of time the client will be drinking more, resulting in significantly greater physical, mental, and spiritual consequences.

The *chronic* nature of the disease signifies that it is ongoing, with no cure in the traditional medical sense (Fisher & Harrison, 2000). Once a person crosses that invisible line into compulsive, addictive use, it is unlikely that he or she will ever drink or use drugs in moderation again. Many addicted clients believe that if they can stop using for a few months or years, they can then safely return to controlled use. More often, they find that within a period of time their use increases, with more serious consequences.

Addiction is potentially *fatal* if left untreated. Individual substance abusers have higher rates of fatal car accidents and death from gunshot wounds as well as more physical problems (e.g., ulcers, digestive problems, cirrhosis of the liver, kidney problems, cognitive decline) related to addictive substance use (Fisher & Harrison, 2000; Kinney & Leaton, 1987).

Finally, addiction is a *symptomatic* illness. According to the *DSM-IV-TR* (APA, 2000) the typical symptoms of substance dependence include an increased tolerance to the chemical, continued use of chemicals despite negative consequences, withdrawal, and repeated unsuccessful attempts to control or stop using the substance.

The following scenario illustrates the disease process:

Fred presented with a ten-year history of addiction to alcohol and marijuana. He is currently in crisis because his wife and child recently left him due to his continuing alcohol/drug use and his verbally abusive behavior. He described prior therapy with a counselor who spent most of the time focusing on early childhood issues, believing that if those issues were resolved, Fred would discontinue the alcohol and marijuana abuse. Fred stated that although he did reduce his alcohol and marijuana intake, he continued to use both substances.

Fred stated that he stopped "cold turkey" two years ago after a drunk driving ticket because he feared that a drug test would come back positive and that he would be sent to jail. He abstained for approximately four months, but on the day of his "graduation" from court-mandated counseling, he celebrated with a twelve-pack of beer. From that time on, Fred increased his alcohol use from four times a week to daily, and up to eight beers each evening. He found that in order to "feel good" he needed to drink and smoke more. At some level, Fred recognized that he was becoming more dependent on the chemicals and more obsessed with drinking and smoking, but he felt enough "in control" not to stop until his wife and children left.

Fred's case exemplifies how central the addiction is to an individual's problems and, ironically, how frequently helping professionals treat clients without directly addressing it. It is clear that Fred's drinking progressed and that the addiction did not disappear. In fact, he presents with symptoms of increased tolerance and preoccupation with his substance use. This scenario also illustrates how it often takes a painful and difficult crisis to force a client to confront his or her extensive addiction denial system and for change to occur.

The typical dynamics of addiction are also illustrated in the case of Steve:

Steve is a twenty-three-year-old male who was referred for counseling by his employee assistance program because he tested positive for marijuana during a routine urine screening. Steve presented, as instructed, saying he was unlucky to get caught, yet also admitting that it may be difficult for him to discontinue his use of marijuana. He also recognizes that if he doesn't, he will lose his job.

The task for the counselor is to utilize this crisis in Steve's life as leverage for change. The choice for Steve is to stop using marijuana, follow through with treatment recommendations, and maintain his job, or choose to continue smoking marijuana and lose his job. Steve's use of chemicals must be a primary focus and he now must confront a long-term dependence on marijuana. A counselor who is aware of the addictive process will proceed by supporting and empathizing with Steve, but will at the same time use this crisis as an opportunity to force Steve to examine his behavior and challenge him to make positive changes in his life.

In some ways this approach differs from other types of crisis intervention in which the crisis counselor's goal is to stabilize and reduce the urgency of the crisis. For example, a crisis counselor working with a depressed client who is contemplating suicide would clearly not want to increase the anxiety or intensify the crisis, but rather would try to stabilize and reduce the emotionality associated with the client's depression and suicidal behavior. Conversely, when working with addiction, the crisis that precipitates a focus on the substance abuse problem can be used as leverage to precipitate change.

TERMS USED IN ADDICTION COUNSELING

The crisis counselor should be familiar with the terms used in addiction counseling. Commonly used terms are defined below.

Addiction/Substance Dependence

Addiction or substance dependence is the compulsive, excessive use of a chemical that continues despite negative consequences and is characterized by an increase in tolerance and symptoms of withdrawal following discontinued use of the chemical(s) (Fisher & Harrison, 2000). According to Morgan and Jordan (1999), addiction is a mental, emotional, physical, and spiritual disease that affects every aspect of the individual. It is a process whereby the individual continues to use a chemical that is slowly affecting every aspect of his or her life despite the negative consequences of continued chemical abuse. One of the hallmarks of addiction is the addict's extensive denial system.

Substance Abuse

Substance abuse, in contrast to substance dependence, does not include the symptoms of tolerance, withdrawal, or a pattern of compulsive use (APA, 2000). Rather, the substance abuse diagnosis includes only the harmful consequences of continued substance use. The diagnosis of substance abuse is usually given to individuals who have just started to use drugs or drink heavily.

Denial System

The denial system of the addicted client develops over years with concomitant distancing from emotions and reality. Individuals in denial do not identify their substance use as problematic, and they blame other problems or people for their situation (Fisher & Harrison, 2000; Johnson, 1973). Ramsay and Newman (2000) cited manifestations of denial including concealment/minimization, rationalization/justification, and resistance. According to this characterization, the substance-abusing client engages in a level of manipulation that includes outright attempts to hide chemical abuse, in arguments that support their continued abuse of chemicals, and attempts to subvert therapeutic efforts on their behalf.

An individual may blame his or her partner, stress in the workplace, or a demanding supervisor as the causal factor that precipitated his or her immediate crisis. The reality, more likely, is that the individual avoids acknowledging the substance abuse and the resulting breakdown of functioning at home and work through an elaborate denial system. He or she may be absolutely certain that abuse is not the problem and may attempt to convince others to share that view. This individual is not lying; rather, he or she is in denial and actually believes the rationalization. Lying may come into the picture, however. For example, when asked, "When was the last time you smoked marijuana?" although an individual may know that it was the night before, he or she may say that it was two weeks ago. In this case, the individual is consciously lying. The difference between denial and lying is that denial is a less conscious deceptive mechanism (Brown, 1985; Wallen, 1993). This distinction is important in the discussion of single-session and crisis counseling strategies later in this chapter.

Continuum of Use

Severity of use is important to assess during a crisis intervention. The addictive continuum begins with no use of chemicals and typically proceeds to use of chemicals, to the abuse of chemicals, and, finally, to the development of addiction. Depending on the person, this process may take years to develop; however, there are individuals who report that from their very first drink they drank "like an alcoholic." There are also people who use and may even abuse alcohol or other drugs and never progress to addiction.

A high school student is caught smoking marijuana in the school parking lot, suspended, and, upon return, is forced to see the school-based drug and alcohol counselor for a substance abuse evaluation.

This student may have just started smoking marijuana or may be abusing marijuana and may be in need of education and counseling because the marijuana use is interfering with performance at school and outside of school. The counselor must understand the continuum of use in order to accurately assess needs and provide the appropriate level of care.

A college student is reported as drunk and disorderly on university grounds for the third time. He is referred to the office of the Dean of Students, where he is given the option of an alcohol and drug assessment or dismissal.

If this student was "caught" three times, the chance is very good that this is routine behavior. Keeping the continuum of use in mind, the crisis counselor must assess the student's alcohol use and related problems in order to accurately identify whether it constitutes abuse or dependence and what level of care will be required to effectively treat him.

Recovery

Recovery is defined as abstinence from alcohol or drugs, followed by changes in thoughts, feelings, and behavior, as well as the potential exploration of spirituality (Gorski, 1989). In recovery the addict or alcoholic can potentially "recover" that which was lost due to addiction. When losses and "damage" cannot be undone, recovery in sobriety must address the loss of relationships, material possessions, or vocational or educational roles. Recovery is a lifelong commitment.

Relapse

Relapse is the part of the recovery process when an individual begins to deny feelings and responsibility again and to rationalize his or her ability to use the substance of choice. It also includes a return to previous addictive behaviors (e.g., going to a bar) and culminates in the actual use of the chemical (Gorski, 1989). Although it is commonly thought that relapse begins with the use of the chemical, in actuality, the relapse process begins at a cognitive level long before an individual starts to use again.

Enabling

Enabling is a behavior other people in the addict's life engage in that protects the chemically dependent individual from the negative consequences of substance abuse (Curtis, 1999). Typically, enabling occurs within a committed relationship;

however, other people in an individual's life, like a friend or parent, may also play this role. For example, the husband of a woman addicted to prescription drugs may call her office to say she has the flu when, in reality, she is high on drugs. He may also bail her out of jail and pay for her lawyer after she is arrested for possession. His behavior prevents her from experiencing the negative consequences of her substance abuse: confinement and financial accountability. He is her enabler.

Codependency

Codependency is defined as a "cluster of symptoms or maladaptive behavior changes associated with living in a committed relationship with either a chemically dependent person or a chronically dysfunctional person either as children or adults" (Gorski, 1992, p. 15). Typically, the codependent is the one closest to the alcohol or drug addict and over the course of time and progression of the disease, becomes enmeshed and inseparable from his or her partner. Characteristics of codependency may include obsessing over attempting to control the addicted person's behavior, measuring self-worth primarily through the approval of others, and significant personal sacrifice (Stevens & Smith, 2000).

MYTHS OF ADDICTION

You can't help an alcoholic or addict who doesn't want help.

False. Most individuals come into treatment through a third-party referral (e.g., school, job, partner, legal system, disciplinary board) because of out-of-control behavior that may have resulted in a relational or legal crisis. Denial protects and defends addicted individuals from their feelings and also from attacks or confrontations about their substance use. When individuals come in for an assessment or in crisis, they do their best to deflect, defend, blame, and avoid questions about or attention on their substance use. Assessment that identifies substance abuse or dependence leads to a referral for appropriate treatment. Group intervention is frequently recommended as most effective for challenging the denial system (Flores, 1988).

Consider Steve, the twenty-three-year-old at risk for losing his job due to marijuana usage. If he were referred to an intensive outpatient program, he might be asked to remain abstinent during treatment, to attend a therapy group, to attend support meetings, and to submit to urine screening on a random basis. For Steve to be able to acknowledge the reality of his marijuana use, he needs to be abstinent and to be around others who have been or are in a similar position. If the treatment is comprehensive and supportive, he stands a good chance of being able to examine his behavior and make changes in his lifestyle. Although he didn't initially want help, he will be able to benefit from the opportunity to learn and take constructive action.

Alcoholics/addicts do it to themselves; they just don't have enough willpower to stop.

False. It would be hard to imagine an addicted client making the statement, "Please, I would like to be addicted to alcohol and crack cocaine. And, by the way, I would like to lose my job, my house, and my family because of it." Addicts don't want to be addicts, yet they continue to use a chemical that slowly or quickly affects every facet of their lives. When individuals begin drinking or using chemicals, their wish or desire is not to become dependent or addicted to the substance. They may start as a result of curiosity, pressure from peers, or exposure to substance use in their family. Regardless of how they begin, their intent is not to be addicted to the substance; yet for millions of individuals the process of addiction unfolds.

Addicted persons may actually have a considerable amount of willpower in that they are usually adamant that "this is not going to beat me" and that "I will win." Paradoxically, it is not until they surrender this sense of control that they can actually begin to recover. Once addicts ingest chemicals, one dose is too many and a thousand are not enough. The compulsion to use them takes over, and the willpower to stop is not active (Alcoholics Anonymous, 1976). The addicted individual, however, does have the ability to avoid people and places associated with using chemicals, the ability and control to attend support meetings and treatment, and the ability to identify and work through feelings related to addiction.

Most alcoholics are unemployed and living on the street.

False. For years many people believed that all alcoholics were homeless and panhandled money from strangers. In reality, most active alcoholics are employed, have homes and families, and function normally. The image of the homeless alcoholic, or the skid row bum, is what may await some addicts who currently have homes and families. The disease of addiction, if left untreated, can take individuals from their homes in the suburbs to jail or onto the streets (Kinney & Leaton, 1987).

Drug addicts and alcoholics are lying thieves who will never change.

True and false. Addicted individuals do lie, cheat, and steal in order to obtain their drug of choice (Alcoholics Anonymous, 1976). Essentially, nothing gets in the way of obtaining the next score, fix, or drink. The addict does whatever needs to be done, regardless of compromised values, societal norms, laws, or disrupted family connections, in order to obtain a high. This is the nature of addiction: For most individuals, it goes against everything that they value.

Steve was raised in a two-parent family that went to church every Sunday. He was taught to be honest, hard-working, and loving. Over the course of his addiction, however, he has lied to almost everyone he knows. He has missed work because of his chemical use, and, on more than one occasion, he has gone to work high. Steve needs to manipulate, hide, lie, or deceive as a means to obtain his drugs and alcohol. During the periods when he sobers up, Steve may recognize his manipulations and deceptions and may feel guilty, ashamed, and remorseful for what he has done.

It is in this recognition and remorse that the seeds of change can be found. Addicts do lie, cheat, and steal; but they can and do change.

Alcoholics/addicts are only hurting themselves; they are not hurting anyone else.

False. Yes, addicted persons are indeed hurting themselves, but they are also negatively affecting their family, workplace, and community. One family member's addiction affects everyone in the family system, and family members often need help as much as the addict (Wegscheider, 1981).

Drug addicts can safely use alcohol because it was not their drug of choice.

False. An addict may be addicted to heroin; however, he or she cannot use other addictive substances safely without potentially developing a coaddiction. Denial of the severity of addiction leads some addicts to contend that they can switch to a different substance safely. What many find is that over the course of time they develop a dependency to alcohol or another drug just as they did to heroin (Fisher & Harrison, 2000). Once intoxicated, it is also easier for addicts to return to their drug of choice. In fact, many individuals who come into treatment for a substance abuse disorder are already abusing more than one substance. Some have a "drug of choice," and others routinely use multiple drugs and/or alcohol simultaneously. Using multiple drugs has become the norm for many young illicit drug-abusing individuals.

DEVELOPMENTAL MODELS OF RECOVERY

In this chapter we have discussed the disease model of addiction, defined terminology crucial to understanding the addiction, recovery, and relapse processes, and presented common myths about addiction. With this information the reader is prepared to consider various developmental models of recovery and how to employ them in working with clients in either single-session or ongoing crisis counseling sessions.

The Brown Model

Brown (1985) posed a developmental model of addiction recovery based on her research with alcoholics. Her model outlines developmental stages and the interacting components that affect recovery within each stage. She suggests that clients can be educated to evaluate themselves using this description of stages and relevant components. This model provides a guide for assessing which treatment or modality is most appropriate for a client.

The first stage Brown identified is called the *drinking* stage. During this stage clients are continuing to drink and/or use chemicals, and are not associating their behavior with any negative consequences. At this time an extensive denial system is in place, which protects individuals from recognizing how their abuse is affecting their lives (Brown, 1985).

During the *transition* stage clients are beginning to connect their drug-taking and drinking behaviors with the problems in their lives. For instance, Fred now sees that his second DUI charge is related to his drinking rather than viewing the officer as out to get him. A paradigm shift occurs when the individual states to him- or herself, "I am an alcoholic or addict and I cannot control my drinking or drugging" (Brown, 1985, p. 32). In the prior stage, the client's frame of reference was, "I'm in control, and I'm not an alcoholic or addict." As the client's thought process transitions from "I'm in control of my use" to "I'm not in control of my use," he or she may also progress from taking no action to taking action to cease use of the substance.

The third stage Brown identified was *early recovery*. During this period individuals are acknowledging their addiction, and are beginning to stabilize and take stock of how their substance use has damaged their lives. They reach out to others for support and, for some time, rely on others in their recovery. Twelve-step programs such as Alcoholics Anonymous (AA) and Narcotics Anonymous (NA) often recommend that participants attend ninety meetings in ninety successive days.

Over time, those who attend twelve-step programs often acquire a personal sponsor in the group as well as the phone numbers of other recovering addicts they can call when necessary. Early recovery is challenging for addicts, as they are quite vulnerable and need to be around supportive people. In this stage, clients are more aware of their behaviors, are not self-medicating, and are feeling the raw emotions surrounding their drug or alcohol use and trying to live substance-free. This is a challenging and painful time for the recovering individual.

In *ongoing recovery* clients are more stable, have support, attend meetings on a regular basis, and attempt to eradicate character flaws and make amends to those who have been harmed by their substance-abusing behavior. Recovering individuals now see recovery as a "problem of living" rather than simply a drinking or drug-taking problem. In ongoing recovery, individuals also often begin to work with others who are just starting recovery, sharing their experience, strength, and hope as others did for them on their own path to sobriety (Brown, 1985).

Brown also identified three components to consider in each stage: the alcohol axis, environmental interactions, and the interpretation of self and others. The alcohol axis focuses on control. Clients in the drinking stage feel in control and not addicted. As the recovery process unfolds and they stop drinking or using drugs, clients begin to look at their lack of control and their inability to use safely, thus changing the alcohol axis to "I'm not in control and I am addicted" (Brown, 1985).

The environmental focus examines the extent to which clients, throughout the transition and early recovery stages, are externally focused and dependent on other people and relationships for support in recovery. Clients usually need a lot of support and encouragement and need to be challenged in order to face their fears and physical cravings while taking responsibility for their behaviors and the people they hurt when under the influence.

The third component pertains to how clients interpret their own thoughts and behavior as they relate to others in recovery. Clients gradually learn to examine how they move in the world, the relationships in which they are involved, and how being in recovery necessitates healthy choices in all spheres of their lives (Brown, 1985).

The Gorski Model

Gorski (1989), a pioneer in the treatment of addiction and relapse prevention methods, also developed a developmental model of recovery. Although the names of the stages differ, his recovery stages parallel Brown's, with additional stages to further delineate the process of recovery.

Gorski's first stage of recovery is the transition stage, which corresponds to Brown's drinking stage. He sees this stage as a time during which the individual continues to use drugs or drink without acknowledging the negative consequences. For a crisis counselor, the goal during this stage is to assist clients to draw the connection between their chemical use and the crises in their lives. Denial is pervasive during this stage and group therapy is believed to be the most effective way to challenge the denial system (Flores, 1988; Yalom, 1995).

Gorski's second stage is stabilization, which is similar to Brown's transition stage. During this stage clients discontinue their use of chemicals and may begin to experience physical withdrawal, in which case medical intervention may be necessary. By this stage, individuals have begun to associate both their withdrawal and their disrupted lives with the substance abuse. At the same time, they must find ways to stabilize their lives and develop support for their abstinence. The counselor's tasks are to evaluate for medical referral and to quickly help the client develop a support network and plan. Cravings, drug-using friends, and environmental triggers (e.g., bars, hot weather, particular neighborhoods) are complicating factors that may require additional supports.

Gorski's stages of stabilization and early recovery are similar to Brown's early recovery stage. During these stages, the reality of how the chemical dependency has affected others becomes clear, and with this insight comes the emotional consequences. As a result, many individuals relapse due to strong cravings, insufficient support, inability to deal with stressful emotions and situations, and residual denial that tempts clients into thinking they can drink or take drugs in a controlled way. As individuals enter early recovery, they are challenged to develop relationships with other recovering people and to develop plans of action to implement when they are under stress or having physical cravings. Utilization of the twelve-step slogans, sponsor contacts, service work within twelve-step meetings, and daily meditations are all critical for individuals moving forward in recovery (Gorski, 1989).

The stage of middle recovery brings new issues and, for many, continuation of efforts to work through the twelve steps. Clients may address character defects, make amends to those they have harmed, and develop meaningful relationships in recovery. Although they may be clean and sober, working through the emotional wounds from years of continuous drug or alcohol use is critical for clients to continue in recovery. These feelings are important for clients to work through, because otherwise they can turn into self-hatred and resentment, which ultimately can result in relapse (Gorski, 1989).

During late recovery, individuals begin to focus on childhood issues that are playing out in their adult relationships. These issues can range from parental alcoholism to childhood abuse, to communication problems. Crisis counselors often see clients who are experiencing crises in their relationships or as the result of resurfacing childhood traumas. It is important for recovering persons to continue attending meetings and working with new members in recovery as they address family of origin issues, for these intense confrontations with their past can also precipitate relapse (Gorski, 1989).

Gorski's (1989) final stage is maintenance, which involves continuing to do whatever works to remain sober. Maintaining recovery means to tend the garden with all of the tools and means available, and not to neglect it. It is when clients neglect their recovery or feel they are "done" that relapse thoughts and behavior can begin to resurface.

The Prochaska, DiClemente, and Norcross Model

Prochaska, DiClemente, and Norcross (1992) proposed a "stages of change" model that was first employed with patients trying to stop smoking cigarettes. Their model similarly describes the process of change relating to addiction recovery. *Precontemplation* is the stage during which individuals are unaware of the need to make changes or of what others perceive as problematic. During the stage of *contemplation,* individuals become aware of problems and consider, or contemplate, making a change. At this stage the individual has collected data, is more aware of his or her addiction, and is thinking about taking action. In the *preparation* stage, individuals with a history of attempts to change their behavior decide that they are going to change their behavior within the next month (thirty days) and are thus ready for change. In the *action* stage, individuals are aware of their addiction and consciously take steps to make changes. They begin to remedy or address the problems before them. During the last stage, which is *maintenance,* individuals continue to maintain their changed patterns of thinking, feeling, and behaving, and consciously evaluate the positive outcomes of continuing with such change (Prochaska & DiClemente, 1995).

TWELVE-STEP SUPPORT GROUPS

Self-help addiction support groups such as Alcoholics Anonymous and Narcotics Anonymous are essential to many individuals' recovery process. The foundation for most of these member-led groups is Alcoholics Anonymous's "twelve steps." Many of the ideas expressed in the developmental models just discussed are also rooted in the assumptions that form the basis of the twelve steps, particularly assumptions about control, powerlessness, and the process of changing addictive thoughts and behavior.

A.A.'S TWELVE STEPS

1. We admitted that we were powerless over alcohol . . . that our lives had become unmanageable.

2. Came to believe that a Power greater than ourselves could restore us to sanity.

3. Made a decision to turn our will and our lives over to the care of God as we understand Him.

4. Made a searching and fearless moral inventory of ourselves.

5. Admitted to God, to ourselves, and another human being the exact nature of our wrongs.

6. Were entirely ready to have God remove all these defects of character.

7. Humbly asked Him to remove our shortcomings.

8. Made a list of all persons we had harmed, and became willing to make amends to all of them.

9. Made direct amends to such people wherever possible, except when to do so would harm them or others.

10. Continued to take personal inventory and when we were wrong promptly admitted it.

11. Sought through prayer and meditation to improve our conscious contract with God as we understood Him, praying only for knowledge of His will for us and the power to carry to carry that out.

12. Having had a spiritual awakening as a result of these steps, we tried to carry this message to alcoholics and to practice these principles in all our affairs.

Spirituality and religiosity are clearly embedded within the AA twelve steps, and for those who find recovery support in this type of program, spirituality either is, or will become, important. The AA philosophy has also been criticized, however, precisely because of its overtly religious focus, and because of the assumption that recovery requires "turning our will and our lives" over to God.

Although AA programs have been useful to many individuals, alternative ways of envisioning twelve-step recovery programs are presented here in order to accommodate the variation in belief systems of crisis clients. The first alternative was proposed by B. F. Skinner (1987) as a "humanist alternative" to the religion-based AA twelve steps.

THE HUMANIST ALTERNATIVE

1. We accept the fact that all our efforts to stop drinking have failed.

2. We believe that we must turn elsewhere for help.

3. We turn to our fellow men and women, particularly those who have struggled with the same problem.

4. We have made a list of the situations in which we are most likely to drink.

5. We ask our friends to help us avoid those situations.

6. We are ready to accept the help they give us.

7. We earnestly hope they will help.

8. We have made a list of the persons we have harmed and to whom we hope to make amends.

9. We shall do all we can to make amends, in any way that will not cause further harm.

10. We will continue to make such lists and revise them as needed.

11. We appreciate what our friends have done and are doing to help us.

12. We, in turn, are ready to help others who may come to us in the same way.

The AA twelve-step program has also been criticized by some feminist addicts and their advocates who assert that many of the recovery principles are gender-biased in that they reflect the experiences and needs of men more than women. In particular, some feminists have suggested that the emphasis on the addict's ego-centeredness that underlies the need to relinquish power and control are gender-biased assumptions about addiction and that women's experience of addiction may be different from men's. Unterberger (1989) proposed an alternative twelve steps for women addicts that incorporate a feminist perspective and understanding of woman's experience of addiction.

The humanist and feminist alternative models differ from the AA model in their de-emphasis of God as the instrument of change. In each of the alternative models, there is an assumption that one can use one's own personal power and agency, not to engage in "controlled" drinking or drug-taking, but to change one's own life patterns with the resources of friends, family, and community.

TWELVE STEPS FOR WOMEN ALCOHOLICS

1. We have a drinking problem that once had us.

2. We realized we needed to turn to others for help.

3. We turn to our community of sisters and our spiritual resources to validate ourselves as worth-while people, capable of creativity, care, and responsibility.

4. We have taken a hard look at our patriarchal society and acknowledge those ways in which we have participated in our own oppression, particularly the ways we have devalued or escaped from our own feelings and needs for community and affirmation.

5. We realize that our high expectations for ourselves have led us either to avoid responsibility and/or to overinvest ourselves in others' needs.

6. Life can be wondrous or ordinary, enjoyable or traumatic, danced with or fought with, and survived. In our community we seek to live in the present with its wonder and hope.

7. The more we value ourselves, the more we can trust others and accept how that helps us. We are discerning and caring.

8. We affirm our gifts and strengths and acknowledge our weaknesses. We are especially aware of those who depend on us and of our influence on them.

9. We will discuss our illness with our children, family, friends, and colleagues. We will make in clear to them (particularly our children) that what our alcoholism caused in the past was not their fault.

10. As we are learning to trust our feelings and perceptions, we will continue to check them carefully with our community, which we will ask to help us discern the problems we may not yet be aware of. We celebrate our progress towards wholeness individually and in community.

11. Drawing upon the resources of our faith, we affirm our competence and confidence. We seek to follow through on our positive convictions with the support of our community and the love of God.

12. Having had a spiritual awakening as a result of these steps, we are more able to draw upon the wisdom inherent in us, knowing that we are competent women who much to offer others.

THE CONTINUUM OF CARE

Crisis workers who work with individuals in crises related to addiction must be knowledgeable about the types of alternative services available. The service programs available to chemically addicted individuals exist on a "continuum of care" wherein a program provides the least restrictive level and intensity of service necessary to match the clients' needs. For example, the needs of a person addicted to the antianxiety agent Xanax® after five years of prolonged usage at high doses are dramatically different from those of a college freshman diagnosed with Substance Abuse Disorder after a drunk and disorderly arrest. Similarly, services provided to systemic members (e.g., partners, children, biological family) in crisis as a result of the addict's substance abuse should also be at a level that addresses identified needs, but interferes as little as possible in the life of the client and significant others.

Many states have developed assessment protocols that are utilized by drug and alcohol agencies to determine the appropriate level of care and type of service to provide to an individual based upon the extent to which his or her behavior fulfills the identified criteria. Before discussing these criteria, the crisis worker should be familiar with the general organization of substance abuse services in the United States. The following system organization chart taken from the Pennsylvania Department of Health/Office of Drug and Alcohol Programs (1997a) is typical of the levels and types of services that are available in most communities nationwide.

Level I	Level II	Level III	Level IV
Outpatient	Day treatment/ partial hospital	Medically monitored inpatient detox	Medically managed inpatient detox
OR	OR	OR	OR
Intensive outpatient	Halfway house	Medically monitored short-term residential	Medically managed inpatient residential
		OR	
		Medically monitored long-term residential	

Reprinted with permission of the Pennsylvania Department of Health/ODAP.

The least restrictive services identified are outpatient and intensive outpatient counseling services, and the most restrictive are medically managed inpatient detox and residential substance abuse treatment services. Historically, the majority of rehabilitative substance abuse treatment services were provided in medically monitored or medically managed residential programs of varying lengths. The operational costs involved in these programs resulted in spiraling costs and accompanying accountability concerns. Today, at least in part due to efforts to control health care costs, there is an increasing emphasis on providing substance abuse treatment in an *intensive outpatient* format. Essentially, individual and group counseling and case management, the types of services that might also be provided in an inpatient/residential setting, are provided to the client on an outpatient basis without the medical management or costs associated with room and board. This translates into longer and more frequent treatment sessions at a lower cost. It is also less restrictive of the individual's ability to continue with normal life activities. Although some helping professionals adhere to the philosophy that hospitalization or residential programs are always preferable, the available data does not support the contention that inpatient care has advantages over other treatment approaches, apart from the ability to provide medical monitoring or care when that is necessary (APA, 2000).

At the next level of the service continuum are *day-treatment/partial hospitalization* services, which are, in essence, inpatient services provided in full-day format but in a community-based setting. The client comes to treatment during the day and returns home at the end of the day. The client can attend the program for up to five days a week, but without the loss of freedom or the cost associated with program residence.

The next level of intervention consists of services provided in a *medically monitored detox program, medically monitored short-term residential program, or medically monitored long-term residential program*. These programs are often located in facilities that are not affiliated with medical institutions. "Medically monitored" usually implies that there is a consulting supervising physician connected with the treatment program in some capacity. The physician's involvement may be limited in time and scope and may vary according to local and state medical practices. Often, programs are monitored by nurse practitioners and/or physician assistants with varying levels of physician supervision.

Medically managed inpatient detox programs and *medically managed inpatient residential programs* are usually programs offered under the direct control of a medical institution. All services are provided under the auspices and direct medical supervision of a physician and/or nurse practitioner or physician assistant. This level of care is appropriate for those clients who require close monitoring and have a high risk of medical consequences due to withdrawal. Program philosophy and practices reflect a physiological/medical model of addiction.

Admission Criteria

In general, decisions regarding the most appropriate setting for an individual depend on the individual's clinical characteristics and treatment needs, the available alternatives, and individual client preferences (APA, 2000). An additional factor is related to financial needs and the availability of medical insurance. Admission to particular types of programs is based upon fulfilling specific criteria using the following six dimensions (Pennsylvania Department of Health/ODAP, 1997b):

1. Acute intoxication or withdrawal
2. Biomedical conditions and complications
3. Emotional/behavioral conditions and complications
4. Treatment acceptance/resistance
5. Relapse potential
6. Recovery environment

THE CRISIS OF ADDICTION

Crisis and addiction can be thought of synonymously. As a result of this dynamic, addicts and alcoholics learn to manage crises in a way that obscures the true nature of their loss of control.

John, an attorney, is continually late for court appearances and meetings with clients because he is hung over. Routinely, John can't get himself going in the morning following his binge the night before. Thus he starts with his schedule in a minor crisis most days. He has learned, however, to make sure that his secretary calls ahead to the court and makes excuses to clients who are waiting at his office. In other words, he has his secretary manage his crises and he is "saved" from having to confront the degree to which his drinking has created his crisis lifestyle.

Alcoholics and addicts usually have developed enabling teams of people who have become accustomed to their behaviors. The full impact of a crisis does not land squarely on the shoulders of the addicted individual, as family, coworkers, and friends handle the brunt of the crisis, enabling the out-of-control behavior to continue. As long as addicted individuals have primary enablers, they can avoid or minimize the full impact of crisis situations (Johnson, 1986).

There are a number of ways addicts or alcoholics can arrive at crises. When members of an enabling team refuse to cover for the addict, he or she must eventually face the current crisis *and* face the enormity and progression of his or her illness. Sometimes counselors recommend a planned intervention with concerned family members, friends, and coworkers in order to precipitate a crisis as the previous enablers confront the addict and communicate their unwillingness to continue to enable his or her behavior (Johnson, 1986).

An *intervention* is a planned group confrontation of the addict or alcoholic that aims to get the person to admit him- or herself to some type of treatment once the person has been able to admit that there is a problem. The process involves significant people in the addict or alcoholic's life (e.g., partners, children, employers, neighbors) confronting him or her as a group in a caring yet firm fashion. The group challenges the addict to look at his or her alcoholic/addictive behaviors, the harm caused to self and others, and the need for behavioral change. Often the message also includes a warning that the addict is risking the loss of relationships.

What is important to note here is that addicted clients initially move into a recovery process *as a result of crisis*. Thus, crisis in the addicted client's life can serve as a reality check; awareness of the connection between the substance abuse and subsequent crises becomes a catalyst to further the addict's movement toward recovery. The client may not initially understand the crisis in this way, which creates a challenging paradox for the counselor. Although the counselor may see the crisis as an opportunity for growth, the client may resist and attempt to avoid the opportunity for growth.

SINGLE-SESSION CRISIS INTERVENTION: SUBSTANCE ABUSE AND ADDICTION

For addicted clients not yet in recovery or for those who find themselves relapsing, crisis is commonplace. The developmental-ecological model of single-session crisis intervention can provide crisis workers with a blueprint for working with this challenging population.

Step 1:
Supportively and empathically join with the client.

Whether the counselor is working with a new client or a client already in counseling, being accurately empathic, genuine, and unconditionally supportive is crucial in developing trust (Rogers, 1957). When addicted individuals' problems reach crisis proportions, their means of coping or managing typically have failed, thus creating an out-of-control situation for which they are in need of assistance.

Addicted clients in crisis typically feel terrified, angry, guilty, ashamed, or embarrassed about their situation. At the same time, they may not associate their substance use with the crisis. The crisis is not only an opportunity for the client to begin connecting the two, but also an opportunity to make behavioral changes. If the individual in crisis is an ongoing client and the relationship of support and empathy has been established, he or she is more likely to be open, willing, and trusting of suggestions and recommendations made by the crisis counselor at the time of crisis.

When meeting with the addicted individual, it is important for the counselor to genuinely hear the story of crisis and to connect with the client's feelings, perspectives, and understanding of the experience. Being open, calm, nonjudgmental, and supportive is key. Even when a client is relapsing for the second, third, or fourth time, the last thing he or she needs to hear is, "I told you so. I knew you were going to relapse." What the crisis counselor may want to share is awareness and empathy with how overwhelming this must be. *"It must be really frightening . . . and frustrating, to find yourself in this place again."* The counselor's empathy may be the only support and validation that the client receives due to the nature of addiction and how it pushes others away.

Many first-time clients suffering from addiction come for crisis counseling at the request of someone else involved in the crisis and often in response to a potential or impending loss (e.g., job loss, suspension from school, loss of a relationship). These losses or potential losses create emotional crises for the addict, but the feelings of fear, vulnerability, and loss are often masked by anger and blame. Clients who come for help in a crisis after losing their driver's license or being threatened with job loss are typically angry at the "system," but at a deeper level they may also be angry with themselves. The crisis worker needs to validate the feelings of vulnerability and loss that accompany losing a job or driver's license or a threatened divorce, but at the same time begin to facilitate a process whereby the individual can accept responsibility for his or her problem. For example, *"It must be very frustrating having to go through this a third time, especially since this time it sounds as though your license is gone. Being without wheels must create overwhelming problems. Seems as though your drinking is really taking a toll on your freedom."* The crisis counselor genuinely validates and empathizes with the client, but also begins to address how the drinking is the catalyst for the cascade of troubles looming in the client's life.

Step 2:
Intervene to create safety, stabilize the situation, and handle the client's immediate needs.

In addition to providing support, the crisis worker must assess the amount of alcohol and/or drugs consumed by the client in order to determine the need for a medical referral. In many cases, when an addict is seen for crisis intervention, he or she has consumed a considerable amount of alcohol and/or drugs. The crisis typically comes when the person is beginning to experience the physical effects of withdrawal. A detailed timeline and assessment of chemicals ingested will help the counselor determine whether a medical referral is warranted. Unless the crisis counselor is part of an inpatient or outpatient medical team, it is important to have a network of physicians knowledgeable about addiction medicine as referral resources. It is also important for the crisis counselor to have connections with structured day treatment, detoxification, or partial programs that can provide individual and group counseling services, as needed.

Following a medical referral, the physician assesses the patient for a history of seizures, delirium tremors, or withdrawal symptoms (Buelow & Buelow, 1998). The client's most recent alcohol and drug use is evaluated, and a thorough physical exam is performed to rule out any comorbid medical problems. The physician also determines whether the client needs detoxification services, either on an outpatient or inpatient basis, and whether the client requires medication for withdrawal symptoms.

If the client does not have a physician or insurance, a referral to the local emergency room can sometimes provide the medical evaluation necessary to initiate detoxification services. The options described above depend upon the setting in which the counselor is working, the severity of the client's addiction, access to medical care, and the continuum of services available in a community.

Crisis workers must be able to recognize withdrawal signs in order to assess the need for a medical referral. Withdrawal symptoms can include small twitches of the facial muscles, alcohol odor, bruises or burn marks on the hands from falls or cigarettes, shakiness of the hands and arms, dryness of mouth, an acetone smell, yellowing of the whites of the eyes, difficulty with speech, sweating, reports of stomach pain, cramping, and vomiting (Fisher & Harrison, 2000). An in-depth chemical history can also reveal patterns of abuse of prescription or illicit drugs or alcohol; however, it may not be possible to obtain a complete history in a single-session intervention. In this case, the crisis worker can arrange a follow-up drug and alcohol assessment if the client is willing.

The crisis client may not be willing to follow through with a referral for a medical assessment. In this case, the crisis worker needs to discuss a backup safety plan should the client continue to have significant withdrawal symptoms. The backup plan can include the client calling the local ambulance service or going to the local emergency room for care.

Addicts in crisis may also have overwhelming medical, legal, financial, and/or relationship problems. It is thus always necessary to think about the physical and emotional safety of the addicted client. Combined losses and reduced functioning often create feelings of hopelessness, depression, and isolation. It is important for crisis counselors to evaluate clients for symptoms of depression, suicidality, homicidality, and potential violence.

Step 3:
Explore and assess the dimensions of the crisis and the client's reaction to the crisis, encouraging ventilation.

As crisis counselors begin to establish a supportive relationship with a client, they simultaneously engage in the process of exploring the problems presented by the client and assessing his or her current needs and strengths. The individual who is addicted to substances frequently does not identify the current crisis as related to their substance abuse and instead focuses on whatever concrete loss or event has precipitated their crisis response. In such cases, close attention to indicators of substance abuse and skillful questioning about the identified problem may reveal the substance use. If identified, it can then become a focus of at least preliminary assessment.

In some situations the substance abuse/dependence is clearly paramount.

Stacey called the twenty-four-hour crisis line clearly drunk and barely coherent. Sobbing, she described her wish to die. She related that earlier in the day she had been in family court, where physical custody of her children had been awarded to her ex-husband because of her continued inability to hold down a job or maintain a home. The court gave her supervised visitation only.

In this case the crisis counselor must explore and assess both Stacey's addiction and her reactions to the current crisis regarding loss of her children. The counselor must consider her affective state, her drinking behavior, and her thoughts and cognitions—in particular, her suicidal ideation. The crisis counselor must also listen for the purpose of comprehending her developmental capacities, especially as they relate to immediate coping and problem-solving capabilities, and explore her social supports and relationship to potential community resources. The crisis counselor's knowledge of the characteristics, dynamics, and developmental stages of addiction and recovery guides the exploration and assessment.

Assisting the crisis client to freely express thoughts and feelings provides emotional release for the individual and allows the crisis worker to empathize and gradually reframe despair and hopelessness as an opportunity to make changes.

Step 4:
Identify and examine alternative actions and develop options.

In addition to considering the need for a medical referral, the crisis counselor must also focus on other options and opportunities that may be helpful. Family members' involvement can be helpful in this process of discussing alternatives, referrals, and backup plans. In some cases, a family member or significant other can help motivate the client to follow through with a physical examination or can accompany the individual to the physician's office or the hospital.

Crisis workers must be familiar with the continuum of services available in their community. They should have some idea of the criteria for admission to different levels of care and should have the phone numbers and know the contact persons at drug and alcohol treatment programs that provide both medical and treatment services. They should also have thorough knowledge of the AA or NA resources that are available in the community.

Crisis counselors should also be familiar with the range of social services available in their communities that addicted clients in crisis could access for help with such things as legal issues, housing, financial needs, and employment. The longer a person remains addicted, the more likely he or she is to be involved with multiple service providers.

Step 5:
Help the client mobilize personal and social resources.

The crisis worker should always encourage addicted clients in crisis to involve a partner or significant other in order to create a support network. Family members, friends, and partners often see the imminent crisis before the client relapses, and usually have pertinent and critical information from which options and stabilization procedures can be drawn. For the relapsing client who has been in and out of treatment for years, obtaining support from family, friends, and employers may be difficult. An individual may have repeatedly promised to change, to repay debts, or to "do things right," but may have continually fallen short on these promises and continued to lie. Thus the crisis counselor may be the only significant support person in the client's life.

John has relapsed intermittently for the past ten years, but was able to string together almost two years of continuous recovery before his current relapse. He has been married for fifteen years and has three children. His entire family is fed up with his drinking and broken promises. Although they participated in three of his previous treatment programs as family participants, this time they are unwilling to get involved and report that they are tired of "wasting their time."

Attempting to involve the family at this time would probably prove unsuccessful although they may support him if he takes responsibility for getting help. As this point, encouraging John to consider involving his sponsor might be the only option.

It may be a different picture for the client who is getting sober for the first time, because such clients usually have considerable support from family members, partners, and coworkers. In this case, the counselor and client can involve as many support people as possible in order to increase the chances of maintaining the connections so important in stabilization and early recovery. In some cases, the individual may not want family or friends involved during the crisis meeting. The crisis worker should explore the client's resistance to involving family members, coworkers, support group members, and sponsors, as they can be vitally important during the crisis and later as the individual tries to maintain or return to sobriety.

The crisis counselor should also seek to obtain releases of information so that information can be shared with referral sources, when appropriate, and with the client's partner or family member(s) in order to maximize the support system. If the client is willing to provide releases, the client and the counselor can work on a plan of action that involves family members and other supports. A client in crisis who is isolated or who has lost relationships or is fearful of losing them may not want to include others in the treatment planning process. Or a client may not be ready to admit a problem to others. For example, a college student who has developed a serious substance abuse problem may have managed to hide the problem from his friends and family back home. He may not be willing to involve them even though he's facing a legal or academic crisis because he does not want them to know the full extent of his addiction.

In some instances a client's support system can paradoxically include probation and parole officers, other treatment providers, or even judges. In many cases the client's crisis is related to a court order, a mandate by a contract licensing board, probation or parole department, or employer. The client may have returned to drinking or using drugs and may be fearful of losing freedom or his or her job. The referring third party, however, can be instrumental in applying the therapeutic leverage that allows the person to continue in the treatment process (Buelow & Buelow, 1998; Flores, 1988). Additionally, twelve-step support groups like NA or AA can provide the structure, support, and fellowship so important in recovery from addiction.

Step 6:
Anticipate the future and arrange follow-up contact.

Although clients in crisis may present as out-of-control and overwhelmed, the nature of addiction is progressive and predictable. The crisis counselor can thus help the client prevent and prepare for future crises. If the client is unfamiliar with the addictive process, it is helpful to provide information that can help him or her recognize their abuse or dependence and take appropriate steps to begin recovery. If the client is already knowledgeable about the process, the crisis worker can help the client in crisis assess what went wrong and what needs to happen next.

Crisis workers should always keep in mind the probability that addicts will not follow through with referrals. It is therefore always prudent to anticipate the need for backup and prevention plans should the chosen alternative not work out effectively. For example, a client who presents with symptoms of withdrawal and wants help, but is unwilling to be seen by a physician for a medical evaluation, is likely to fail. The crisis counselor knows from experience that the client's addiction is likely to override any good intentions of discontinuing substance use. The counselor should explore a backup plan with the client and make a follow-up appointment if possible.

After a client has been given a referral, and if the client has agreed to release information, it is crucial that the crisis worker follow up with the person the client has been referred to in order to provide critical assessment information. For example, knowing that a client has discontinued the use of Xanax (a highly addictive antianxiety medication with potentially life-threatening withdrawal properties) would be very important when a treatment team determines a detoxification protocol for a specific client.

Crisis Intervention with Partners and Family Members

Alcoholism and drug addiction can affect families and every relationship of the addicted person (Wegscheider, 1981). Viewing the family of the addicted person as a system in which a delicate balance of power and control is played out on a daily basis can be helpful in understanding addiction. Even in the most chaotic families, a type of homeostatic balance emerges which can perpetuate dysfunctional behaviors of its members. Most addicts would be unable to continue their addictive use of substances if the people around them did not act in ways that permitted their continued addictive behavior. A family member drawn into an enabling role protects and takes responsibility for the consequences of an addicted person's behavior and thus cushions the emotional, physical, and financial impact of addiction. For example, the wife of a cocaine addict may hold down a second job in order to pay the household bills because her husband spends the bulk of his paycheck on cocaine. The crisis counselor is always advised to involve the partner or family in treatment, if possible.

Although the family or partner may be supportive, they may not truly understand the nature of the illness. Some families do not see addiction as a disease, but rather, as purposeful and intentional behavior that the individual could control with strong will and conviction. Thus family members can benefit from education about the disease of addiction. The counselor might refer them to a support group like Al-Anon or Co-Dependents Anonymous, or provide them with reading material on addiction and the enabling process.

Crisis for the addict often comes in the form of loss of relationship or family support. Sometimes, the family members experience more of a crisis than the addicted loved one. The addicted individual may not be as upset or as aware of the negative impact of his or her behavior on others. For example, an alcoholic mother may believe that her drinking has not negatively affected her children because she thinks they have never actually observed her taking a drink. Her denial system prevents her from acknowledging the negative effect her intoxicated behavior has on her children, and thus, the children experience the crisis of her drinking more than she does.

Partner and family responses vary depending on how many relapses their loved one has had, how much support the family or partner has had as they lived with the addicted individual, and how they understood addiction. The first time a chemically dependent client comes in for a crisis session, their family or partner is generally very supportive and relieved that their loved one is seeking help (Johnson, 1986). With each relapse there is likely to be less support and more frustration and hurt. By treating the crisis as a systemic issue, the counselor can simultaneously address the enabling behaviors, the client's addictive behaviors, and other associated situational crises.

In the same way that addicts or alcoholics can be in denial about the extent and negative consequences of their substance abuse, family members or partners may also be in denial. In some families one family member may recognize the problem of addiction whereas others do not. For instance, in a family of four in which the mother is the alcoholic, the husband and one child may not see the alcoholism, whereas the other child may see it very clearly. And, in some cases, partners or family members understand what their loved one needs to do, yet when the counselor makes suggestions about their own recovery process, their defensiveness increases and they deny the necessity for such focus (Wallen, 1993).

Support groups such as Families Anonymous can help parents gain support and perspective on issues their young children or adolescents are facing in their lives. Al-Anon is a group for the support of friends and family members concerned about the alcoholic. Nar-Anon is a similar support group for family and friends of addicts. All support groups provide literature, support, and the fellowship of others. Additionally, counselors can encourage partners and other family members to attend open AA or NA meetings in order to understand the nature of addiction and how recovery looks and feels, which may provide them both hope and understanding.

Family members or partners can also benefit from reading about addiction and/or participating in counseling groups. Sometimes, referring family members or partners to individual counseling can help them understand the impact of addiction on their lives and how their own behaviors can be a consequence of involvement with the loved one's addiction. The counselor should thoroughly expose the counterproductive nature of this interaction for the addicted client and the family member and provide treatment.

ONGOING CRISIS COUNSELING FOR SUBSTANCE ABUSE

To reiterate a point, clients suffering from addiction will not voluntarily come for help unless their behavior with alcohol or drugs causes a crisis. When addicted individuals reach out for help, it is usually because their lives are out of control and they are overwhelmed with the emotional, social, and relational consequences of their substance abuse. Another way to view an addict's substance abuse is that the person is self-medicating anxiety, depression, anger, or other unacceptable emotions. At the addict's point of reaching out for help, self-medication is no longer working or is no longer regarded as a tenable means to manage those unacceptable emotions.

The crisis usually involves a third-party referral, although some individuals seek treatment in crisis, recognizing that they are sick and tired of being sick and tired. The following examination of ongoing crisis counseling goals and processes provides a format for working with substance-abusing and substance-dependent individuals, whether self- or other-referred, over time.

The Counseling Relationship and Addiction

Crisis is a time of great vulnerability for clients and an opportunity for crisis counselors to connect with the pain and suffering of their clients. Virginia Satir described her clinical focus during first sessions as connection with the spirit and essence of the person (Loeschen, 1997). Unless an addicted individual comes into crisis counseling shortly after a crisis occurs, it is unlikely that he or she will voluntarily pursue ongoing counseling. Thus it is important for crisis counselors to see individuals as soon as possible following a precipitating event in order to take advantage of the crisis-precipitated window of therapeutic opportunity. Addiction is an insidious illness in which addicts believe that they are not ill and that they can handle their substance use despite the increasing severity of consequences. When a crisis occurs there is a period of disequilibrium and potential self-awareness. After the crisis subsides, however, the addict begins to feel better and begins to believe again that he or she can handle things without help.

When a crisis counselor meets with an addicted client, it is vital to create an atmosphere of support and understanding. If a client has relapsed, the counselor can help him or her understand how the relapse process began and examine aspects of recovery that had not been addressed prior to the relapse. The goal is always to help individuals proceed through the recovery process by helping them take action that they did not take before. Knowledge of the stages of recovery can provide a guide to this process.

Counselors can also strengthen the helping relationship over time by not becoming angry or blaming clients when they fail. Rather, counselors must show unflinching support of clients' efforts to return to sobriety. Ongoing affirmation provides critical positive reinforcement to the crisis client who is trying to abstain.

Assessment of Addiction

When an addicted client is seen for crisis counseling, the counselor needs to explore and identify the details of the specific crisis event as well as the areas of psychosocial functioning affected by substance abuse. As long as the addicted client continues drinking or using drugs, resolution cannot occur. Therefore, it is necessary for the crisis counselor to evaluate the various levels of the addiction's impact and help the client begin to examine options for resolution.

Assessment includes evaluation of how the chemical use affects or has affected the client emotionally, behaviorally, cognitively, spiritually, developmentally, physically, relationally, financially, and legally. The goal of assessment is to identify the multiple areas of the client's life that have been negatively affected by the addiction, and also to identify personal strengths and other resources that the individual can draw on to conquer the addiction and resolve related issues. The crisis counselor also assesses the dimensions of the precipitating crises.

Greg physically abused his wife while drinking and was arrested after his wife called the police. Upon being released he learned that his wife and children were in a shelter and that a judge had issued a restraining order that prevented him from having any contact with his family.

Although relationship violence may occur only when an individual is drinking, it would be an error to assume that Greg's drinking is his only problem. It may appear that his current family crisis is a consequence of his drinking, but his drinking behavior may only serve to lower his impulses or increase his irritability. He probably also has problems associated with his need for power and control. The crisis counselor needs to simultaneously assess the family crisis precipitated by the domestic violence and the individual who perpetrated the violence. His drinking behavior, although important, may be only one part of the picture.

When assessing an addicted client who has been experiencing either a situational crisis or a crisis directly related to the substance-abusing behavior (e.g., an individual who has just been released from a six-month jail term for reckless endangerment), it is helpful for the crisis counselor to utilize the stages of recovery models presented earlier in this chapter. Familiarity with those stages can alert the counselor to the types of emotional, cognitive, behavioral, and relational issues and needs that an individual is likely to have at different stages of his or her recovery from addiction.

Goals and Processes of Ongoing Crisis Counseling with Addicted Individuals

Affect stability:
Assist the client to express and process his or her emotions related to the addictive behavior and related crises.

Initially, the crisis counselor needs to explore the newfound feelings that have emerged for the client surrounding the precipitating crisis. Crisis events are potentially moments of truth for addicts because their defenses begin to collapse. Helping the client identify his or her feelings in an honest and undefended fashion allows him or her to begin to feel the pain related to drinking or using drugs and the resultant losses.

Research suggests that ongoing substance abuse can actually create changes in the way the brain processes emotion. These neurological changes impair emotional resilience and also create unpredictable emotional reactions to normal stressors (Koob & Le Moal, 1997; Nesse & Berridge, 1997). Emotions are thus a critical focus of working with addicted individuals.

When addicted individuals stop using substances, they often become aware of many emotions that they had hidden and denied. As they cognitively connect those feelings to their addiction and to the consequences of their substance-abusing lifestyle, they finally begin to acknowledge the emotional impact of their alcohol and/or drug consumption. That emotional awareness combined with the cognitive appraisal that their life is out of control may be enough to motivate them to stay clean and sober while dealing with the crises their addictive behavior has created. Because of their high affective arousal, and their impaired emotional resilience and ability to cope, however, this is likely to be a very difficult process, often experienced as one emotional crisis after another.

Ramsay and Newman (2000) noted that, even for experienced crisis counselors, the high level of affect and agitation presented by the substance-abusing client can be disconcerting. It can be particularly difficult for counselors when clients direct their emotional outbursts toward the counselor, for example, responding with unreasonable anger to a perceived slight or to their fear that the counselor will betray them to legal authorities or employers. Ramsay and Newman also identify the high potential for relapse, parole violation, and/or suicidal behavior when substance-abusing clients present with spiraling and unmodulated emotions.

The denial system of addicts and alcoholics is a complex array of minimizing, excuse-making, rationalizing, and blaming processes, which all serve to protect them from having to face the fact that they are addicted to chemicals and that their lives are out of control (Fisher & Harrison, 2000). Their defenses also protect and defend them from the emotional pain related to the various losses created by their substance use and, for some individuals, the underlying pain that their substance use is designed to manage. For example, for individuals like Rose, described at the beginning of the chapter, addiction and the defenses surrounding the addictive behavior make it possible to numb oneself as a way of guarding against the emotional scars of childhood trauma and abuse. Although the substance abuse was clearly not a healthy form of coping and, in reality, created many additional problems for Rose, it was an effort at coping. When individuals, like Rose, are able to begin to let down their defenses, usually because they are struggling with sobriety and no longer self-medicating, all of their denied feelings begin to surface.

Many addicts have perfected the art of avoiding their emotions. In some ways the addiction process is self-reinforcing because as the substance abuser causes more and more damage to him- or herself and others, more and more feelings have to be denied. The addict's learned response to those painful feelings is to push them away through the continued use of alcohol or drugs.

When addicts take their first steps toward sobriety, they become more familiar with those feelings. As crisis counselors assist them with recovery, those feelings become a critical focus. This means supporting sobriety and facilitating clients' awareness and expression of emotions. Counselors must help addicted individuals develop a different set of skills or self-management strategies and create an ongoing healthy support network. As Ramsay and Newman (2000) described, however, given the high emotional arousal and lability in the early stages of crisis counseling, "simply managing the crisis without a worsening of the relapse is a therapeutic success" (p. 141).

Behavioral adjustments:
Assist client to make and sustain necessary behavioral changes.

As crisis counselors work with addicted clients, client behavior is always a primary focus, as ending substance use is necessarily a critical goal. Problematic behaviors of the addict and alcoholic include all of the behaviors related to their drinking or drug-using style (e.g., do they drink alone or with others? do they party when high? do they drink to get drunk?) and all of the behaviors that occur as they cope with the problems their drinking or drug-using creates including verbal and/or physical aggression, missed time from work or school, and neglected family responsibilities. Ideally, clients in crisis counseling following situational crises precipitated by substance abuse are willing to examine and discontinue substance use behaviors and substitute regular support group attendance and continuing individual crisis and addiction counseling. Learning a new set of skills to manage life stressors is essential for the recovering individual. This behavioral change is fundamental and necessary in order to correct the myriad imbalances in the addict's life.

As the substance-abusing behavior ends, the crisis counselor can also help clients focus on healthy actions or behaviors that they were unwilling to try in the past. This often includes taking action to create support for sobriety.

Scott has been sober for over a year and has been sporadically attending AA meetings. He attends weekly group addiction counseling and sees his individual counselor relatively consistently. . . . Scott has resisted obtaining a sponsor in AA, however, because he feels that what he is doing is working and that he doesn't need "some other drunk telling me what to do." Following a conflict with his girlfriend, Scott became angry and depressed and ended up having a couple of beers at the local bar. Two beers turned into fifteen beers, which, in turn, resulted in public intoxication and assault and battery charges for hitting his girlfriend. The following day, he returns to see his counselor.

This is an example of a time when the crisis counselor, in addition to being empathic, must focus attention on both the problematic behavioral responses to anger and on new actions and behaviors that Scott may want to consider, which he was not willing to risk before. In this case, the counselor might strongly encourage Scott to obtain a sponsor who has successfully struggled with addiction and remaining sober. The counselor might encourage him to "cope" by calling his sponsor to talk about his feelings and his impulse to drink rather than by drinking and behaving aggressively.

Almost always, there is a set of "I'm not ready to do that yet" behaviors that significantly contribute to relapse potential. For example, consider a counselor who has been working with a male client who is struggling with sobriety. The client has been attending AA meetings twice a week and an addictions support group run by the counselor in addition to his individual sessions. The client reports to his group that he continues to go to the local bar where he used to drink. He states that he has no intention of drinking and that he goes to the bar to throw darts with his friends because he loves to throw darts. This is a major relapse issue for this client. Although he has not yet picked up a drink, he goes to a bar where he drank for years. Not surprisingly, when the client drank alcohol for the first time in more than six months, he did so at the bar where he'd been throwing darts. Following this relapse, his counselor may be able to motivate him to stop going to the bar and to replace that leisure activity with another. His willingness to take new actions or try new behaviors is directly related to the current crisis. This time, as a result of his relapse, he not only lost his relationship with his girlfriend and the trust of his family, but was also charged with drunk driving.

With an addicted individual, behavioral change always includes both ending problematic behaviors and identifying and committing to new behaviors. The process of recovery ultimately requires taking action—action that results in a substance-free lifestyle. The goal, however, is not just the absence of problematic drinking or drug-taking behaviors. Rather it is to create a life that is rewarding and full without alcohol or drugs.

Cognitive mastery: Assist the client to examine and reformulate beliefs about him- or herself and the substance abuse/dependence, as well as beliefs and personal meanings that have been threatened by the addiction.

After binging on alcohol, Mary reports to her counselor that she feels guilty and that she thinks that her life will never work out. Her core belief about herself, reinforced by successive failures, is that she will never be successful in anything she attempts. Alcohol initially allowed her to feel more social, more at ease around people, and to take more risks. Following a major crisis, Mary began to acknowledge that her drinking was only making her feel worse. Yet she continued to drink.

Mary's cognitions, or core beliefs about herself, must be a focus in crisis counseling. Two questions that crisis counselors need to ask their addicted clients are *"What does drinking or drug-taking allow you to do or become?"* and *"What does drinking or drug-taking allow you to escape or avoid?"* If Mary is able to identify the cognitions that support her drinking, she may be able to work on coping strategies that are more constructive and useful. Cognitions such as "I'm not good enough" probably existed long before the drinking started. Being high allowed Mary to ignore her self-doubts and insecurities. When drinking she believed that she was better able to relate spontaneously and with fewer self-doubts, thus leading to the conclusion that she was "OK."

As Mary's example illustrates, beliefs and perceptions about self, relationships, and life are often critical areas of focus when working with addicted individuals. Similar to the role the substance plays in allowing individuals to deny their emotions, substance use also enables individuals to avoid confronting dysfunctional beliefs. At the same time, the addiction cycle contributes to the development of a host of dysfunctional cognitions that serve the purpose of denying consequences and responsibility.

The core belief system surrounding a client's relationship with the substance of choice is at the heart of the relapse process. A client may begin the process of relapse weeks, if not months, before his or her actual use of the substance (Gorski, 1989). The crisis counselor needs to help the client identify the thought processes that lead or led to reinitiating use of the substance.

Addicted people function in a crisis mode most of the time, thus in addition to the crisis that precipitates their entrance into crisis counseling, they frequently present with ongoing crises that they describe with a palpable sense of urgency, abetted by catastrophic thinking (e.g., "I've blown it; I'm never going to make it"). Such catastrophic thinking patterns may lead individuals to exaggerate the hopelessness of a specific crisis and minimize or overlook the progress they are making. Crisis counselors can help addicted clients avoid their "all-or-nothing" patterns of thought and recognize both their strengths and the "up and down" reality of long-term sobriety (Ramsay & Newman, 2000).

It is also useful to help clients make connections between their patterns of thinking, their emotional responses, and their addictive behavior. Recognizing these relationships can bolster the client's ability to manage current crises and also teach them a self-monitoring skill that they can employ in the future.

For many individuals in recovery, AA's twelve steps provide a new way of thinking that is essential in their efforts to get sober. Each step entails a statement of beliefs that stand in stark contrast to the belief system that allowed the addict to deny, conceal, and minimize his or her addiction.

Step 1 asks individuals to admit to themselves that they are powerless over alcohol and that their lives have become unmanageable as a result of their drinking. Steps 2 and 3 ask individuals to accept the belief that one can turn one's will and life over to a power that is "greater than oneself" in order to restore sanity. These first three steps challenge the client's thoughts about control and introduce the role of spiritual belief. The humanist and feminist alternative steps similarly introduce new ways of thinking that are designed to assist the individual in recovery. Crisis counselors working with addicted individuals need to assess each client's receptivity to these alternative belief systems and work with the ones that are best suited to each client.

<u>D</u>evelopmental mastery:
Assist the client to examine the impact of addiction on his or her ongoing development.

When working with addiction, "development" refers to both individual development (e.g., psychosocial, emotional, moral, cognitive) and the addiction recovery process itself. The counselor can assess the developmental stage of the client in recovery using the models discussed earlier in this text. Careful examination of whether the crisis is a result of developmental deficits or situational factors is also an important aspect of developmental assessment.

It is also important to be cognizant of the client's earlier developmental stages in order to help the client with developmental tasks that he or she did not address in childhood or while addicted (Wallen, 1993). Looking at a combination of human developmental discontinuities and recovery deficits allows counselors to construct targeted treatment plans that address both psychosocial development and recovery-based skills training.

A situational crisis can have a significant impact on a client's development. For example, consider a woman who has been in recovery for eight years who begins to drink again after the death of her husband. The crisis situation (the death of her husband), which is not alcohol- or drug-related, affects her recovery as well as the developmental tasks she is facing at that time in her life. Counseling for this client would need to address the loss of her husband at a time in her life when she and her husband had been planning to retire. They had planned to do some of the things in retirement that they had been unable to do when she was drinking. Helping the client with the impact of her husband's death on her emotions and her life stage would be critical. She would also need to acknowledge the fact that her sobriety came too late to affect her future with her husband.

Tom is a thirty-two-year-old man who started using alcohol on a regular basis at age thirteen. For nineteen years Tom medicated himself with alcohol. Although he is thirty-two years old, emotionally he operates on the level of an adolescent. His alcohol use has contributed to his difficulties with intimacy, trust, and autonomy.

Many addicts experience developmental stagnation as the result of their substance abuse. In the example of Tom, the crisis counselor would need to assess the impact that his drinking has had on his educational and vocational development in addition to his social and emotional development. The counselor would then assist Tom in identifying appropriate developmental goals in each of these areas.

<u>E</u>cosystem healthy and intact:
Assist the client to make changes in his or her personal ecosystem in order to reestablish connection and community.

Calvin is a thirty-year-old client who is recovering from alcohol and cocaine addiction. He grew up in an inner city and spent most of his life on the street. He has been in prison and is currently living with his mother while working part-time at a convenience store. He is frustrated with not making enough money to get out on his own and states that he could make much more money by selling drugs. At this point in his recovery he has been attending AA and NA meetings regularly on a weekly basis. As a result of his frustration about his inability to get out on his own, he begins to sell drugs and eventually starts using them again. He is arrested for possession with intent to distribute.

Addressing Calvin's environment would be a critical factor in his recovery process. He lives in a depressed area with minimal employment opportunities for a high school dropout. His support comes primarily from his mother, on whom he has been economically dependent for his entire life. The counselor should try to involve Calvin's mother in the crisis management plan and recovery process because of her significant status in his life.

The drug charge would likely be followed with prison time. Nevertheless, during the period that Calvin is out on bail, he could begin evaluating his options for training both in prison and in the community. In addition to the other domains of concern (e.g., behavioral changes, thought processes, and developmental issues), the crisis counselor needs to consider the environment and culture in which Calvin lives, including the significance of his mother in his life. A failure to address the cultural aspects of Calvin's family and the impact of his environment would adversely affect the entire scope of his recovery and crisis situation. The crisis counselor may also work directly with the court and/or probation and parole officers.

Working with interpersonal relationships is always important when providing crisis counseling to addicted individuals. The addict's behavior may have damaged his or her relationships, and many relationship losses may be unrecoverable. Many addicts also need to develop new relationships that support a sober and clean lifestyle. Thus an adolescent who was using drugs and who was a member of a drug-using crowd is going to have to find a new circle of friends. For young people in a closed environment, where reputations and which group you belong to have powerful ramifications, this can be a difficult task. But ultimately, it is a task that every addicted individual must address. Self-help groups like AA and NA, in addition to providing direct support, can also be helpful in introducing the addict to others who are similarly committed to recovery and to social experiences (e.g., dances, picnics) that are drug- and alcohol-free. The client's relationship with the crisis counselor and with other people in recovery is an important first attempt at developing honest, open relationships.

CASE EXAMPLE: CONNOR

Single-Session Crisis Intervention

The counselor on call receives Connor's crisis telephone message saying that he has relapsed and needs to talk with someone. Connor has been drinking for the past two weeks, has just discontinued his use, and is worried about withdrawal.

The crisis counselor surmises that Connor is very anxious, not only from the withdrawal, but also from accumulated misfortunes that have resulted from his drinking.

Connor is a sixty-year-old male, well known to local drug and alcohol workers, who has been attempting to get sober for many years. He has been in and out of alcohol and drug treatment programs most of his adult life, achieving six to nine months of sobriety before he relapses. The crisis precipitating his current involvement in counseling was the suspension of his license to practice law. The licensing board stipulated ongoing supervision for the next five years, with urine tests, attendance at AA meetings five times a week, group therapy once a week, and regular contact with his sponsor. He was also required to keep an ongoing journal of the meetings he attends and note his gains and losses. After three years, Connor will be able to petition the licensing board for a temporary license to practice law.

After six months in the counseling group, Connor started coming late and eventually started missing groups. His wife of thirty-five years left him and he is surviving by doing some paralegal work under the table. Convinced that he can control his drinking, he drives by his local "watering hole" and stops in for a few beers, which eventually leads to a bender that lasts two weeks, culminating in a crisis call to the center. The crisis counselor's first concern is to validate Connor's decision to call. With each statement, he strives to provide hope, support, and empathy. As the crisis counselor listens to Connor, he tries to identify the process that led to his relapse and possible alternative actions Connor can take now that he may have been unwilling to take before. He will also try to evaluate Connor's recovery process prior to the relapse. Was Connor calling his sponsor? Was he attending and becoming involved in meetings? When was he having the urge to drink? What can he do now that he wasn't willing to do before?

Connor: I am really, really scared. I stopped drinking two days ago and am starting to feel nauseous and agitated. What should I do? I can't go to the ER.

CW: *You sound pretty upset. Give me a little more information so I can try and help you out.*

Connor: I've been drinking. Daily for the past two weeks. A pint of vodka and a six-pack or two every day. I drink. All day when I'm not sleeping or out of it.

CW: *Sounds as though your body's missing the booze and you may be into the start of a pretty serious withdrawal. You're digging out of a hole again, Connor—there's a lot on the line. Something tells me you're also worried about how it's going to affect getting your license back.*

Connor: You got it. I'm not sure I can go to any detox. I'll lose my job, as shitty as it may be. It's my only source of money.

CW: *Makes me wonder if you're not missing time at work already, Connor. Pretty overwhelming.*

Connor: I'm not really sure what to do. I've been here before. Lots of times, it seems. I know I need to get detoxed but I'm tired of starting over. I just wanna give up.

CW: *Sounds as though you're trying to convince yourself of something, Connor. As though you're hopeless—so you can just throw in the towel. How hopeless are you?*

Connor: I am living by myself in a 10-by-10-foot room at the Y, with no family or friends, and I drink. No booze for two days and I'm climbing the walls. I can't take it much longer.

CW: *Why call tonight, Connor? You know the drill. Why tonight?*

Connor: I'm afraid I'm not going to make it this time. So sad and alone . . . like no matter what I do . . . it just gets screwed up.

CW: *Yeah, you've been around this way once or twice. But you did reach out for help, Connor. You're not gone yet. You've still got guts and, down deep, you keep trying. That says a lot. I can't quite shake the feeling though that you're thinking about hurting yourself tonight. What's that about?*

Connor: Well, I'd be out of my misery, once and for all. But I keep thinking about my wife and my kids. Even though no one wants anything to do with me. I've got grandchildren I've never been able to see. Can you believe that? I know I'm better when I'm sober. . . . I know I'm better when I do a meeting a day. . . . I know I feel better when I get through the first week. I know I can be happy. . . . I want a life.

Connor presented symptoms of withdrawal that the crisis worker deemed as requiring a controlled intervention setting. The crisis worker also noted the isolation and hopelessness in Connor's voice and assessed for suicidal ideation, intent, and plan. Based on Connor's response, the crisis worker determined that there was loose suicidal ideation but no intent or plan, so the goals for the interaction became ensuring the client's continued physical safety, supporting the client's mastery of the current situation, and reconnecting the client with formal and informal supports. Hearing that Connor was isolating himself, the crisis worker also wanted to encourage the client's efforts to reconnect with his sponsor and other supportive relationships. The crisis worker made a concerted effort to provide a supportive yet confrontational sounding board for Connor.

CW: *I hear that loud and clear. You can function and you can stop drinking. Have you talked to your sponsor lately or seen anyone you know from meetings?*

Connor: No, I haven't called Bob or seen anyone I'd want to talk to. Yeah, I still have Bob's number. He's Mr. AA and probably at a meeting right now.

CW: *So why haven't you called him?*

Connor: I feel like I'm wasting his time. I'm a drunk. Why would he waste time on a screw-up like me? He's a great guy and stood by me a couple of times, but how much can people take?

CW: *He must have seen something in you. Bob's a pretty experienced sponsor. I can't imagine he would have taken you on if he didn't think you were worth it* *or at a point where you were ready. It's pretty hard to bite the bullet and swallow your pride.*

Connor: You read me well, I can tell. I'm pretty good at throwing a pity party. So you think I should call Bob, right?

CW: *Well, it's not really important what I think, Connor. You're the one with the problem. I feel for you but I also know you know yourself. I think you need a detox just to be sure you make it through the tough part but I also think you need more than just detox and counseling. I think you know you need support. The type of support a home group and a sponsor can give you. People who know and care about you. So . . . what's the next move?*

Connor: Do you think I really need a detox?

CW: *I think you know that answer, Connor. Your body's screaming for booze. You get crazy in the beginning and you need some extra help then. Why don't you call Bob and see what he thinks? Talk with him about going to St. John's Detox.*

Connor: I really don't want to go, you know.

CW: *I hear that, Connor, and I know you're worked up. But I also know you're taking some big chances here, physically going cold turkey. Will you call him?*

Connor: All right, but what if I can't get hold of him?

CW: *If you can't get in touch with him, you need to find someone else. Someone in AA or a friend who can take you.*

Connor: Not sure I can do that, but I'll try. There is another guy in AA that I used to hang out with. I think he is still sober. I guess I could call him.

CW: *Sounds like a plan. After you have talked with them, call me back. In the meantime, I'll reserve a spot at the hospital for you. No names, just a bed in the agency's name. I'd really like someone to go with you. Someone you know. If that doesn't work, you can always drive or take a taxi.*

Connor: Like I said, no booze in two days. I'm shaky but I drove this afternoon to get some cigarettes and coffee. I guess I could go to the hospital myself now if I wanted to.

CW: *It's up to you.*

Connor: Let me call my two numbers first and see if they're there. If they're not, I'll call you back and let you know.

Connor: Hey, what is your name, anyway?

CW: *My name is John.*

Connor: Well John, regardless of whether I go to detox tonight or not, you have been helpful. Thanks.

CW: *Connor, come on, man. Sounds like you've already made up your mind not to go. I thought we had a plan?*

Connor: All right. All right. We have a plan. I'll call you back. For sure.

CW: *It's up to you, Connor. I hope I hear back.*

Connor: Thanks, John, be in touch . . .

Although Connor perceived himself as isolated, he did have previous connections with individuals in AA whom he could contact. John also wanted to help Connor make a tentative plan and keep him in the loop. Based on Connor's statement that he hadn't been drinking for two days and that he had driven a car to get coffee and cigarettes, the worker suggested that the client might drive himself to the hospital. It is possible that Connor was lying and that he was, indeed, still drinking. That is why John suggested calling two other AA members first, in the hope that one of them might drive him to the hospital. Another option was for Connor to call for a taxi to take him to the hospital. John did not, however, tell Connor to just drive over to the hospital because he could detect some resistance in Connor's voice. What he wanted Connor to do was to continue reaching out for help so that he might be more willing to go the hospital as a result of talking with another individual in AA. He also contracted with Connor to hold him responsible to his word, which created some structure and a bit of levity at the end of the conversation.

Crisis Counselor Wellness

Crisis intervention with an addicted population is emotionally taxing work yet can also be very rewarding. Intervention with this population is fraught with ongoing crises and relapse. Although single-session crisis intervention is limited in time, crisis counseling with an addicted population requires a great deal of time, patience, and knowledge about addiction and recovery. Suggestions for crisis workers engaged in counseling addicted clients include:

1. Understand that relapse is often part of the process of getting clean and sober.
2. Be aware of your own personal and professional limitations and acknowledge your own powerlessness over the addict or alcoholic.
3. Maintain a sense of humor.
4. Develop your own support network (i.e., therapy, supervision, consultants).
5. Know when to refer a client to alternative levels of care.
6. Be patient with both yourself and your client.
7. Take time to relax, meditate, exercise, eat, and so on.
8. Take time off.
9. Maintain and grow with relationships in your own life.
10. Teach by your own example.

Working with crisis day in and day out can be draining and intense; however, if the counselor is able to develop and maintain a balanced lifestyle, work with this population can be extremely powerful and rewarding. Humility, honesty, and humor will also serve you well.

DISCUSSION QUESTION

1. The disease model of addiction is widely accepted, yet this chapter focused on addiction and crisis. Discuss how and where substance use can precipitate crisis.

EXERCISES

1. Although the American Medical Association designated alcoholism as a disease in 1956, the disease concept continues to be controversial. Divide the class in half and have one side take the position that alcoholism is a disease and the other half take the position that it is not. Each group should also address the impact of its position on crisis intervention.

2. Create an in-class group in which members make a commitment to abstain from the use of a particular substance or activity for a period of two weeks. The substance or activity must be one that group members engage in frequently and that gives them pleasure. The other members of the class are the support group. Members who are abstaining can call and/or e-mail each other and members of the support group for encouragement, if needed. Students should monitor the ABCDE assessment domains during the two-week time period and report back to the class.

REFERENCES

Alcoholics Anonymous World Service. (1976). *Alcoholics Anonymous* (3rd ed.). New York: Author.

American Psychiatric Association. (2000). *Diagnostic and statistical manual of mental disorders* (4th ed., Text Revision). Washington, DC: Author.

Brown, S. (1985). *Treating the alcoholic: A developmental model of recovery.* New York: John Wiley and Sons.

Buelow, G. D., & Buelow, S. A. (1998). *Psychotherapy in chemical dependency treatment: A practical and integrative approach.* Pacific Grove, CA: Brooks/Cole.

Curtis, O. (1999). *Chemical dependency: A family affair.* Pacific Grove, CA: Brooks/Cole.

Fisher, G. L., & Harrison, T. C. (2000). *Substance abuse: Information for school counselors, social workers, therapists, and counselors* (2nd ed.). Needham Heights, MA: Allyn & Bacon.

Flores, P. J. (1988). *Group psychotherapy with addicted populations.* New York: Haworth Press.

Gorski, T. T. (1989). *Passages through recovery: An action plan for preventing relapse.* Center City, MN: Hazelden.

Gorski, T. T. (1992). Diagnosing codependence. *Addiction and Recovery, 12,* 14–16.

Institute of Medicine. (1990). *Broadening the base of treatment for alcohol problems.* Washington, DC: National Academy Press.

Johnson, V. E. (1973). *I'll quit tomorrow*. Toronto: Harper & Row.

Johnson, V. E. (1986). *Intervention: How to help someone who doesn't want help. A step-by-step guide for families and friends of chemically dependent persons*. Minneapolis: Johnson Institute Books.

Kinney, J., & Leaton, G. (1987). *Loosening the grip: A handbook of alcohol information*. St. Louis, MO: Times Mirror/Mosby College.

Koob, G. F., & Le Moal, M. (1997). Drug abuse: Hedonic homeostatic dysregulation. *Science, 278*(5335), 52–58.

Loeschen, S. (1997). *Systematic training in the skills of Virginia Satir*. Pacific Grove, CA: Brooks/Cole.

Morgan, O. J, & Jordan, M. (Eds.). (1999). *Addiction and spirituality: A multidisciplinary approach*. St. Louis, MO: Chalice Press.

Nesse, R. M., & Berridge, K. C. (1997). Psychoactive drug use in evolutionary perspective. *Science, 278*(5335), 63–66.

Newman, C. F., & Wright, F. D. (1994). Substance abuse. In F. M. Dattilio & A. Freeman (Eds.), *Cognitive-behavioral strategies in crisis intervention* (pp. 119–136). New York: Guilford Press.

Pennsylvania Department of Health/Office of Drug and Alcohol Programs. (1997a). *Pennsylvania client placement criteria for adults*. Harrisburg, PA: Author.

Pennsylvania Department of Health/Office of Drug and Alcohol Programs. (1997b). *Admission criteria "checklist"* (Form #HD1024-F). Harrisburg, PA: Author.

Pipes, R. B., & Davenport, D. S. (1999). *Introduction to psychotherapy: Common clinical wisdom* (2nd ed.). Needham Heights, MA: Allyn & Bacon.

Prochaska, J. O., & DiClemente, C. C. (1995). An empirical typology of subjects within stage of change. *Addictive Behaviors, 20*(3), 299–320.

Prochaska, J. O., DiClemente, C. C., & Norcross, J. C. (1992). In search of how people change: Applications to addictive behaviors. *American Psychologist, 47*, 1102–1114.

Ramsay, J. R., & Newman, C. F. (2000). Substance abuse. In F. M. Dattilio & A. Freeman (Eds.), *Cognitive-behavioral strategies in crisis intervention* (2nd ed., pp. 126–149). New York: Guilford Press.

Rogers, C. (1957). The necessary and sufficient conditions of therapeutic personality change. *Journal of Consulting Psychology, 21*, 95–103.

Royce, J. E. (1989). *Alcohol problems and alcoholism: A comprehensive survey* (Rev. ed.). New York: Free Press.

Skinner, B. F. (1987). A humanist alternative to A.A.'s twelve steps: A human centered approach to conquering alcoholism. *The Humanist, 47*, 5.

Stevens, P., & Smith, R. (2000). *Substance abuse counseling: Theory and practice* (2nd ed.). Upper Saddle River, NJ: Merrill Prentice Hall.

U.S. Department of Health and Human Services. (2001a). *Illicit drug use*. Retrieved June 23, 2002, from http://www.samhsa.gov/oas/NHSDA/2kNHSDA/chapter2.htm

U.S. Department of Health and Human Services. (2001b). *Alcohol use*. Retrieved June 23, 2002, from http://www.samhsa.gov/oas/NHSDA/2kNHSDA/chapter3.htm

Unterberger, G. (1989). Twelve steps for women alcoholics. *Christian Century*, 1150.

Wallen, J. (1993). *Addiction in human development: Developmental perspectives on addiction and recovery*. New York: Haworth Press.

Wegscheider, S. (1981). *Another chance: Hope and health for the alcoholic family*. Palo Alto, CA: Science and Behavior Books.

Yalom, I. D. (1995). *The theory and practice of group psychotherapy* (4th ed.). New York: Basic Books.

CHAPTER 9

Chronic and Terminal Illness

ELIZABETH J. JACOB
THOMAS M. COLLINS

Jane is a thirty-six-year-old married female who was recently diagnosed with breast cancer. Jane has been married to Steve for five years, has a two-year-old son, and works full time as a human resources manager for a successful corporation. Jane found a lump under her right breast while showering a few months ago. Her family physician recommended a mammogram. The mammogram results suggested the need for a biopsy, which came back positive for breast cancer.

Following surgery, an appointment was scheduled for Jane with an oncologist. The oncologist recommended chemotherapy followed by intensive radiation, with the possibility of starting chemotherapy in the office the same day. Jane broke down into uncontrollable sobbing and was unable to regain control. The oncologist called one of the mental health counselors on staff at the medical practice to speak with her. Jane, overwhelmed with emotions and feeling pressed to make an immediate decision, agreed to talk with the counselor.

Being diagnosed with a chronic or terminal illness is often accompanied by immediate and ongoing crisis responses. Health crises affect individuals of all ages across the life span and can trigger different types of reactions and responses, not only for the patient, but also for his or her related social network. Estimates indicate that the number of people in the United States diagnosed with chronic health conditions is expected to increase from 99 million people in 1995 to a projected 134 million people by the year 2020 (Goodheart, Marganoff, & Ricketts, 1997). Mental health providers will increasingly need to work with medical personnel to integrate physical and psychological health factors in the treatment of chronically and terminally ill individuals. Patients will need crisis workers to assist them in coping with both the shock of diagnosis and the accompanying crises of illness management.

Ozer (2000) suggested that knowledge of pathophysiology (underlying biological process) is as important for clinicians focused on biopsychosocial issues as it is for other health care providers. A contextual approach to both medical and psychosocial intervention highlights the importance of assessing the environment in which the person with the disease functions. Crisis intervention with patients facing health crises involves managing the ways in which the patient's life is affected with an ultimate goal of being able "to add life to years" (Ozer, 2000, p. xiii). Focus must be on both the progression of the specific illness and on the extent to which the client reaches an acceptance of having the illness and can cope constructively.

This chapter focuses on understanding chronic and terminal illnesses as potential crisis moments in individuals' lives and on the process of crisis intervention with individuals diagnosed with serious illnesses. The diagnosis of a serious illness can be considered a health crisis for an individual and a family, with related concerns including acceptance of a diagnosis, coping and adjustment issues, and coming to terms with the long-term impact of the illness on quality of life. According to Marcus and Bernard (2000), individuals who are diagnosed with serious illness often experience helplessness and questions about their ability to "influence events related to the illness" (p. 188). Multiple dimensions of crisis responses include emotional, cognitive, behavioral, developmental, and relational components. Interventions using a crisis response framework that addresses biopsychosocial dimensions may help patients learn to cope and accept a life-altering situation.

Given the range of possible health crises, the nature of the specific illness also influences the psychological adjustment of the patient. With certain types of serious illnesses patients may experience complete remission of symptoms, yet their quality of life may still be negatively affected. The continuum of possible outcomes ranges from complete remission to death if the illness is diagnosed as terminal. Serious illness has similarities to other types of crises as well as unique biopsychosocial dimensions that counselors must take into consideration.

DEFINING CHRONIC ILLNESS

The concept of chronic illness comprises a wide range of medical diagnoses that can affect the life of an individual across the life span. Chronic illnesses are "diseases that are perpetual, permanently affecting, and disruptive. Patients are faced with incurable, sometimes debilitating illnesses with potential for physical disabilities, disfigurement, and a shortened life" (Garrett & Weisman, 2001, p. 120). Symptoms vary according to the nature of the illness, with the patient most likely experiencing significant decreases in level of functioning. The patient's quality of life is inevitably affected, but because each chronic illness has different symptoms, and because individual responses vary, the ramifications differ for each patient. Health-related *quality of life* refers to the extent that a person's satisfaction with various domains of life (physical, emotional, relational, social well-being) has been affected by illness or its treatment (Wilson & Cleary, 1995).

According to Garrett and Weisman (2001), patients seek counseling services for psychosocial problems resulting from chronic illnesses including cancer, human immunodeficiency virus-positive status (HIV+), multiple sclerosis (MS), epilepsy, Parkinson's disease (PD), diabetes, and cardiovascular disease. The symptoms of each of these diseases are unique, with patterns of remission and relapse continually disrupting the life of an individual. The nature of onset may itself lead to a complex and difficult diagnostic process and an emotional roller coaster for the individual because of the difficulty of diagnosing and determining the prognosis for many chronic illnesses. The patient's physical condition affects multiple levels of psychological functioning, and the individual's ongoing adjustment and acceptance of his or her diagnosis, in turn, affect all dimensions of treatment.

Within a cultural context, societal emphasis on individual responsibility can create additional difficulties for a patient in coping and dealing with loss of control in one's life. Although a chronic illness presents with specific symptoms, all are rooted in societal concepts that place value judgments on sickness and health (Garrett & Weisman, 2001). This can often leave a patient feeling doubly stigmatized by the diagnosis and make it more difficult to accept and cope with the illness. Emerging research with ethnic minorities suggests that one's culture also influences coping and adjustment to the diagnosis of a chronic illness (Betancourt & Fuentes, 2001; Chazin, Kaplan, & Terio, 2000; Markowitz, Spielman, Sullivan, & Fishman, 2000). Crisis counselors working in health care settings must be attentive to the role of cultural issues in the life of a patient because culture can affect health behavior and influence the treatment process. The following example illustrates how cultural factors can influence a patient's ability to accept the diagnosis of a serious illness.

Marco is a twenty-eight-year-old, single, Catholic, gay male, born in Puerto Rico. Marco, who recently tested HIV+, just lost his partner of five years to AIDS. Marco and his partner lived a very closeted life, at least in part to hide his homosexuality from his parents and extended family, who continuously pressure him to get married and start a family. Marco's family believed that his partner was his long-term roommate. They felt sad about his roommate's death from pneumonia but don't quite understand why Marco is so upset. They are continuing to pressure him to settle down and start a family, suggesting that Marco should start looking for a Puerto Rican woman to marry.

Marco has isolated himself from his family and friends and refused to see a doctor since receiving his HIV+ diagnosis. Marco suspects that his HIV+ status is punishment for being gay. He has become increasingly suicidal, thinking that he is better off dead than having his family find out that not only is he gay, but HIV+. Marco believes that he deserves to die because he has humiliated his family and he is not a real man because he has disgraced his parents and family.

A crisis counselor working with Marco would need to understand the role of cultural issues on his ability to accept his diagnosis. The role of familial ties and the cultural notions of *respecto* and *machismo* found in his culture may shed light on Marco's worldview and beliefs about his HIV+ status. A crisis counselor would also need to understand Marco's suffering and inability to publicly grieve the death of his partner because he has hidden his sexual orientation from family and friends. The psychosocial stressors of bereavement and difficulties with his primary support network are intertwined with cultural dynamics. Understanding the cultural context of Marco's worldview and lifestyle would be essential in helping him resolve loss issues and accept his HIV+ status.

Crises may occur at any point in the disease trajectory from the moment of diagnosis to the loss of physical functioning, to the traumatic experience of specific medical procedures, to the loss of important social roles. The nature of crisis intervention varies based on the unique complexities of each type of chronic illness and each individual's psychosocial responses. Knowledge about the specific illness a patient is experiencing as well as understanding its unique symptomatology and diagnostic implications are essential. Regardless of the type of chronic illness a patient is experiencing, crisis counselors must help the patient cope with the common emotional, cognitive, behavioral, and social implications of being diagnosed with a serious chronic illness. Importantly, though not specifically addressed, accidental injuries that result in chronic pain and/or long-term impairment may have similar implications for survivors and crisis workers who may provide assistance.

Types of Chronic Illnesses

This section describes specific types of chronic illnesses in order to identify the unique dimensions of each disease as it shapes a patient's experience and thus the counseling process. It is not possible to discuss the diagnostic and medical aspects of every chronic illness, so only a brief overview of selected illnesses is provided. The descriptions illustrate some of the similarities in coping and adjustment issues faced by patients who are diagnosed with a chronic illness. Crisis workers who regularly work with patients with a specific illness (e.g., cancer, kidney failure, MS) must develop a detailed knowledge base regarding specific etiology, nature of the illness, disease trajectory, and treatment implications.

This chapter presents specific illustrations of some commonly diagnosed chronic illnesses to demonstrate crisis intervention with health crises. Crisis workers, however, must remain cognizant that different types of chronic illnesses not discussed comprehensively here also present unique crisis moments for patients. Although we do not discuss cardiovascular disease (CVD) in this chapter, it is important to note that it has been the number one killer in the United States since 1900 (American Heart Association, 2002). In addition, there are over 17 million people (6.2 percent of the population) in the United States who have diabetes, including Type 1 diabetes, Type 2 diabetes, and gestational diabetes. Type 1 diabetes usually occurs during childhood or adolescence; Type 2 diabetes is the most common form of the disease, usually occurring after age forty-five; and gestational diabetes affects women halfway through pregnancy, caused by excessive hormone production in the body (American Diabetes Association, 2002).

Cancer   The literature on coping with chronic illnesses is replete with information and strategies on how to facilitate psychosocial adaptation to both sudden and gradual onset of chronic illness. According to Livneh (2000), cancer is one of the most comprehensively researched chronic illnesses. The course of the illness, or its "trajectory," provokes distinct concerns for an individual diagnosed with cancer. Coping and psychosocial adaptation issues vary based on the type of cancer an individual has (e.g., breast cancer, ovarian cancer, lung cancer, prostate cancer), with different disease progressions, prognostic indicators, treatment modalities, and psychosocial reactions for patients (Livneh, 2000). Breast cancer is utilized both as an example in this section and as a case example at the end of this chapter.

Women of all ages, races, ethnicities, socioeconomic statuses, sexual orientations, and geographical locations (and even some men) are afflicted by breast cancer. According to Hoskins and Haber (2000), more than 182,000 women in the United States were diagnosed with invasive breast cancer in the year 2000. A National Cancer Institute (2002) report, based on cancer rates from 1997 to 1999, estimated that roughly 1 in 8 women in the United States (approximately 13.3 percent) will develop breast cancer during their lifetime. Even though 90 percent of breast cancer patients survive for five years or longer, the emotional toll the disease can take is considerable. Even if the breast cancer is treated with invasive surgical procedures (e.g., lumpectomy or mastectomy) and/or radiation or chemotherapy that results in remission of the cancer, the patient is often left with the uncertainty of recurrence and fears about what may happen in the future. The dilemma is captured by a survivor quoted in Hoskins and Haber's (2000) article on surviving breast cancer: "Once you've had cancer, whenever you feel another pain, your response is never quite the same again. It's never a case of, 'I'm getting old; there's a pain in my back.' There's always that little voice in the back of your mind that says, 'Oh, no, has the cancer returned? Is it growing somewhere else?" (p. 26).

The degree of psychosocial distress and adjustment varies for the individual as well as for members of her family and support network depending on the nature of the particular breast cancer (e.g., stage, recovery status following surgery, symptoms), perceptions and felt meaning of the illness, and methods of coping. Individuals utilize familiar coping mechanisms when dealing with life stressors and unpredictable life changes. When a problem's scope exceeds a patient's ability to cope using those familiar strategies, crisis responses may result.

Often a patient is most anxious when she experiences uncertainty or is in transition (e.g., waiting for diagnosis/test results, treatment protocol changes). In the case of breast cancer, psychosocial adjustment may also be influenced by treatment protocols that have cosmetic implications in a society where standards of beauty often dictate how women perceive themselves and their breasts. In addition, the emotional stress of cancer may alter a woman's body image and make her feel that she is no longer a "whole" woman, especially if there is the possibility of disfigurement. Some cancer patients may associate disfiguring treatment with sexual problems. They may need to contend not only with discomfort and/or disability but also with the impact of physical changes on their self-image. Crisis workers must recognize that over the course of the disease trajectory, women may feel less sexually attractive, which can disrupt romantic relationships and precipitate sexual problems with a partner or spouse.

All chronic illnesses should be thought of as "family illnesses" in that every individual diagnosed with a chronic illness functions as a member of a larger network of relationships that are invariably influenced by the crisis of illness. Breast cancer is no exception. The cancer disease trajectory not only influences the patient's psychosocial adjustment but the family's as well.

Hoskins and Haber (2000) identified specific phases of illness with corresponding unique physical and emotional sequelae. The phases include (1) the diagnostic phase, which can trigger shock and disbelief when a patient has to make immediate treatment decisions; (2) the postoperative phase, which includes coping with bodily changes and potential life-role transitions; (3) the adjuvant therapy phase, which involves making informed ongoing treatment decisions (e.g., chemotherapy) along with symptom management; and (4) the ongoing recovery phase, which can trigger fears of recurrence, ambivalence about ending treatment, and apprehension regarding reentry into mainstream life.

Phases of adjustment can be stressful in different ways (e.g., in the diagnostic and adjustment phases) and disruptive (e.g., in the ongoing recovery phase when one is living with uncertainty and the fear of recurrence) in the lives of individual patients and families. A particularly significant phase in the cancer disease trajectory is the terminal phase, as patients and their families struggle to accept the patient's impending death and experience anticipatory grief. Bereavement is a potential final phase, as patients and families cope with grief and loss responses on multiple levels (e.g., emotional, physical, spiritual, and social).

Psychosocial adjustment is unique to the person with cancer as well as to the family of the person with cancer. Counselors can assist patients and their families to identify the specific psychosocial stressors they are facing and intervene accordingly. Psychosocial problems common among cancer patients and families include quality of life, adjustment to the diagnosis and illness, marriage and family disruption, varying emotional responses, sexuality and fertility, changes in body image, rigorous and intrusive treatment protocols, and financial concerns (Holland & Rowland, 1990; Hoskins & Haber, 2000; Spiegel & Diamond, 1988).

Not all patients or families require intervention, but psychosocial interventions have been found to be useful for many cancer patients and their families (Hoskins & Haber, 2000). The psychosocial dimensions of a cancer diagnosis frequently lead to understandable and common difficulties in patients' adjustment and/or acceptance. For example, breast cancer can significantly alter the relationship between the patient and her romantic partner. Because the cancer patient's needs become the focus, a partner's needs may go unrecognized, changing the relationship and affecting the psychosocial adjustment of both individuals.

Research has suggested a blurring of the boundaries between psychosocial and biomedical interventions through the positive impact of psychosocial support on both the quality and longevity of life for women with advanced breast cancer and for patients with melanoma (Fawzy, Canada, & Fawzy, 2003; Fawzy, Fawzy, Hyun,

Elashoff, Guthrie, Fahey, & Morton, 1993; Spiegel and Diamond, 1988). Psychosocial support has been consistently found to facilitate the psychological adjustment of patients with cancer; more recent research is attempting to study the relationship between psychological adjustment and physical health. There is a clear need for ongoing collaborative work with physicians and medical personnel.

HIV+/AIDS   Another chronic disease that frequently precipitates crisis responses is HIV infection and/or AIDS. The needs of people living with AIDS (PLWAs) and the realities of the disease have changed dramatically over the past two decades. Recent pharmacological advances have changed the perception of HIV+/AIDS from a terminal illness to a chronic illness (Holt, Houg, & Romano, 1999). Etiologically, AIDS is precipitated by an HIV retrovirus that causes progressive deficiency in CD4+ T-lymphocytes and resultant vulnerability to serious opportunistic infections and cancers. The HIV virus can be transmitted through sexual contact, blood or blood products, breast milk, or from mother to fetus during pregnancy (Nelson, 1998). The progressive nature of AIDS leads to successive potential crises for patients, including psychological adjustment problems, neurobehavioral problems, and existential concerns.

As the demographics of people contracting HIV shift, a more diverse group of people living with AIDS has emerged. Because there is still stigma attached to the diagnosis of AIDS, PLWAs often experience more losses than people with other chronic or terminal illnesses. These include "losses inflicted from societal prejudices, stigma, fear of exposure, and the effects of the disease on the patient's sexual and social identities" (Bonde, 2001, p. 84). In addition to the societal stigma of living with AIDS, patients also face potential rejection or condemnation by family and friends. The fear of familial rejection can lead to complications in adjustment.

The overlay of societal stigma and misperceptions of AIDS as a "gay" disease may lead individuals to hide their diagnosis in order to prevent rejection by family and friends. The case example of Marco illustrates the plight of a Puerto Rican male responding to powerful homophobic messages rooted in his culture and Catholic upbringing. Similarly, familial issues and stigma may arise for heterosexual individuals due to the assumption that one became infected through drug use or sexual promiscuity with same-sex and opposite-sex partners (Holt, Houg, & Romano, 1999). Stigmatization and moral judgment precipitate adjustment differently as they exacerbate social isolation and loss issues.

Research has identified numerous common psychological responses of individuals when first diagnosed with the HIV virus, including anxiety, depression, social isolation, and anger (Holland & Tross, 1985; Nelson, 1998). Crisis counselors should always assess the potential for lethal behavior, as the risk and incidence of suicide among people living with AIDS is elevated (Nelson, 1998). Immediate crisis responses can also include sexual acting out by an individual who is angry upon hearing the initial HIV+ diagnosis. Crisis counselors should routinely screen for and conduct ongoing assessment of suicidal ideation and level of lethality. Risk factors for suicide for newly diagnosed patients include lack of social support and social isolation along with serious psychological reactions such as shock, denial, depression, anger, shame, and guilt.

Nelson (1998) suggested that there are three distinguishable phases of HIV illness. The psychosocial difficulties experienced by the HIV-infected individual vary with, or reflect, the specific phase of disease progression. It is important for crisis counselors to be familiar with the phases of the disease progression in HIV+/AIDS patients because presenting issues and thus the types of appropriate intervention may differ.

The *initial phase* of progression of AIDS is the period of acute infection that occurs around the time of seroconversion, when the HIV infection is diagnosed either by detection of antibodies to HIV or by direct detection of the virus. The crisis counselor can help the newly diagnosed patient cope with a range of emotional responses to the diagnosis (e.g., denial, depression, anger) in addition to providing education about the disease and helping the patient identify available social supports. These supports allow the individual to disclose his or her HIV+ status and receive emotional support during the initial phase of the disease trajectory.

The *middle, chronic infection phase,* is a time when the patient may be relatively symptom-free, yet still HIV+. During this phase, crisis counselors may encounter patients dealing with ongoing practical disease-related issues, treatment options, quality-of-life and lifestyle changes, relationship concerns, disclosure to family and friends, ongoing grief and loss issues, and "learning to live with" the disease. The *end phase* occurs as immune function gradually deteriorates. During this period, the individual begins to experience more HIV-related symptoms (e.g., HIV-associated dementia) over the course of a period of chronic infection estimated to last approximately ten years. New drug protocols continue to influence these phases, as individuals may remain in the middle, chronic infection phase, but be relatively symptom-free for longer periods of time. Similarly, individuals may experience intermittent bouts of HIV symptoms, but successfully manage them by following a new drug protocol. Crisis counselors may encounter patients experiencing concerns related to death and dying, treatment compliance/side effects of medication, pain management, and potential cognitive impairments from HIV-associated neurocognitive changes.

The crisis counselor might encounter a person during any of these phases of the illness for either brief, single-session crisis interventions or for ongoing crisis counseling. As noted, however, some phases of the disease progression are particularly traumatizing yielding potential diagnostic levels of response. There is a range of emotional reactions at the moment of diagnosis, so it may be difficult to predict how an individual will respond or what his or her counseling needs may be. When a recently diagnosed individual is seen in crisis, it is important for the counselor to allow the individual to vent his or her feelings about the diagnosis, to offer emotional support, and to provide as much information about both the disease and available resources as possible.

According to Nelson (1998), it is important, however, not to overwhelm the HIV-infected individual in the initial health crisis moment. The impact of the diagnosis of HIV infection is captured by Elia's (1997) reflections, "The instant the client receives test results showing infection, the client becomes a participant in an ongoing grieving process. This individual immediately grieves the loss of his or her HIV-negative status. Now he or she is living with HIV, and the future, as previously imagined, is changed forever. Concurrently, the individual has to begin the process of integrating the new status—'HIV-positive'—into his or her psychological world" (p. 67).

Research with HIV+/AIDS patients has suggested seven potential crisis points: (1) learning one's seropositive status, (2) receiving the diagnosis of AIDS, (3) beginning a new treatment, (4) discontinuing treatment, (5) the appearance of new symptoms, (6) recurrence and relapse, and (7) terminal illness (Flaskerud, 1995). Crisis counselors may find themselves in contact with patients and their families at several crisis points over the span of the disease process, and intervention with family members or partners can often continue beyond the patient's death.

Parkinson's disease   Chronic neurological conditions include Parkinson's disease (PD), which affects approximately 200,000 individuals each year (Ozer, 2000). Recognition of the severity and extent of the problems surrounding PD has resulted in increased attention to the availability of short-term and ongoing crisis intervention services as well as management and care services for persons living with the disease.

Parkinson's disease is a type of progressive movement disorder. Symptoms of Parkinson's include rigidity (muscular stiffness), bradykinesia (slowness in carrying out motor functions), instability in postural movements, resting tremors (a regular, rhythmic, involuntary to-and-fro movement affecting a limb), and motor fluctuations with increasing symptoms over the course of the disease trajectory (Duvoisin, 1991; Pincus, 2000). PD results from the degradation of the nerve cells that produce dopamine in the subtantia nigra part of the brain for unknown reasons (Pincus, 2000). Dopamine functions in the nervous system as a chemical messenger transmitting impulses from one nerve cell to the next and is deficient in Parkinson's disease. The undetermined cause of PD adds to the confusion in understanding the impact of the disease on the lives of patients.

The progressive nature of the disease process results in ever-changing treatment options. This necessitates adjustment to different stages of the illness and to the interactive changes in both treatment effectiveness and level of functioning over time. As Pincus (2000) remarked, "To add complexity, a patient may at first have symptoms that respond fully to dopamine replacement and then, in time, develop other symptoms that do not" (p. 214). The reality is that even though treatment is readily available, the progressive nature of PD precipitates several crisis moments in the life of the patient that can have profound psychological implications.

Research has shown a differential age-of-diagnosis impact on how patients cope with a diagnosis of PD, because it is primarily (but not exclusively) a disease that appears in older adults (Ozer, 2000). According to Pincus (2000), on the average PD begins at age fifty-nine and affects approximately 1 percent of the population over age sixty. The progressive nature of the disease along with concomitant dementing processes and nonresponsiveness to dopamine negatively alter the quality of life for older adults. Furthermore, associated movement impairment causes significant difficulties, especially in an elderly population.

Because the disease rarely affects people under the age of forty (Duvoisin, 1991), a diagnosis of early-onset PD can lead to unique implications and difficulties in coping with the diagnosis and progressive nature of the symptoms. The dearth of research on how PD affects younger patients further hampers effective intervention. Not only the patient, but medical personnel also experience confusion and difficulty in understanding the disease progression, which inevitably complicates adjustment.

A unique aspect of PD, which in itself may contribute to a crisis response, is that the first symptoms of PD do not appear until at least 80 percent of the dopaminergic neurons have been lost (Pincus, 2000). This statistical reality means that the patient first learns of the disorder when it is already quite advanced, and because PD is a progressive illness, the symptoms may worsen quickly. Medication can control or delay the onset of certain symptoms but there is no cure for the disease. The adjustment for a patient with PD often varies based on the stage of the disease. Dopamine deficiency has several stages that can be differentiated by patient response to treatment protocols.

In stage I, over 80 percent of dopaminergic cells are deficient and the patient is only mildly symptomatic. This stage lasts for an average of five to ten years, but PD may advance more quickly when there is early onset (in the forties or fifties). Stage II's moderate PD is characterized by a "wearing-off phenomenon." Stage-related fluctuations in motor movement are related to the administration of medication and symptom management. During this phase, a patient is able to recognize both the duration of the medication's therapeutic effect and its diminishing returns, or "wearing off." Stage III is the end stage of PD and is characterized by the "on-off" phenomenon. During this final phase, the patient has virtually no dopamine storage capacity in the brain. The only dopamine in the brain is provided by medication and any delay in the supply of dopamine precipitates movement impairment and bradykinesia.

This freezing of motor movements is known as an "off" period. As PD worsens, patients begin to experience more frequent alternating periods of being "off" (Parkinsonian) and "on" (mobile) (Pincus, 2000). Although the disease is not primarily considered terminal, its progressive nature leads to a gradual lack of responsiveness to the dopamine agonist treatment protocols, and the resultant possibility of complete physical disability and thus unpredictability in the lives of patients and families. Rate of progression varies for individuals with PD, necessitating ongoing shifts in the care and management of this chronic neurologic illness.

According to Dreisig, Beckmann, Wermuth, Skovlund, and Bech (1999), "Psychological reactions most frequently observed in Parkinson patients include anxiety, worrying, depression, a sense of isolation, alienation, hopelessness, frustration with regard to the presence of and failure to acknowledge impaired memory, reduced libido and potential for work, impulsiveness, and self-esteem" (p. 217). Changes in tremors, movement rigidity, bradykinesia, cognitive impairments, and worry about disease progression can provoke short-term and ongoing health crisis moments in a patient's life. For example:

Dianna is a thirty-two-year-old single, professional woman with no significant prior medical history. She first presented to her family physician with symptoms of "weakness and the shakes" in her left arm. After several months of ongoing and intensive testing that included magnetic resonance imaging (MRIs) of the brain and spinal cord, nerve conduction testing, blood tests, an electroencephalogram (EEG), along with numerous consultations with neurologists and specialists at movement disorder clinics, Dianna was diagnosed with early onset PD. She was devastated, especially because physicians were initially cautious about making the diagnosis of PD, given her age and health status up to that time. The overwhelming effect of Dianna's initial dilemmas and her intense emotional reactions of denial and anger led her to speak with a crisis worker at the clinic where she was diagnosed.

Several weeks later, Dianna faces making a decision about starting the recommended treatment protocol. She fears starting medications yet the symptoms have been affecting her work and daily level of functioning. Dianna is especially frustrated by and struggling with the decision to begin a research trial-based treatment protocol of a dopamine agonist (stimulator) because the consulting physicians are uncertain about the nature of the side effects she may experience. Since the moment of diagnosis, Dianna has been unable to imagine integrating the reality of the PD diagnosis into her active professional and personal lifestyle. She recognizes the need for more ongoing crisis counseling at this time to help her not only accept the diagnosis of PD but to make decisions regarding medical interventions.

Multiple sclerosis   Multiple sclerosis (MS) is a chronic, degenerative neurological disease of the central nervous system affecting an estimated 350,000 people in the United States (Anderson, Ellenberg, Leventhal, Reingold, Rodriguez, & Silberberg, 1992; Mohr & Cox, 2001). The disease, usually diagnosed between the ages of 20 and 40, affects approximately twice as many women as men (Allen, Landis, & Schramke, 1995; Mohr & Cox, 2001). It is an inflammatory and demyelinating disease of the central nervous system (Mohr, Boudewyn, Goodkin, Bostrom, & Epstein, 2001) with common physical symptoms (e.g., loss of function in the limbs, debilitating fatigue, sexual dysfunction), cognitive impairments, and psychological difficulties (e.g., depression, anger, anxiety). The age of onset is older in men, with the course of the disease becoming more progressive. The diagnosis of multiple sclerosis can precipitate a health crisis because it frequently affects young adults in the prime of life and has an often unpredictable and progressive course.

The pathogenesis of MS has not been clearly defined (Krupp, 2000; Mohr & Cox, 2001). No single factor completely accounts for the disease, although most research suggests an origin based on immunologic, genetic, and environmental factors. As the disease progresses, neurotransmission within the affected areas of the central nervous system (CNS) becomes impaired, leading to ongoing disruptions in sensory and motor functioning and related symptoms (Mullins, Cote, Fuemmeler, Jean, Beatty, & Paul, 2001). Uncertainty about disease progression is partially due to the heterogeneity of symptoms and the complex nature of multiple sclerosis as a disease. Evidence, however, suggests that the disease course typically consists of periods of exacerbation and remission of symptoms, with exacerbations gradually becoming more disruptive based on the disease subcategory.

Two subcategories of disease course have been identified. The relapse-remitting course, affecting 80 to 85 percent of individuals diagnosed with MS, is characterized by acute exacerbations and clinically significant symptoms. The second subcategory is the chronic-progressive course, exhibited by 15 to 20 percent of individuals, in which the disease progresses steadily without periods of remission (Allen et al., 1995; Krupp, 2000; Mohr & Cox, 2001). The uncertainty and unpredictability of the course of the disease highlights potential courses of adjustment.

Krupp (2000) indicated that a vital aspect of accurately diagnosing MS is recognizing that manifestations of the disease vary dramatically and temporally. The diagnosis is often based on a thorough medical history and ongoing evaluation by a neurological specialist. The process of evaluation in itself is stressful. Krupp (2000) asserts that a physician should never deliver a diagnosis of MS to a patient over the telephone but should always deliver it in person. Because individuals are frequently overwhelmed and devastated to hear this diagnosis, they may not be able to take in much information immediately, thus follow-up appointments may be required in order to further explain the diagnosis and answer any questions. Patients and family members need clear, understandable information about the disorder as well as referrals to additional support services and sources of assistance.

MS is considered a chronic illness, and effective treatment protocols have been developed; however, there is no cure. Despite the multiple symptoms experienced by MS patients, approximately 85 percent of MS patients have normal life expectancies (Allen et al., 1995). Crisis counselors can assist patients in coping with specific psychological symptoms and maintaining a good quality of life. Symptoms of MS can be very severe, but the disease itself is not terminal in most cases (Mohr & Dick, 1998).

The course of the disease can vary dramatically from patient to patient. The following illustration captures some of the dimensions of MS in a newly diagnosed young woman:

Susan is a twenty-five-year-old woman, recently diagnosed with relapsing-remitting MS. The initial symptom that led Susan to consult her family physician was unsteadiness when standing and walking. Her family physician conducted numerous tests and referred her to a neurologist for a follow-up consultation. An MRI revealed multiple brain lesions, and the neurologist discussed the possibility that she had MS. Susan's immediate concern was to try to understand what having MS would mean to her life. Her primary goal was to address any immediate symptoms that might interfere with her career as a nurse. Her recurring questions are: How is she going to continue working if neurological functioning is disrupted?

And, having been married less than a year, how will this impact her future as a wife and mother because she and her husband have been thinking of starting a family?

Physical, cognitive, psychological, social/relational, and developmental dimensions and disease course-related symptoms result in the need for short-term and ongoing crisis intervention with patients and families. Mohr et al. (2001) indicated that the rate of depression is higher for MS patients than for patients with other chronic illnesses or neurological disorders. Contributing factors to depression include the unique physiological changes associated with this disease and the concomitant changes in mental processes associated with brain lesions. Fatigue is a classic clinical feature of MS, with both physical and mental aspects, and may overlap with depressive symptoms (Krupp, 2000). Other contributing factors to depression include multiple changes in social role functioning. In the example of Susan, a particularly difficult issue for her may be that pregnancy is contraindicated for individuals with MS, as hormonal changes associated with pregnancy can exacerbate symptoms. Additional factors may include loss of social support and inadequate coping skills.

Crisis counselors who intervene with individuals with an MS-related crisis must be familiar with the etiology and pathophysiology of MS as well as the course of the disease. Crisis counseling is a critical component in the continuity of care for the patient adjusting to living with multiple sclerosis. Unfortunately, crisis counseling opportunities may not occur in some cases until cognitive impairments begin to show; the referrals initiated by primary care physicians are usually for neuropsychological assessment rather than for assistance with the broader array of psychosocial needs (Mohr & Dick, 1998).

Dynamics and Impact

The illustrations of chronic illness in this chapter indicate unique disease-specific components as well as common psychological dimensions experienced by patients diagnosed with a serious illness. A recurring theme in chronic and terminal illness is loss. Patients living with chronic illnesses experience many losses associated with their specific disease and its often life-altering consequences. These losses affect not only the patient but also the patient's entire social system. For many, these losses begin with diagnosis and continue to emerge and change over the course of their lives and the progression of the illness. A professional literature associated with the nature of grief and loss has begun to emerge for people with chronic and serious terminal illnesses, such as HIV and AIDS (Bonde, 2001; Elia, 1997), cancer (Hoskins & Haber, 2000; Livneh, 2000), and neurological disorders such as PD and MS (Krupp, 2000; Ozer, 2000; Pincus, 2000).

Kubler-Ross (1969) suggested that the grief process following diagnosis of a terminal illness consisted of five stages, each characterized by different responses to impending death. This model has been applied to grief associated with other types of losses as well. Kubler-Ross identified five sequential stages: denial, anger, bargaining, depression, and acceptance.

Denial and isolation occur when the initial moment of diagnosis results in shock and numbness. When first hearing a diagnosis that portends potentially permanent changes in physical functioning, many individuals cope by psychologically denying the reality of the news. The denial can be a necessary buffer for coping with the initial shock. This can be a time when individuals isolate themselves, not wanting others to view them differently, or begin searching for "proof" that the diagnosis is not accurate (e.g., ongoing consultation with specialists; ignoring the recommended treatment protocols). The stage of *anger* occurs when patients move beyond denial. As patients begin to recognize the reality of the diagnosis they often express anger that this is happening to them. Individuals in this stage may be emotionally overwhelmed with intense resentment, bitterness, and rage. Expression of anger is a healthy way of moving toward acceptance yet can become problematic if individuals get "stuck" in anger and related ineffective coping mechanisms (e.g., excessive alcohol or substance use). *Bargaining* may be clearly evident, as patients try to hold on to hope that there will be a cure or an extension of life in the case of terminal illness. It is a natural aspect of grieving the loss of physical health and the uncertainty that accompanies disease progression in chronic illness. Patients may experience depression throughout the course of the disease trajectory, and depression is often a symptom of specific chronic illnesses (e.g., fatigue for individuals with MS). Acknowledgment of one's diagnosis and prognosis is often a response to a decline in physical functioning. *Acceptance* is a personal and reflective process for patients and family members who may deal with the implications of the illness differently. As they move through the grief process, individuals gradually reconcile themselves to the reality of the disease and accept their situation. Efforts to address lifestyle and quality-of-life issues differ with changes in the level of acceptance patients experience during different phases of the disease trajectory (e.g., accepting the initial diagnosis versus changes in treatment as the disease progresses). It is important to remember that the stages do not necessarily occur in linear fashion; rather, individuals may loop through the stages because confronting the grief and loss associated with illness is often a multidimensional and complex process. Crisis counselors must understand the dynamics of the grieving process and its implications for both patients and family members.

Other common dimensions of chronic and terminal illness also increase the risk of crisis responses. The trajectory of the illness is a prime influence on the development of adjustment difficulties. The patient's and family's psychosocial adjustment to a serious chronic illness can vary according to the phases of the disease and accompanying life-role transitions, as previously depicted in Hoskins and Haber's (2000) model of breast cancer adjustment. Although their typology primarily addresses the phases of adjustment to breast cancer, generalization to other chronic illnesses is useful. Physical and emotional adjustment issues vary during the different phases of chronic illness. In the case of terminal illness, the loss of hope for a long life complicates the adjustment process further. It may be very hard for both the patient and family members to accept the fact that death is the inevitable outcome of some disease trajectories.

Specific symptoms of a chronic illness are often physically and emotionally disruptive yet are not always readily apparent to others in the patient's life. Family, friends, coworkers, and even life partners may not fully comprehend or appreciate the patient's discomfort, limitations, and emotional distress (Krupp, 2000). Moments of crisis for someone with a chronic illness may occur in discrete periods of time over the disease trajectory or in an ongoing way as the symptomatology associated with the illness progresses. Decision making (e.g., about treatment options) and adjustment to physical and social changes precipitated by the disease can trigger crisis responses. In the case, described earlier, of Susan, who was diagnosed with MS, her first crisis moment was coping with her diagnosis and making a decision about treatment options including the pharmacology protocol and adjunctive services such as outpatient physical therapy. Her concerns could be explored in a single-session crisis intervention focused on the need to make an immediate decision and to address her initial fears regarding the potential disruption of her career and family plans. She may also benefit from ongoing crisis counseling as she copes with her later issues.

CRISIS INTERVENTION

As described, the diagnosis of a serious and chronic illness is a potential health crisis in the life of an individual. Because patients and their families have both short-term and long-term emotional, cognitive, and behavioral responses to illness, it is important for crisis professionals to be familiar with both immediate and ongoing dynamics. Crisis counselors must also be comfortable responding to the uniqueness of a situation and a specific chronic illness.

To address the impact of different psychosocial problems, a comprehensive patient-oriented approach to chronic illness is necessary. This approach stresses the need for collaboration between different professionals working on a team as opposed to the traditional fragmented approach to patient care (e.g., the physician and medical personnel treat a patient's physical problems, while the counselor addresses the psychological issues). Comprehensive care approaches highlight the importance of interdisciplinary teams to address the multiple and interconnected needs of patients with chronic and terminal illnesses and the types of interventions necessary to assist them (Allen et al., 1995).

Crisis workers share the responsibility of ensuring effective collaboration with medical personnel. Effective collaboration is enhanced when the counselor recognizes that for most patients, their medical status is the primary reason they are seeking help, and psychosocial intervention must reflect that reality (Collins, Barrow, & Haupt, 1999). The counselor must function as part of the medical team. Being part of a team that attempts to address the biopsychosocial (physical, psychological, and social) needs of patients is more efficacious than counseling alone.

When providing services in a medical setting, the crisis worker must be able to intervene quickly and knowledgeably (Collins, Greenwald, & Greenwald, 1998).

Most of the clinical literature exploring the role of counseling with people diagnosed with chronic illness focuses on enhancing coping through skills training, emotional expression, enhancement of social support, and pharmacological intervention (Mohr & Cox, 2001; Pincus, 2000). Psychoeducational components can be a critical aspect of crisis intervention with chronic illnesses. Interventions can focus on clarifying key issues surrounding symptoms of the disease, the nature of the chronic illness, and treatment options and side effects.

For example, patients with Parkinson's disease can present with wide-ranging deficits in cognitive functioning (Brown, Rahill, Gorell, McDonald, Brown, Sillanpaa, & Shults, 1999) that can disrupt overall functioning and result in recurring crisis moments. Educating the patient with PD about the nature and progression of the cognitive shifts that may occur can help the patient understand the specific dimensions of these symptoms. It also enables individuals to feel more in control of decision making and to cope more effectively with traumatic cognitive changes.

The primary purpose of single-session crisis interventions is to help the individual regain a sense of control and mastery, whereas the goals of ongoing crisis counseling are to help the patient and family members cope over the long term with multiple potential psychosocial difficulties and adjustment to the nature of the disease and the disease trajectory.

SINGLE-SESSION CRISIS INTERVENTION IN HEALTH CRISES

Initial professional contacts for an individual diagnosed with a chronic illness are with physicians, specialists (e.g., neurologists, oncologists), and other medical personnel involved in the diagnosis and delivery of medical services and treatment. Although some outpatient clinics and health care facilities have established psychosocial services, including crisis intervention, those services are more often provided in institutional settings. Thus, unless a person seeks out help via a hotline or crisis center, crisis workers may not encounter a newly diagnosed patient unless they are employed in a health care setting. Regardless of where the contact is, the crisis counselor must assess the client's affective, cognitive, and behavioral responses and attend to the developmental and social/relational factors affecting the client's functioning.

Although responses by patients diagnosed with a chronic or terminal illness vary, the goals of short-term, or single-session, crisis intervention are always to ensure that the client is safe, composed, at least in the short term (e.g., overwhelming emotional distress has been regulated), and feels a sense of control in the situation (e.g., has identified what steps are necessary to gain a sense of control). The crisis counselor also needs to provide information to the patient and help him or her connect with informal and formal support systems so that the patient does not experience social isolation and disconnection. Identifying resources and increasing access to supportive resources (e.g., community support groups) can reduce the risk of recurring crisis, decrease feelings of helplessness, and increase a sense of control for patients at a time when emotional distress is likely to be high (Hoskins & Haber, 2000).

Step 1:
Supportively and empathically join with the client.

Crisis counselors engaged in single-session crisis interventions with patients dealing with chronic or terminal illness must communicate acceptance, caring, and high levels of empathy. The client may be feeling completely alone or may be in shock following an initial diagnosis, and just talking may be difficult. It is vital to quickly establish rapport and to create an environment in which the client feels safe and that he or she is not being judged. If indicated, the counselor should address the patient's physical comfort level immediately (e.g., offering a couch or chair with a legrest for a patient whose motor functioning is impaired). The counselor must also address the issue of confidentiality so patients are aware of any relevant limits to confidentiality (e.g., the counselor may have a duty to warn or to take preventive action following disclosures of suicidal ideation).

Because the initial contact is often brief, crisis counselors should identify themselves, clearly describing their role and the nature of their interactions with patients, as well as answer questions. The crisis counselor should immediately strive to build an alliance with the patient, conveying respect, authenticity, and genuineness, whether interacting with the patient and/or his or her significant others. Working with a client who has just received an initial diagnosis necessitates an alliance that can provide an environment for the client to express intense emotional reactions (e.g., shock, anger, disbelief, rage, denial). The primary goal is to provide a safe setting for the patient's emotional expression without attempting to provide immediate solutions or extensive education about the chronic illness.

Step 2:
Intervene immediately to create safety in the environment.

Crisis counselors may encounter patients during different phases of a chronic or terminal disease when assessment of immediate safety is critical. In the initial moment of diagnosis, emotional distress can lead to escalating psychological disorganization and a sense of chaos. Patients may feel hopeless and helpless in the face of a diagnosis of chronic illness because they often experience it as a death sentence. In single-session interventions, it is important for crisis workers to intervene immediately to stabilize patients, de-escalate the situation, and help patients regain a sense of control at a time when they perceive that they have no control.

The diagnosis of a chronic or life-threatening illness can interfere with an individual's ability to make effective decisions about immediate concerns. Of course, this ability is partially dependent on premorbid levels of functioning and utilization of effective coping strategies. A patient's health locus-of-control beliefs, a set of beliefs about one's personal influence over the course or outcome of an illness, may also affect the patient's struggle to accept and adjust (Williams & Koocher, 1998). Numerous clinicians and researchers have noted that when people believe that their actions can have an impact on improving a situation, they are more likely to engage in effective problem solving and experience less subjective distress (Nezu, Kalmar, Ronan, & Clavijo, 1986; Thompson & Collins, 1995).

Crisis workers must help patients focus on the specific dimensions of their immediate concerns. In health crises, this includes identifying immediate causes of psychosocial distress and helping patients address a specific problem so that they can regain a sense of control. If an individual is experiencing complicated grief reactions to a diagnosis, there may be evidence of self-destructive impulses (e.g., alcohol or drug abuse) or suicidal ideation. Providing information to stimulate clearer thinking can help stabilize the client and create a sense of safety.

The crisis worker can correct discrepancies in understanding or thought processes and provide accurate information about treatment options. Dispelling misconceptions can instill hope and facilitate effective decision making. Crisis workers must structure interventions according to the specific needs of the patient and family members.

Step 3:
Explore and assess the dimensions of the crisis and the client's reaction to the crisis, encouraging ventilation.

Through an ongoing process of observing, listening, and integrating information, crisis workers assess the patient's affective, behavioral, and cognitive reactions, as well as his or her relevant developmental issues and ecological situation (ABCDE). They also strive to develop a sense of the individual's premorbid (prediagnosis) level of functioning. The patient's premorbid level of functioning gives the crisis worker an idea of the level of functioning that the patient will be able to attain again. The overarching goal of this evolving assessment is to construct an integrated picture of the patient and the patient's crisis response.

The crisis worker also continues to listen with empathy and support while encouraging expression of overwhelming emotions. The crisis worker should encourage the patient to tell his or her story and vent as needed. For example, a patient may be feeling angry and enraged or may be questioning the fairness of life. Questions like "Why is this happening to me?" and "What did I do to deserve this in my life?" are common.

Each dimension of the ABCDE assessment framework is briefly examined in the following discussion. This information is applicable to crisis workers intervening in either single-session or ongoing crisis counseling. In single-session intervention, the assessment process is truncated, whereas in ongoing crisis coun-seling assessment can be more in-depth and evolves over the course of contact.

Affect

According to Garrett and Weisman (2001), "Regardless of the specific diagnosis, chronic illness may produce uncertainty and anxiety, which heightens the poten-tial for depression, emptiness, despair, isolation, and disillusionment" (p. 119). Crisis counselors must assess the immediate emotional responses and concurrent suicidal ideation to ensure physical safety in the case of a patient who may be overwhelmed with emotions or experiencing extreme despair. The reality is that, in all cases, chronic illness precipitates a merger of physical and emotional re-sponses that transforms repeatedly over the course of a disease.

In working with patients confronting serious illnesses, it is important for crisis counselors to differentiate affective responses due to psychological distress from neurological and/or physiological shifts in functioning. Many chronic illnesses produce affective and cognitive changes due to pathophysiology of the illness that mimic psychiatric symptomatology. This can result in misdiagnosis if the coun-selor does not conduct a thorough assessment. This caveat reaffirms the need for crisis workers to understand the etiology of specific serious illnesses as well as the disease trajectories and specific symptomatology. For example, depression, anxi-ety, euphoria, and affective disturbance are salient features of MS (Allen et al., 1995); thus crisis workers must distinguish between affective disorders and emo-tional disturbances resulting directly from an underlying pathophysiological pro-cess. In the later case, pharmacological treatment may be the first-line interven-tion, and crisis workers can arrange a referral to address this physiologically based affective problem.

Behavior

In assessing patient's behavior, it is important to consider both what patients are doing and what they are not doing, as it relates to their sense of being in crisis. Chronic illnesses usually disrupt patients' lives, and the diagnosis often requires many immediate behavioral changes. For example, patients may need to follow a very strict regimen of medication (e.g., HIV+ patients) or may benefit from regu-lar moderate exercise and healthy eating habits (e.g., patients with early-stage MS).

Restrictions associated with illness can create barriers to social activities as well as difficulties in interpersonal relationships. Individuals may be unable to engage in activities they previously enjoyed and may need to identify new leisure activi-ties. Individuals may also isolate themselves or withdraw from activities or rela-tionships in response to depression or other difficulties in coping. In the case of cancer, as the ability to cope with the disease decreases, the patient may withdraw from social networks with associated problematic decreases in social interaction (Rokach, 2000).

Crisis workers must also be aware that assessing behavioral changes includes understanding physical symptoms and potential deterioration in levels of functioning. For example, individuals with MS must adjust their behavior in response to exacerbation of the disease. During an exacerbation, individuals must rest, perhaps taking time off from work, and may have a more difficult time taking care of themselves. Similarly, persons diagnosed with PD may experience decreased physical capacity with resultant changes in behaviors related to mobility and self-care.

Cognition

Crisis workers must always consider the interconnection between affect, behavior, and cognition when working with patients in health crises. It is also necessary to consider disease-related physiological changes. As noted, researchers have begun to document a relationship between coping behaviors and both quality and longevity of life for people with serious chronic illnesses. How people think about their disease and what meaning they attribute to it and to its accompanying life changes are major influences on coping behavior. For example, a diagnosis of cancer may lead to the conclusion "I'm going to die," which can trigger emotional reactions of fear, anger, or hopelessness. The individual may take action in response to his or her thoughts and emotional reactions. Even lack of action is a decisive response to thoughts and feelings. The mental status of the individual and the behavior he or she engages in may, in turn, directly or indirectly affect the physical disease process (e.g., worsen symptoms, precipitate an exacerbation). Cognitions can be considered the fulcrum upon which the cycle of effective or ineffective coping balances.

Some authors have suggested that there are several important aspects of cognitive orientation that affect how an individual copes with a serious illness (Nezu, Nezu, Friedman, Faddis, & Houts, 1998). *Problem perception* refers to the recognition of specific problems as they emerge. For example, an individual may not perceive a job as overly stressful until he or she suffers a complete physical collapse. Problem perception also entails utilizing emotions as cues that a problem exists.

Problem attribution refers to the process of ascribing blame or making attributions regarding the causes of a particular problem. For instance, in the case example, Marco attributed his HIV+ status to his being sinful. Nezu, Nezu, Friedman, Faddis, and Houts (1998) contended that a general style of blaming oneself leads to ineffective problem solving and coping.

Problem appraisal refers to the way individuals evaluate how significant a problem is to them. If an individual views a problem as "the end of my life," emotional distress will inevitably follow. There are two issues of importance related to problem appraisal. One is the importance of addressing the unique or idiosyncratic importance that an individual may attribute to an event. The second relates to the possibility of misjudgments. For example, an individual may misjudge a temporary period of decreased functioning as signaling inevitable and continuing decline.

Personal control beliefs refer to individuals' beliefs about whether they can solve a problem and whether they are capable of coping. The expectancy of coping behavior has a direct effect on actual coping. Each of these cognitive processes directly affects *problem solving* as a coping process, and extensive research suggests that effective problem solving decreases the amount of distress individuals experience in coping with serious illness (Nezu et al., 1998).

Crisis workers must also attempt to understand the patient's premorbid level of cognitive functioning because of the prevalence of cognitive impairments in chronic illnesses due to either progression or treatment of the disease (e.g., dementia, medication, surgery). In specific chronic illnesses, it may be difficult to accurately determine which cognitive effects are due to the physiology of the disease and which are due to the patient's thought patterns and perceptions of the illness.

It is always critical to consider the meaning that patients have attributed to their illness, its impact on their lives, and what core beliefs it may threaten. In health crises the moment of diagnosis often leads to cognitive dissonance, shattering patients' beliefs about life and fairness and their sense of control. Spiritual beliefs also affect the way many people cognitively cope with health crises; counselors must consider patients' spiritual beliefs as a potentially important ongoing support in a patient's life.

Development

It is always important to consider the developmental continuum when responding to patients in health crisis. Different aspects of a disease affect individuals differently as they move though phases of the disease. The impact of the disease as a whole and the specific stage-related changes are mediated by factors such as age of diagnosis, gender, and life-span milestones. For example, a diagnosis of MS might affect a woman who has completed childbearing differently than one who, like Susan, has not yet begun. The diagnosis of MS will also affect males and females differently as it relates to the issue of reproduction.

Developmental coping and adjustment to a chronic illness are also affected by the course of the disease trajectory and what the progression of the disease means to the individual and his or her support network. For example, a diagnosis of cancer in a child has a different impact than the diagnosis of cancer in a seventy-five-year-old man. Similarly, the disease trajectory of PD has significantly different ramifications in the life of a person with early onset than for an older person.

According to Rankin and Weekes (2000), "While many families have the ability to incorporate changes initiated by chronic illness and to accomplish individual and family life-span developmental tasks, others become fixed in their developmental trajectories, and long-term developmental needs are not met" (p. 355).

Ecosystem

Individuals diagnosed with a serious chronic illness are members of families and social support networks and, although it is the individual who is directly affected, families and friends are affected as well. Crisis counselors must assess potential social supports including family, friends, coworkers, and other community resources, as they have a critical impact on the individual's coping and adjustment.

It is also important for crisis workers and patients to collaboratively assess the larger community within which the individual resides. For example, an individual who lives in a small, rural town may have to travel out of his or her geographical region to obtain expert, high-quality medical treatment (e.g., specialists, hospitals). Access to support resources (e.g., support groups for cancer patients) may be unavailable within a small community. Crisis workers can help patients identify potential resources and provide information about how to access them.

There are often real and/or perceived barriers or difficulties within a patient's ecosystem that the counselor must assess. A patient may have concerns about medical insurance coverage for ongoing medical treatment and services. In an era of managed care and restricted health care options, a patient may need help sorting through insurance policies and coverage limitations, which can often be overwhelming and frustrating. Patients and their families may have concerns about depleting their financial resources; the ongoing nature of chronic illness often involves expensive treatment protocols and procedures not covered by health insurance. Similarly, individuals may lack needed transportation or live in an environment that provides limited or no accessibility for people with disabilities.

When crisis counselors identify insurance or financial needs, they can collaborate with patients to develop creative strategies for meeting those needs and provide useful referral information and supportive assistance. For example, one of the authors worked with a wheelchair-bound patient. Living alone, dependent on Social Security disability insurance, and lacking the financial resources to make her home accessible severely restricted her ability to leave her home or even take a shower. She contacted a local home improvement supply store and asked if there was any way they could help her. In response to her request, the store donated both materials and labor to construct a ramp, widen doorways, and build her a wheelchair-accessible shower.

Step 4:
Identify and examine alternative actions and develop options.

Crisis workers help patients examine alternatives in order to cope with their illness. Patients need to engage in effective problem solving to determine what their options are and make decisions about how to address their immediate needs. Crisis workers must keep in mind that priorities and decisions will vary for patients and family members, depending on the phase of the illness and the patient's adjustment to it. For example, a patient in the postoperative phase of breast cancer faces different issues and different alternatives and will make different decisions than an individual in the diagnostic phase. In the postoperative phase, a patient may be facing the stress of meeting with an oncologist (e.g., making decisions about chemotherapy and/or radiation treatments) and alterations in her family and work roles (e.g., inability to care for young children).

The psychosocial problems that the counselor and client identify as causing the immediate distress must be the primary focus in single-session intervention. These problems might include how an individual can continue university course work or who will care for a patient's children while she undergoes surgery. The crisis counselor's tasks include exploring possible alternatives with the patient while continuing to monitor levels of emotional distress that might signal that the patient is becoming overwhelmed and immobilized by the process. The crisis counselor must encourage the patient in crisis to explore a wide range of options, being careful not to impose his or her recommendations about how the patient should proceed.

Step 5:
Help the patient mobilize personal and social resources and connect with community resources.

One important function of the crisis worker is to provide information and access to resources that may help the client with ongoing coping. Because education is a critical aspect of crisis intervention with patients diagnosed with chronic illnesses, this may also include providing information about where to get additional information, for example, referrals to Web sites, books, organizations, or agencies. There are national organizations that collect and distribute information about all of the major diseases discussed here, which can be useful ongoing sources of information. Many local communities also have support groups for individuals afflicted with some of the illnesses discussed here, including cancer support groups and groups for people living with AIDS.

Helping patients mobilize personal resources also entails assisting them to recognize the strengths and skills that they have developed in other areas of life. Belief in one's ability to cope is a primary resource, as it can lead to active problem solving rather than avoidance or being overwhelmed by emotional distress. Helping patients mobilize resources involves motivating them to dig deep into their personal coping reserves in order to meet the challenges they face as the result of illness. It simultaneously involves helping family members focus on meeting the patient's specific needs rather than succumbing to their own fears and anticipatory grief.

Crisis workers may not have the opportunity to meet with a patient again due to the nature of single-session crisis intervention; thus, providing referral information is vital. Crisis workers must be sure to inform patients about their limited role in assisting them in the immediate crisis. As the single-session intervention ends, both patient and crisis worker should have a clear understanding of which follow-up services can be provided by the organization that the worker represents. For example, the crisis worker employed in a hospital setting might refer a patient to an ongoing support group or might follow up by talking to the patient's physician and providing feedback to the patient.

Step 6:
Anticipate the future and arrange follow-up contact.

In single-session intervention with patients in health crisis, anticipating the future does not mean examining the specifics of the disease progression in depth. It does mean assuring that the individual leaves the session with the resources necessary to cope with the immediate issue causing distress. It may also mean gently assuring the individual that although additional challenges will arise in coping with an illness, you believe that he or she has the resilience and resourcefulness to meet those challenges. Assuring individuals that they will not be alone in that process if they utilize sources of support is also helpful. Reaching out for help the first time is a sign of strength and determination, not weakness.

In addition to ensuring that individuals have access to relevant resources that can provide additional assistance, it is helpful to make plans for a follow-up contact with the individual if he or she is receptive. The crisis worker might offer to telephone the patient the next day or might even arrange a return visit for the patient to "touch base" and meet the leader of a support group. It is helpful to communicate that you will be thinking of the patient and would like to know how he or she is doing.

Alternatively, the crisis worker could arrange a follow-up telephone call a week later in order to check on how the patient is doing in following through with selected alternatives. For example, a patient might have agreed to contact his or her physician and be more assertive in asking difficult questions. The crisis worker could make a follow-up call to determine whether the patient was able to talk to the physician and obtain the information he or she was looking for. Continued expressions of interest and concern are valuable, as is a direct offer to be available in the future, if needed. The crisis worker can end a single-session intervention with a statement reassuring the patient that it is normal to periodically feel overwhelmed when facing difficult challenges and emphasizing the importance of reaching out for help at those times.

ONGOING CRISIS COUNSELING FOR PATIENTS WITH A CHRONIC OR TERMINAL ILLNESS

Ongoing crisis counseling can vary depending on the specific nature of an individual's illness, yet there are features common to chronic and terminal illnesses. Certain stressors in patients' lives are also similar despite the differences related to specific chronic illnesses. Similarly, serious illness has a common cascading impact on family members and other significant persons regardless of the specific type of serious illness. Feelings of helplessness and lack of control over life choices routinely arise for patients and their significant others. The shock of diagnosis can lead to denying the existence of the disease due to the gravity of a chronic/terminal illness (Livneh, 2000; Marcus & Bernard, 2000; Ozer, 2000). As a chronic illness progresses, patients and families are confronted with emerging and often complicated issues that can reciprocally influence the nature of psychosocial difficulties and quality of life. Even if a serious illness is not diagnosed as terminal, individuals may experience an underlying and unexpressed concern with death (Marcus & Bernard, 2000).

Crisis counselors must recognize that the onset of a chronic illness always affects more than just the patient's physical being. There is always an emotional response—sometimes expressed, sometimes not expressed—by the patient. Factors such as age, medical history, developmental background, prior ways of coping with crises, and familial patterns of dealing with stress influence the way individuals react to a chronic illness (Marcus & Bernard, 2000). The nature of available support networks and the quality of community and familial interactions also impact the adjustment and coping process. Questions and uncertainty will continue to emerge because treating a chronic illness does not often result in a cure or remission. Medical treatment is often aimed at controlling or delaying the onset of symptoms and the course of the disease. The nature and course of crisis counseling is ultimately driven by multiple factors associated with the illness, the patient, and the patient's ecosystem.

The goals of ongoing crisis counseling are different from the goals of single-session crisis intervention. Achievement of crisis counseling goals with chronically or terminally ill patients mandates an ongoing assessment of functioning within the ABCDE framework, often including family members. Patients and family members may require assistance with *affective* stability, *behavioral* adjustments, *cognitive* mastery, *developmental* continuity, and *ecosystem* utilization.

Crisis workers need to be both sensitive and flexible in their interactions and interventions with patients and families. This can be challenging yet meaningful, given that the overarching goal of crisis counseling is to help patients survive, thrive psychologically, and integrate the chronic or terminal illness into their lives so that they can continue to live the highest possible quality of life.

The Counseling Relationship and Patients with Chronic or Terminal Illnesses

The need to establish a trusting, empathic therapeutic alliance is critical regardless of the therapeutic endeavor. Crisis counseling involves a considerable amount of contact with patients over time, which allows for the development of a therapeutic alliance that should be carefully nurtured. A supportive and empowering counseling relationship is essential for chronically ill patients with ongoing adjustment problems. The crisis counselor enters the biopsychosocial world of the patient and becomes part of a larger ecosystem that includes the patient, the patient's family, the medical team, and the overall community in which the patient resides. Joining with each component of this ecosystem increases the complexity of the counselor's involvement and the amount of time required. Many treatment plans have failed because of lack of attention to developing relationships across the patient's ecosystem.

Preliminary and Ongoing Assessment of Patient Adjustment

Ongoing crisis counseling should focus on a patient's adjustment to his or her illness and the patient's efforts to maintain quality of life. Even if treatment or surgical procedures have controlled or cured the illness (e.g., cancer that is in remission), the potential for recurrence or residual side effects always remains. This uncertainty can continue to generate dissonance for the patient and family members. The lack of predictability makes it difficult for patients to regain the feeling of control over their lives and the disease process, and is often described as "being on an emotional roller coaster" (Williams & Koocher, 1998). The reality is that after a person is diagnosed with a chronic or terminal illness, life will never be the same. A patient of one of the authors referred to his disease as "an unwanted guest at the table who never leaves." A return to life as it was before the diagnosis is impossible, and efforts rooted in denial to recapture a sense of control are doomed to frustration and failure.

This is not to say that a patient should not fight the disease or its effects. Contrary to that notion, crisis counselors can instill a fighting spirit for survival but encourage selectivity regarding the battles to wage. Efforts based on denial only serve to drain valuable psychic and physical energies at a time when they are needed most.

Some patients may experience ongoing suicidal ideation or a tendency to sink into despair that increases the risk of suicide. Crisis counselors must be aware of the particular stresses faced by individuals experiencing chronic illness. For example, many clinicians believe that the suicide rate among chronically ill patients is considerably higher than reported because drug overdoses can be intentionally or unintentionally misperceived as accidents.

The Goals and Processes of Ongoing Crisis Counseling with Chronically or Terminally Ill Patients

Affect stability:
Assist patients to express thoughts and feelings associated with their illness.

The crisis counselor should encourage patients to express their emotions about their illness; however, the counselor should not expect that every person is going to feel the need to emote at every moment. People display their emotions in different ways based upon many factors (i.e., past history, age, gender). Sometimes, patients and family members only want to talk about positive feelings and ideas and do not want to talk about fear, sadness, or anger. Sometimes family members believe that they are being positive for the sake of the patient. Sometimes patients believe that they are being positive for the sake of their families. The unwritten rule in these situations is that expressing negativity will lead to bad things in the future. "If you worry about dying, you'll die sooner." "If you get upset, your tumor will grow faster." Some authors have described this phenomenon as becoming "prisoners of positive thinking." If anything, what we know from repeated studies is that the expression of emotions (even negative ones) not only results in a positive psychological outlook but also appears to be related to longevity (Fawzy, Cousins, Fawzy, Kemeny, Elashoff, & Morton, 1990; Spiegel, Bloom, Kraemer, & Gottheil, 1989).

Processing memories and associated emotional responses in the context of a patient's health crisis usually occurs when a patient and his or her family are anticipating the patient's death. Reminiscing about the past can be helpful in validating good experiences of the past but also in allowing the patient and family members to come to terms with unfinished business that they may want to bring to a close before the patient dies.

Behavioral adjustments:
Assist patients to make and sustain necessary behavioral changes.

The patient with a chronic or terminal illness may have to comply with medical recommendations that involve cessation of behaviors that are dangerous to his or her health (e.g., a lung cancer patient may have to stop smoking, a patient may have to stop drinking because of the interaction of prescribed medications and alcohol). At the same time, the patient may be encouraged to engage in behaviors to promote health (e.g., exercise, nutritious diet, yoga). Crisis counseling can help patients manage these lifestyle behaviors that are frequently difficult to change.

The lives of chronically or terminally ill patients revolve around their illness. Their contact with medical facilities and staff may have increased to the point where they feel that their job has become being a compliant patient. Patience with the process of ongoing medical treatment is essential if the person is not going to succumb to the illness and its effects. Crisis counseling can help patients become actively rather than passively involved in their medical care. The crisis worker can encourage the patient to function as the treatment "team leader" as a means of coping and maintaining control of what otherwise often feels like an out-of-control process.

Cognitive mastery:
Assist patients to examine and reformulate beliefs about themselves and their illness as well as beliefs and personal meanings that have been threatened by the illness.

The nature of the illness and disease trajectory can trigger existential questions and doubts for patients about themselves, others, spirituality, and so on. For family members, trying to make sense of the chronic illness as it affects the life of a loved one, coupled with the long-term implications of care giving and disruptions in family members' lives, creates emotional distress.

For example, cancer becomes a family issue, as normal family functioning is disrupted during the health crisis. Each family member has different needs and may react differently along the disease trajectory. Ongoing crisis counseling must address family members' responses to the cancer (e.g., fear of death, helplessness, shifts in individual roles). The crisis worker's assessment must include how the patient and each family member is reacting and coping with the disruptions in the familial and social system. The meaning of the cancer will be different for each member of the family (e.g., patient, partner, parent, children), with the nature of the emotional, behavioral, and cognitive responses depending on the phase of the illness (e.g., moment of diagnosis, postoperative phase) and the nature of the disease progression (e.g., remission, recurrence/metastasis, terminal).

For example, in the terminal phase of cancer, crisis counselors need to help the patient and/or family members cope with anticipatory grief and end-of-life decision-making processes. A spouse may begin to emotionally withdraw from his wife as a way of dealing with the reality of her impending death. His difficulty in accepting that his wife is going to die affects his ability to let go and say good-bye. Grief is a unique process for each individual in the family. The crisis counselor may need to intervene with other family members as well. In the case of the husband withdrawing from his wife, crisis counseling can help him deal with his grief and loss responses and find a way to accept his wife's impending death both for his own well-being and so he is able to better meet his wife's needs.

Coping with a chronic or terminal illness also triggers issues related to spirituality or religion for many clients and families. Holt et al. (1999) examined the counseling issues surrounding spiritual wellness with HIV+ clients and their families, finding that spiritual issues are critical to examine as individuals struggle to integrate the diagnosis into their lives. The existential issues may become even more complex in cases of terminal illnesses, when patients have to integrate their impending mortality. According to Yalom (1980), terminally ill clients may need to examine three vital issues: (1) fear of death, (2) the need for hope, and (3) creation of life meaning.

In the process of examining and reframing core beliefs, expectations, and personal meanings, crisis workers must assess the relevance of spirituality and religion in the life of the patient and in the process of coping with the chronic or terminal illness. Being diagnosed with a chronic or terminal illness often leads to an ongoing examination of spiritual and personal connections and reconnections in the individual, familial, and cultural contexts of clients. The crisis worker may be able to utilize clients' religious and spiritual connections as a useful coping tool in health crises.

Developmental mastery:
Assist patients to examine the impact of their illness on their ongoing development.

Crisis workers must be cognizant of the developmental implications of a health crisis in the lives of patients. Chronic and terminal illnesses disrupt the lives of patients and their support networks (e.g., partners, parents, children, siblings, friends) permanently, often dramatically altering normal individual and family life passages. For example, chronic illness may precipitate increased involvement of family members and others in the lives of patients who need care or who have impairments that affect their functioning. Grown children may become dependent on their parents again, seemingly in the prime of their lives. They may find themselves prematurely requiring the care of others.

Crisis workers must help patients and family members explore and find ways to cope effectively with this developmental impact. An important goal is to assist patients and families to find ways to live and grow as much as possible in developmentally expected ways, despite the changes precipitated by illness. When a family member is diagnosed with a chronic illness, a framework that links life-span development theory to family developmental changes can be useful in ongoing assessment and intervention.

Life-span development and families   Rankin and Weekes (2000) proposed four life-span development themes in working with chronically ill individuals and their family members. The first theme is that "conjoint occurrence of a major illness with a major life transition is positively related to loss of individual and family coherence and adaptability" (p. 366). The case of Dianna discussed in the illustration of PD earlier in this chapter can be understood in this context. A young woman, thirty-two years old, is likely to have more difficulty adapting to the diagnosis of Parkinson's disease because of expected developmental transitions affected by the early onset of a disease normally diagnosed in older adults.

The second is that "the greater the concurrence between the social environment of the family and the developmental needs of its members, the better is the adaptation to the onset of a non-normative event such as chronic illness" (p. 367). Both the patient and the family must continue to master developmental milestones and tasks in spite of the illness. Consider a twenty-year-old college sophomore diagnosed with cancer whose parents begin to make all of the treatment decisions for him without his consent. A young adult male of twenty is usually grappling with relationship issues and career goals and, by sophomore year in college, he has defined himself as a separate individual requiring little parental guidance or control. Similarly, his parents are at a point in their lives as adults when they have their own developmental needs. Most of the time, neither the patient nor family members want to do anything that would be a burden to others in the family system. A system that can allow its members to nurture each other yet still pursue their own lives is healthy and can rise to the occasion even in times of increasing demands.

The third theme proposed by Rankin and Weekes is that "in middle-aged families with adolescents where a member has a chronic illness, decreased family unity and cohesiveness affect achievement of family and individual developmental tasks" (p. 368). For example, in a family in which the mother is diagnosed with breast cancer, there may be changes in roles, as an adolescent daughter assumes caretaking responsibilities for her mother. The needs of the healthy children or family members may be forgotten or ignored, which can often disrupt normative developmental tasks and milestones for individual family members. Care must be taken to nurture cohesion through the continuation of family-centered activities.

The final theme in the model is that "the older the family, the less is the disequilibrium caused by illness of a member" (p. 369). An older family has achieved more developmental milestones than a younger family, so family members may not have the same perception of being cheated of time and pleasure. Thus, it may be easier for a family to accept an older adult being diagnosed with a serious illness than a young child or adolescent.

Realistically, crisis counseling must assist individuals with chronic illnesses to both identify and take action to attain those developmental milestones that are important to them and achievable. This might mean identifying a creative support system and/or accommodations so that an individual can continue to work or helping individuals accept the fact that tasks may take more time to accomplish. Crisis counseling must also assist families to provide needed support to the patient, but also recognize that family members will sometimes stumble, fall, and pick themselves back up.

Ecosystem healthy and intact: Assist patients to make changes in personal ecosystems in order to reestablish connection and community.

Relationship and lifestyle changes are inevitable for patients and their family members. Sometimes these changes result in difficult but necessary role reversals, at least during times when the patient is incapacitated (e.g., a partner who must return to the work force in order to obtain health insurance for the family). The patient may no longer be able to fulfill responsibilities that are necessary for family functioning, which may necessitate reassignment of responsibilities or alternative means of fulfilling responsibilities (e.g., visiting nurses) that have systemic ripple effects. Such changes can be difficult to accept. For example, some individuals are uncomfortable with the thought of having a stranger in their home.

Crisis counseling with patients and their families helps patients make connections with various resources and overcome the personal barriers that might otherwise impede their ability to utilize available formal supports. Counselors can also encourage patients and loved ones to become involved in support groups. Research in living with chronic illnesses suggests that psychosocial support can be a critical factor in moderating the effects of life stressors (Spiegel & Diamond, 1988). Members of a support group are all experiencing the same challenges. Support groups can mediate the potential for denial and social isolation that may occur either initially upon diagnosis or as the disease progression results in physical changes that threaten or shatter one's self-image. They can also provide opportunities for sharing and support to family caregivers.

Crisis counseling should also attempt to link patients to other community groups that can be additional sources of support and information and also provide a sense of meaning and accomplishment. For example, cancer survivors may become involved in fundraising events to raise money for ongoing research or in grass-roots efforts to improve the quality of life for cancer patients.

PERSONAL RESPONSES TO HEALTH CRISES

Health crises present unique and common challenges for crisis counselors in both single-session crisis intervention and ongoing crisis counseling. As crisis counselors, our first reaction to working with health crises begins before we interact with the first patient. Our own feelings about serious illness, our own personal experiences with illness, and our own cultural socialization can have a major impact on how we perceive our role in working with sick people. When confronted with our first crisis involving a chronically or terminally ill patient, all of these influences rush to the foreground as we grapple with our own responses.

Bonde (2001) examined the impact of clinician loss and grief dynamics in working with people who are HIV+ or living with AIDS. Confronting the losses associated with chronic illness and impending death in cases of terminal illness may trigger thoughts of one's own mortality. It may also force crisis workers to grieve the loss or impending death of their clients. According to Bonde (2001), ethically it is important for clinicians to acknowledge the losses and personal impact of the grief process. Crisis workers must be able to identify their own symptoms of loss and grief so that they can take active steps to prevent or handle burnout. Suggestions for crisis counselors include seeking the support of coworkers, actively seeking supervision or additional training, and taking care of oneself even if it means taking a break from working with clients coping with chronic and/or terminal illness.

It is also important to dispel the common misunderstanding among professionals new to working with seriously ill patients that crisis counseling primarily consists of existential discussions about life, death, meaning, and purpose. Of course, one can interpret anything through an existential lens, but the reality of most work with chronically and terminally ill patients and their ecosystems is far removed from this vision. Seriously ill patients have surgeries and invasive procedures. They experience times of great joy and great sorrow. Their lives are different from the moment of diagnosis onwards. But after patients have been diagnosed with a chronic illness, or even a terminal illness, they still have to live. The amount of time they have left to live may be truncated, but they continue living to the moment they die.

The point is that not all crisis counseling is focused on life and death issues. Many of the issues that patients and family members raise have to do with normal relationship concerns and other everyday concerns. The diagnosis of a chronic or terminal disease may precipitate at least four types of systemic responses: emergence of problems in response to the diagnosis, exacerbation of problems already in existence prior to the diagnosis, resolution of problems in existence prior to the diagnosis, or no change at all. Obviously, the systemic influences that crisis counselors encounter most often in the lives of people who seek crisis counseling are those involving the emergence or exacerbation of problems. Further, the crises faced by patients with chronic or terminal illnesses and their families may be similar to crises encountered in the general healthy population. A patient's illness affects these problems in a unique way, but the problems and crises are the problems and crises of living, not just of dying or struggling with disease.

CASE EXAMPLE: JANE

Single-Session Crisis Intervention

Jane has recently been diagnosed with breast cancer and has had a lumpectomy. Her surgeon referred her to an oncologist. While meeting with him, she began to feel distressed. When Jane agreed to speak to the crisis counselor, the oncologist called him and asked him to join them in his office. After introducing Jane and the counselor and saying a few words about Jane's medical condition, he left the room. The counselor escorted Jane down the hall to his office and offered her a seat. After explaining his role at the clinic, he began to engage Jane, empathizing with her obvious distress.

CW: *It looks as if you've been having a pretty hard time dealing with all this. How are you doing now?*

Jane: I guess that I'm OK. *(looking down at the floor)* That meeting with Dr. Greenberg . . . it was just too much . . . that *(voice trailing off, tears welling up again)* I don't know.

CW: *It must have been a difficult journey getting to this point.*

Jane: Yeah, it has been. It felt weird coming into this office today. Because you see all of these people, you wonder what is going on with all of them. Some people look really ill . . . and I don't want to be here.

CW: *I know a little bit about your illness from what Dr. Greenberg said, but can you tell me in your own words what you know?*

Jane: Well *(pauses and swallows)*, well, a few months ago, I felt a lump in my left breast. And I do the exams pretty regularly. I have the yearly appointments. I do my Pap smears. I am pretty healthy. I don't smoke; I don't drink excessively. I don't know why this happened to me *(shaking her head, tears welling up again)*. But I found this lump and I didn't go to the doctor right away. I was busy and I let it go and then I finally went to my family doctor. She recommended that I get a mammogram. That was just a few weeks ago. I got the mammogram and then she was concerned about the mammogram. They had me contact a surgeon, who did a needle biopsy of the lump and also of *(sighs)* some lymph glands. The biopsy came back malignant; the lump from the breast was malignant. The lymph gland was OK. And then I had a lumpectomy.

CW: *And the surgeon recommended that you see an oncologist, that you see Dr. Greenberg?*

Jane: Yes. I had the lumpectomy a week and a half ago. They recommended that I come see Dr. Greenberg. I guess what you are supposed to do is have chemotherapy, and they recommended radiation, too *(stated in a low, matter-of-fact tone)*. Dr. Greenberg wanted to start *(chokes back tears)* . . . he wanted to start today.

CW:: *It sounds like it's been a bit of a roller coaster ride so far and now you have to make some more treatment decisions on top of it all.*

Jane: Yeah, I'm not sure. . . . I'm not sure what I'm feeling.

CW: *I hear a lot of feelings as you're telling me about what's been happening to you so far.*

Jane: I just wanted it not to be. Part of me knew that I should have gone to see the doctor. I have a two-year-old. A stepmother who is dying of cancer. I've only been married five years at this point. I just can't believe that this is happening to me! *(begins sobbing quietly for a few seconds)*

The crisis worker was silent and allowed Jane some space to express her emotions. As she regained composure he spent a few minutes talking with Jane about her family's reactions. Her father and stepmother live in town, and she has one sister who also lives close by. Another sister lives out of state. As she spoke, the crisis worker began to get a sense of who were the possible supports in Jane's life and how they were responding so far.

CW: *So it's your older sister who's here with you today?*

Jane: Yes, my sister Susan. She's been great. She offered to come with me today. She's out in the waiting room right now. My husband is working *(pauses)* and my son is in day care.

CW: *How is your husband handling what's happening?*

Jane: Well he is. . . . Phil just says that we will get through this. He is being supportive. Being positive. He keeps . . . *(voice trails off)*. I'm not sure how he's dealing with it, to tell you the truth. But it seems like he wants me to keep going. He wants me to do all of this. He hasn't been upset, not crying or anything like that. He is trying to be upbeat, I think. Just carrying on as if everything is just normal.

CW: *Jane, you have been going through a lot in the past few weeks. From the moment that you found the lump to right now. Things have been happening quickly for you and you're faced today with making some decisions . . . at a time, I imagine, when it feels as if your world could fall apart under the pressure. What are you doing to take care of yourself?*

Jane: I have always taken care of myself. *(voice quivering with emotion and tears in her eyes)* That's one of the things that bothers me about this. . . . I have done everything. My stepmother has cancer but she is not a blood relative to me.

CW: *Feels pretty unfair that this is happening to you right now.*

Jane: Yeah, I guess. I've got mixed feelings. I'm angry because I did everything right. I exercise, I eat right, take care of myself. But at the same, I don't know how this could have happened!

CW: *I'm glad you're here, talking to me right now. When you make big decisions, it's natural to question things as you begin to try and make sense of what's happening. It's an important part of making decisions like the one you're trying to make right now. And it seems as though you're making it alone.*

Jane: Everyone in my family is walking on eggshells around me. No one is mentioning the C word. I don't know . . . it's all screwed up.

CW: *Do you want to talk about it with them?*

Jane: I do want to talk to them about it *(pauses and swallows)*, but I don't want to burden anyone, bum anyone out with my problems. I don't want people treating me differently, because of the diagnosis. It's there, I have cancer. *(tone of resentment in her voice)*

CW: *In many ways, cancer is a family illness. It affects members of a family, often in different ways. What does it mean for you to say you have cancer, and know it's true?*

Jane: I'm worried. I have a two-year-old little boy. I don't want to be pessimistic.

CW: *It's hard not to be pessimistic when you're feeling so much. It's overwhelming. Plus, it's hard not to look at cancer as the "Big C." You probably grew up with that idea because everyone else around you saw it that way, too. Cancer used to be viewed as a one-way ticket out of here instead of as a chronic illness. You've already been through some pretty big challenges—you've experienced the diagnosis of cancer and you've been through the surgery. But now there's more, because Dr. Greenberg is recommending chemotherapy followed by a series of radiation treatments. And you're not sure what to do.*

Jane: I know what I have to do. I hate being nauseated, and I am afraid of the chemo and being nauseated. I know that I am going to lose my hair—I just know it, and I am not sure how to deal with that. I'm not sure about a lot of different things. I don't know how it's going to affect my relationship with my husband, my relationship with my son, my family, everybody.

CW: *There's a lot of uncertainty about the effect this is going to have on you and your family. Unfortunately you can't answer all those questions in advance. What you can try to figure out, though, is whether you want to start chemo—today, later, or not at all.*

Jane: Yeah. Dr. Greenberg wants me to go to the chemo rooms so the nurses can start it today. I don't know what I was thinking, but I was not ready to start it today. On the other hand, if the cancer is in my body right now, I want to get rid of it—now *(said with determination)*.

CW: *Even though it is not easy for you, it sounds as though you know what you have to do.*

Jane: I know . . . I know. I just wasn't ready. Dr. Greenberg told me there are medications to help me with the side effects and . . . but it's so strange to think that I am going to start this treatment, that I am a cancer patient, and having cancer is what drives my life right now.

CW: *The cancer has changed a lot in your life. You don't have to deal with all of it right now. People deal with cancer differently. How you do it will be your way. The steps you take to manage the whole process are yours to take. You're in charge.*

Jane: I have to do what I have to do right now. I don't really want to, but I know that I have to do it because I'm not going to let the cancer beat me. I've got too much to live for. Do you think my sister can come back into the chemo room with me?

CW: *Absolutely. You'll see lots of family and friends in the chemo room. And that will give you and Susan a chance to break the "don't talk about the cancer" rule (smiles).*

Jane: Will you be there as well?

CW: *You bet. I'll be dropping in to see you each time you come for treatment. And if you like, we can talk again. In fact, what do you say we set up an appointment for some time next week before your next treatment? I want to keep close contact with you, especially until you get a little more used to this whole process. And if you'd like to bring you husband along, it might help you both to have him with you.*

Jane: OK. I think I would like that. It is good to be able to finally talk about the cancer with someone who is not walking on eggshells around me.

CW: *Good. And let's try to get rid of some of those eggshells. We'll pick up your sister on our way back to the treatment room and we can bring her up to speed on what's happening. How does that sound?*

Jane: OK. . . . Yes, I guess I am as ready as I can be right now.

The crisis counselor escorts Jane out to the waiting room, where he is introduced to Jane's sister, Susan. After speaking for a few moments about Jane's decision to start her chemotherapy, he contacts the nurse from the chemo room and introduces both Jane and Susan.

In this short exchange the crisis worker established a beginning relationship, helped Jane express some of her thoughts and feelings about what she's been going through since being diagnosed, and helped her focus on the immediate decision that she was facing—whether to start chemotherapy. He assessed that Jane was a resourceful and determined young woman, but also that, so far, she seemed to be mostly going it alone. She had managed so far, but the reality of beginning chemotherapy was too much for her and she fell apart.

It was clear to the crisis worker that Jane needed to be able to rely on her family for support and needed to be able to talk about what she was experiencing. He also assessed that some of her family members, especially her husband, may need help in facing her condition and in being there with her. He gently suggested ways of bringing both Susan and Jane's husband, Phil, into the foreground of her support system. Knowing that this was just the beginning of what could be a tough couple of months while she received chemotherapy, he also arranged a follow-up appointment. He also followed up that same day, checking in to see Jane before her treatment was over. At that time she was composed and able to smile and even laugh as the crisis worker lightly joked with her, her sister, and the nurse.

This was not an atypical intervention in a busy oncology practice. Patients may experience momentary or ongoing crisis responses that interfere with their ability to cope with the medical decisions and treatments they face. Crisis intervention, when the counselor is part of the medical team, assists patients, but it also enhances the overall delivery of medical services.

EXERCISES

1. Empirical studies have consistently validated the role of supportive expressive therapies in facilitating psychological adjustment to illness. Yet many patients become "prisoners of positive thinking" and believe that any negative thoughts or emotions will worsen their illness. Engage in a role-playing activity with a fellow student in which you provide crisis counseling to a patient who is resistant to discussing any thoughts or feelings that are not optimistic or positive. Alternate roles after ten minutes.

2. After a series of invasive examinations and medical procedures, you are informed by your treating physician that you have a terminal illness and a life expectancy of six months to two years. Reflect on how you would spend your remaining days, and share your plans with a small group of classmates.

DISCUSSION QUESTIONS

1. Select a chronic or terminal illness not discussed in this chapter and identify the symptoms, underlying pathophysiology, and stages of the illness. Discuss the specific emotional reactions that a patient might experience over the course of the illness. Compare and contrast these reactions to those experienced by patients with other chronic or terminal illnesses.

2. Discuss the role of the crisis counselor in multidisciplinary medical settings. How would you explain your role to other medical professionals? How would you explain your role to patients and their families?

REFERENCES

Allen, D. N., Landis, R. K. B., & Schramke, C. J. (1995). The role of psychologists in the treatment of multiple sclerosis. *International Journal of Rehabilitation and Health, 1*(2), 97–123.

American Diabetes Association. (2003). *Basic diabetes information.* Retrieved from http://www.diabetes.org/info/diabetesinfo.jsp

American Heart Association. (2002). *Heart and stroke statistical update.* Dallas, TX: Author.

Anderson, P. B., Ellenberg, J. H., Leventhal, C. M., Reingold, S. C., Rodriguez, M., & Silberberg, D. H. (1992). Revised estimate of the prevalence of multiple sclerosis in the United States. *Annals of Neurology, 31,* 333–336.

Betancourt, H., & Fuentes, J. L. (2001). Culture and Latino issues in health psychology. In S. S. Kazarian & D. R. Evans (Eds.), *Handbook of cultural health psychology* (pp. 305–321). London, ON, Canada: Academic Press.

Bonde, L. (2001). The effects of grief and loss on decision making in HIV-related psychotherapy. In J. R. Anderson and R. L. Barret (Eds.), *Clinical decision making in complex cases* (pp. 83–98). Washington, DC: American Psychological Association.

Brown, G. G., Rahill, A. A., Gorell, J. M., McDonald, C., Brown, S. J., Sillanpaa, M., & Shults, C. (1999). Validity of the dementia rating scale in assessing cognitive function in Parkinson's disease. *Journal of Geriatric Psychiatry and Neurology, 12,* 180–188.

Chazin, R., Kaplan, S., & Terio, S. (2000). The strengths perspective in brief treatment with culturally diverse clients. *Crisis Intervention and Time Limited Treatment, 6,* 41–50.

Collins, T. M., Barrow, R. A., & Haupt, C. H. (1999, April 15). *The professional counselor in outpatient medical oncology.* Presented at the World Conference of the American Counseling Association, San Diego, CA.

Collins, T. M., Greenwald, C. S., & Greenwald, D. W. (1998, February 8). *Psychosocial intervention in outpatient medical oncology.* Presented at the Midwinter Convention of the American Psychological Association, Divisions of Psychotherapy, Family Psychology, and Independent Practice, La Jolla, CA.

Dreisig, H., Beckmann, J., Wermuth, L., Skovlund, S., & Bech, P. (1999). Psychologic effects of structured cognitive psychotherapy in young patients with Parkinson disease: A pilot study. *Nordic Journal of Psychiatry, 53*(3), 217–221.

Duvoisin, R. C. (1991). *Parkinson's disease: A guide for patient and family* (3rd ed.). New York: Raven Press.

Elia, N. (1997). Grief and loss in HIV/AIDS work. In M. G. Winiarski (Ed.), *HIV mental health for the 21st century* (pp. 67–81). New York: New York University Press.

Fawzy, F. I., Canada, A. L., & Fawzy, N. W. (2003). Malignant melanoma: Effects of a brief structured psychiatric intervention on survival and recurrence at 10-year follow-up. *Archives of General Psychiatry, 60,* 100–103.

Fawzy, F. I., Cousins, N., Fawzy, N., Kemeny, M., Elashoff, R., & Morton, D. (1990). A structured psychiatric intervention for cancer patients: Changes over time in methods of coping and affective disturbance. *Archives of General Psychiatry, 47,* 720–725.

Fawzy, F. I., Fawzy, N. W., Hyun, C. S., Elashoff, R., Guthrie, D., Fahey, J. L., & Morton, D. (1993). Malignant melanoma: Effects of an early structured psychiatric intervention, coping, and affective state on recurrence and survival 6 years later. *Archives of General Psychiatry, 50,* 681–689.

Flaskerud, J. H. (1995). Psychosocial and psychiatric aspects. In J. H. Flaskerud & P. J. Ungvarski (Eds.), *HIV/AIDS: A guide to nursing care* (3rd ed., pp. 308–338). Philadelphia: Saunders.

Garrett, C., & Weisman, M. G. (2001). A self-psychological perspective on chronic illness. *Clinical Social Work Journal, 29*(2), 119–132.

Goodheart, C. D., Marganoff, P., & Ricketts, K. S. (1997). Integrated disease management: Psychology and medicine. *Behavioral Health Management, 17*(4), 16–21.

Higgins, T. (2002). *Brittle diabetes mellitus.* Retrieved October 22, 2002, from http://www.bouldermedicalcenter.com/Articles/brittle_diabetes_mellitus.htm

Holland, J., & Rowland, J. (Eds.). (1990). *Handbook of psycho oncology: Psychological care of the patient with cancer.* Newark, NJ: Oxford University Press.

Holland, J. C., & Tross, S. (1985). The psychosocial and neuropsychiatric sequelae of the acquired immunodeficiency syndrome and related disorders. *Annals of Internal Medicine, 103,* 760–764.

Holt, J. L., Houg, B. L., & Romano, J. L. (1999). Spiritual wellness for clients with HIV/ AIDS: Review of counseling issues. *Journal of Counseling and Development, 77*(2), 160–170.

Hoskins, C. N., & Haber, J. (2000). Adjusting to breast cancer. *American Journal of Nursing, 100,* 26–33.

Krupp, L. B. (2000). Management of persons with multiple sclerosis. In M. N. Ozer (Ed.), *Management of persons with chronic neurologic illness* (pp. 199–212). Boston: Butterworth Heinemann.

Kubler-Ross, E. (1969). *On death and dying.* New York: Macmillan.

Livneh, H. (2000). Psychosocial adaptation to cancer: The role of coping strategies. *Journal of Rehabilitation, 66*(2), 40–49.

Marcus, M., & Bernard, H. S. (2000). Group psychotherapy for psychological traumata of prolonged, severe, and/or terminal illness. In R. H. Klein & V. L. Schermer (Eds.), *Group psychotherapy for psychological trauma* (pp. 188–208). New York: Guilford Press.

Markowitz, J. C., Spielman, L. A., Sullivan, M., & Fishman, B. (2000). An exploratory study of ethnicity and psychotherapy outcome among HIV-positive patients with depressive symptoms. *Journal of Psychotherapy Practice Research, 9*(4), 226–231.

Mohr, D. C., Boudewyn, A. C., Goodkin, D. E., Bostrom, A., Epstein, L. (2001). Comparative outcomes for individual cognitive-behavior therapy, supportive-expressive group psychotherapy, and sertraline for the treatment of depression in multiple sclerosis. *Journal of Consulting and Clinical Psychology, 69*(6), 942–949.

Mohr, D. C., & Cox, D. (2001). Multiple sclerosis: Empirical literature for the clinical health psychologist. *Journal of Clinical Psychology, 57*(4), 479–499.

Mohr, D. C., & Dick, L. P. (1998). Multiple sclerosis. In P. M. Camic and S. J. Knight (Eds.), *Clinical handbook of health psychology: A practical guide to effective interventions* (pp. 313–348). Kirkland, WA: Hogrefe & Huber.

Mullins, L. L., Cote, M. P., Fuemmeler, B. F., Jean, V. M., Beatty, W. W., & Paul, R. H. (2001). Illness intrusiveness, uncertainty, and distress in individuals with multiple sclerosis. *Rehabilitation Psychology, 46*(2), 139–153.

National Cancer Institute. (2002). Surveillance, epidemiology, and end results (SEER) program publication. *SEER Cancer Statistics Review, 1973–1999.* Retrieved October 22, 2002, from http://cis.nci.nih.gov/fact

Nelson, W. L. (1998). Human immunodeficiency virus infection and acquired immunodeficiency syndrome. In P. M. Camic and S. J. Knight (Eds.), *Clinical handbook of health psychology: A practical guide to effective interventions* (pp. 271–312). Kirkland, WA: Hogrefe & Huber.

Nezu, A. M., Kalmar, K., Ronan, G. F., & Clavijo, A. (1986). Attributional correlates of depression: An interactional model including problem solving. *Behavior Therapy, 17,* 50–56.

Nezu, A. M., Nezu, C. M., Friedman, S. H., Faddis, S., & Houts, P. S. (1998). *Helping cancer patients cope: A problem-solving approach.* Washington, DC: American Psychological Association.

Ozer, M. N. (Ed.). (2000). *Management of persons with chronic neurologic illness.* Boston: Butterworth Heinemann.

Pincus, J. H. (2000). Management of persons with Parkinson's disease. In M. N. Ozer (Ed.), *Management of persons with chronic neurologic illness* (pp. 213–236). Boston: Butterworth Heinemann.

Rankin, S. H., & Weekes, D. P. (2000). Life-span development: A review of theory and practice for families with chronically ill members. *Scholarly Inquiry for Nursing Practice: An International Journal, 14*(4), 355–373.

Rokach, A. (2000). Terminal illness and coping with loneliness. *The Journal of Psychology, 134*(3), 283–296.

Spiegel, D., Bloom, J. R., Kraemer, H. C., & Gottheil, E. (1989). Effects of psychosocial treatment on survival patients with metastatic breast cancer. *The Lancet, 2,* 888–891.

Spiegel, D., & Diamond, D. (1988). Psychosocial interventions in cancer: Group therapy techniques. In S. Taylor and G. Dakof (Eds.), *Social support and the cancer patient* (pp. 215–233). Newbury Park, CA: Sage.

Thompson, S. C., & Collins, M. A. (1995). Applications of perceived control to cancer: An overview of theory and measurement. *Journal of Psychosocial Oncology, 13,* 11–26.

Williams, J., & Koocher, G. P. (1998). Addressing loss of control in chronic illness: Theory and practice. *Psychotherapy, 35*(3), 325–335.

Wilson, I. B., & Cleary, P. D. (1995). Linking clinical variables with health-related quality of life: A conceptual model of patient outcomes. *Journal of the American Medical Association, 273,* 59–65.

Yalom, I. D. (1980). *Existential psychotherapy.* New York: Basic Books.

CHAPTER 10

The Crisis of Death

JOHN W. KRAYBILL-GREGGO
MARCELLA J. KRAYBILL-GREGGO
THOMAS M. COLLINS

No one ever told me that grief felt so like fear. I am not afraid, but the sensation is like being afraid. The same fluttering in the stomach, the same restlessness, the yawning, I keep swallowing. At other times it feels like being mildly drunk, or concussed. There is sort of an invisible blanket between the world and me. I find it hard to take in what anyone says. Or perhaps, hard to want to take it in . . . yet I want [the] others to be about me. I dread the moments when the house is empty. If only they would talk to one another and not to me. There are moments, most unexpectedly, when something inside me tries to assure me that I don't really mind so much. . . . Love is not the whole of a man's life. . . . I've plenty of what are called "resources." People get over these things. Come, I shan't do so badly. One is ashamed to listen to this voice but it seems for a little to be making out a good case. Then comes a red-hot memory and all this "commonsense" vanishes like an ant in the mouth of a furnace. On the rebound, one passes into tears and pathos . . . and no one ever told me about the laziness of grief. Except at my job . . . I loathe the slightest effort. Not only writing but reading a letter is too much. Even shaving. What does it matter now if my cheek is rough or smooth?

C. S. Lewis (1961) *in* A Grief Observed

• • •

Dave's eldest son, James, who was six years old, was pinned against a tree outside the family home by a car that rolled backward in their driveway. James and his younger brother were playing in the car when the car began to move. Dave ran outside when he heard his youngest son screaming and moved the car, freeing James. The ambulance arrived and transported James and Dave to the hospital emergency room. On the way to the hospital, James died.

• • •

Marlene's husband of ten years died in an industrial accident, leaving her with two young sons (ages five and seven) and no viable means of support. When she was going through his personal effects, she discovered letters from a woman with whom he was apparently having an affair.

The study of death and human responses to death has preoccupied scholars of many disciplines for centuries. Words and phrases like *bereavement, grief,* and *mourning* have become part of our everyday language. More and more families have utilized hospice services, where the terminally ill receive care focused on pain management and quality of life rather than invasive medical procedures to prolong life in the final stages of their illness. Also, many individuals have established living wills and advanced directives so that if or when they become seriously or terminally ill their stated wishes about the type of care they receive will be respected by the medical community. According to the most recent National Vital Statistics Report (Centers for Disease Control, 2001), in the previous year, 97,860 individuals were killed in various types of accidents, 725,192 individuals died from heart disease, 549,838 individuals died from cancer, and 167,366 individuals died from strokes. Additionally, 29,199 died as a result of suicide attempts and 16,889 individuals were victims of homicide.

One might assume that given the pervasiveness of death in our lives people would have become adept at adjusting to death. The reality is that despite the prevalence of death, its occurrence causes tremendous disruption in our lives. Social scientists have studied our reactions to death and tried to discern patterns of behavior in human responses to death, but the range of responses is quite variable and the uniqueness of individual responses depends upon many factors. In this chapter, we identify the commonalities of reactions to the death experience, examine the factors that contextualize and affect this experience, and describe interventions with individuals experiencing crises related to loss and grief. Although loss is a concept and grief is a process that can be used to understand many other crisis events, including divorce, our attention here focuses solely on loss and grief precipitated by death.

DEFINITIONS OF TERMS

Bereavement refers to the loss of a loved one by death. Most definitions of bereavement refer to the state of having suffered a significant loss (Cook & Dworkin, 1992; Rando, 1984, 2000).

Grief is the deep and personal distress caused by bereavement. Rando (1984) defined grief as "the process of psychological, social, and somatic reactions to the perception of loss" (p. 15). In her seminal work on grief and death, Rando implied that grief was a natural adjustment to the loss experience that can pervasively influence our thinking, our interactions with others around us, and our bodies. Key to understanding grief is the recognition that there are many types of losses: death-related losses, loss of physical health, loss of relationships through separation and divorce, loss of employment, and abandonment by caregivers. Many experiences in life can be best understood from a loss perspective. Wolfelt (1992) viewed grief as the "composite of thoughts and feelings about a loss that you experience within yourself," or "the internal meaning given to the experience of bereavement" (p. 8). For the purposes of this chapter, *grief crisis counseling* will be limited to those reactions associated with loss from death.

Mourning refers to the expression of grief and sorrow, often by engaging in a culturally defined mourning practice. Rando (1984), building on Bowlby's (1980) definition of mourning as an intrapsychic process precipitated by loss and her own view of mourning as the "cultural response to grief," used *mourning* interchangeably with *grief*. Mourning, according to Wolfelt (1992, p. 8), is "when you take the grief on the inside and express it outside of yourself," or, in other words, "grief gone public."

It is important to recognize that bereavement and corresponding grief and mourning are considered to be normal in most cultures around the world. The way grief is expressed, however, depends on the cultural context. For example, a common employee benefit in the United States is funeral leave for the death of a close relative (e.g., parent, spouse, child). Usually, this benefit extends to five days of leave from one's place of employment. The inherent reasoning is that in this time the bereaved individual should be able to achieve a sufficient level of adjustment to return to work—a clear cultural expectation of how much time people need to return to a satisfactory premorbid level of functioning.

Uncomplicated grief is just that: grief that is expressed with no extenuating circumstances that might preclude a person's ability to mourn. If a ninety-two-year-old grandmother dies of congestive heart failure after a long stay in a health care facility, family members may grieve her death but also may find solace in reflecting on the richness and longevity of her life. By contrast, if a family member is murdered in the course of a robbery, surviving family members may have a much more difficult time accepting the loss. The circumstances of the death can weigh heavily on the minds of surviving family members and interfere with their ability to integrate the death experience.

The example of a murdered family member cited above may result in a *complicated* grief response. Rando (1993, 1996) identified seven high-risk factors for complicated mourning: (1) sudden, unanticipated death; (2) death from an extremely lengthy illness; (3) loss of a child; (4) the mourner's perception of death as preventable; (5) a premorbid relationship with the deceased that was either angry, ambivalent, or dependent; (6) a prior history of unresolved losses or mental health problems; and (7) the mourner's perceived lack of social support.

There are numerous factors to consider when assessing a complicated grief reaction. Worden (1991) outlined several of these factors: relational, circumstantial, historical, personality, and social. In viewing *relational factors,* the crisis worker needs to assess the nature of the relationship the client had with the deceased, understanding that an ambivalent relationship can inhibit grief and produce excessive anger and guilt. Parkes and Weiss (1983) referred to this as "conflicted grief." A death can also cause the bereaved person to revisit prior losses and traumas, for example, when an adult loses a parent who neglected him or her in childhood. Previous patterns of coping and perceptions of self and others may emerge as a result. In these situations, individuals may experience a double loss: the deceased as well as their hopes and dreams for a better relationship with the deceased. Finally, highly dependent relationships can also be difficult to grieve and can cause a shift in one's self-image (Worden, 1991).

The *circumstances* of death may also make it difficult to grieve, in that individuals may not have had the opportunity to say good-bye to a loved one or gain a sense of closure with the deceased. Circumstances in which a loss is uncertain (e.g., if a loved one is lost at sea or a soldier is missing in action) can also make it difficult for the survivor to mourn. Circumstances in which one experiences multiple losses can overwhelm one's response to grief, such as the employee who called in sick to her job at the World Trade Center on the morning of September 11, 2001, and later grieved the loss of dozens of coworkers. *Historical factors* also need to be considered in assessing for complicated grief. Those who have had previous complicated reactions to loss are more likely to have them again. *Personality factors,* including coping style and self-concept, can lead to vulnerabilities for complicated grief. Those who tend to "go it alone" may be unable to cope with the debilitating feelings commonly experienced by the bereaved and may not know how to ask for support. *Social factors* surrounding a death, especially whether there is social disapproval of it (e.g., suicide) also need to be considered (Lazare, 1979, cited in Worden, 1991). Additionally, a lack of a social support complicates one's reaction to a loss.

Disenfranchised grief, as Doka (1989, 1996) called it, can also complicate one's reaction to grief. Disenfranchised grief occurs when one's grief cannot be "openly acknowledged, publicly mourned, or socially supported" (Doka, 1996, p. 14). Grief may fall into this category when, for example, the bereaved cannot acknowledge a relationship (e.g., a gay man whose partner has died) or when people believe that the bereaved person cannot experience grief (e.g., a recently widowed man in the early stages of Alzheimer's disease). Particular forms of death—such as suicide and homicide, in which survivors experience a societal stigma—can also be disenfranchising. The difficulty for the bereaved in seeking and receiving social support in these and other situations is discussed later in this chapter.

Sudden Loss Versus Anticipatory Mourning

The crisis worker must consider both the form and circumstances of death in responding to the bereaved. Whether a death is sudden or anticipated influences the process of an individual's mourning. Thus, one of the most important considerations in the death of a loved one is whether or not the death was expected (Rando, 1988, 1993).

There has been growing awareness and examination of the process of *anticipatory mourning* experienced as individuals anticipate the death of a loved one (Rando, 2000). It is helpful to view the anticipatory mourning process as preparation for the impending loss rather than as a process in which one accepts in advance how she or he will feel when the loss actually occurs. It is especially crucial for crisis workers frequently exposed to anticipatory mourning, for example, those in health care settings, to attend to the developmental variables (i.e., pending role transitions) and ecological variables (i.e., the degree of social support) that also influence the experience of anticipated grief. An individual mourning a natural death following a chronic illness may experience a qualitatively different reaction from an individual grieving a sudden loss. Doka (1997) points out that some survivors of an anticipated loss experience a sense of emancipation and relief at the time of death related to the end of caregiving responsibilities and the loved one's suffering. It is also common for survivors to feel guilty about these feelings as well as about the quality of care provided during the illness.

Sudden loss Sudden deaths often leave survivors with a sense of "unreality." Also common are exacerbated guilt feelings surrounding the death, a need to blame someone or something for the loss, the frequent involvement of medical and legal authorities, a sense of helplessness, agitation, and unfinished business, and an increased need to understand why the death occurred (Worden, 1991). Survivors' coping abilities are often diminished and overwhelmed by the shock of losing somebody suddenly (Rando, 1988).

Complications in mourning may arise in response to a sudden natural death when the mourner believes that the deceased could have prevented his or her death (e.g., a heavy smoker who dies from a fatal heart attack) or that the mourner's acts of omission or commission were responsible for the death (e.g., "I should have made sure she went to the doctor regularly"). When the death is related to an acute illness (e.g., heart attack or stroke) rather than a prolonged illness, the survivor may experience shock, disbelief, and a palpable sense of the lost opportunity to say good-bye (Hersh, 1996).

Doka (1996) identified six factors that influence the way survivors respond to sudden loss. Each factor is located on a continuum, with the location on that continuum important to understanding the grief response of the survivor:

1. Natural—Human-made (tornado versus September 11 attacks)
2. The degree of intentionality
3. The degree of preventability
4. Suffering
5. Scope (the number of people affected by the loss)
6. The degree of expectedness

Survivors of sudden loss are at risk for complicated mourning because the suddenness and shock make it difficult for the mourner to make sense of the loss. Additionally, the lack of closure, complicated further if the survivor's last interaction with the deceased was negative, and having multiple secondary losses (e.g., social roles, economic security) can increase the risk (Rando, 1993).

Accidental death can be sudden or anticipated in that a person may die at the time of the accident or later, as a result of injuries. In either situation, mourners often experience confusion, anxiety, incomprehensibility, self-reproach, and psychological and physical shock. Given that many accidental deaths are violent and mutilating, mourners often also experience feelings of vulnerability, fear, and insecurity (Rando, 1993).

PROCESS MODELS OF GRIEF

"Time heals all wounds." Most people who have experienced the death of a loved one have heard those words. Although well intentioned, such platitudes provide little relief or support to the grieving person. The phrase "time heals all wounds" implies that with the passage of time, the severity of the grief will lessen and the person will "get over it." This may be true for some, but during the times of intense grief, the idea that one will "get over it" doesn't help.

It is true that the experience of grief changes over time, although not always in a linear fashion. Each person experiences grief differently, and grief is a process rather than a static response. Since Lindemann's (1944) groundbreaking study of tragedy survivors, theorists have attempted to develop models that track this process. Lindemann noted the characteristics of grief as somatic distress, preoccupation with the image of the deceased, guilt, hostile reactions, and loss of familiar patterns of conduct. "Grief work," or the tasks of grief, occurred as the person experienced the following responses in successive stages: shock and disbelief, acute mourning, and resolution of the grief process.

Bowlby (1961) suggested that the grief process consisted of the urge to recover the lost object, disorganization and despair, and reorganization. Building on this early work, Parkes (1974) refined the model to encompass numbness, yearning and searching, disorganization and despair, and reorganization. Kubler-Ross (1969) delineated a model based upon her pioneering work as a psychiatrist working with dying patients that included the sequence of denial, anger, bargaining, depression, and acceptance.

A number of contemporary theorists (Parkes & Weiss, 1983; Rando, 1988, 1993; Worden, 1982, 1991) have also outlined the tasks, phases, and/or processes of grief. Commonly identified phases include the initial struggle to recognize and acknowledge the reality of the loss, the intense experience of the pain associated with the loss, and finally, the gradual accommodation to a changed life and changed relationships. Wolfelt (1992) expressed concern over the use of terms in some grief models that suggest that the bereaved reach a sense of "resolution" (or ending) of their grief. He introduced the concept of "reconciliation" as a final phase to reflect the reality that one never "gets over" grief, but rather accepts the loss and learns to move forward in life.

FACTORS AFFECTING REACTIONS TO LOSS

In order to understand loss, one must appreciate its multidimensional nature. Common psychological, behavioral, social, and physical responses to loss include deep sorrow, anguish, anxiety, fear, yearning, powerlessness, guilt, regret, anger, despair, loneliness, frustration, apathy, and abandonment (Rando, 1993). The intensity and manner in which survivors express these responses varies. Additionally, survivors may experience confusion, preoccupation with the loss, and dissociation from and depersonalization of the loss. They may also demonstrate a number of psychological defenses in attempting to cope, engage in searching behavior (for the deceased), increase their intake of medicine and/or psychoactive substances, and suffer from decreased interest and initiative. For survivors, a general lack of interest can include lack of interest in other people and one's usual activities due to feeling alienated, detached, or estranged from others (Rando, 1993). As poignantly described by C. S. Lewis (1961) in the quotation at the beginning of this chapter, grief can also have physical manifestations including fatigue or exhaustion, restlessness, and various somatic complaints.

It is important for the crisis worker to remember that grief is a uniquely personal experience that is influenced by many factors. For example, a young widow with three children may be influenced psychologically by how untimely her husband's death is, by the presence of concurrent stressors, and by secondary losses (e.g., loss of the coparent, loss of the home due to financial constraints). Other psychological factors that influence how she responds to this loss include her own mental health, coping style, previous experience with loss, and religious or spiritual orientation. The extent of her social support system as well as her openness to it, the meaning she ascribes to and the comfort she draws from the funeral ritual, and her socioeconomic status also influence her response. Her health and her ability to take care of herself (e.g., rest, eat balanced meals) also affect her. Although grief can exact a cumulative physical and psychological toll, mourners often fail to attend to their physical health needs.

Finally, people experience loss and grief within the context of a given cultural milieu. The way an individual understands loss and grief depends on his or her beliefs about life, death, and afterlife. Similarly, there are religious and cultural mourning rituals.

TYPES OF LOSSES

Although there are common reactions experienced by the bereaved in response to a death, there are also reactions idiosyncratic to the type of loss. Crisis workers may intervene with individuals experiencing one of many types of losses. This section summarizes some of the common reactions related to the death of a spouse, child, parent, sibling, or to perinatal loss (e.g., through miscarriage, stillbirth, or sudden infant death syndrome), as well as deaths by suicide and homicide.

Death of a Spouse

The death of a spouse often means the loss of multiple, interrelated types of support including social, economic, emotional, and physical support (McCrae & Costa, 1993). Although married people know intellectually that loss of their spouse is inevitable, most widows and widowers are unprepared for it. Except in the case of unnatural death (e.g., accident, disaster, double homicide) when both spouses die, the surviving spouse not only has the task of grieving but must often assume the roles and responsibilities of the deceased. When parenting and other family duties are extensive, there may be a diminished opportunity to attend to one's own grief. This may be particularly true for a parent attempting to help children make sense of their loss while minimizing disruption in their lives.

The survivor often confronts issues such as a changing identity, loneliness, and adjustment to widowhood. Married people often define themselves within the context of the couple. One approaches decisions, establishes social connections, assumes various roles, and addresses life on a day-to-day basis with awareness of oneself as part of a couple. When a partner dies, one's identity is lost and one must now interact with the world as an individual. The security and validation provided by the relationship are also lost. The couple that acted as a unit no longer exists. The survivor can feel lonely when those around him or her have difficulty relating to the individual who is no longer a part of the couple and vice versa. Adjustment to widowhood often centers on the assumption of new and unfamiliar roles and responsibilities. Women may be affected by additional factors—greater financial problems, economic discrimination, lower remarriage rates, and a diminished social life in widowhood (Rando, 1988).

Survivors whose marriage could be characterized as tense, hostile, or ambivalent may be at risk for "conflicted grief" (Parkes & Weiss, 1983). Also, older survivors may experience greater degrees of loneliness due to other lost relationships (e.g., friends and family who have either died or moved away) and role adjustments related to prior "traditional" role assignments (Lund, Caserta, & Dimond, 1993). Issues of loneliness and adjustment are also common when a death occurs in gay-lesbian-bisexual-transgender (GLBT) relationships. In such cases, the crisis worker must also be sensitive to the family dynamics in the deceased's family, especially when the family does not include the bereaved partner in mourning rituals for fear that others may discover that the deceased was a gay male or lesbian (Cook & Dworkin, 1992).

Death of a Child

The death of a child is commonly recognized as one of the longest-lasting, most heart-wrenching, and complicated types of grief to address, particularly for the parent. The parent-child relationship, originating before birth, is the closest and most intense relational bond for many people. As a result, parents are extremely vulnerable to experiencing complicated grief in this type of loss, particularly because a child's death feels "unnatural." Common wisdom assumes that children should survive their parents. Regardless of the age of the child, bereavement for parents can be long lasting, have a powerful influence, and involve complex processes of coming to terms with the child's death. A parent's experience of this type of loss is related more to the parenting role than to the child's age at the time of death (Rando, 1993).

When a child dies, a parent loses hopes, dreams, plans, and visions for who that child would become. Parents may also feel that they have lost a part of themselves. Additionally, the death of a child involves a loss of family membership and constellation, as well as a loss of prospects for the parents' future. According to Rando (1993) the loss of a child is considered the worst possible violation of the assumptive world of the mourner. One grieving father stated, "Life has stopped for one—and for a time it seems to stop for others. Or at least one wishes that it would" (Nisly, 1992, p. 23).

As noted earlier, the age of the child does not have an impact on parental grief per se. The age of the child, however, does reflect the developmental issues that may have been present in the parent/child relationship at the time of loss (Rando, 1993). Developmental stages determine the types of issues that parents must face in the bereavement process. The pain experienced in child loss differs depending on the developmental tasks expected of the parent.

When a young child dies, the loss affects the entire family system. Although the child's life may have been short, many hopes, aspirations, feelings, and styles of relating are deeply embedded in family life. The family has to renegotiate plans for the future in order to integrate their new reality. An additional challenge with the death of a young child may involve the amount of time outsiders have had or have not had to bond with the child (Rando, 1993). Well-meaning outsiders may unintentionally invalidate the grief experienced with this type of family loss, which can increase the parents' risks for social isolation. Later in the chapter we discuss the effects of the loss of pregnancy and newborn children, a situation in which families often struggle with feeling "overlooked" in their grief.

Parents who have lost an *adult child* are a growing segment of the population due to longer life expectancies. This bereaved population has unique risk factors. Due to the nature of the parental role in later life, the parent is probably less involved in the adult child's daily life. As a result the grief needs of the parent may not receive much attention, as support is typically extended primarily to the immediate family rather than to an older surviving parent. Research suggests that this lack of social support is particularly detrimental to fathers who have lost an adult child because fathers experience more intense grief for this type of loss (Rando, 1988, 1993).

Mediating factors in parental grief of an adult child include the impact of the psychological relationship between the parent and child before the death, as consistent with Worden's (1991) relational factors to consider in assessing for complicated grief. The relational components that classified the level of closeness and distinctiveness prior to death are the same components that may make grief and loss more difficult (Rando, 1993). For example, when the relationship was very close, as when a mother and daughter communicated daily and the family had dinner together every Sunday, the mother is likely to experience the loss of her daughter intensely and experience an extensive period of great emptiness.

Death of a Parent

As with other types of loss, the developmental stage of the survivor plays an important role in responses to the loss of a parent. For children, the death of a parent can be life transforming and disruptive as few other events can be, as the child feels the impact within multiple dimensions and revisits it during different developmental periods. The developmental stage of the child at the time of a parent's death influences both the tasks of grief and the losses sustained.

Worden (1996) asserted that the way children learn of their parent's death (e.g., when, from whom, how they are told/not told) and the circumstances of the death are critical in shaping their response. When children are not told directly, gently, or in a developmentally appropriate way, complications may arise. Funerals and other family rituals can assist the surviving child to acknowledge the parent's death, honor the life of the parent, and provide support and comfort to the child (Worden, 1996). It is important for many children to establish an ongoing relationship to the deceased parent. This may include thinking of the parent as being "in heaven," dreaming about the parent, speaking with the parent at the gravesite or when feeling sad, reminiscing about past times together, or keeping an object close at hand that reminds the child of the parent (Silverman, Nickman & Worden, 1992; Worden, 1996).

When adults lose a parent, many factors affect their response: the quality of the relationship both historically and in the present, their expectations about how one should grieve this type of loss (i.e., "I shouldn't feel this strongly, especially as a forty-year-old . . . I'm not a kid anymore"), and the meaning ascribed to the parent-child relationship (i.e., the loss of connection to the past and to childhood) (Rando, 1988). Myers (1986) asserted that the meaning of the loss of a parent across the stages of adulthood varies based on the developmental tasks at hand for the survivor; for example, the tasks will be different for an adult child in early adulthood attempting to establish a new marriage and an adult child in later adulthood adjusting to retirement and his or her own health concerns.

Death of a Sibling

As with any type of grief, in looking at the impact of sibling loss, the counselor must assess the impact of culture, family roles, gender, age, and sexual orientation as well as multiple other diversities. Also, as with other bereavement crises, the morbid relationship between siblings influences sibling loss.

In order to appreciate the experience of sibling loss, it is useful to clarify what has been lost (Rando, 1988). First, a "shared history" that others may or may not fully understand or know is lost. For example, a boy whose only brother dies loses a shared understanding of childhood stories and experiences. Second, a child's position in the family may change, for example, when the second oldest child becomes the oldest child and assumes the weight and cultural responsibility of that role. Third, a "constant" in one's life is now gone. For example, even siblings who lived on different continents may have always known that they could call upon the other sibling, and now this support is gone. Fourth, a shared understanding of family dynamics and aging parents is lost. For example, a lesbian who loses her supportive brother has lost not only a sibling but her family advocate and ally as well. Fifth, one's sense of immortality has been violated. When a sibling who was close in age dies, for example, when a twin is killed in a car accident, the remaining sibling's death may seem more real and inevitable.

Worden (1996) described additional behavioral and cognitive concerns in sibling loss. For example, a surviving younger brother may attempt to "replace" his deceased older brother, perhaps responding to a projective need of his parent. Adepending on the developmental stage of the remaining sibling, a parent may be overly protective of the child, interfering with the child's normal development. Alternatively, a surviving sibling may be angry and blame the parent for not "saving" the dying sibling, which may be manifested as detachment or independent behavior. Troubling cognitions may include survivor guilt experienced by the sibling who asks, "Why not me?" or has regrets about words he or she said or did not say prior to the sibling's death.

Environmental stressors to assess in crisis work with sibling loss involve the level of functioning of the family system as well as the degree to which remaining family members are linked with social supports within their community. With multiple sibling deaths, surviving family members may face even greater difficulties such as media coverage and public knowledge of their losses (e.g., a house fire that has taken the lives of three children).

Miscarriage, Stillbirth, Neonatal Death, and Sudden Infant Death Syndrome

Perinatal grief and loss   Pregnancy is a normal developmental process involving major life role changes. When a pregnancy does not come to full term, there is an interruption in this developmental process. Not only do physical change and loss occur with a truncated pregnancy, but emotional and psychological shifts occur as well. Parents may begin to feel attached to their offspring long before the actual birth occurs. For both parents, but especially for the mother, attachment occurs when the baby is in utero. Loss of a pregnancy is deeply disappointing for most prospective parents. Whether it is through miscarriage, abortion, or stillbirth, the loss presents unique challenges.

To more fully understand the impact of loss during pregnancy one needs to understand the physical and psychological changes that occur throughout gestation. Costello, Gardner, and Merenstein (1988) suggested that there are a series of psychological and emotional tasks within each trimester of pregnancy that influence attachment including, in the first trimester, acceptance of the gradual identification of the fetus as separate, in the second trimester, fantasizing about what the child will be like, and, in the third trimester, the gradual preparation for both the birth and the parents' future relationship with the child.

Miscarriage most frequently occurs during the first trimester of pregnancy. This type of loss may be complicated by the fact that there may be no visible signs of pregnancy. Because the mother experiences the fetus as part of her and not yet as a separate entity, it is common for women to feel guilt and to blame themselves after having a miscarriage (Costello et al., 1988). "If only I had or had not . . ." are common sentiments expressed by women following a miscarriage. Feelings of isolation can also accompany this type of grief, with partners experiencing the loss differently (Rando, 1988). Women may also fear being unable to ever carry a newborn to full term.

Additionally, when a miscarriage occurs, if the pregnancy has not been previously announced, the couple may feel a sense of alienation, as others may not be aware of their loss. The level of attachment that the parent or parents had to the pregnancy also has an impact on grief (Rando, 1988). Was the baby a planned addition to the family, to whom many hopes and dreams had been attached? Had fertility treatments and considerable amounts of time and effort gone into the pregnancy? Was the pregnancy expected? A sensitive crisis worker must listen carefully to the meanings parents attach to their loss.

The deeply painful experience of *stillbirth* typically occurs within the last trimester of pregnancy. Developmentally, at this point in the pregnancy the parent typically has formed a significant bond with the nearly developed child (Rando, 1988). The parent has usually set up a nursery, selected a name, and is happily awaiting the birth of the child.

One particularly painful aspect of this type of loss is the knowledge, sometimes a few days prior to delivery, that the child that the mother is carrying is no longer living. The emotional impact of this knowledge can be excruciating. Additionally, the parent(s) need to make a number of decisions: Whom should they tell? Should they hold a funeral? Whom should they invite, and how will they respond? Should they give the child a name? If there are other children, who will inform them of the baby's death and how will they tell them? These decisions need to be made at a time when it is difficult to make decisions.

The biological shift for the body may also be a difficult developmental task to navigate, as the mother's body has already prepared for nursing (Rando, 1988). Postpartum depression and irritability as well as feelings of powerlessness and anger are common (Rando, 1993). The crisis worker who can provide affective, behavioral, cognitive, developmental, and environmental supports has an important role to play. It is particularly important to look at the level of the parents' attachment to the pregnancy and the number of social supports that exist for the family. Stillbirth may also be a difficult type of loss for labor-and-delivery staff, who may need a special crisis response (Costello et al., 1988).

Sudden Infant Death Syndrome (SIDS), the death of a child within the first year of life, is another deeply painful loss that may trigger a crisis for both the parent(s) and other family members. As the parents have attached to the child not only in utero but during the child's short life, the loss can be disorienting and incapacitating. Mothers, in particular, may be temporarily unable to care for other children (Rando, 1988). The family life of the bereaved has experienced a tragic violation of form. Family members may deal with the loss in different ways depending on their age, developmental stage, and coping mechanisms prior to the child's death. Additionally, parents not only have to face the immediate tragic reality of life without their baby but may also be vulnerable to what Ostfeld, Ryan, Hiatt, and Hegyi (1993) referred to as shadow grief, "the sense of loss parents will retain throughout their lifetime, [which] can recede or intensify as a function of immediate events in the parents' lives" (p. 160). Reminders of this shortened life, either by anniversaries or by "would have been moments," can retrigger earlier grief.

A number of support groups have emerged for parents dealing with this type of painful bereavement. Special support may be essential during the initial phase following an infant's death, as law enforcement or child protective service staff often need to investigate the death (Rando, 1988). An investigative inquiry can add to the pain and guilt of surviving family members if questions of neglect are raised. A supportive spouse has been identified as a critical component in the healing and adjustment phases of this grief process (Ostfeld et al., 1993). The effective crisis worker can also help identity other environmental supports including extended family, religious communities, and neighborhood groups. Special attention needs to be given to social supports for single mothers and to the role that pediatricians may play in bringing medical knowledge to this painful experience (Ostfeld et al., 1993).

Suicide

The death of a loved one by suicide leaves many unanswered questions and countless emotions. Stillion (1996) and others have suggested that those who experience the death of a loved one to suicide have qualitatively different grief reactions than those whose loved ones died from natural or accidental causes and are at a heightened risk for complicated grief reactions. Complicating psychological reactions include increased feelings of anger, guilt, and shame, concern, and fear over one's own suicidal tendencies in response to the suicide of a loved one, the agonizing effort to understand why the suicide occurred, feelings of rejection, and unfinished business caused by the suddenness of the death and the inability to say good-bye. Familial and social reactions that contribute to complicated mourning include social isolation (feeling cut off from potential sources of support), societal stigma (feeling harshly judged by one's community), the projection of guilt and blaming others for the suicide, and scapegoating (Rando, 1993; Stillion, 1996). Given the stigma and isolation survivors often experience, crisis workers should be sure to assess the amount of social support survivors are receiving.

Violent Death

Violent death refers to death caused by an act of homicide. Survivors grieving this type of death are at risk for complicated bereavement reactions as they struggle to understand what seems to be an incomprehensible act. Factors that may complicate mourning after homicide include its suddenness and randomness; the violence, trauma, and horror inherent in the act of murder itself; and the mourner's belief that he or she could have prevented the homicide somehow (Rando, 1993).

Survivors of violent death are often unable to accept the news even in light of incontrovertible information. They may experience a desire for revenge or recurring fears about their own safety. They may receive less social support due to the stigma often attached to murder, and they may struggle with their own feelings of shame (Redmond, 1996). Survivors may also have horrifying images of the pain and suffering experienced by their loved one.

It is important for crisis workers to be aware that, although feelings of anger, guilt, and self-blame are common reactions to other types of loss, they are likely to be intensified in response to homicide. A survivor's grief may also be exposed to the public due to the involvement of the criminal justice system and media attention (Redmond, 1996). An additional complicating event in surviving a loved one's death by homicide is when one family member is murdered by another, thrusting the entire family into the criminal justice system and under the media's spotlight.

Crisis workers need to be prepared, both in assessment and intervention, for intense affective expression, the possibility that family members may continue to search for their loved one even after the body has been recovered, the likelihood that survivors will have persistent cognitive images of both the suffering of their loved one and their own fantasized (or actual) violent retaliation against the murderer, the realization that survivors have suddenly lost known social roles (e.g., the parent who loses an only child to an act of homicide), and the possibility that the survivor's social support system may pull away due to the societal stigma attached to homicide.

Death of a Pet

The loss resulting from the death of a pet is often underestimated and neglected in discussions of loss. The human to pet relationship, however, is a twenty-four-hour-a-day bond that is often experienced as mutual unconditional love and devotion. Myers (2000) described the loss of an animal companion as an experience of disenfranchised grief due to the frequent lack of social acknowledgment.

The death of an animal affects individuals differently depending on their age and developmental stage, their current life situation, concurrent life disruptions, the length of time with the animal companion, and the availability of environmental supports regarding the loss (Myers, 2000). A child who loses a pet may be experiencing death for the first time, and a person with a visual impairment who loses a guide dog may experience the primary loss of the animal companion as well as secondary losses involving mobility and independence.

It is important for a crisis worker to understand the type of relationship that the person or family had with the animal, including when the animal came into the family, the circumstances of the animal's death, and what part a child may have had in caring for the animal. The way the worker refers to the animal is important; the term *animal companion* may be the most respectful way to represent the relationship. Finally, because society does not have a socially sanctioned forum for honoring and saying goodbye to animals (e.g., a wake or funeral), the crisis worker may encourage exploring ways to meaningfully acknowledge the loss. This might include writing a death announcement or poem or creating a photo album or memory book (Myers, 2000).

Other Losses

Many profound and powerful loss experiences not related to death occur over the course of one's life span. Many of these losses are due to severed attachments, life transitions, aging and health processes, and changes in the social roles people fill. Although a detailed review of these types of losses is beyond the scope of this chapter, it is vital for the crisis worker to assess and be aware of an individual's loss history as well as any concurrent losses experienced by a survivor while he or she is grieving the death of a loved one. For example, a recently retired and recently widowed woman is not only adapting to the loss of her husband but also to the loss of long-term known social roles, changes in the composition and accessibility of her social support system, a shifting self-image, and an unfamiliar daily routine. It would be an incomplete response if the crisis worker focused only on the immediacy of the death of her husband without assessing for these concurrent developmental-related losses.

When people experience a death, they revisit their personal history with loss on a conscious and unconscious level within the grief process, and the crisis worker can address this history in the course of the intervention. Previous loss informs responses to current loss. A common loss that adult survivors may have experienced is that of separation and divorce. The survivor's history of coping with this severed attachment may affect their ability to cope with an attachment that has been severed by death. Coping may be even more complicated if the deceased is a former spouse or separated partner. In such cases, the crisis worker needs to assess whether the survivor is experiencing conflicted grief.

DEVELOPMENTAL ASPECTS OF GRIEF

Child and Adolescent Grief

In order to effectively address the bereavement experience of children and adolescents, the crisis worker must have a working knowledge of normal developmental tasks for each age group. Grief crises may interrupt age-appropriate activities and force a child or an adolescent to address issues for which he or she is not developmentally prepared. Some authors report that in working with bereft young people, cultural imprinting can affect a young person's understanding of death and violence as much as his or her developmental stage (Irish, 1995).

No matter what the young person's developmental stage, having an available adult in his or her life is the single most important determinant of a positive outcome of the grief process (Worden, 1996). Although much has been written about the potential developmental impact of grief on children and adolescents, young people are remarkably resilient in the face of adversity. The crisis worker seeks to tap into this reservoir of resiliency.

The emotional components of grief for young people vary across a broad range, including sadness, anger, anxiety, and guilt (Worden, 1996). The way a young person handles and "acts out" each emotion varies depending on his or her developmental stage. Grieving children *are* our teachers. For example, after crying over "not seeing mommy," a young child may go off and play for a period of intermittent forgetting, a common developmental expression of sadness. Anger due to feeling abandoned and forgotten by the deceased parent is a common reaction in children whose egocentrism makes them think their parent did this to them. Anxiety after a death, commonly experienced as the fear of losing the other parent to death or as fears for one's own safety, is expected and developmentally appropriate, because if one unexpected death occurred, another could as well. Additionally, the experience of guilt for a child may include wishing that he or she had appreciated the parent more while the parent was alive and regretting an expression of anger before the parent's death. Participating in risky behavior such as dangerous climbing or fast driving can be a manifestation of the guilt that a young person may experience in grief as well, as the young person may attempt to punish him- or herself for something left undone or unsaid, or even for the death itself (Worden, 1996).

Because their language skills are typically less developed, children and adolescents often externalize their emotions through behaviors that reflect their internal conflict (Worden, 1996). It is therefore important for crisis workers to assess a bereaved young person's body language, as behavior and affect can inform an intervention with individuals who "act out" their issues developmentally. Play therapy, art therapy, or a sand tray, if within the worker's realm of expertise, may therefore be the most effective therapies with this younger population. A child's angry outburst may be less about what is occurring in the immediate environment and more about what he or she is attempting to address internally. Internal preoccupation with grief manifests itself behaviorally as well, frequently noted as "absent-mindedness" in school and evaluated as "poor academic performance." An additional behavioral manifestation of a preoccupation with grief may be accident-proneness in children and youth (Worden, 1996).

The developmental stage of children or adolescents at the time of death predicates the components that they need to adjust to and grieve. The ability to comprehend and make sense of the death, the development of coping mechanisms, and the capacity to access environmental supports may all vary depending upon the age of the young person when confronted with the crisis of death (Rando, 1984). For example, a six-year-old may have a better cognitive understanding of death than a three-year-old but still has not developed the coping skills to deal with the intense emotions elicited by the loss; whereas during early adolescence generally there is a deeper understanding of death and more effective coping skills (Worden, 1991).

The impact of the crisis of death may continue to influence adjustment developmentally in significant ways. A young boy who loses his mother may need to adjust to a bedtime routine without mom reading a storybook and giving him a goodnight kiss. Similarly, a teenage girl's adjustment to the death of her mother may include not being able to get her father's opinion on the boyfriend she wants to date. The child or adolescent may need to continually readdress life without the deceased and make new adjustments as he or she encounters different developmental challenges. Learning to drive without the help of a deceased older brother, or facing the anxiety over the onset of menstruation without mom available to talk to are examples of ongoing grief work young people may contend with.

When working with grieving adolescents, crisis workers must provide ample opportunity for death-related questions. Although a youth may feel the need to "act grown up," she or he may be emotionally overwhelmed. Additionally, the death of a peer can be particularly devastating to a young person who is at a developmental stage characterized by using friends as a reference and identity group (Cook & Dworkin, 1992). Because of this, with the increase of violent death among youth, increased attention must be given to understanding and responding to the expression of grief in response to traumatic situations such as episodes of school violence.

Important questions to ask in these situations include: Did the youth have an opportunity to express his or her connection with the deceased in a socially sanctioned forum such as a funeral (Cook & Dworkin, 1992)? Rituals that honor the relationship one had with the deceased are important in the process of saying good-bye. Additionally, with young people of any age, and particularly with adolescents, the crisis worker must assess lethality and be attuned to suicidal behavior and intent to harm self or others (Cook & Dworkin, 1992).

An Elderly Adult's Grief

The longer one lives, the more acquisitions and losses one experiences. Acquisitions include life experiences, relationships, memories, material goods, accomplishments, and spiritual realizations, whereas losses include health, independence, known social roles, loved ones, and familiar living environments. It is common in later life to engage in a life review process to determine whether one has lived life well (Erikson, 1968). If we view development as continuous and lifelong, then aging involves changing. In assessing the grief experiences of elderly persons, the crisis worker should gain an understanding of the acquisitions, losses, and changes they have experienced.

Features of grief among the elderly include interdependence, experiencing multiple losses, awareness of the inevitability of one's own death, loneliness, dislocation, and role adjustment. Elderly men, however, may experience role adjustment as more disruptive on a day-to-day basis than women, and at the same time they may have greater difficulty in connecting with social supports (Worden, 1991).

For some elderly, the death of a spouse after a marriage of several decades may highlight specific roles and activities for which they depended on their deceased spouse. The grandmother of one of the authors had never driven a car or balanced a checkbook during her marriage, which made it difficult for her to get around and manage her finances when her husband died. For other elderly, managing grief related to multiple losses is a common experience. These losses may include relationships (e.g., family or friends who have died or moved away), social roles (e.g., retirement), physical health, or cognitive functioning that may negatively affect the elderly person's ability to grieve the death of a loved one. As a result, many elderly people have a heightened awareness of their own mortality. The crisis worker must be willing to explore this and be prepared to address concurrent existential or spiritual crises.

The Family as a Unit

If a crisis worker is intervening with a bereaved family, it is essential to understand two key points: (1) the family is an interactional unit (or system) attempting to maintain a sense of equilibrium with change in one component (i.e., a family member's death) causing change in the rest, and (2) not all family members will have the same experience of grief. Walsh and McGoldrick (1991) asserted that the adaptation of the family to a death occurs through both immediate and long-term reorganization. The crisis worker engaged in ongoing crisis counseling should be aware of what Bowen (1985) called the "emotional shock-wave," the "network of 'after-shocks' of serious life events that can occur anywhere in the extended family system in the months or years following serious emotional events (i.e., a death) in a family" (p. 325).

In assessing grief and the family system, Worden (1991) outlined three areas for the crisis worker to evaluate: (1) the functional role of the deceased, for instance, a parent, and how he or she fulfilled it; (2) how able the family is to assist one another in coping with the loss; and (3) what the family does or does not do to facilitate emotional expression. Walsh and McGoldrick (1991) identified two central tasks for the family: (1) developing a shared acknowledgment of the reality of the death and shared experience, which can be facilitated by open communication, and (2) reorganizing the family system and reinvesting in other relationships and life pursuits, with family cohesion and flexibility necessary for this stabilization to occur. The crisis worker needs to assess the numerous factors (e.g., manner of death, timing of loss, family and social network) that influence how the family adapts and accomplishes these tasks and intervene accordingly.

In working with a bereaved family, the crisis worker must be aware that there is also a loss of family subsystems. This loss may be related to the special bond shared by all the siblings, or the role and connection a parent had with a particular child. When families prepare for the impending death of a terminally ill family member, not only are they experiencing anticipatory grief for the loss of that person but also for the family they have known and experienced (Rando, 1984, 1993).

Special consideration is necessary in responding to a family when there are either multiple deaths (e.g., two siblings killed in a plane crash) or when the death of a family member is directly or indirectly caused by another family member. When multiple losses occur it may be difficult for the family to address each loss separately without feeling overwhelmed by the grief. The crisis worker must assist the family to experience and to acknowledge the pain associated with each loss.

SPIRITUALITY AND THE CRISIS OF DEATH

In the crisis of death, clients frequently must come to terms with the existential question, "Why?" Questions of ultimate significance, motivation, and purpose often surface, and even the most resilient survivors may struggle with questions that challenge their prior beliefs. "How could something as horrific as an airplane crash take the life of my beloved?" "Why was this tragic accident that took the life of our child allowed to happen?" "How could this heart-wrenching miscarriage be a part of the 'big picture plan' when the pregnancy itself felt like a gift from the Creator?" Crisis counselors must be sensitive to the spiritual beliefs, nuances, and resources in a client's life. In assessment, it is also important to broaden the focus on the client's environment to include the spiritual realms of beauty, music, and nature as well as the client's beliefs about a higher power or what is sacred (Canda & Furman, 1999).

Existential and transpersonal theories highlight the importance of attention to the realms of meaning that are significant to the client. These frameworks address how one comes to terms with "the human condition of impermanence, suffering, death, and the inhumanity of human beings" (Canda & Furman, 1999, p. 157). Inviting discussion, dialogue, and permission to explore disillusionment and confusion can be critical in validating the full impact of loss and grief. Helping the bereaved to identify and address unhelpful cognitions and the resultant behavior that the loss may have triggered provides a safe forum for the legitimate search for meaning and reconstruction of reality within the therapeutic relationship. The crisis worker is also ethically bound to make responsible referrals to local resources within the client's spiritual or cultural community. Examples of this might include referring a priest to a Catholic client who wishes to take Communion as part of the healing process or referring a tribal healer to a grieving Native American.

A spiritually sensitive crisis worker must also be attentive to the interplay of spirituality and culture. It is important for the crisis worker to assess and understand how culture and beliefs about the spiritual inform and interact with each other in the life of a client (Fukuyama & Sevig, 1999). The crisis worker must be aware of the mores, norms, and traditions that affect beliefs about the meaning of death and the possibility of an afterlife, and rituals and beliefs about mourning. As noted, this may also include referrals to spiritual leaders and traditional healers, when appropriate.

INTERVENTION

Helping professionals working in varied settings find themselves responding to the crisis of death. The specific setting, context of practice, and professional role of the crisis worker influences the nature of the intervention. For example, there will be a different frequency, intensity, and duration of contact for a hospice worker helping a family that is experiencing anticipatory grief as they prepare for the death of a terminally ill parent and an emergency room crisis worker responding to a family whose loved one was brought to the hospital near death who has since died from a gunshot wound. The role of the crisis worker and the setting in which he or she works, by their very nature, influence the types of loss the professional is exposed to. These factors determine whether the model is applied to a single-session crisis intervention or to ongoing crisis counseling.

The crisis worker must also remember that individuals have unique reactions to the crisis of death. In addition to some of the common manifestations of grief outlined earlier in this chapter, the type of loss, the manner of death, and the developmental ages of the deceased and of the survivors must be considered when applying the developmental-ecological model of crisis intervention. In the following section we apply the model and highlight a number of examples. The chapter concludes with an expanded crisis counseling case example.

SINGLE-SESSION CRISIS COUNSELING

In responding to the crisis of death the crisis worker needs to establish an immediate empathic helping connection and be prepared for the possibility of an array of intense emotional reactions by the survivor. During a single-session crisis intervention contact, there are three essential goals. First, the crisis worker must secure the immediate safety of the survivor and assess lethality, especially if the death has occurred due to suicide, homicide, accident, or disaster. A violent death may trigger the survivor to express suicidal thoughts or thoughts of retaliation, or the survivor may be in an unsafe physical environment (e.g., in the aftermath of a disaster or at the scene of a violent crime). This goal also includes reducing the survivor's emotional distress. Second, the survivor must attain short-term mastery of the crisis situation in order to deal with the immediate concerns that arise in the aftermath of a death (e.g., arranging a funeral, contacting friends and relatives). The crisis worker focuses on enhancing the survivor's immediate coping skills. Third, the crisis worker must make the survivor(s) aware of the social, spiritual, and community supports available to them. There will be differences in how survivors utilize support, but the crisis worker must be prepared to provide information regarding possible resources and/or to broker these connections. In order to fulfill the goal of helping clients connect with support systems, the crisis worker may first need to assist clients in identifying their need for support. It is not atypical for one family member to be the "rock" of support for others while being unable to verbalize his or her own needs. The impact of shock, especially after sudden death, can make the process of identifying their own needs even more difficult for survivors.

Although the steps of the single-session crisis counseling model are presented here in a linear fashion, they are not necessarily sequential. It is also important to remind readers that the process of assessment is ongoing throughout the intervention.

Step 1:
Supportively and empathically join with the survivor.

The crisis worker may intervene very soon after the actual loss of the loved one and in or near the setting where the death occurred, highlighting the critical need for an authentic and empathic approach. Survivors may experience bewilderment, depersonalization, shock, and numbness in the aftermath of a death and, as a result, may have difficulty processing information provided to them by health professionals, law enforcement personnel, or disaster relief workers.

Envision walking into the waiting area of an emergency room to meet with a family that has only been told that their loved one was rushed to the hospital after being shot outside of his car when leaving work. Absorbing the environmental stimuli while obsessing about the limited information they have received, the family may not necessarily even remember who has already spoken to them, what that person's role was, or perhaps even who said what. In this type of situation, the family's sense of control is fleeting, at best. How might the crisis worker begin to join with this family? The crisis worker can start by clarifying his or her role and purpose in providing the family with an idea of what is happening at the moment (e.g., "I am a social worker here in the ER and would like to talk with you about your son"). The crisis worker should also find a private location in which to speak with the family. The crisis worker must also be aware of the tone and volume of his or her voice as well as body language and eye contact. Actively listening to the family's spoken and unspoken concerns is vital. Avoiding the use of professional jargon and indicating acceptance of the family's emotional expression are additional ways to demonstrate respect for the family.

Recognizing the uniqueness of each person's expression of grief, acknowledging and validating the various emotions expressed (e.g., anger, sadness, shock, and numbness), and normalizing these reactions give the family permission to feel and convey both acceptance and warmth. In order to effectively do this, the crisis worker must be comfortable with tears, the expression of anger, and silence, which can be the response when there is either an absence or an overwhelming number of emotions.

In the case of the crisis with the family in the emergency room, the family may feel some urgency to share the way they heard the news, "to tell their story," and to process what they have experienced since hearing the news. It is important to allow them to do so rather than immediately engaging them in problem solving. Joining, or developing a working alliance with, clients requires the crisis worker to communicate recognition of their predicaments and their related distress, to be emotionally moved or touched by the clients' experiences, and to demonstrate a commitment to collaborate with the clients to help them change their situation (Teyber, 2000).

Given the intensity inherent in responding to a grief crisis, and the importance of establishing effective working alliances with the bereaved, it is essential for crisis workers to have looked inward to address their own losses and related stressors in order to avoid burnout or unresolved grief experienced as a result of the work they do (Cook & Dworkin, 1992). If crisis workers have not done their own "grief work," the task of joining with the bereaved and forging an alliance may be mitigated.

Step 2:
Intervene to create safety in the environment, stabilize the situation, and handle the survivor's immediate needs.

Crisis workers sometimes need to take concrete steps to calmly assume control of the immediate environment either at the scene of death or surrounding the "news" of the death. For example, the survivor at the scene of an automobile accident who is trying to "free" the trapped body of his or her deceased spouse may be at risk for injury by getting in the way of fire, rescue, and police personnel. In this case, the crisis worker may need to remove the survivor from the immediate scene. An example of creating contextual safety in response to the news of a loved one's death might be for the crisis worker to escort the devastated parents out of the morgue after they have identified the brutally beaten corpse of their missing son. In a case such as this, the crisis worker might try to arrange an opportunity for the family to spend time with the body after the parents' initial overwhelming feelings have stabilized somewhat.

A calm and supportive approach on the part of the crisis worker can help to gradually stabilize the parents' overwhelming feelings, ranging from extreme anguish, rage, and powerlessness to guilt and regret. Assisting the parents in giving voice to the injustice of their child's disappearance and death, conveying understanding that their whole world seems out of control and that they feel powerless over it, and accepting their intense, wide-ranging, and sometimes incongruent feelings can serve to stabilize and lessen the intensity of the emotional response. This approach can bring "calm control" to an otherwise escalating situation.

Similarly, a crisis worker intervening with the parents of a child who died of SIDS would need to listen to and understand their feelings of guilt and blame, which might be accentuated by the presence of police investigators. By normalizing their feelings, and informing the parents that police involvement is common protocol, the crisis worker can help de-escalate the situation.

The immediate needs of those dealing with the aftermath of loss are often logistical. Providing as many facts as possible regarding the circumstances of the death may offer a renewed yet limited sense of control to the bereaved. Subsequently, the need to notify others (e.g., family, friends, neighbors) as well as to begin thinking about funeral arrangements may be pressing. Preliminary decision making may provide the bereaved with an increased sense of power and control over themselves and their situation. There may be special concerns in relation to the impact of the news on those who need to be notified (e.g., an aging grandparent in poor health or a mentally ill sibling). Discussions focused on whom to contact and how to communicate the news can be a helpful support to the survivor.

Step 3:
Explore and assess the dimensions of the crisis and facilitate the ventilation of emotions.

In this step the crisis worker explores and assesses the dimensions of the crisis situation and provides many opportunities for the survivor to ventilate. Due to high levels of physical and emotional arousal, the survivor may have an overwhelming need to talk about what has happened. If the crisis worker empathically joined with the survivor earlier through active listening, at this point he or she can encourage the survivor with gentle probes to "tell" and "retell" the story about what has happened. Specific emphasis should be placed on the feelings and emotions associated with the loss. With survivors who are unable to ventilate due to shock, numbness, or overwhelming feelings that may have led to silence, the crisis worker can ask detail-oriented questions that focus on how they heard the news or ask them to share their thoughts. It is also important for the crisis worker to assess the potential for suicidal or violent behavior, especially in the aftermath of the suicide or violent death of a loved one.

Assessment utilizing the ABCDE framework occurs simultaneously, as the crisis worker assesses the survivor's affective, behavioral, and cognitive states as well as his or her developmental issues and ecological situations. We have reviewed various types of loss and the resultant responses in this chapter. For illustrative purposes, using the example of the parents whose missing child has been found beaten to death, the crisis worker doing a single-session crisis intervention one week after the identification of the body should conduct the assessment as follows:

Affect

Provide parents the opportunity to express the wide range of emotions and feelings they are experiencing. Encourage this expression with the goal of affect stability. The crisis worker should be prepared in this case for extremely intense emotional reactions, including rage, and perhaps frightening impulses to locate and murder those responsible for the death. These feelings may intermittently be replaced by feelings of excessive guilt and self-blame.

Behavior

The crisis worker should explore whether the parents have engaged in searching for their child (e.g., as if their son were still missing) or if they have experienced restlessness, sleep or appetite disturbances, or increased safety concerns.

Cognition

These parents may not quite believe that their son is dead, even in the face of compelling factual information (i.e., having identified the body). They may also struggle with ongoing imagery of their son's pain and suffering. The crisis worker can invite the parents to share any spiritual questions they may have regarding the injustice of the death—questions about "why God let this happen"—and talk about the potential internal conflict this form of death creates with their core values and beliefs about the world.

Development

Specifically, the crisis worker should assess the impact on the family unit of this crisis event. It is also important to assess whether these parents are currently able to meet the task of parenting their remaining children. The developmental age of the child who was killed and his or her position in the family unit are also factors to consider, as are the ages and developmental stages of the surviving siblings.

Ecosystem

It would be essential, given the manner of death, for the crisis worker to assess what types of social support (e.g., extended family, friends, spiritual community) to which these parents have access. The family's privacy may be compromised as law enforcement investigations and media coverage expand. These factors coupled with the societal stigma associated with homicide may cause some members of their support system to withdraw.

Step 4:
Identify and examine alternative actions and develop options.

Although the crisis worker and survivor have previously addressed immediate needs in the aftermath of the death (e.g., whom to notify, how to make funeral arrangements), the task of identifying the "next steps" in determining priorities and the most pressing issues to address is an essential collaborative process. Often, due to disorientation, preoccupation with the loss, and intense emotions, the survivor may have great difficulty making decisions and a limited sense of what options exist. Brainstorming about the next steps will expand the range of alternatives and solutions for the survivor to consider. This process does not focus on long-term solutions (e.g., dealing with secondary losses that impact the survivor's ongoing financial situation) but rather on immediate needs (e.g., a supportive companion for the coming days, for making funeral arrangements, and simply for keeping the survivor company). It is important to identify obstacles (e.g., schedule of the companion) and assess the survivor's ability to carry out the assigned tasks (e.g., can the survivor cope with making the funeral arrangements?).

Step 5:
Help the survivor mobilize personal and social resources.

The crisis worker must assist survivors in identifying both internal and external resources (e.g., social networks including family and friends) to be mobilized in response to their loss. Initially, the bereaved may want others to be present but may not have the energy, interest, or desire to emotionally connect with them or even talk to them. In mobilizing the survivor's internal resources, the crisis worker needs to assess his or her precrisis level of functioning. Components of this assessment include the survivor's coping style, mental health, level of maturity, and previous experience with loss, as well as the degree to which the survivor has accommodated the loss (Rando, 1984, 1993). Connection with formal and informal support systems is often critical. Given the numerous religious and spiritual questions that may arise for survivors, brokering a connection with the survivor's faith community, an available chaplain, or another resource to address his or her spiritual concerns can be critical.

The counselor must also consider other community resources including support groups. The parents of the murdered child described earlier might benefit from a referral to a support group such as Compassionate Friends, a support group for parents who have lost a child, or a support group for survivors of violent death. In the area of bereavement, however, it is not generally recommended that survivors immediately join a bereavement or support group. The intensity of the normal manifestation of survivors' grief reactions in the immediate aftermath of a loved one's death may not be suitable for group participation in the initial weeks after the loss.

Assisting survivors in identifying and utilizing their own internal resources, coping strengths, and resilience is also essential. It may be more difficult for survivors to identify their strengths in the immediate aftermath of the loss, especially if they are experiencing shock. It can be useful, however, to review the strengths they have already demonstrated in responding to this loss as well as how they may have coped with previous or recent losses.

Step 6:
Anticipate the future and arrange follow-up contact.

Because the manifestation of grief in the immediate days and weeks following a loss can be immobilizing and leave one with little energy or interest in one's former routine or roles, it is important for the crisis worker to let survivors know that what they are experiencing is normal. This may assist survivors in identifying their feelings and experiences, and may decrease fear. Some survivors may want to return to work and their former routines as quickly as possible in order to demonstrate that they are coping. Discussing survivors' expectations regarding the mourning process, such as how long they believe it will take and how much time they will permit themselves, can assist survivors in making realistic adjustments to their routines. In doing so, they can work toward a balance of meeting their responsibilities while allowing themselves to grieve.

Follow-up plans may include follow-up contact. In some practice settings (e.g., a hospice program), the provision of follow-up bereavement counseling is common protocol. In other settings the crisis worker needs to develop a plan for follow-up contact with the survivor. Safety planning with survivors may be necessary with certain types of loss. Fears regarding suicidal behavior among those surviving the loss of a loved one to suicide are common. The crisis worker must assess the lethality of suicidal ideations and engage in safety planning if the situation warrants it. The crisis worker must also assess lethality with survivors of violent death who are experiencing homicidal impulses or fantasies.

If the single-session crisis intervention does not occur soon after the loss but is rather an "anniversary reaction" to the loss, the crisis worker can follow the steps outlined, explaining that this is a common experience for survivors. Additionally, follow-up planning should include an assessment for the presence of complicated grief reactions or forms of "disenfranchised grief" that the survivor is just getting in touch with. In those cases, referrals for ongoing crisis counseling as well as for a support group would be indicated.

ONGOING CRISIS COUNSELING

As we have noted, survivors of loss are often at risk for complicated grief reactions that may last for months or years after the loss of a loved one with little relief of emotional pain and ongoing difficulty accommodating to the loss. In those cases in which complicating circumstances interfere, ongoing crisis counseling can focus on the longer-term process of adjusting to and reconciling with the loss. This section provides an overview of the goals and processes of ongoing developmental-ecological crisis counseling with those experiencing the crisis of death. It concludes with a case example.

Establishing a Supportive and Empowering Counseling Relationship

When an individual seeks counseling for bereavement issues, special consideration must be given to creating a safe, supportive environment in which the raw, vulnerable, and violated feelings that are often associated with the death of a loved one can be expressed. When the loss of the beloved was sudden and unexpected, the survivor may feel stripped of power and control, making it critical to create an empowering environment in which he or she can feel safe to grieve. Additionally, acknowledging early in the working relationship that no feeling is "off limits" and that any expression of felt loss can be given voice is important for the development of trust and the experience of support. In creating a supportive milieu, it is also important to help the survivor feel in control of the pace of the grief process. This ownership of control and the regaining of self-efficacy in the face of what may feel like betrayal and violation also aids in building an empowering rapport with the bereaved.

Assessment

The crisis worker's counseling must assess and address the client's unique grief process, which in some cases may be fraught with denial. If the presenting issue has not been overtly stated as grief over a death, but rather as vague signs of grief such as ongoing and disruptive crying, the crisis worker must explore with the client what may be triggering the crying. If the crisis of death is uncovered through collaborative exploration, the counselor can support the survivor through the often circuitous process of coming to terms with the reality of his or her loss.

Educating the client regarding the normal stages of grief, including denial and tears, can illuminate and clarify the next steps that might be needed to reconcile and integrate the death. The counselor can offer the grieving client patience, sensitivity, and compassion, as grief work is not linear but rather cyclical in nature. In the case of complicated grief, perhaps due to the nature of the premorbid relationship or due to the disenfranchised nature of the grief, special supports and education may be needed to address being stuck in a particular aspect of the grief process. For example, in the case of a lesbian whose life partner was tragically killed in a car accident who never felt free to publicly grieve her loss, giving her a forum to express her pain, isolation, and loneliness can help her come to terms with what this loss meant in her life. This expression of the normal feelings of loss that have been truncated because social contexts did not permit their expression can lift the burden of unshared grief and facilitate the continuance of the grief process.

Utilizing Wolfelt's (1992) "criteria for reconciliation" as one measurement in assessing stability, adjustment, and mastery, the crisis worker can help the survivor conceptualize the criteria for determining whether goals have been achieved. These criteria include the renewed capacity to enjoy experiences in life that are normally enjoyable, the ability to establish new and healthy relationships, the attempt to plan one's life for the future, being comfortable with the way things are rather than trying to make things as they were, acknowledging new parts of oneself that have been discovered in one's grief journey, being compassionate with oneself when intense grief recurs (e.g., holidays, anniversaries), and having the capacity to acknowledge that the pain of loss is an inherent part of life resulting from the ability to give and receive love.

Ongoing Crisis Counseling Goals and Processes

Affect stability:
Assist survivors to express and process memories and emotions related to the crisis of death.

Asking the survivor to repeat the story of how the death occurred can alert the counselor who listens carefully to possible "sticking points." Points in the story-telling when the survivor gets choked up or cannot recall or drastically distorts details, either by overemphasizing or underemphasizing them, can alert the counselor to possible areas for future sensitive work. Verbal and nonverbal "listening" is critical in hearing the full impact of the crisis. The survivor who wraps her knees up under her lap as she recalls the horrifying details of her loved one's death is informing the counselor of important feelings. Gradually, individuals must be assisted to express the range of emotions (e.g., anger sadness, guilt) that they previously experienced as intolerable and debilitating.

Behavioral adjustments:
Assist survivors to make and sustain necessary behavioral changes.

Specific behaviors can be constructive or destructive to the grief process and/or to the survivor's functioning. Behavior is thus an essential domain to assess as survivors share the story of their loss and describe their subsequent efforts to cope with the reality of a changed life. For example, in the case of a survivor who has been identified as a recovering alcoholic, the effective counselor will ask about the void that has been created by the loss of a loved one, in part to identify the risk of relapse. The counselor should attempt to determine what the survivor is doing constructively and/or destructively as he or she attempts to fill the void created by the loved one's death. A referral to specifically address maintaining sobriety or a referral for drug and alcohol treatment may be a critical component of that survivor's healing process.

Concomitantly, individuals must be assisted to resume and/or create new healthy behaviors that can help them heal. This might include improved eating and sleeping patterns or seeking assistance with parenting if the responsibilities of parenting have become overwhelming.

Cognitive mastery:
Assist survivors to utilize beliefs, expectations, and personal meanings that optimize understanding and reconciliation of the death.

As a survivor "tells the story" of the death crisis, assumptions about responsibility and the meaning of life and death may arise that the counselor and survivor must explore together. For example, when a counselor is working with a child whose parent was killed in an automobile accident, a child might say, "If I hadn't been mad at my mom and *wished that she were dead* the day before the accident, then maybe she would still be alive today." The cognitive developmental stage of this child has contributed to a distorted belief about personal responsibility for a death over which, in reality, the child could have no influence or control. Explaining and clarifying the facts of the accident can help alleviate irrational guilt based on faulty assumptions and developmentally immature cognitions.

Additionally, as the story unfolds from the viewpoint of the survivor, the sensitive crisis worker makes note of a belief system or worldview that may be troubling to the client. The concept of God being a "just and fair God" may be difficult for the parent addressing the loss of a newborn baby. Helping the client to identify and name this internal dissonance and to have the courage to wrestle with it can be a sensitive yet important component of grief work. Workers must be aware of their own comfort and competency level in this domain, and be able to make knowledgeable referrals to respectable spiritual resources. Clarifying one's values and beliefs can be an important task of healing.

Developmental mastery:
Assist survivors to examine the impact of the death crisis on their stage-of-life needs and to make healthy adjustments.

At what developmental stage was the survivor at the time of the death crisis? How is the survivor reintegrating the deceased into his or her current stage of life? The crisis worker must assess which normal developmental tasks are being attained and which are not, possibly due to the impact of bereavement. A female teenager who has difficulty leaving her mother's side after the sudden death of her father six months before may be struggling with the normal individuation process, which has been thwarted due to the overload on her normal coping skills. The effective counselor strives to address this loss in a manner that honors the present, teaches skills for the future, and acknowledges and remembers the past.

Ecosystem healthy and intact:
Assist survivors to examine and make healthy changes in their personal ecosystem.

Assisting clients to utilize local resources such as support groups, religious affiliations, or community groups is critical for building the alliances that can sustain individuals over time. Grief can be triggered again throughout the life span, particularly at times of major life events such as marriage, childbirth, and retirement. For survivors, having a supportive community can be a source of buoyancy and "emotional health insurance" for navigating life's normal transitions. Particularly true in cases of disenfranchised grief, whether the death of a companion animal or an elderly parent's loss of an adult child, finding supportive resources can help establish connections and alliances that reduce the risk of social isolation and solitary pain during periods of intensified grief.

Discussion with the bereaved about what to expect "down the road" with their grief can be helpful in facilitating the future management of grief. Assisting the survivor to develop tools to manage and process grief such as journaling, drawing, and/or writing a letter to the deceased can help the client feel empowered to manage grief in the future. It is also important to help the survivor identify the signs and symptoms of grief, which can alert the survivor to the need to take care of him- or herself and for possible professional support in the future.

CASE EXAMPLE: MARLENE

Ongoing Crisis Counseling

Marlene's husband, Andy, died one year ago in an industrial accident, leaving her to raise two young daughters (ages five and seven) with no viable means of support. She had been married for ten years and was a full-time homemaker and mother prior to her husband's death. When she met with the crisis counselor for the first time, she described the first year after Andy's death as "living in a fog." Marlene was overwhelmed with the details of the funeral, her daughters' daily needs, decisions about education and/or work, and pursuit of a wrongful death lawsuit against her husband's employer. On the first anniversary of his death, she decided it was time to finally begin to sort through and pack his clothes and belongings for storage. As she went through his personal effects, Marlene discovered numerous cards and letters from a woman with whom he had apparently been involved in an affair. Since that time she has told no one about her discovery and she has been crying uncontrollably, not participating in her vocational retraining, and becoming progressively more depressed. Finally, realizing that she was heading for a breakdown, Marlene decided to seek crisis counseling. She is furious with her husband for his deception, deeply hurt by his apparent unfaithfulness, and preoccupied with memories of the funeral and the fact that she couldn't bring herself to cover her husband's face with the casket blanket before the casket was closed. She is angry that God would punish her with this fate. There are no indications of suicidal ideation, intent, and/or plan.

Intervention

Marlene arranged an appointment with a crisis counselor known for specializing in working with clients who have experienced loss. In the first session, the crisis counselor began to establish a supportive and empowering relationship with Marlene by employing active listening skills and making supportive statements while Marlene related the events of the past year. She reported the "roller-coaster" nature of her feelings toward her husband, describing how in one moment she could be missing him intensely, and then in another feeling so angry and hurt at him for having the affair that she would yell out loud how glad she was that he died. She then acknowledged that these outbursts were followed by guilt and sobbing over expressing anger toward her deceased husband. She also presented her belief that she is a bad mother because she has been irritable with her daughters and engaged in confrontations with them over their chores. Marlene told the counselor that she wanted to stop feeling so "up and down," to be a better mother to her daughters, and to remember only the good things about her marriage with Andy.

The counselor's assessment was that Marlene was still in the earliest phase of grief resolution. She neither appears to have been able to accept the reality of her husband's death nor has she allowed herself to experience the corresponding emotions. From a behavioral adjustment view, although she has managed to perform the necessary activities (e.g., running the household, paying bills) of the last year, she has engaged in a level of compulsive overworking and "busy-ness" that has not allowed time for thinking or feeling and, ultimately, grieving. If anything, her level of activity has contributed to physical and emotional exhaustion that has been recently exacerbated by the revelation of her husband's affair.

From a cognitive mastery standpoint, she has been unable to engage in the process of integrating her husband's death or the totality of the marriage experience. At this point in her grief, she has been unable to attribute any acceptable meaning to her husband's death, and she is struggling with her spirituality. Core beliefs about her life, purpose, and religion have come into question for her. The cognitive dissonance she has suffered in the year since his death has intensified with the evidence of her husband's relationship with another woman, calling into question her beliefs and memories about her marriage.

From a developmental mastery standpoint, she has pursued needed vocational retraining but remains stagnated in regard to both her relationship needs and proactive planning for her future as a single parent. She has experienced a significant and disruptive discontinuity in her development, as what she expected to be the normal progression of her life has been altered permanently by the loss of her husband and the loss of her identity as a wife and mother.

From an ecosystemic standpoint, she has begun to isolate herself from her family of origin and from her deceased husband's family, which has resulted in a lack of support for herself and her children. She has also been hesitant to burden her friends with her grief for fear of alienating them or causing discomfort. The isolation she has experienced since the funeral has served to widen the gap between Marlene and the interpersonal supports she desires. Although she has sought out environmental resources for vocational retraining, she has yet to draw on other resources such as partner grief groups or women she knows whose partners have also died.

As part of the first session, the counselor briefly described the "normal" grieving process and suggested to Marlene that her grief was complicated by the way her husband died, the "fog" of the first year following his death, and the recent revelation of Andy's affair. Marlene and the counselor ended with an agreement to work on helping her resolve her husband's loss and the surrounding issues.

In the second session, the crisis counselor began by asking Marlene to describe her emotional response to the first session.

CW: *Marlene, it's been a week since our first session and I just want to start out by asking your reaction to the first session.*

Marlene: I have mixed feelings. On one hand, it felt good to share my feelings because nobody in my family and none of my friends want to hear about Andy, and I couldn't bear to hurt them by telling them things that would only hurt them more. I should be over this by now. Everyone tells me how well I did, how well the girls look, and how well I look. But they're wrong. I'm not doing OK, and I know I'm not doing it right.

CW: *What is it that you're not doing right?*

Marlene: *(a long pause followed by her eyes filling with tears).* I'm not being an adult. I see other women who have lost their husbands and they go on. They even get married again. Why can't I get over this?

CW: *Something is stopping you from getting over Andy's death?*

Marlene: I feel as though I've been trying to do that but it doesn't work. I just want it to be over with.

CW: *Marlene, I've noticed that you seem to have a hard time saying that Andy is dead. I notice you use words like "passed" and "lost," and that you don't say the word "died."*

Marlene: I know he's dead but. . . . *(Marlene continues to cry)*

CW: *Part of me wonders whether you ever got a chance to even cry at Andy's funeral.*

Marlene: I couldn't. I had too many people to meet. Andy's mother was a mess, and the girls kept running around with their cousins. I had to take care of everything.

CW: *And taking care of everything hasn't stopped until recently.*

Marlene: I figured keeping busy was good. If I kept doing things, I wouldn't feel depressed. If I kept moving, I wouldn't have to . . . I wouldn't have to . . . *(begins to sob again).*

CW: *You wouldn't have to grieve Andy's death.*

Marlene: Yes . . . yes . . . yes. Why do you keep making me say he's dead? Why do you want me to keep admitting he's dead?

CW: *I think you've held your feelings back for such a long time in order to protect yourself from the reality of Andy's death. You've held them back and it may have allowed you to get through the first year, but I think you recognize that burying your feelings is not working anymore. If anything, the feelings seem to be overflowing. I believe that you're capable of handling these feelings and I also believe that the grieving process will not go forward until you acknowledge Andy's death and allow yourself to feel it.*

Marlene: I couldn't pull the blanket over him before they closed the casket. I just couldn't.

CW: *It sounds almost as though you didn't want to say good-bye.*

The case of Marlene is an example of an ongoing crisis counseling intervention in the grief process associated with her husband's sudden and violent death. As the counselor meets with Marlene, he utilizes empathic and empowering interventions as he strives to deepen the trust and relationship connection with Marlene. He is aware that helping Marlene resolve the complicated grief she is experiencing will require a significant level of trust, especially when the focus shifts to her husband's affair. Based on what Marlene has revealed about the first year after her husband's death, the counselor hypothesizes that Marlene did not have an unfettered opportunity to grieve and determines that he must help her face her husband's death and the painful feelings that emerge. He believes that Marlene will be unable to go on with her emotional life fully unless she is finally able face the reality of his death. Asking Marlene to say and listen to the words *death* and *died* over and over again cements this reality and helps her avoid words like *passed* or *lost,* which imply temporary absence. Denial of her husband's death (even subtle denial) only perpetuates the unresolved issues surrounding his death and stops Marlene from expressing her feelings and confronting the irrational beliefs she has come to have about herself and her marriage. The counselor viewed her preoccupation with her inability to pull the casket blanket over his body as a metaphor for her difficulty in saying good-bye to her husband and adjusting to a world in which he is no longer present.

In the following set of interventions, the crisis counselor attempted to help Marlene examine her core belief system, expectations, and personal meanings, which have been threatened by Andy's death:

CW: *Marlene, you mentioned feeling angry with God over Andy being taken from you. Can you tell me a little more about that?*

Marlene: I am angry with God. I went to church regularly. I brought my children up believing in God. We've been a good family. Andy was a good man. How could God treat me this way?

CW: *Is it OK for you to be angry with your God?*

Marlene: I know that people say that God only gives us what we can handle, but why do I have to go through this? Why do my girls have to go through life without a father?

CW: *You're angry that you've done everything in your life as best you can and it feels as though you're being punished for something you didn't do.*

Marlene: Right. I haven't been back to church since Andy died. Neither have the girls. My in-laws want to take them but I won't hear of it.

CW: *It seems it would be helpful if you could find some way to understand Andy's death. A way of making sense of his loss to you and the girls. Andy's death has caused you to question many things that seemed so fundamental before.*

Marlene: Yeah, it has. It's too much. I've had to learn how to do everything on my own . . . like changing tires, mowing the lawn, and all of it. And take care of everything and everyone else at the same time.

CW: *It makes sense to me that you want to find some answers and that you're searching for some meaning or truth or just an answer of some sort. Have you found any?*

Marlene: No . . . I haven't, even when I talk to my minister. I just don't want to hear about God's will and that Andy's in a better place and that I'll see him when I die. I want answers down here. I want answers that don't require waiting. Nothing seems to help.

CW: *It's almost as if the constant search for answers makes life harder and in some ways keeps you chasing your tail. Does that make sense when I say it that way?*

Marlene: A little. I don't know how to stop it. My mind just keeps on going from the moment I wake up until the moment I go to sleep.

CW: *I'm wondering if you can begin to see that this type of searching for answers is part of the grieving process. I've talked to a lot of people through the years whose loved ones have died and I've had people who were dear to me die, too. It seems as though we always ask, "Why?" We try to make sense out of something that hurts us so deeply. Almost as if there has to be a reason. And when we don't find any answers, we start to question the whole shooting match: ourselves, our lives, our thoughts, and our feelings. Everything ends up under the microscope.*

Marlene: I have to make sense of Andy's death. And his life.

CW: *I agree. But it seems as though the harder we try, the worse we feel. As if we're trying to push the process. And truthfully, I'm not sure about the quality of our thinking when we're grieving. Grief is a process that is unique to each of us. No one can tell you how to do it or how long it's going to hurt.*

Marlene: I just want it to be over. I want my life back. I know Andy and I. . . . I know my life will never be the same. I just want to be happy at least part of the time.

CW: *I agree, Marlene. Life will never be the same. At the same time, the past and what you had with Andy will always exist in your memories, in your children, and in your heart. You'll never forget him. It doesn't work that way.*

Marlene: I'm afraid of that. It's almost as if some people have forgotten him already, and they want me to forget him. They tell me that it's time to move on. Time to go out and get a father for my girls. I just can't do that.

CW: *And there's no reason you ever have to do anything you don't want to. The way you live your life is up to you.*

The crisis counselor opened up the discussion of Marlene's beliefs, expectations, and personal meanings that have been threatened by asking directly about her spiritual conflict. Many clinicians are averse to talking about anything associated with a client's spiritual or religious beliefs. Spiritual beliefs, however, are central to many clients' lives and a counselor can assist a client in exploring these beliefs, especially when they concern the grieving process. As demonstrated above, a crisis counselor can encourage a client's reflection without revealing his or her own values or steering the client in a particular direction.

Throughout the previous set of interventions, the crisis counselor was empathic and empowering to Marlene. Appropriate self-disclosure can be helpful because clients can see that you have struggled with a crisis similar to the one they are experiencing. The counselor attempted to normalize Marlene's reactions by suggesting that she view her questioning as part of the grieving process experienced by many people whose partners have died. He went on to further suggest that Marlene's grieving process is unique to her and, even more important, determined by her. This empowering position affirms Marlene's grief as individual and normal. Grieving people become hypersensitive to how others react to their expressions of grief and tend to make assumptions that are often not borne out by reality. For example, Marlene feels uncomfortable sharing her reactions with anyone close to her for fear of rejection, overwhelming others, or being perceived as not getting on with her life. Affirming her individual grieving process entitles her to her own feelings, her own timetable, and her right to grieve in her own way. She can choose what to share as well as when, where, to whom, and how to share it. She doesn't have to compare her grief to other people's grief. She doesn't have to feel any less entitled to her feelings. Reaffirming grief as a process also provides the crisis counselor with a context for normalizing the many reactions the client will have on the road to grief resolution. The crisis counselor's empowerment of Marlene extends to the developmental tasks that she will eventually need to master if she is going to continue to grow and change as an individual, as a mother, and as a potential partner in future relationships. There is an inherent recognition of a future for Marlene and a recognition that she will decide when to broach new ground.

In the following sequence, the crisis counselor confronts the issue of her husband's affair and attempts to help Marlene process her emotions regarding that relationship and suggests ways that she can resolve the conflict that has precipitated the current crisis.

CW: *Marlene, an issue that has been looming in the background since we first started working together was your finding the cards and letters that Andy apparently had hidden from you. When you read those cards and letters, you concluded that he had been seeing another woman and was, in fact, still having an affair at the time that he died.*

Marlene: I have no doubt of it. When I start to piece together some of the things he said and did in the months preceding his death, it becomes even more obvious.

CW: *How did you feel when you first came across the cards and letters?*

Marlene: How do you think I felt? *(begins to tear up and cry)* I'm crying my eyes out as I gather his things together so I can save things for our girls and keep things that were important to both of us, and I find cards and letters from someone else telling Andy how much she loves him and describing their love-making. *(sobbing and trembling)* I loved him so much and this is what he leaves me with. I gave him everything and he stabbed me in the back. I can't live with knowing that.

CW: *Your realization of his betrayal is overwhelming.*

Marlene: *(continues to sob heavily for a few minutes and repeats her husband's name)* Andy . . . Andy . . . Andy . . . Andy . . .

CW: *It was hard enough losing Andy, but it seems as though now you have experienced a double loss.*

Marlene: Yes . . . my husband died, but now my trust in him has also died. My marriage died. I'm so angry at myself for not seeing it. For not knowing something was up. I'll never trust another man in my life, so help me, God.

CW: *It sounds as if one of the big things you're questioning is whether the marriage and your relationship with Andy was a sham.*

Marlene: Yes.

CW: *You're questioning whether he really loved you and the girls.*

Marlene: I know he loved the girls. They were his pride and joy. He always talked about them and always looked forward to spending time with them whenever he could. I know he loved the girls.

CW: *You're just not sure whether he loved you. Do you know if you loved him?*

Marlene: The relationship changed over the years and there wasn't the same old spark we used to have in the beginning, but I know that I still loved him. I'm angry with myself for loving him at all.

CW: *Why is that?*

Marlene: How can you love someone who doesn't love and respect you back?

CW: *Sounds as though you're pretty clear that he didn't love you or respect you.*

Marlene: You don't respect someone you're supposed to love when you do what he did.

CW: *It's hard to remember anything good about your marriage to Andy, given what you found out.*

Marlene: I try to keep focused on good things that happened in our marriage but the thought of him being with someone else just keeps coming into my head.

CW: *Those thoughts interfere with your ability to feel good about your life with Andy or to believe in his love for you.*

Marlene: To make matters worse, I keep pulling out the cards and letters and rereading them. When I go out of my house, I look around to see if anyone is staring at me because I think I'm going to figure out who she is.

CW: *So you're really doing a job on yourself. Not only do you torture yourself with the thought of Andy betraying you, but you put salt in the wound by going over and over the cards and letters.*

Marlene: Sounds pretty sick, doesn't it?

CW: *I'm not sure "sick" is the right word, Marlene, but it certainly doesn't seem to be doing you any good. Would you agree?*

Marlene: Definitely.

CW: *Yet something keeps you coming back to them.*

Marlene: I keep wanting to believe that it's not true. That they're someone else's letters. That it's someone else's life. I guess I just don't want to accept it.

CW: *Makes sense, because if you accepted it, then what?*

Marlene: *(pauses for a minute)* If I accepted it, then I'd have to live with knowing that Andy did that to the girls and me. I'd have to accept that there were good things about him and pretty rotten things about him. I'd have to accept that he wasn't all that I thought he was.

CW: *Does it make you love him any less?*

Marlene: No, I was never unfaithful. I gave him everything I had . . . and then some. I never lied to him. Never.

CW: *So what I hear you saying is that other than not knowing about Andy's relationship with this other woman, you have nothing to feel guilty about. Nothing to feel ashamed of. In fact . . . everything to feel good about when it comes to your being a good wife and partner.*

Marlene: I guess so, when you put it that way.

CW: *Is there some reason or need for you to punish yourself, Marlene?*

Marlene: No. There's no reason. And there's no reason I need to keep hurting myself with these cards and letters. *(pulls cards and letters from her purse)* What do you think I need to do with them?

CW: *I'm not sure, Marlene. What would give you a sense of closure to this aspect of Andy's death?*

Marlene: I think I need to start fresh. Not forgetting . . . but I need to start living without these reminders. I don't want to tell anybody about Andy's affair and I especially don't ever want the girls coming across them. Ever. Their relationship with their dad is totally separate from this.

CW: *Sounds as though you just want to say good-bye to this memory and move on without the reminders.*

Marlene: You're right. *(begins to rip up the cards and letters and throws them in the wastebasket)*

The crisis counselor tapped into the difficult subject of Andy's affair, which precipitated the current crisis for Marlene. By not taking a judgmental position and not trying to convince Marlene to take a particular viewpoint, the counselor helped empower her to draw her own conclusions about the affair. The counselor assisted her to consider the self-destructive aspects of her ruminative behaviors (thinking about the affair and rereading the cards and letters). In addition, the counselor helped Marlene recognize the connection between the way she tortured herself with reminders of Andy's transgression and her inability to move forward. As their session continued, Marlene began to conclude that Andy had strengths as well as weaknesses. Some of those weaknesses were quite painful to her, but she gradually began to see shades of gray instead of polar opposites. She also began to acknowledge that to engage in self-destructive behavior that made her feel worse was her choice rather than something over which she had no control. The crisis counselor made that choice clear, and the client decided to terminate that behavior. In assisting Marlene to express and process her feelings regarding her deceased husband's affair, the counselor encouraged her not to be afraid of her feelings and affirmed the worthiness of expressing them. Marlene then was more able to examine painful issues and to reframe generalizations she made about herself or her life.

In a later session, the crisis counselor worked with Marlene to begin making changes that optimize her personal and social functioning in her own ecosystem:

CW: *Marlene, I felt very good about the work you did in our last session. I feel that we broke some new ground and that you freed yourself from some thoughts and behaviors that have held you back.*

Marlene: I agree. I felt much lighter all week and slept a lot better.

CW: *How do you explain that?*

Marlene: I feel as though I'm starting to come out of the fog and I'm starting to believe that I can do something to reclaim my life . . . and my future. I was beginning to believe that there was no future.

CW: *That's great. Why don't we spend some time looking at some steps you might take in that direction?*

Marlene: Baby steps, right?

CW: *Only the steps you feel ready to take and where you feel that it's worth the effort.*

Marlene: Where do you think I need to be able to go?

CW: *Good question. What do you think you need at this point in your life?*

Marlene: I need to be around other adults, and I need the girls to be around other kids who can understand what it's like to lose a parent.

CW: *You want the girls to be in an environment where they can interact with other kids who have also gone through losing someone close to them. I guess I also hear the same thing holds true for you.*

Marlene: Yeah . . . I don't want to have to explain everything that's happened, but I also don't want to feel as though I'm from outer space if I do begin to talk about Andy or anything connected to him.

CW: *Have you thought about anyplace where you can do that or where the girls can do that or even where you can do that with the girls?*

Marlene: I have a friend who went through a tough divorce two years ago and was left with a son who's in the same grade as Leah, my older girl. She's been trying to get me to go to Parents Without Partners (PWP) with her. I just haven't felt up to it.

CW: *How do you feel about it at this point?*

Marlene: I think it would be good for me. I think it would be good for the girls. She told me there are other parents whose spouses have died, too. They meet once a month and usually it's some type of family activity. I just don't want to be hit on and I certainly don't want to get involved with someone who has a bunch of kids who need a mother. *(laughs out loud)*

CW: *Just what you need, huh? I guess you could try it out and see how it goes. Knowing someone in PWP certainly doesn't hurt. Sounds as if it could be fun.*

Marlene: When I think about it, I realize that I do have friends and family who care about me. As much as I'm angry with God right now, our minister has called me to check in on me pretty regularly. Even without my going to church. I've been thinking of calling him and seeing if it's too late to get the girls involved in some youth group activities.

CW: *Those all sound like helpful ideas. What are you going to do for yourself?*

Marlene: Well, those things are for me, too. In some ways, I think I've been over-involved with the girls and just trying to make sure that everything always goes right.

CW: *That's a lot of pressure. On you and on the girls, too.*

Marlene: I suppose you're right. I need time away from them as much as they need time away from me. I'm back at school and I'm actually liking it. That's for me. Long after the girls are gone, I'll still need to fend for myself financially.

CW: *That sounds like a good start. Is there anything else you need to be doing?*

Marlene: If you mean dating, no, I'm not ready for that. The girls aren't either.

CW: *No, I didn't mean that, but I guess I hear that it's not out of the question . . . at some point! At some point you might be willing to entertain the thought.*

Marlene: I suppose. I certainly miss being held and cuddled. I guess that's a good sign. Isn't it?

CW: *Sounds pretty normal to me.*

Crisis counseling with Marlene took place over a three-month period. As the crisis abated, Marlene was able to begin to think more clearly about her past and her future. She began to acknowledge her own needs as being important and to acknowledge that her girls' needs sometimes extended beyond what she alone could realistically provide for them. She will become increasingly more drawn to the external world as her needs emerge and as she begins to get back on track developmentally. The crisis counselor encouraged her to think of options and to weigh them carefully in terms of cost versus benefit. As individual counseling ended, Marlene had made significant inroads toward reconnecting with friends, family, and other support systems. Her involvement in PWP and a grief support group and her use of other community resources for herself and her family will continue to improve her level of personal and social functioning through increased interpersonal relationships.

Case Synopsis

The goals of the crisis counseling intervention model include affect stability, behavioral adjustment, cognitive mastery, developmental mastery, and a healthy and intact ecosystem. When the model is applied to Marlene's case, the following conclusions could be drawn as crisis counseling was terminated.

Affect stability

Marlene is more able to openly discuss her husband's death and the affair with a tolerable and appropriate range of emotion. From a grief resolution standpoint, she can more easily allow herself to experience the range of emotions associated with her husband's death, but then bring them to a close until the next time she decides to revisit her loss.

Behavioral adjustment

Marlene has become acutely aware of some of the self-destructive behaviors that she engaged in as a result of unresolved conflict and complicated grieving. She is aware that working too hard can interfere with her relationship with her daughters and her own free time to think and mourn her husband's death. She has also been able to stop torturing herself by rereading the cards and letters from her husband's affair. She has returned to her educational training and has ended her self-imposed isolation from family and friends.

Cognitive mastery

Marlene has reframed her thinking about the affair and has gained some perspective on her marriage and her roles as wife and mother. There are some initial indications of a renewed optimism for life and a renewed commitment to her core beliefs.

Developmental mastery

Marlene has begun to refocus on the life tasks of a young woman and is beginning to make plans that hold potential for her future as employee, mother, and partner. The discontinuity she experienced with her husband's death and the perpetuation of that suspended state of development exacerbated by her deceased husband's affair has become less significant in her life and she is more able to continue her path of normal development.

Ecosystem healthy and intact

Marlene is once more beginning to engage with the outside world. The pursuit of activities for her girls, for her family as a unit, and for herself is occurring on several different fronts including PWP, her church's youth group, and her continued involvement with a grief support group. Her gradual reconnecting with friends and family will provide many more options for obtaining support.

DISCUSSION QUESTIONS AND EXERCISES

1. Identify a personal experience of grief, whether through death or another type of loss, and reflect on the effect of this loss on the various domains of your life: friendships, family, neighbors, finances, behavior, belief systems, thought patterns, values, and so on. In what ways might your own grief experience affect your work with clients experiencing the crisis of death?

2. Make a list of the common, or "pat," answers that are often offered to a person experiencing the crisis of death. What are the potential unintended consequences of these "heard messages" and how might they impede the process of mourning? List six therapeutically effective counseling responses to the crisis of death. What are the consequences and "felt messages" that might support both crisis counseling and mourning?

3. In groups of three, take turns playing the role of crisis counselor, client, and observer. Role-play a case in which an aging father has recently experienced the death of his adult male child or create a case of your own choosing. Have each participant choose a different goal of ongoing crisis counseling: affect stability, behavioral stability, cognitive mastery, developmental mastery, or ecosystem stabilization. Then, in fifteen-minute increments, take turns role-playing this specific crisis counseling goal. After each role-play, take five minutes to discuss it and give constructive feedback to the crisis counselor regarding application of the crisis counseling model.

REFERENCES

Bowen, M. (1985). *Family therapy in clinical practice*. New York: Jason Aronson, Inc.

Bowlby, J. (1961). Processes of mourning. *International Journal of Psycho-Analysis, 42,* 317–340.

Bowlby, J. (1980). *Attachment and loss: Vol. 3. Loss: Sadness and depression*. New York: Basic Books.

Canda, E. R., & Furman, L. D. (1999). *Spiritual diversity in social work practice: The heart of helping*. New York: Free Press.

Centers for Disease Control. (2001, September 21). *National vital statistics report for 1999*. Atlanta: Author.

Cook, A. S., & Dworkin, D. S. (1992). *Helping the bereaved: Therapeutic interventions for children, adolescents and adults*. New York: Basic Books.

Costello, A., Gardner, S. L., & Merenstein, G. B. (1988). Perinatal grief and loss. *Journal of Perinatology, 4,* 361–370.

Doka, K. J. (Ed.). (1989). *Disenfranchised grief: Recognizing hidden sorrow*. Lexington, MA: Lexington Books.

Doka, K. J. (1996). Commentary by Kenneth J. Doka. In K. J. Doka (Ed.), *Living with grief after sudden loss: Suicide, homicide, accident, heart attack, stroke* (pp. 11–15). Washington, DC: Hospice Foundation of America.

Doka, K. J. (Ed.). (1997). *Living with grief when illness is prolonged*. Washington, DC: Hospice Foundation of America.

Erikson, E. H. (1968). *Identity: Youth and crisis*. New York: W. W. Norton.

Fukuyama, M. A., & Sevig, T. D. (1999). *Integrating spirituality into multicultural counseling*. Thousand Oaks, CA: Sage.

Hersh, S. P. (1996). After heart attack and stroke. In K. J. Doka (Ed.), *Living with grief after sudden loss: Suicide, homicide, accident, heart attack, stroke* (pp. 17–24). Washington, DC: Hospice Foundation of America.

Irish, D. P. (1995). Children and death: Diversity and universality. In E. Grollman (Ed.), *Bereaved children and teens: A support guide for parents and professionals* (pp. 77–91). Boston: Beacon Press.

Kubler-Ross, E. (1969). *On death and dying*. New York: Macmillan.

Lazare, A. (1979). Unresolved grief. In A. Lazare (Ed.), *Outpatient psychiatry: Diagnosis and treatment* (pp. 498–512). Baltimore: Williams and Wilkens.

Lewis, C. S. (1961). *A grief observed*. New York: Seabury Press.

Lindemann, E. (1944). Symptomatology and management of acute grief. *American Journal of Psychiatry, 101,* 141–148.

Lund, D. A., Caserta, M. S., & Dimond, M. F. (1993). The course of spousal bereavement in later life. In M. S. Stroebe, W. Stroebe, & R. O. Hansson (Eds.), *Handbook of bereavement: Theory, research, and intervention* (pp. 240–254). Victoria, Australia: Cambridge University Press.

McCrae, R. R., & Costa, P. T. (1993). Psychological resilience among widowed men and women: A ten-year follow-up of a national sample. In M. S. Stroebe, W. Stroebe, & R. O. Hansson (Eds.), *Handbook of bereavement: Theory, research, and intervention* (pp. 196–207). Victoria, Australia: Cambridge University Press.

Myers, E. (1986). *When parents die: A guide for adults*. New York: Viking.

Nisly, P. W. (1992). *Sweeping up the heart: A father's lament for his daughter*. Intercourse, PA: Good Books.

Ostfeld, B. M., Ryan, T., Hiatt, M., & Hegyi, T. (1993). Maternal grief after sudden infant death syndrome. *Journal of Developmental and Behavioral Pediatrics, 14,* 156–162.

Parkes, C. M. (1974). "Seeking" and "finding" a lost object: Evidence from recent studies of the reaction to bereavement. In *Normal and pathological responses to bereavement (Series on attitudes toward death)*. New York: MSS Information Corporation. (First published in *Social Science and Medicine*, 1970, 4, 187–201.)

Parkes, C. M., & Weiss, R. S. (1983). *Recovery from bereavement*. New York: Basic Books.

Rando, T. A. (1984). *Grief, dying and death: Clinical interventions for caregivers*. Champaign, IL: Research Press.

Rando, T. A. (1988). *Grieving: How to go on living when someone you love dies.* Lexington, MA: Lexington Books.

Rando, T. A. (1993). *Treatment of complicated mourning.* Champaign, IL: Research Press.

Rando, T. A. (1996). Complications in mourning traumatic death. In K. J. Doka (Ed.), *Living with grief after sudden loss: Suicide, homicide, accident, heart attack, stroke.* Washington, DC: Hospice Foundation of America.

Rando, T. A. (Ed.). (2000). *Clinical dimensions of anticipatory mourning: Theory and practice in working with the dying, their loved ones, and their caregivers.* Champaign, IL: Research Press.

Redmond, L. M. (1996). Sudden violent death. In K. J. Doka (Ed.), *Living with grief after sudden loss: Suicide, homicide, accident, heart attack, stroke* (pp. 53–71). Washington, DC: Hospice Foundation of America.

Silverman, P. R., Nickman, S., & Worden, J. W. (1992). Children's reactions in the early months after the death of a parent. *American Journal of Orthopsychiatry, 62,* 93–104.

Stillion, J. M. (1996). Survivors of suicide. In K. J. Doka (Ed.), *Living with grief after sudden loss: Suicide, homicide, accident, heart attack, stroke* (pp. 41–51). Washington, DC: Hospice Foundation of America.

Teyber, E. (2000). *Interpersonal process in psychotherapy: A relational approach* (4th ed.). Belmont, CA: Wadsworth/Thomson Learning.

Walsh, F., & McGoldrick, M. (Eds.). (1991). *Living beyond loss: Death in the family.* New York: W. W. Norton & Company.

Wolfelt, A. D. (1992). *Understanding grief: Helping yourself heal.* Levittown, PA: Accelerated Development.

Worden, J. W. (1982). *Grief counseling and grief therapy: A handbook for mental health.* New York: Springer Publishing Company.

Worden, J. W. (1991). *Grief counseling and grief therapy: A handbook for the mental health practitioner* (2nd ed.). New York: Springer Publishing Company.

Worden, J. W. (1996). *Children and grief: When a parent dies.* New York: Guilford Press.

CHAPTER 11

Crisis Intervention with Abused Children

MICHELE A. TAVORMINA

Henry, age seven, was physically abused by both his mother and his father. Not believing what his parents did was wrong, he protectively said, "They said I was bad. They had to hit me for being bad. They wouldn't hit me so hard if I wasn't so bad." (broken arm and bruises in various stages of healing)

• • •

Matthew, age eleven, was sexually abused by his basketball coach. Fearful of what would happen if he told anyone or if his friends found out, he did not tell anyone until two years after the abuse ended. He said, "You didn't argue with Coach. He didn't like no talkin' back. He's really strong and yelled a lot. You did what he said." (sodomy)

• • •

Amanda, age thirteen, was sexually abused by her stepfather. A sexually explicit note to her stepfather was discovered by her mother, who reported the abuse to Child Protective Services. Amanda testified against her stepfather in criminal court, which resulted in his being sent to jail. Subsequently, she reports feeling forced to admit to the sexual abuse and states that she still feels she betrayed her abuser. She angrily recounts, "He was better to me than my mom. He took me places, bought me stuff, and talked to me. I didn't mind what we did. I felt like a grownup. He didn't treat me like I was a dumb kid to be bossed around. He bought me cigarettes and let me drink beer." (vaginal intercourse)

The belief that all children have basic human rights including protection from abuse, neglect, and exploitation is a relatively modern concept. Societal definitions of child abuse have varied throughout history and across cultures. It is only during the last twenty-five years that abuse of children has become a primary focus of attention by mental health and social service providers and researchers.

Child maltreatment, particularly physical and sexual abuse, has been studied, diagnosed, and treated with increasing frequency over the past two decades. It is now recognized that the problem of childhood physical and sexual abuse has a profound impact not only on those directly victimized but also on the family unit and on society in general. Therefore, treating survivors of childhood abuse effectively and comprehensively is a proactive measure to help prevent a number of individual, social, and community problems.

Prevention of Child Maltreatment

There are three types of programs geared toward preventing childhood abuse: primary, secondary, and tertiary. Primary prevention strategies typically seek to educate the public about problems of child abuse and may focus on one particular facet of prevention such as providing parenting classes or "safe touch" programs to prevent sexual abuse of children. Secondary prevention is usually geared toward identifying those at risk of abusing and often includes providing individualized supportive services such as home visits, counseling, education, or self-help groups like Parents Anonymous. Unlike primary and secondary prevention, tertiary prevention takes place after child abuse has occurred in the family. Its goal is to prevent the further abuse of children, often with the involvement of Child Protective Services (CPS) and a multidisciplinary team to assist the family (Videka-Sherman, 1991). Crisis interventions with abused children most commonly occur at the tertiary level.

Sociopolitical View

Popular perceptions and stereotypes, even when inaccurate, often influence and shape the development and implementation of social policies. It is a popular myth that those who are disadvantaged, victimized, handicapped, or disabled are solely responsible for their condition, and that if they were "stronger" people they would not be in a dependent position (Jansson, 1997). This stereotypic view also impacts the advice and information that people are given about the problem of childhood abuse.

Many abusive parents want to be caring parents to their children but lack the resources, supports, education, and therapeutic services that might assist them to parent their children in appropriate ways. Although having the desire and motivation to change is critical to stopping abusive behavior, tools and resources need to be available to assist families in making needed changes. Our society tends to view social problems like substance abuse, poverty, domestic violence, and child abuse as private problems of particular individuals or families. This blaming viewpoint can deter people from seeking help and perpetuate denial of the problem.

Marginalizing child abuse as a problem that only affects "deviant or socially unacceptable" families grossly misrepresents the scope of child maltreatment in our culture. If one views child abuse as someone else's problem, it is easier to view the individuals involved with contempt rather than as individuals needing assistance. Abuse of children is precipitated by many social and environmental factors including poverty, substance abuse, inadequate social and community supports, educational deficits, environmental stressors, and societal tolerance of violence. The stigma of child abuse leads to secrecy and shame for victims and their families.

PHYSICAL AND SEXUAL ABUSE DEFINED

Federal Government Definitions

Child abuse and neglect are defined by the federal Child Abuse Prevention and Treatment Act (CAPTA), which was first enacted in 1974. The Child Abuse Prevention and Treatment Act is also the primary federal mechanism for the appropriation of funds to support state efforts to prevent, assess, investigate, prosecute, and provide an array of treatment services geared toward the problem of child maltreatment (U.S. Department of Health and Human Services, 2002a).

Although each state's definition may vary, the National Clearinghouse on Child Abuse and Neglect Information (U.S. Department of Health and Human Services, 2002b) identifies four main types of child maltreatment:

Physical abuse is characterized by the infliction of physical injury as a result of punching, beating, kicking, biting, burning, shaking, or otherwise harming a child. The parent or caretaker may not have intended to hurt the child; rather, the injury may have resulted from over-zealous discipline or physical punishment.

Child neglect is characterized by failure to provide for the child's basic needs. Neglect can be physical, educational, or emotional. *Physical neglect* includes refusal of, or delay in, seeking health care; abandonment; expulsion from the home or refusal to allow a runaway to return home; and inadequate supervision. *Educational neglect* includes allowing chronic truancy, failure to enroll a child of mandatory school age in school, and failure to attend to a special educational need. *Emotional neglect* includes such actions as marked inattention to the child's needs for affection; refusal of or failure to provide needed psychological care; spousal abuse in the child's presence; and permission of drug or alcohol use by the child. The assessment of child neglect requires consideration of cultural values and standards of care as well as recognition that the failure to provide the necessities of life may be related to poverty.

Sexual abuse includes fondling a child's genitals, intercourse, incest, rape, oral sex, sodomy, exhibitionism, and commercial exploitation through prostitution or the production of pornographic materials. Many experts believe that sexual abuse is the most underreported form of child maltreatment because of the secrecy or "conspiracy of silence" that so often characterizes these cases.

Emotional abuse (psychological abuse/verbal abuse/mental injury) includes acts or omissions by the parents or other caregivers that have caused, or could cause, serious behavioral, cognitive, emotional, or mental disorders. In some cases of emotional abuse, the acts of parents or other caregivers alone, without any harm evident in the child's behavior or condition, are sufficient to warrant Child Protective Services (CPS) intervention. For example, the parents or caregivers may use extreme or bizarre forms of punishment, such as confining a child in a dark closet. Less severe acts, such as habitual scapegoating, belittling, or rejecting treatment, are often difficult to prove and, therefore, CPS may not be able to intervene without evidence of harm to the child. (pp. 2–3)

Mandated Reporters of Child Abuse

More than one-third of states mandate that all individuals, regardless of profession, report suspected child maltreatment. Although anyone can, and arguably should, report suspected child abuse or neglect, people who work with children or who are in a helping profession are usually mandated by state reporting laws that have penalties such as fines or imprisonment for failing to report known or suspected child maltreatment. Mandated reporters usually include (1) health care professionals, (2) school personnel, (3) mental health professionals, and (4) law enforcement officers and officials.

MANDATED REPORTERS

1. Health care professionals, such as:

   | nurses | physicians |
   | dentists | hospital personnel |

2. School personnel, such as:

teachers	administrators
bus drivers	guidance counselors
school nurses	coaches
teacher's aides	day-care providers

3. Mental health professionals, such as:

counselors	psychologists
therapists	caseworkers
social workers	psychiatrists

4. Law enforcement officers and officials

Definitions and criminal codes for child abuse and neglect vary from state to state because each state enacts legislation to define child abuse and neglect and to establish laws within its respective jurisdiction. Helping professionals should be familiar with the laws governing child abuse and neglect in their state because these laws dictate their responsibility to report suspected child maltreatment and the conditions necessary for intervention by juvenile or family courts on behalf of children.

PREVALENCE OF CHILD ABUSE

Although the true extent of childhood maltreatment is unknown, research indicates that, tragically, it is and has been common in American society. Official reports on child abuse, which reflect only cases reported to child welfare agencies, vary dramatically from information gained from victim surveys. Statistical data presented in this section was compiled by the U.S. Department of Health and Human Services Administration for Children and Families (2001).

Collection of Data

The Administration on Children, Youth and Families (ACYF) Children's Bureau, in partnership with the states, sponsors the National Child Abuse and Neglect Data System (NCANDS), which collects data on the maltreatment of children from each state to disseminate to professionals and the interested public. State data is compiled by local Child Protective Service agencies. CPS agencies exist in every state and are governed by federal and state laws to investigate and report data on referred cases of child abuse or neglect and provide a variety of preventative and protective services including out-of-home placements in foster care when necessary. There are two components of the NCANDS data collection system: (1) the Summary Data Component (SDC), which surveys and collects aggregate data from the states, and (2) the Detailed Case Data Component (DCDC), which collects data at the case level for analysis of multiple variables.

Statistics on Total Initial Referrals

In 1999, CPS agencies received almost 3 million family-based referrals of child abuse and neglect (which may include abuse or neglect of more than one child in the family), of which nearly 1.8 million (60.4 percent) were screened for investigation, meaning that the agency personnel responsible for screening reports concluded that the call met the criteria for further investigation. Approximately one-half million (29.2 percent) of these referrals were deemed either "substantiated" or "indicated" child maltreatment. Approximately one million (54.7 percent) referrals were found to be unsubstantiated—meaning that there was not enough evidence under state law to substantiate. The remaining 16.1 percent were either closed without a finding or categorized as "other," "unknown," or "in need of services."

Statistics on Substantiated or Indicated Referrals

In 1999, approximately 826,000 children were identified as victims of indicated or substantiated maltreatment, which is a rate of 11.8 victims per 1,000 children in the population. Of these, 58.4 percent suffered from neglect; 21.3 percent suffered from physical abuse; 11.3 percent suffered sexual abuse; and 35.9 percent were categorized as victims of "other or additional types of maltreatment." Percentages total more than 100 percent because each child is counted under each type of maltreatment and could be counted more than once. Fifty-two percent of all victims were female. The age group of zero to three years had the highest rate of maltreatment; it must be noted, however, that reports of abuse involving young children are much more likely to be indicated or substantiated given the higher risk assigned to the case because of younger children's greater vulnerability.

Perpetrators

According to 1999 data, 61.8 percent of all perpetrators were females and 38.2 percent were males. For the three main categories of maltreatment, parent perpetrators victimized 91.8 percent of all neglected children, 85 percent of all physically abused children, and 50 percent of all sexually abused children.

Fatalities

In 1999, the national estimated fatality rate of child victims of abuse or neglect was 1.66 per 100,000 children in the population, with male and female deaths nearly equal. This equates to approximately 1,100 child deaths nationally per year or three children each day. Children who died due to child abuse or neglect were usually very young, with deaths declining as age increased to age eight. Almost 43 percent were one year old or younger, and approximately 86 percent were younger than six.

Research on the Prevalence of Childhood Sexual Abuse

Childhood sexual abuse can occur at any time from infancy to late adolescence. Children between the ages of eight and twelve years have a heightened risk for sexual abuse, as extensive research has identified this age group as most vulnerable to sexual victimization (Briere & Runtz, 1988; Briere, Smiljanich, & Henschel, 1994; Finkelhor, Hotaling, Lewis, & Smith, 1990). Some experts suspect the actual onset of sexual abuse may be earlier than the research suggests due to lack of recall of very early sexual victimization (Courtois, 1988; Russell, 1986). Females are almost three times more likely than males to experience some form of abuse, and twelve times more likely to be sexually victimized than males (Silverman, Reinherz, & Giaconia, 1996).

DYNAMICS AND IMPACT

Dynamics and Impact of Physical Abuse

Physical abuse of children includes bruises; burns; head, eye, and abdominal injuries; fractures; and broken bones. Children can sustain permanent physical damage including scars; vision and hearing loss; or brain, organ, or bone damage. And, as previously documented, many children die as a result of child abuse.

The diagnosis and treatment of physical injury is primarily handled by medical personnel, but social service workers often assist in collecting information, working collaboratively with family members and Child Protective Services, and assisting the child cognitively and emotionally in the aftermath of the abuse through counseling and other supportive services.

Although physical injuries resulting from abuse may be treated and healed, the psychological and emotional impairment from the abuse may have a more long-standing and significant impact. Infants or toddlers are most vulnerable to child abuse by caretakers because (1) they are almost entirely dependent on adults for their care and protection; (2) they have limited, if any, cognitive or verbal skills to know the abuse is wrong or to tell someone who could protect them; and (3) the constant demands of caring for an infant or toddler can be particularly frustrating for ill-equipped, immature, overstressed, or substance-abusing caregivers.

Many factors influence how a child copes and heals in the aftermath of physical abuse. Counselors need to obtain information about the family and the extent of maltreatment in order to gain a complete understanding of the child's specific traumas and to assess ways to help the child and the family. Because child abuse is a family problem, family involvement is a key component of preventing further episodes of child abuse and changing the family dynamics that put the child at risk for abuse. Very detailed information about the family system is often sought from a variety of sources involved with the child, including (1) immediate and extended family members, (2) formal and informal caregivers for the child, (3) school personnel, and (4) medical or helping professionals involved with the child or family.

The initial evaluation should include (1) a thorough description of the abuse that has occurred, (2) information pertaining to the individual characteristics of family members, (3) a detailed description of the family system and collective family functioning, (4) a risk assessment of the potential for further harm to the child, and (5) recommendations and requirements for interventions and treatment of the child and family. A comprehensive assessment is often the product of a multidisciplinary team including medical professionals, Child Protective Service workers, school personnel, and mental health providers (Jones, 1997a, 1997b; Pearce & Pezzot-Pearce, 1997).

It is also essential to identify family strengths. For example, positive and growth-enhancing relationships are important sources of assistance for the child and family, as evidenced in the following case:

Tina, age eight, was physically abused for six months by her mother. The abuse mostly consisted of excessive use of force during periodic spankings that often left her buttocks badly bruised and marked. During a Child Protective Services investigation, Tina reported, "I know my mom's not supposed to do that. She didn't spank me like that 'til we moved out of grandma's house. I like it better living with grandma. There was no hitting at grandma's. I was happy there."

Tina's example illustrates the benefits of a natural support system. Tina experienced a positive and nonabusive relationship with her grandmother, who helped protect her from abuse by her mother, and who apparently assisted the mother as well when the family resided together.

Due to physical abuse and comorbid psychological trauma, the emotional needs of chronically abused children are not met. The need for consistent and predictable nurturance, soothing, protection, and comfort from caregivers is typically ignored. A child abuse survivor may thus struggle or fail to synthesize a firm concept of loved ones who provided nurturance, protection, and kindness. This loss impacts both the child's ability to internalize a positive self-image and the child's ability to cultivate nurturing qualities within themselves (Beebe & Lachmann, 1988; Mahler, Pine, & Bergman, 1975; Winnicott, 1953, 1958).

The external world can seem hostile, dangerous, and unpredictable to an abused child. As a result, the child is forced to devote significant emotional and psychological resources to maintain survival and basic functioning, which, in turn, diminishes the resources available for normal developmental tasks.

Tommy, age fifteen, recounts, "It wasn't a day if I didn't get beat. I knew it was coming. I just didn't know when. I thought about when it was coming a lot when I was little. Most other kids think about stupid stuff like being popular, getting girls, or doing well in school. I think about how I'm gonna stay out of the house so I don't get my ass kicked."

Over time, the disorganizing effects of severe child abuse can erode the child's ability to cope with the psychological trauma and may result in mental health impairments including attachment problems, posttraumatic stress, depression, anxiety, dissociation, and developmental or conduct disturbances (Jones, 1997a, 1997b; Pearce & Pezzot-Pearce, 1997; van der Kolk, 1999).

Long-term effects of child abuse   Children experience a variety of long- and short-term impairments due to maltreatment. Abused children may have problems behaving in socially acceptable ways and in relating to peers, and may thus be rejected for seeming different. They may also isolate themselves from peer encounters, be removed or aloof from others, have unstable relationships, or have heightened dependency needs in relationships (Jones, 1997a, 1997b; Martin, 1976; Pearce & Pezzot-Pearce, 1997).

Abused children may also struggle to relate with adults in a healthy and positive manner because the dynamics of abuse contribute to distrust, which, in turn, can lead children to be fearful or overly suspicious of adults (Helfer, Kempe, & Krugman, 1997; Pearce & Pezzot-Pearce, 1997). Abused children may mimic the way their primary role models express their feelings and how they put those feelings into actions. Children may have learned that it is "OK" to hit when they are mad or to hurt people or objects when they have been "wronged." An abused child may have a distorted perception of how to express thoughts and emotions. Because a caregiver may have been caring one moment but abusive the next, the child may have a difficult time knowing what to expect in interactions with others. Thus the child may be overly attuned to and responsive to certain cues. For example, if an adult raises his or her voice, the child may expect an act of violence and experience a strong fear response.

Maintaining self-esteem and a sense of self-worth is a challenge for abused children who may have been told they were worthless and deserved their abuse. Further, being victims of abuse may have reinforced the belief that they are not worthy of care and protection. Abused children often feel helpless and powerless and try to shield themselves from situations and opportunities that would require them to take initiative or risks (Helfer et al., 1997; Pearce & Pezzot-Pearce, 1997). A child may believe that the consequences of failure outweigh the potential gains.

Abused children often have difficulty putting their feelings into words at the appropriate developmental level. It is often helpful to use therapeutic games and educate them about feelings to help them communicate their thoughts and feelings. Abused children may not have mastered developmentally appropriate problem-solving skills and behaviors because they may have had to devote so much emotional and psychological energy to coping with the abuse. They may behave in a regressed manner or have insufficient coping abilities to mange expected stressors (Helfer et al., 1997; Pearce & Pezzot-Pearce, 1997).

Characteristics of abusing families   Abusing families often experience multiple environmental and intrafamily stressors that impair family members' coping abilities and the overall functioning of the family system. Common environmental problems found in families that mistreat children include unemployment, financial hardship, poverty, and absent or inadequate social support systems. Common intrafamily stressors include substance abuse, domestic violence, a family history of victimization, difficulties during pregnancy, becoming a parent at a young age, adult or child medical problems, a perception that a child has temperamental difficulties, and impairments in normal attachment (Videka-Sherman, 1991).

Dynamics and Impact of Sexual Abuse

Historically, most people have believed that sexual abuse, especially incest, was rare and that children who claimed to be sexually abused were making up their allegations (Courtois, 1988; Herman, 1992). Armstrong (1982) termed the period from the early twentieth century until the late 1970s the "age of denial" because, due to the influence of Freud's theories, little serious attention was given to the problem of childhood sexual abuse.

Considerable research with victims has since documented the prevalence of childhood sexual abuse, a form of abuse dramatically underestimated in official data. Based on victim reports, it is estimated that 20 to 30 percent of all adult women experienced some form of sexual abuse in childhood (Cosentino & Collins, 1996; Finkelhor, 1984; Russell, 1986). In light of these startling statistics, those who treat survivors of childhood sexual trauma recognize the need to advocate for a social and clinical milieu that validates rather than disparages the veracity of sexual abuse survivors' experiences.

It is now widely recognized that individual treatment of childhood sexual abuse requires (1) helping to facilitate short- and long-term safety from abuse; (2) helping the survivor talk about the abuse; (3) validating the survivor's experience and feelings; (4) helping to correct misperceptions of blame and responsibility for the abuse; (5) prioritizing and addressing co-occurring problems such as substance abuse, self-mutilation, suicidal behavior, or psychiatric disorders; and (6) encouraging survivors to reach jointly identified goals geared toward individual coping and healing (Courtois, 1988; Helfer et al., 1997; Herman, 1992; Kirschner, Kirschner, & Rappaport, 1993; Pearce & Pezzot-Pearce, 1997).

The vast majority of perpetrators are known and trusted by the child. These perpetrators deliberately exploit and distort their relationship with the child, capitalizing on the child's natural curiosity and trust. As a result, the victimized child frequently misinterprets his or her victimization because the child "didn't stop" or "allowed" the perpetrator's sexual advances. But this type of reaction to adult manipulation should never be confused with giving consent. Children cannot give consent to sexual exploitation by an adult because they do not have the cognitive or emotional capacity to make an informed choice.

Although some victims of childhood sexual abuse are also physically abused, many children are not beaten, tortured, or threatened with physical harm in order to get them to submit to sexual exploitation. This level of force is often unnecessary to coerce a child into engaging in sexual behavior with an abuser. A child can be a victim of multiple types of abuse, including sexual and physical abuse, but the physical abuse may not be aimed at getting the child to submit to the sexual abuse. Children desire love, approval, and attention from adults. Their innocence makes them easy targets for sexual abuse, and for the psychological and emotional manipulation designed to keep them from telling anyone about the abuse.

It is common for children to think they are willing participants in the sexual abuse or that they are responsible for the abuse. Some children believe that aspects of the sexual abuse were "good" because they may have enjoyed activities leading up to the abuse, like playing or cuddling with the abuser. Some parts of the sexual molestation may cause a child to have involuntary physiological responses that can lead to pleasurable sensations, not to be confused with adult sexuality. This does not mean that the child "likes" the abuse; any attempt to cultivate sexual behavior in a child is exploitative.

It is now understood that childhood sexual abuse survivors, and particularly incest survivors, may disavow that their abuse was traumatic or aberrant due to the power of forced silence, denial, self-blame, or the family's collusion with the abuser. Immense psychological pressure is often placed on victims to invalidate the reality of their trauma, blame themselves, and protect the perpetrator. This does not necessarily change for adult survivors.

Sue, a twenty-eight-year-old married woman with two young girls, presents as a cordial, reserved, and extremely agreeable woman. She lives in a middle-class neighborhood, is married to a professional man, and works in her home. Upon entering therapy, her complaints were vague but she sought help for overwhelming feelings of depression and anxiety. She felt dissatisfied with her marriage, thought she was a poor mother, and experienced little happiness or pleasure in life.

In therapy, discussions of her past history revealed that she was a childhood victim of severe physical and sexual abuse by her alcoholic father. Sue feels that it is likely that her mother knew of the sexual abuse but did nothing about it until Sue disclosed the abuse to a social service worker at age twelve. She was then placed in foster care until her father was "rehabilitated." When she returned home several months later, the abuse resumed and her mother refused to protect her or discuss what was happening.

In adulthood, when Sue tried to confront her mother about her abuse, her mother consistently told her, "That was in the past. You should forget about it. Stop bringing it up. It doesn't matter now." Consequently, Sue has internalized the belief that she should forget her abuse and not discuss it. She feels threatened and is reluctant to process her victimization because she fears that facing those experiences and feelings will rupture her current relationship with her mother and her family of origin, a terrifying thought for her.

Effects of childhood sexual abuse on the child's development   Many sexually abused children have been taught to believe that sexual activity between children and adults or other children is an appropriate way to show love and affection, and that a normal way to receive nurturance, affection, and love is through sexual activity. Therefore, children may develop sexually inappropriate behaviors such as making sexual advances toward other children or adults, which places the children at risk for further victimization and increases the risk of victimization of other children in the community (Gold, Hughes, & Swingle, 1996; Mandell, Damon, Castaldo, Tauber, Monise, & Larsen, 1989).

Sexually abused children are often threatened, bribed, or coerced into silence about the sexual abuse. As a result, they often experience fear, anxiety, and other emotional and physical distress when processing the victimization due to internalized feelings of shame, blame, and stigmatization. Children do not have the cognitive or emotional skills to effectively cope with being in the role of a sexual partner or with the intense emotions that result from sexual exploitation. Sexually abused children often experience sleep disturbances, psychosomatic symptoms, fatigue, anxiety, poor impulse control or poor concentration, and depression (Finkelhor, 1981). They often have poor grades in school, frequent absences, problems interacting with peers, and disciplinary problems, which contribute to their feelings of alienation and low self-worth, all of which impair their chances of success in adulthood (Finkelhor, 1984).

Sexually abused children must deal with a premature loss of innocence about sexual activity and may feel alienated from their friends and different from their peers who are naive about sexual activity. Some sexually abused children become fearful, anxious, or repulsed by normal and appropriate forms of affection, such as hugging, because the boundaries between appropriate affection and exploitation are blurred as a result of the abuse. Because healthy displays of affection may have preempted the molestation, normal displays of affection could feel threatening.

Adolescents who were sexually abused as children are more likely than adolescents who were not abused to experience clinical levels of depression, attention and thought problems, aggressive behavior, social problems, somatic complaints, suicidal thoughts, and suicidal behavior (Silverman et al., 1996).

Long-term effects of childhood sexual abuse   The long-term negative sequelae of childhood sexual abuse are well documented. The symptomatology includes a tendency for self-sabotage and self-destructiveness, trauma repetition and resistance to change, and revictimization. Additional common symptoms include somatization with an array of physical complaints and medical conditions, repression and denial, eating and substance abuse disorders, vivid flashbacks, sexual difficulties, intense body memories, depression, suicidal behavior, nightmares and sleep disturbances, difficulty trusting others, impairments in attachments to others, social isolation, poor self-esteem and self-efficacy, feelings of helplessness and powerlessness, and hypervigilance and hyperarousal (Briere & Runtz, 1988; Cosentino, & Collins, 1996; Courtois, 1988; Finkelhor et al., 1990; Gold et al., 1996; Kirschner et al., 1993; Neumann, Houskamp, Pollock, & Briere, 1996; Roche, Runtz, & Hunter, 1999; Runtz & Roche, 1999; Russell, 1986).

Childhood sexual abuse has a long-term impact on the survivor's cognitive, physical, emotional, and social development in adulthood, with significantly decreased mental health for many adult sexual abuse survivors. In addition to the symptomatology described above, survivors are more likely to have inpatient psychiatric hospitalizations, first pregnancies prior to age nineteen, declines in socioeconomic status, and decreased likelihood of graduating from high school or obtaining additional career skills than women who were not sexually abused in childhood (Mullen, Martin, Anderson, Romans, & Herbison, 1996).

Also, child sexual abusers are more likely to have been sexually victimized as children themselves. A generational cycle of sexual abuse can exist in families when sexually abused children grow up and become adults who sexually abuse their own children or become perpetrators by omission, by not protecting their children from incestuous family members. These adults grew up in family systems that actively or passively condoned the sexual exploitation of children and did not model parental skills that proactively sought to keep children safe from sexual victimization.

Increased symptoms of dissociation, symptoms of PTSD, and Disorder of Extreme Stress Not Otherwise Specified (DESNOS) are common for survivors of sexual abuse (Zlotnick, Zakriski, Shea, & Costello, 1996). Significant associations between female childhood sexual abuse and anxiety, anger, depression, interpersonal problems, obsessions, compulsions, dissociation, posttraumatic stress responses, and somatization have been found (Neumann et al., 1996).

Sexual abuse survivors have significantly more negative perceptions of their sexuality, are less assertive about using birth control and rejecting unwanted sex, have more incidents of sexual victimization in adulthood, expect negative responses from partners regarding protected sex, have higher levels of substance usage, and have more feelings of powerlessness about HIV prevention (Johnsen & Harlow, 1996).

Factors related to childhood sexual victimization such as age of onset, frequency, severity, and duration of abuse, number of perpetrators, and use of force are important variables that can have an impact on victims. The level of severity of the sexual abuse (e.g., rape or intercourse as opposed to fondling) is significantly associated with mental health problems such as dissociation, anxiety, depression, sexual dysfunction, and sleep disturbances for both men and women (Heath, Bean, & Feinauer, 1996).

SINGLE-SESSION CRISIS INTERVENTION

There are wide variations in the ways children are physically or sexually abused, and multiple types of abuse frequently occur at the same time. Emotional and psychological abuse invariably contribute to the child's feelings of self-blame, shame, fear of telling, and feelings of responsibility for the abuse.

Crisis counseling with children necessitates special considerations. First, because childhood and adolescence are periods of constantly evolving cognitive, emotional, and physiological development, each child is unique in his or her developmental mastery. As noted, trauma and abuse can impede and derail a child's ability to successfully master necessary developmental tasks. Crisis counselors must therefore always be attuned to the developmental abilities of the child. Compounding factors such as preexisting developmental, cognitive, or emotional disabilities also affect crisis counseling, as do social, cultural, and religious differences.

Second, the context in which children are likely to be seen is unique because they are unlikely to contact crisis centers or community services themselves. Child victims are most often initially seen in their school, a child care center, a hospital emergency room, a police station, or a Child Protective Services agency. First contact with a Child Protective Services investigator might also occur in the community, for example, at a friend or neighbor's house or even in the child's own residence. Often school counselors, social workers, Child Protective Services workers, police, or hospital personnel are the first persons to talk with a child following a disclosure of abuse.

Because abused children may have developed significant problems related to their school, home, or community environments, they may already be involved with human service professionals such as counselors, social workers, or psychologists, or they may be receiving mental health services provided by paraprofessionals such as mental health technicians or therapeutic support staff. Being involved with a safe, caring, interested, and empathetic adult may facilitate the abused child's "telling the secret" of his or her victimization. After reporting this information to Child Protective Services, these professionals can assist the child if a crisis ensues after "telling the secret."

The goals of crisis intervention with child abuse victims focus on (1) ensuring the victim's present physical safety; (2) helping the child cope with the immediate aftermath of the disclosure, both emotionally and cognitively; (3) facilitating any time-sensitive or involuntary interventions required such as medical examinations or police interviews with the child; and (4) aiding the child in reconnecting with appropriate social supports and resources (e.g., nonabusive loved ones) or helping to link the child to necessary supports and resources (i.e., temporary foster care or referral for counseling services). "Single-session" crisis interventions with abused children may consist of one contact with the child, as in the case of hospital personnel, or may entail several time-limited meetings with the child. In either case, the goal of short-term crisis intervention focuses on safety and short-term stabilization, not on achieving a resolution to the problem.

Because children are often ill prepared for the events that transpire following disclosure or the discovery by others of the abuse, they can be traumatized not only by the impact of the abuse but by subsequent protective actions taken such as medical procedures, interviews with investigators, or removal from the home. This is likely to be a very emotional time for a child, who may feel overwhelmed, confused, and frightened. The child may have been given distorted information by the abuser(s) and have misperceptions about his or her role in and responsibility for the abuse. Because a maltreated child may be especially sensitive to being blamed for the abuse or "getting in trouble," crisis workers must be careful not to blame the child and should emphasize that he or she is not responsible for the abuse.

Although gathering information about the abuse may be necessary for reporting laws and ensuring the child's safety, a crisis worker needs to be of immediate assistance to the child in a real and genuine relational capacity. Focusing too much on documentation and fact-finding may alienate the child and prevent the crisis worker from being empathically present with the child in the moment. When working with an abused child, a crisis worker must always be actively listening and seeking to understand the child's frame of reference regarding feelings, thoughts, and behaviors while constantly assessing how the child is responding emotionally, behaviorally, cognitively, and interpersonally.

Step1:
Supportively and empathically join with the child.

It is important for the child victim to perceive the crisis worker as nonthreatening, compassionate, and willing to listen. A maltreated child may have been coerced into silence, blamed for his or her victimization, and threatened verbally or physically not to tell. The child may be afraid of discussing what happened and feel confused, powerless, and uncertain about what to say. The child may also be afraid of getting the perpetrator(s) in trouble for the abuse, and feelings of betrayal or guilt may emerge.

When working with child survivors of sexual abuse, treatment protocols recognize that genuineness, warmth, empathy, and active participation are essential, and that a technically neutral, bland, or removed stance is contraindicated. Child survivors of trauma might interpret a therapist's neutrality as uncaring and hostile, and might associate a therapist's long silences and contained affect with the secrecy and stonewalling they experienced in their abuse, which could contribute to retraumatization and decompensation (Kluft, 1993; Putnam, 1989a, 1989b; Ross, 1989).

The crisis worker should foster an atmosphere of safety and trust to encourage the child to begin sharing thoughts and feelings. If possible, find a place that is private and child-friendly such as a quiet, comfortable room that has toys or games available for the crisis worker and child to play together. The younger the child, the less likely that he or she will be comfortable sitting in a chair talking directly with a counselor for a significant period of time. Playing with a child offers a powerful venue for the worker and child to create a therapeutic alliance that is sensitive to the particular interests and desires of the child. It also helps to break down the barriers between traditional adult and child roles that might impede a supportive and empathic joining.

A child usually feels more comfortable on his or her "home turf," which may be sitting on the floor and talking while playing with blocks or drawing pictures. Counselors should be flexible about how the child prefers to join with the crisis worker; for example, the child may want to write down responses to questions instead of saying them aloud or to draw a picture to express his or her feelings.

Crisis counselors who intervene with abused minors must be astute regarding ethical and legal considerations. As noted, all helping professionals are mandated reporters according to both state child abuse reporting laws and professional ethical guidelines. This means that if a child reveals previously undetected abuse or abusers, the counselor must report that information. During initial counseling contacts, crisis counselors must be sure to carefully explain to children the limits of confidentiality and the duty to report. Further, if the counselor must make a report while engaged with a child, he or she must carefully explain and process that, too.

Crisis counselors must also be vigilant in their choice of words when probing and or responding to children's concerns. The counselor should use the individual child's language when describing body parts and/or sexual behaviors and be sure not to assume or assert physical or sexual abuse.

Step 2:
Intervene to create safety in the environment, de-escalate and stabilize the situation, and handle the child's immediate needs.

Intervene to create safety in the environment If a child has been the victim of abuse or is at risk of being a victim of abuse, the counselor's first priority is to ensure that the child is not at further risk of harm. This requires immediately notifying appropriate authorities such as Child Protective Services and/or the police of suspected abuse and taking the necessary steps to keep the child safe from danger. It is not solely the crisis worker's responsibility to take all of the steps necessary to keep a child from harm. Unless the crisis worker is also in protective services, he or she will not have the legal authority to take protective custody of a child or have the specialized training to make a detailed child abuse risk assessment and service plan. But the crisis worker is responsible for contacting and working with Child Protective Services and/or the police and helping the child reach or stay in a safe location until further assistance can be provided. Also, the crisis worker may need to help the child attain sufficient emotional control to stay in a safe location, put his or her feelings and thoughts into words, and not escalate behaviorally or emotionally.

Jimmy, an eleven-year-old boy with chronic conduct problems, got into a fight again at school and was called to the vice principal's office, where he was informed that he would be suspended for three days. The vice principal told Jimmy that he had called his father to notify him of his suspension. Jimmy was visibly shaken and became distraught. He begged the vice principal to call his father back and tell him it was a mistake. After a period of angry outbursts and tears, he told the principal he feared that his father would really hurt him when he got home because his father had beaten him before for fighting and threatened to really give him a lesson if he got in trouble again at school. Just as Jimmy was saying this, the bell rang for school to be dismissed. Jimmy said his father worked the night shift and would be waiting for him when he got home from school.

Allowing Jimmy to take the bus home to meet his father would have removed him from the safe environment of school and put him at risk of physical harm. The vice principal asked Jimmy to remain at school until someone from Child Protective Services arrived to speak with him. He escorted Jimmy to the guidance office to talk with the school counselor until the protective services worker assessed Jimmy's risk of abuse if he were to return home.

De-escalate and stabilize   A child may experience a variety of feelings following an incident of abuse or the discovery by others that abuse has occurred. Many variables such as the child's age and developmental level, history of abuse(s), relationship to the perpetrators(s), and family supports affect the child's response and ability to de-escalate and stabilize. Children usually feel overwhelmed and may have high levels of emotionality, most often sadness, anger, confusion, anxiety, and fear. Some children are prone to behavioral disturbances and tend to "act out" their feelings instead of putting them into words.

The crisis worker needs to maintain a positive and caring stance toward the child even when the child is not behaving reasonably. The crisis worker should be empathic and caring but should not absorb the child's level of distress. The crisis worker's calmness and stability can help the child to regain control. Children look to adults to confirm their feelings; therefore, it is important to validate the child's pain without inadvertently sending the message that the crisis warrants a panic response.

A crisis worker should be sensitive and attuned to the child's needs and preferences in order to foster an atmosphere conducive to stabilization. In Jimmy's case, he initially went willingly to talk with the counselor and was cooperative but kept his responses brief and formal. Jimmy did not particularly like the guidance office because he had often been called to the office because he was in trouble. After about thirty minutes in the guidance office, he became agitated, started pacing around the room, and wanted to leave. The full impact of the fact that he would be talking to someone from Child Protective Services who could "get his dad in trouble" or "take him away" started to overwhelm him.

He reported feeling "trapped" in the office. The counselor asked Jimmy if he would like to walk around the outside track and talk. Jimmy enthusiastically went outside, stating that he "felt better just being out of the school." He began to talk more spontaneously and was more receptive to the counselor's efforts to provide support, empathy, and validation.

The crisis worker needs to assist the child to regain appropriate cognitive, emotional, and behavioral control, which, in turn, helps empower the child to cope with the present situation. It is a good idea to ask which types of activities the child would find comforting (e.g., drawing, walking, or throwing a ball together), as this usually increases the child's ability to soothe him- or herself, de-escalate, and feel a sense of control.

Handle immediate needs   An abused child may need immediate medical treatment or may need to be taken into protective custody. In such cases the crisis worker can foster the child's adjustment to these circumstances. Assisting the child to understand what is happening at the moment or what is going to happen helps the child prepare for it and anticipate future needs, and gives the child an enhanced feeling of control.

A crisis worker can meet an abused child's immediate need for information by clearly, calmly, and in understandable language explaining to the child what types of medical procedures will be done, what the tests or procedures will be like, why they need to be done, and how long they should take and inviting the child to ask questions or raise concerns. The crisis worker may not have all the answers to these questions but should be able to collaborate with medical personnel to obtain the answers for the child.

Within appropriate limits, the crisis worker should inform the child about the Child Protective Services investigation. The reasons should be clearly explained to a child if he or she will be unable to return home. If it is unclear whether a placement will be long or short term, the crisis worker should not try to comfort the child with an idealized description of what will happen. It is important to validate the child's feelings and empathize with his or her grief and dismay, but it is never acceptable to foster unrealistic expectations. No crisis worker can predict in the midst of a family crisis whether a parent will stop abusing substances or stop physically harming the child, or if a sexual abuse perpetrator will be removed from the home permanently. A child may try to obtain promises or strike a bargain with a crisis worker, but the crisis worker should never make false promises; if broken, they will only result in the child's feeling betrayed again. Most children love their parent(s) even though the parent(s) may have repeatedly hurt them. Validation of the child's bond with their parent(s) is thus important.

With these cautions in mind, it would not be appropriate to say to a child, "You can't go home now because when mommy drinks too much, she leaves you alone. But mommy is going to stop drinking, and then you will be able to live with mommy." It would be appropriate to say, *"You can't go home now. One reason is that when mommy drinks too much, she leaves you alone. I am going to try to help mommy get the help she needs. But mommy has to make some changes, like not drinking and leaving you alone. If mommy can make the changes she needs to make for you to be safe, I want you to be able to go home."*

The crisis counselor should help foster feelings of hope and recovery. The crisis could be an opportunity for positive growth and family strength. The crisis situation may lead to interventions and plans that increase family cohesiveness and positive adjustment.

Some abused children have basic, concrete needs for physical objects, especially objects associated with comfort and self-soothing. Whenever possible, crisis workers should make efforts to reconnect a child with loved objects or to propose a substitute for those objects. The crisis worker can ask a child what possessions (e.g., a stuffed animal, blanket, favorite toy, beloved photograph, soothing music, art supplies) he or she may find comforting during times of stress.

The crisis worker should also inquire about the child's physical needs, for example, whether the child is thirsty, hungry, or needs to use a bathroom. Even children who are not traumatized often need to be reminded of these needs, but a traumatized child may be even more overwhelmed and distracted.

Children often want to be reunited with their family. Nonabusing relatives and caregivers may be able to help the child regain control and comfort the child. The crisis worker should make every effort to link the child with supportive persons known to the child, but if an active CPS investigation is occurring, CPS must be involved in determining whether this is possible.

Step 3:
Explore and assess the dimensions of the crisis and the child's reaction to the crisis and encourage ventilation.

Each abused child has a unique story. It is important for the crisis worker to convey interest in hearing about the child's world from the child's perspective. Assuming the role of the expert or the person who has all the answers is counterproductive. Rather, a crisis worker needs to encourage and find ways to assist the child to share what he or she is thinking and feeling by asking what happened, who was involved, and how the child feels. Some children may appear numb or disinterested in talking about a crisis. Other children may be more willing to talk about the details of the abuse, but may struggle to put feelings and thoughts about what happened into words. Young children typically do not have the introspective capacity to talk about feelings or thoughts in great depth, but it is important for them to express themselves within normal developmental limits. The crisis worker should provide the child with opportunities to talk about what has happened and should respond in ways that communicate that someone is really listening and understands.

A five-year-old boy may say he does not like it when he gets hit and "it hurts to be hit." The crisis worker can support and validate his feelings and perceptions of being hit. The crisis worker could also empathize with the child by stating, *"It can be difficult and painful to be little when big people can hurt you, and there is not much a little person can do to stop it."* The child's verbal and nonverbal behavior provides important cues for the crisis worker to further explore the child's thoughts and assist the child in expressing his or her feelings.

The resilience children exhibit and the heroic feats of adaptation they are capable of should be openly appreciated; active efforts to cultivate positive coping abilities can further enhance functioning. Many children have survived unimaginable traumas with a paucity of support. Some children have an ability to reflect upon their abuse with profound wisdom and clarity. Lisa, a thirteen-year-old female, was subjected to heinous neglect and physical and sexual abuse by numerous perpetrators until age eleven. During her first meeting with a crisis worker, Lisa made the following poignant analogy when describing how she perceived her abuse:

I am like a bucket of water. I came full of water but every time I got hurt, I spilled some water. I got hurt again and again and again until there was no water left inside. I am now an empty bucket. I want to get over my past so I can trust and love people again. I need to put water in my bucket. I can't stay like this forever. I can be happy if I find a way to fill my bucket. I want to get to the other side of my life and not be the robot I am now.

Lisa describes herself after an onslaught of abuse has "emptied her bucket" but not drained her capacity to hope for love and trust and to try and get what she needs from the world. She knows now that she is functioning in a robotic state, devoid of the energy to feel and to nurture herself. Her spirit of perseverance shows as she aspires to get to "the other side of her life," where she hopes there may be water for her bucket.

An abused child may have attempted to internalize feelings of power, strength, and potency by identifying in thought, behavior, or outlook with the abuser(s) (Benjamin, 1990; Davies & Frawley, 1994). It should be recognized that the child may have had little experience with healthy nonexploitive role models and may struggle with the perception that people are either abusers or victims (Benjamin, 1990; Davies & Frawley, 1994). Especially in cases of incestuous abuse, a female child may come to internalize a belief that femininity equates with masochism, subjugation, powerlessness, and submission to male authority (Benjamin, 1990; Chodorow, 1989).

This belief can result in an abused child internalizing some of the perpetrator's abusive and exploitative characteristics, which helps the child vicariously feel the sense of power, control, and domination held by the perpetrator (Davies & Frawley, 1994). The crisis worker should model nonexploitive personal power rather than taking on the persona of a covictim or someone who is angry at the abuser(s) and would like to punish the abuser(s) for their wrongdoing.

Crisis workers must understand that some cultures encourage masculine power or adult authority over children to an even greater extent than is considered acceptable in the United States. Some maltreated children may not perceive that they were abused. In helping children talk about physical or sexual abuse, it is not appropriate to discount their perceptions and to attempt to convince them that they were abused if they deny this. Crisis workers can be clear and honest about their own viewpoints, but children should have the first opportunity to share what the event meant to them. Lecturing a child almost never assists the child in disclosing personal information, especially if the child sees things differently. Perez-Foster (1997) encouraged clinicians to be sensitive to survivors' cultural norms and to inquire about and be knowledgeable about a variety of potential cultural influences.

Step 4:
Examine alternative actions and develop options.

In cases of reported child abuse, Child Protective Services is usually involved, and a multidisciplinary effort is often the best means to assist the child and family in crisis. Because a comprehensive family needs assessment is time-intensive, the single-session crisis worker is limited in exploring long-term alternatives or options for the child or family system. In single-session interventions, the focus is on exploring possible solutions to immediate and short-term problems.

For abused children, short-term immediate needs may include finding safe shelter for the night, obtaining clothing or toiletries, making a phone call to a friend or loved one, contacting a sibling or supportive relatives, writing a note to a favorite teacher explaining why they will not be in school the next day, arranging for a pet to be cared for, or getting needed medications. The crisis worker and the child should explore the child's needs together, without the crisis worker assuming a position of authority. It is the collaborative process of exploring needs and making choices that is restorative and empowering for the child.

Inevitably, the crisis worker must ensure the priority order in which needs are addressed. For instance, the child may feel it is more important to get a favorite pair of sneakers than to find a way to get needed asthma medication. Most children, however, respond to commonsense explanations of what must come first. Children cannot be expected to think of all the things they may need during a crisis; therefore, the crisis worker should be knowledgeable about the types of things that may be helpful and discuss them with the child. Because children like to play games, creative problem solving and brainstorming that has elements of fun can encourage more active participation from the child.

Step 5:
Help the child mobilize personal and social resources and connect with community resources, as needed.

Although an abused child's primary caregivers may be an inappropriate support network in the midst of the abuse crisis, the crisis worker should determine whether there are appropriate and nurturing loved ones (e.g., extended family members) who can assist the child in coping. It should not be assumed that all natural family members pose a risk to the child's safety. Sometimes one or both parents report the suspected abuse and experience the crisis with the child. The comfort and support that a parent, grandparent, or close family member can provide can help the child restore equilibrium.

Children may be more likely to confide in someone they know and trust, so they may be more comfortable talking with the crisis worker with a loved one present. If such an individual is available, it may be appropriate to include them in the crisis session, always keeping in mind, however, that the child is the focus rather than the other adult. Adults have a tendency to talk to each other and not talk to a child in their company. The best way to tell children that adults are interested in them is to show interest in them.

Step 6:
Anticipate the future and arrange follow-up contact.

Anticipate the future   The first component of this step is to prepare the child for what will happen next. This may require helping the child prepare for a medical examination, an interview with the police, a move to foster care, or the return home. The crisis worker should be informed and should help the child anticipate fully the next step.

Removing the child from the home, at least until his or her safety can be ensured, is an understandable action from an adult perspective. For the child, however, it often feels like punishment. It is difficult for children to understand why they are being taken from their home, school, community, friends, and loved ones and to believe that it is not a punishment. The paradox continues when a child discovers that the perpetrator is still living in the home, enjoying all the rights and privileges that the child is being denied. Even though the perpetrator's presence in the home is the reason the child cannot be at home, it often does not make sense to the child. It is important to explain to children both the positive and negative experiences they may have.

Frank, age fifteen, had a long history of conduct problems and delinquent behavior. While in juvenile detention he disclosed sexual abuse by his much older stepbrother. The police had difficulty accepting the credibility of his accusations and had no other evidence to proceed with charges so they asked him to take a lie detector test. Frank was angry that the police didn't believe him. On the one hand

Frank wanted to "prove" that the abuse really happened, but on the other hand he was angry that the police believed he was a "liar." He did not want to cooperate just because they wanted him to.

The crisis worker helped Frank get information about the procedure and how it might support or not support his statements. The crisis worker did so with Frank's consent and did not try to persuade or dissuade him to take the test. Once Frank got the information necessary to anticipate what the test would be like, he was able to make an informed choice.

The crisis worker should have a way of saying good-bye to the child when the session is over, especially if he or she is unlikely to see the child again. Because the child needs to feel that the crisis worker genuinely cared about the child during the time of crisis, it is important to avoid a hurried or premature good-bye, which might cause the child to doubt that the crisis worker cared about him or her. It is a good idea for the crisis worker to inform the child at the beginning of the session how much time the crisis worker will be spending with him or her.

For instance, shortly after meeting a child, a hospital social worker could say:

"I work here at the hospital. My job is to help children talk about what happened to them and why they are at the hospital. I like it when children ask me questions. I want to help you understand the kinds of things the doctors or nurses may need to do in order to help you. I get to stay with you while you are in the emergency room, which may be a long time, even hours. My job is to help children who come to the emergency room. This is where I stay and help children. I will not be able to go with you when you leave the hospital. I may not even get to see you again after you leave, yet I will remember you and hope you are well. Sometimes we only get to be with someone for a short time, but that time can be very special."

The child may be having difficulty comprehending new information because of feeling overwhelmed by the crisis. It is helpful to say things several times using slightly different words, seeking feedback from the child to assure that he or she understands what is being said as you go along, and not to say everything all at once. It may be helpful for the crisis worker to give the child a small memento when he or she says good-bye. The memento could be a card with a handwritten note, a pin with a nice message, a stuffed animal, or even the pen the crisis worker used to take notes during the session so the child can write down his or her feelings at a later time.

Arrange follow-up   The crisis worker is responsible for arranging to follow up with the child. Children often like to get telephone calls and letters addressed just to them. Depending on the child's age, the crisis worker may need to get their consent for follow-up. A follow-up contact can (1) reinforce to the child that the worker was someone who cared, (2) briefly reinforce the goals of the crisis meeting and provide appropriate reminders (e.g., *"You said you would take your allergy medicine when you got home"*), and (3) provide further assistance and additional referrals, if necessary (e.g., *"The doctor needs you to come back to the hospital for some more tests,"* or *"Do you remember the emergency telephone number we talked about to call any time that you feel as if someone might hurt you?"*).

The crisis worker should also ensure that the child and family, if appropriate, have access to other community services.

ONGOING CRISIS COUNSELING WITH CHILDREN

Special Considerations

For a child, there is a triple jeopardy associated with disclosing familial abuse. First, the relief and healing that can occur after disclosing the secret of the abuse is a process that unfolds, not an immediate outcome of disclosing the abuse. Second, the system's response to a child can traumatize the child again. And third, the child's relationships with other loved ones may suffer.

Disclosure and subsequent crises   Disclosure is the first step toward a child receiving help, yet it can also be the catalyst for subsequent crises. It is inaccurate to assume that a child will be somehow magically "freed" by disclosing abuse, despite the fact that telling may bring about feelings of relief and validation by others. The child may continue to experience negative feelings including ambivalence, guilt, disloyalty, anger, confusion, fear, anxiety, worry, and distrust.

System processes can retraumatize   The system's needs and responses to a child's disclosure of abuse can retraumatize and disempower the child. The child may be required to describe the abuse to a number of professionals within a short period of time. The child may first disclose to a trusted family member, school professional, family friend, or peer but then have to talk to a protective services caseworker and then to the police. A child may also need to have a medical evaluation and talk to numerous medical personnel. It is not uncommon for all of this to take place within the same day.

An abused child may be involved in civil and/or criminal legal actions. Family court proceedings aim to protect the child from further abuse by mandating certain child protective services such as protective custody with an out-of-home placement. This happens most often when primary caregivers have not agreed to receive child protective services or are grossly unreliable in following family service plans. It is common for children in a civil court proceeding to have to testify about their abuse although the requirements for child testimony in civil court are not as stringent as they are in criminal court.

Protective custody hearings result in court orders that can require parents to meet certain criteria deemed necessary for their child's welfare such as drug testing, parenting classes, or home visits by Child Protective Services workers. If the parents fail to comply with these orders they can lose custody of their children temporarily or permanently.

Criminal action is geared toward prosecuting the abuser for a crime or crimes against the child. Many cases of child abuse do not meet the legal criteria necessary for criminal prosecution of the offender. If criminal action is taken against the abuser, children may have to recount their abuse to a prosecuting attorney, often several times, as preparation for court may be necessary. They may also need to testify as a witness and be cross-examined by a defense attorney. And, all too often, they may find that the perpetrator "does not get in trouble" (i.e., is not found guilty, serves no jail time for his offense, or goes to jail for only a brief period).

Abused children are frequently referred to mental health centers, but these centers often have high employee turnover rates and multiple treatment team service providers. Children may end up meeting so many people and telling the story of their abuse so many times that the meaning, effect, and impact of the events seem unimportant. It may seem as if reporting the details and events is all that matters to the adults who are supposed to help them. A child cannot be restored or cured by disclosure alone, or even by multiple disclosures. Only organized and consistent supports, resources, and enrichment can provide the assistance necessary to facilitate restoration and adaptation.

Relationships are jeopardized   After disclosure, a child's relationships with known and trusted loved ones are often immediately jeopardized or impaired. This is due to many factors: the inevitable disruptions to relationships experienced by a child placed in foster care, family dynamics that change as some relatives support the perpetrator for various reasons (often because of denial and disbelief), and the need to protect the child from contact with certain family members. Even sympathetic family members are often insensitive to the trauma of abuse; they may passively or actively encourage the child to hide his or her pain and forget about the abuse, or they may treat the child differently than before.

Because children do not have the verbal or cognitive capacity to express their thoughts and feelings in the same way that adults express themselves, assessing conduct may be the best way to understand what a child is feeling and trying to express. Children have less impulse control than adults and are more likely to act out their feelings rather than simply discuss them. An abused child who may have appeared to cope adequately during or shortly after the crisis event may develop behavioral problems months or even years after the abuse.

Crisis counseling and other service providers   After addressing the crisis that brought the abuse to light, the overall goal is to keep the child safe from further abuse and to foster long-term health. This is a collective effort that may involve ongoing assessment and interventions by multiple service providers. Whenever possible, reunification or preservation of the family system should be the primary goal. Family preservation and reunification efforts seek to rehabilitate abusive family practices; teach parents appropriate parenting strategies; and provide guidance, support, and role models in hopes of creating healthier family dynamics. Parent education is a core component of these efforts, with individual and family counseling sometimes included to improve family cohesiveness and lend support to the family system. The time frame for achieving these goals may be short or long, and there is no assurance that they will be achieved or maintained.

According to Jones (1997b), treatment goals for the abused child and the family should include (1) ending the abuse or neglect; (2) ensuring that the child receives satisfactory care; (3) fostering positive interpersonal relationships in the child and family members; (4) treating any symptoms of psychological disorder; and (5) ensuring that the child is not the direct object of any "sexually aggressive, violent, or exploitive behavior" (p. 524). Jones further describes the treatment process for families that mistreat children as a three-stage interrelated and circular process. The three stages include parental acknowledgment of the abuse and its impact on the child and family, development of increased parental competence and sensitivity to the child, and resolution (Jones, 1997b).

Not all abused children are abused by family members, but in cases of familial abuse, family preservation or reunification efforts can occur concurrently with individual counseling aimed at helping the child heal and cope in the aftermath of the crisis event. Not all cases of abuse result in family preservation efforts, particularly if the abuses were chronic and escalated over time. When children are placed in long-term "out-of-home" care because of abuse, they must begin to build a new life, heal from their abuse, and regain a sense of normal childhood.

Facilitating a Trusting and Empowering Relationship

Abused children who have been through the Child Protective Services system may initially be quite guarded about talking to another adult about what has happened to them. Children may have met with other caseworkers, social workers, or counselors whom they didn't like or who left them abruptly during treatment. It is not uncommon for a child in long-term placement to have lived in numerous foster homes and to have had several caseworkers prior to meeting with a crisis counselor. Children may have been in a residential treatment facility or psychiatric hospital or may know that they are facing the possibility of inpatient treatment if their behavior does not improve.

Due to these complicating factors in addition to their abuse, it is understandable that traumatized children may be cautious about trusting another adult and may feel that they have little personal power or control over what happens to them. Therefore, helping to empower an abused child can be a difficult task. Timothy's case illustrates the many challenges and barriers that can exist in helping an abused child regain a sense of personal power, fostering connections to others, and encouraging positive personal growth.

Timothy, age nine, was sexually and physically abused by his parents. At age six he was placed in foster care. Both his parents served jail time for their offenses and were not considered suitable for family reunification. Parental rights for Timothy were eventually terminated and he became "available" for adoption. Due to his age, previous history of residential treatment for conduct problems, and multi-

ple failed foster care placements, no suitable adoptive parents were found. Timothy knows that he could be adopted if a family "wanted him" and hopes to be adopted by his current foster parents. Timothy feels frustrated, angry, and powerless to get what he really wants in life—to be adopted.

First, the crisis worker needs to earn the child's trust by being reliable, real, nonjudgmental, compassionate and by believing in the child's ability to grow and change. An empowering relationship could help the child (1) move toward making good choices, (2) express feelings and thoughts in more constructive ways, and (3) accept and grieve losses.

In Timothy's case, the crisis worker could help empower Timothy by providing him with a safe and supportive place where his thoughts and feelings will be heard and respected. For abused children, the process of communicating with an adult who openly listens with interest and concern, believes that they are important and valuable individuals, and recognizes their positive qualities, which may have been overlooked or discounted by others, can empower children to begin to see their own strengths.

Assessing Resolution of Multiple Crisis

One of the most difficult challenges in assessing crisis resolution for a severely maltreated child is the multiple crises that child may have faced. In Timothy's case, for example, potentially traumatizing experiences requiring assessment include (1) the experience of physical and sexual abuse by his parents; (2) being removed from his family and placed in foster care; (3) testifying in criminal court against his parents; (4) the knowledge that his parents were placed in jail "because of him"; (5) coping with the fact that his parents' parental rights were terminated, which left him "available" for adoption; (6) the knowledge that no one is interested in adopting him; and (7) the disruption and losses he has experienced from numerous failed foster care placements. This list by no means includes all of the possible crises Timothy has experienced, but it illustrates the complexity of assessing crisis resolution for a chronically abused child.

One crisis event often precipitates another, which builds upon the earlier crisis. As previously noted, assessment does not occur in a linear fashion, and crisis events do not affect all areas of psychosocial functioning (ABCDE) to the same degree. Maltreated children usually have limited insight into how their traumatic experiences are related to their current difficulties.

For instance, Timothy openly verbalized a desire to "get help" with his behavior problems, which he believed were due to his "always being bad," which he perceived as "his fault," as if he had a character defect. Timothy's goal was to improve himself enough to be adoptable. His immediate struggle was the crisis of being available for adoption with no interested parties. Clearly, the multiple crises he has suffered are interrelated and led to his current status, but *his* primary concern was that his "bad behavior" would precipitate removal from his foster home.

To effectively intervene with Timothy, the crisis worker must assess each specific area of his psychosocial functioning. The crisis worker might begin to help a child like Timothy understand the ways his difficulties are connected by making a statement like the following: *"All people, big or little, can get upset when things happen to them. When something happens that makes us feel sad, mad, or scared, things can feel different inside of us. Some people get a bellyache when they are scared. Some people cry when they are sad. Some people yell when they are mad, but others get really quiet. It can be different for everyone. What we feel can change when we are upset. What we think about can change when we are upset. What we do or want to do can change when we are upset. I would like to know what it is like to be you when you are really upset about something. If I could pretend to be you when _____ happened, what would that be like? How would I feel? What would I think?"*

The crisis worker needs to help the child understand that it is normal to feel lots of different things when a crisis occurs and that it is OK, even good, to let others know about it. Some children will express that they are upset through inappropriate angry behaviors. In such cases, interventions should be geared toward helping children express themselves in more behaviorally appropriate ways that still allow them to "vent," as in drawing a "mad picture" instead of breaking toys.

It helps children to understand that their crisis experience may cause them to feel, think, or behave in different ways from nontraumatized children but that it is OK to be that way. For example, a teenager who was abused as a child may still need to sleep with a nightlight on, but may feel ashamed or embarrassed about it. The crisis worker can help the teenager accept that this is understandable and appropriate due to his or her experiences.

Goals and Processes of Ongoing Crisis Counseling with Child Abuse Victims

Affect stability:
Help children to express and process their memories and emotions related to the abuse.

Helping children work through the aftermath of crisis so they do not feel they are still victims or that they deserved to be victimized is an important part of the healing process. Children who have experienced maltreatment may experience a wide array of symptoms and problems. Assisting children to express and process their memories and emotions related to the trauma can assist them in coping with victimization.

For instance, a child may have persistent nightmares with themes of abuse or exploitation and flashbacks of traumatic incidents. Also, sights, smells, and sounds may trigger powerful recollections of the abuse, which can be very frightening to the child.

The crisis worker can help the child express feelings and thoughts as well as correct cognitive distortions about the events (e.g., that he or she is at fault for the abuse) and to express grief and loss. Abused children will not get over abuse by pretending that it did not happen. Denial and secrecy perpetuate the abuse of children, especially sexual abuse, and complicate the child's efforts to make sense of what happened.

Abused children need assistance in finding ways to express their memories of crisis events in order to help them (1) decrease feelings of responsibility, (2) understand that their feelings are accepted and respected, (3) begin to reframe distorted thinking and perceptions, and (4) develop healthy ways to soothe themselves during times of distress. Most abused children struggle with maintaining a positive sense of self-worth and self-esteem and benefit from positive reinforcement and from being perceived as someone who is worthy of compassion, care, and attention.

Prior to encouraging a child to describe trauma experiences and the feelings related to them, the crisis worker should assess whether the child is capable of handling what may be very intense feelings without decompensating to the degree that his or her safety is jeopardized. An emotionally fragile child may need treatment that touches upon the crisis events very slowly and gently in order not to overwhelm the child with intense feelings. It is disempowering for survivors to feel flooded by the trauma and to be unable to cope with their recollections and the enormity of their responses.

Children should be willing participants in processing their feelings and memories and also should be aware that they can stop talking or refuse to answer any questions if they feel uncomfortable or distressed. Children need to be informed, however, that the crisis worker wants to hear their story and is willing and able to help them process painful events. The following example illustrates what a crisis worker can say to help children understand this process:

"I am here to help you with things that have happened to you that were hard for you. I know painful and scary things can be hard to talk about. You will not be forced to answer any questions. I will not make you tell me about anything you don't want to, but part of my job is to help you let out things you may be thinking or feeling that you are keeping inside.

Lots of people keep stuff inside when something bad happens. A lot of the time it only makes it worse when you don't talk about it. People can only keep so much inside before they get full of stuff and they have to let some out and share it with someone. I want to be a person you can talk to about the tough stuff.

This can be hard sometimes but we can do this together. Part of my job is to ask hard questions and part of your job is to try to answer them if you can. I need to know when you can't talk about something so I won't bug you too much about it. But I may ask you again at another time because it helps me to help you when I know as much as you can tell me. We can make up a code word or a hand signal that you can use to let me know when you want to stop talking about something, or you can just say 'stop.'"

Allowing children to say stop can be empowering because they had little power or ability to say stop to their abusers. Children feel more trust and safety with the crisis worker, knowing that they have a voice that will be heard and respected.

Behavioral adjustments:
Help children to make healthy behavioral changes.

Assisting a child to reach optimal functioning is an integral part of working through a crisis event. For example, crisis counseling with a child at risk of residential placement due to conduct problems should include behavioral interventions geared to helping the child regain adequate behavioral controls. Problems such as substance abuse, self-mutilation, truancy, delinquency, suicidality, or violence toward others may be the first focus in working with an abused child.

Although these problems will probably not be completely resolved prior to work on other phases, the crisis worker should make substantial efforts to help the child learn and use alternative coping skills to reduce maladaptive behaviors. Teaching children problem-solving skills and self-soothing strategies can help them react to problems more effectively and thus prevent more destructive consequences.

The crisis worker can help the child to identify triggers or cues that lead to maladaptive responses. The child may need to learn about the interaction between feelings, thoughts, and behaviors in order to be more equipped to appropriately handle situations. For example, a simple analogy about the process of getting dressed for school in the morning and how feelings, thoughts, and behaviors interact can be useful.

"People have to think about what they are going to wear before they go about the act of getting dressed. Depending on how they feel that day, they may choose a bright color or a favorite outfit depending on their mood. They should think about what the weather is like outside (their environment), for example, if it is hot, cold, or rainy, so they can make a good choice about what to wear. Then they have to act out that choice by getting their clothes and putting them on.

Just as the act of getting dressed in the morning involves more than just putting on clothes, the behavioral problems the child may be experiencing involve more than just the problematic behavior. Crisis workers can use interesting, fun, and understandable analogies to assist children to make connections between feelings, thoughts, and behaviors. They can also help children improve their coping skills by developing or "inventing" new ways to deal with old problems and role playing those responses during counseling sessions.

Cognitive mastery:
Help children to examine and reformulate beliefs about themselves and reframe beliefs distorted by crisis events.

In order to fully understand what children think about a crisis event, the counselor must invest time and energy to find out how they perceive their overall world, including how they view adults, peers, home, school, and their community environments. Over time, cognitive distortions about people, the abuse, or other events will emerge. As part of the abuse, children are often conditioned to believe that they are bad or at fault. The conditioning process may have entailed verbal messages or overt and covert behaviors that reinforced distorted perceptions of their abuse. The crisis counselor may need to use a variety of strategies to help the child reformulate beliefs about their abuse. Because abuse often gets progressively worse over time and can be long lasting, counselors must recognize that children may need to both experience and hear many times and in many ways that they are not to blame and that they are valuable and important and deserving of care and respect. A positive and nurturing support system can be invaluable to the abused child; the more loved and trusted adults who treat the child kindly and compassionately, the less inclined the child will be to blame him- or herself and tolerate abuse.

An abused child may also need to be educated about what types of discipline or treatment are considered abusive. Especially in cases of sexual abuse, the child may need to learn "right" touch and "wrong" touch, along with ways to assert appropriate boundaries with other adults and children. A sexually abused child may have internalized the belief that "if you love someone, you let them touch your private parts." The counselor may need to show the child in numerous ways (e.g., verbally, with psychoeducational tools like books or games, or through group therapy) that certain types of adult behaviors are abusive and not "OK." There are many resources available geared toward various ages and developmental levels to help clinicians provide this type of education.

Developmental mastery:
Help children to examine the impact of abuse on their stage-of-life needs and tasks and to make healthy adjustments for ongoing developmental mastery.

Abused children are only able to process their victimization within the context of their current developmental level. An eighteen-year-old who was physically abused until age seven may experience a crisis when he finds out that he is going to be a father because he fears that he will abuse his child the way he was abused by his father. Abused children view their victimization through different developmental lenses as they grow and develop the capacity to understand the complexities of thoughts, feelings, and behaviors.

Mindy's mother gave birth to her at age fourteen. Mindy was physically and sexually abused by both her mother and her mother's paramours until she was placed in foster care at age six. Mindy consistently verbalized intense anger, dislike, and hatred toward her mother. When she turned fourteen herself, she was able to imagine in a different way what it would be like to be on the streets, alone, with a child.

Mindy said, "I didn't care when everyone said my mom was just a kid herself when she had me. It only made me madder to hear excuses for what she did to me. I always saw her as a grownup in my head. Then I turned fourteen and it really hit me. I thought, 'Wow, I'm the same age my mom was when she had me.'

I started thinking about what it would be like to have a kid at my age and be all alone. I couldn't stop thinking about it . . . how I would never want to go through that. . . . I can't even drive yet. . . . I still hate her, but now I feel sorry for her, too, which feels weird."

Abused children may have resolved much of the impact of their crisis at a specific age but may need to return to counseling at a later time, as their development progresses and other issues related to the trauma emerge within the context of their continued maturation. The view through a different developmental lens may create another crisis for the child and cause them to cognitively and emotionally view their victimization differently.

Interventions must reflect the crisis counselor's awareness of and sensitivity to these developmentally influenced understandings. The crisis counselor can help the child recognize that thoughts and feelings can change as people grow and that growth is a continual process. The child or adolescent may not understand that his or her perception of the abuse was limited by his or her life experiences, development, and lack of maturation. The crisis counselor can help the child contrast the changes in his or her perceptions of the abuse and learn to view them in a positive light.

Ecosystem healthy and intact:
Help children to examine and make necessary changes in their personal ecosystem and advocate for change when necessary.

Because children live within the environmental context of home, school, and peer group, it is important for an abused child to have the opportunity to have socially and educationally rewarding interactions in the school environment. Interventions can be geared toward helping children acquire the necessary socialization skills to have meaningful peer relationships. Group counseling can be particularly helpful with peer socialization.

Children may also need assistance in gaining access to special educational services and supports such as tutoring or individualized educational plans to help them reach their academic potential, or they may need guidance or encouragement to participate in extracurricular activities such as sports, music, drama, or art. Connections to an enriching ecosystem further support and cultivate positive experiences of self for the child while diminishing the overall negative impact of their trauma. Positive experiences foster feelings of empowerment, self-worth, and pride in oneself.

Abused children may need encouragement to take risks such as inviting peers for a birthday party or going on an outing with friends. Especially if children perceive themselves as unpopular, they may assume that no one will want to be their friend and may refuse to take chances to make new friends.

A crisis worker should be knowledgeable about the types of services and opportunities available for children in their community. An abused child may greatly benefit from going to a summer camp, having a mentor like a big brother or big sister, or doing volunteer work that gives them the opportunity to help others or care for animals.

Positive relationships with family and friends should be encouraged and fostered whenever possible. Appropriate family members should be included in the crisis counseling process. The crisis counselor can also assist family members to encourage the child to make growth-enhancing personal ecosystem changes and be an advocate for the child when necessary. A child survivor of trauma *can* reclaim his or her childhood.

The Importance of Termination with Abused Children

Saying "good-bye" to the working relationship with an abused child should be carefully and jointly planned. Good-bye will probably be more like *"We'll say good-bye for now but I'll be here if you need me"* because the child may need reassurance that the counselor will be there if things get difficult. If the child has a trusting and positive relationship with the counselor, the child may struggle to understand why it is necessary to stop working together even if he or she is functioning well.

The child may perceive counseling as enjoyable and consider the counselor a friend. It is useful to gradually decrease sessions from weekly, to biweekly, to monthly, as this enables the child to still check in with the counselor and receive support and validation for his or her accomplishments. Even infrequent counseling sessions can serve as a psychological safety net for the child while providing supportive maintenance. Prior to termination, treatment planning should be geared toward fostering and cultivating a safe and supportive natural helping network for the child to assure his or her continued access to needed emotional and psychological sustenance.

A determination about when to terminate should consider (1) what current benefits the child is receiving, (2) whether the benefits warrant continued treatment, and (3) the availability of these benefits in the child's natural environment. Ideally, termination should not have a negative impact on children. It should give the children a say in how and when to say good-bye, along with a feeling of accomplishment based on the progress and growth they have made during treatment. Counselors should remind children of their achievements or provide a certificate of achievement and have some type of celebration at the last session, complete with a reward or prize.

Group Support for Abused Children

Improving socialization skills   A primary goal of group interventions with abused children is to help improve socialization skills with peers. Group objectives often seek to introduce concepts such as sharing, helping, compromising, conflict resolution, team work, appropriate physical boundaries, appropriate verbal communication, anger management, and following rules. Group facilitators assist the children in practicing newly learned social skills in a variety of situations including dialog, therapeutic games, role-playing, free play, storytelling, and drawing.

Maltreated children can develop strategies to cope with uncomfortable aspects of social involvement including choosing appropriate friends; forgiving; apologizing; handling ridicule; teasing; peer alienation; managing feelings of anger, sadness, disappointment, and fear pertaining to social situations; and understanding appropriate ways to compromise and deal with conflict and disagreement. Group members are encouraged to explore and use new behavioral skills in a variety of social situations such as making new friends and interacting with teachers, parents, other authority figures, siblings, and peers.

The group can be a forum to learn and practice social skills and achieve better social competency. Group peer members can help each other by explaining to each other, in their own language, why certain behaviors are appropriate or inappropriate. Helping each other can contribute to a greater understanding of appropriate social behaviors and also increase feelings of self-esteem and self-efficacy as children experience themselves as able to help others.

Improving self-esteem, self-worth, and self-efficacy   Group interventions can also focus on improving feelings of self-esteem and self-efficacy. Group objectives should encourage the group members to explore and appreciate their individual talents, capabilities, and resources. Group facilitators can design activities that enable children to formulate and build upon existing strengths, to increase their capabilities and achieve greater feelings of competency and self-worth, and to validate and support each other.

Group members can explore and conceptualize goals and plans for their futures while formulating realistic strategies to achieve those goals. Facilitators can provide children with a host of self-esteem-building exercises and activities that include setting goals, establishing plans to meet goals, identifying needs versus wants, communicating feelings to others, learning how to make choices and handle mistakes, understanding feelings such as guilt, anger, and sadness, and understanding ways to maintain one's self-worth despite obstacles.

Identifying and exploring feelings and processing the effects of abuse   Group interventions can also assist children to process the aftereffects of the abuse. A primary objective is for group members to explore and identify their feelings through discussions so they can understand the common feelings that accompany abuse. Facilitators can encourage children to conceptualize all feelings as acceptable and to understand that feelings are neither right nor wrong.

Children experience relief in learning that they are not alone in their feelings or in the many difficult situations they have encountered, such as physical or sexual abuse; being in foster care; having contact with numerous professionals such as caseworkers, therapists, psychiatrists, and advisors; having previous psychiatric hospitalizations; not being able to live with siblings; or not having contact with parents or other family members. These experiences are uncommon for most children; therefore, abused children have difficulty finding understanding, acceptance, and support from peers who may not be able to comprehend their life experiences.

In the group setting, children have the opportunity to process as much of their abuse as they are cognitively, emotionally, and developmentally able to. Children should never be forced or coerced into participating in a group or discussing their abuse experiences, however; rather, they should be welcomed into a group setting that fosters an atmosphere of trust, safety, and belonging. This provides the opportunity to share the secret of the abuse in a safe, noncoercive, and accepting atmosphere. The group validates and supports the child and explores strategies to assist members to take care of themselves physically and emotionally.

The group facilitator assists the children to understand the abuse and its impact, and to design their own safety plans in case they ever feel at risk of revictimization. Each child's plan includes a list of people and telephone numbers to call, along with a safe way to exit the threatening situation. Empowerment strategies are incorporated to help group members acquire the skills they need to protect themselves from revictimization.

CASE EXAMPLE: CASEY

Single-Session Crisis Intervention

A Child Protective Services agency received a referral from a local elementary school guidance counselor who reported suspected childhood sexual abuse of one of her students, Casey, age nine. That morning, Casey told her counselor her secret that her father "does bad things to me and I'm not supposed to tell what he does." Upon further inquiry by the counselor, Casey disclosed that her father regularly "did it to me" (referring to having intercourse with her).

An intake caseworker from Child Protective Services was immediately sent to the school to investigate the referral. The caseworker's interview with Casey took place in the guidance office during school hours. Casey was initially shy when talking with the caseworker but became more verbal and cooperative as the interview progressed. Casey finally disclosed to the caseworker the details of being severely sexually abused by her father "for as long as I can remember" and stated that her mother "didn't believe" or "didn't care" that it was happening. The caseworker decided to take emergency protective custody of the child and arranged to coordinate these efforts with the police.

Casey willingly agreed to go back to the caseworker's office with her when the caseworker told her that she would need to tell some other people, like a police officer, about what happened to her. During the ride to the office, the caseworker told Casey that she would have to go to a foster home, at least for a little while, until it could be determined that it was safe for her to return home. When hearing this, Casey became progressively more distraught and agitated (i.e., crying, screaming, cursing, begging to go home, refuting the allegations of sexual abuse).

When they arrived at the office, Casey refused to get out of the car, became more agitated, began kicking the back of the seat, and started screaming that she wanted to go home. Despite the caseworker's attempts to console her, she refused to get out of the car. The caseworker arranged for a crisis counselor known for her specialty in working with children who have been sexually traumatized and children who have been in foster care to talk to Casey, who was still refusing to get out of the car.

Prior to meeting with Casey, the crisis worker obtained as much information as possible via a telephone consultation with the caseworker. She obtained information regarding Casey's age and grade in school and a brief overview of her family constellation. The crisis worker obtained information about the details of the protective services intake interview including the disclosure of sexual abuse and how Casey's emotional state decompensated after being informed she would be going to foster care.

The crisis worker arrived in the parking lot of Child Protective Services and requested to speak with Casey alone in order not to further overwhelm or agitate her. The crisis worker walked slowly up to the side of the car and stood about six feet from the passenger-side rear window. She bent down to see Casey sitting in the back seat staring straight ahead, appearing not to notice anyone. Her eyes looked red from crying and her hair was disheveled. Her affect was blunt and she appeared to be dazed.

In this case, the crisis worker would (1) seek to help Casey increase her capacity to soothe herself and regain appropriate behavioral control; (2) strive to be a person that Casey could trust with her feelings of loss, sadness, and anger; and (3) be truthful and honest with Casey regarding the necessity to remove her from her home. Ongoing assessment would seek to gauge her risk to self or others. It would be important to help Casey feel a sense of control and choice whenever possible to reduce her feelings of helplessness and powerlessness over her current situation.

CW: *(speaking slowly and loudly because Casey is in the car)* Hi, Casey. My name is Michele. *(waving hello)* I want you to know that I am not going to come any closer to the car unless you tell me I can. I was hoping we could talk about why you don't want to get out of the car.

Casey: I want to go home and they won't take me! *(There is the sound of Casey kicking the seat. She still has not looked at the crisis worker but she appears angry.)*

CW: It sounds as though not being able to go home is really making you mad. I bet if the back of that seat could talk, it would say, "She's really, really, really, mad. I should know. I've been getting kicked by her for over an hour!" *(in a playful voice, in a kind tone, with a slight smile)* What do you think the seat would say?

Casey: *(pause)* It would say, "Take her home and everything will be OK." It would say *(pause)* "You should have shut up and not told!" *(Casey looks at the seat and talks to it)*

CW: *Why would the seat not want you to tell? (sounding very curious and perplexed)*

Casey: Because telling—telling is going to put me in foster care—I don't want to go there! *(she gives the seat a slight kick and looks briefly at the counselor)*

CW: *I am really confused now. Could you roll down the window a bit so I could hear you better? (Casey rolls the window down halfway.) Thank you. You know, I thought I heard you say that you thought telling about what happened is putting you in foster care? (sounding genuinely confused)*

Casey: Yeah. *(sounding sarcastic)* He said if I told I'd get in trouble and have to go to foster care. I thought I was going to talk to the police and he'd get in trouble. *(pause)* They just lied to me to get me in the car and take me away! *(eye contact with counselor is improving)*

CW: *(looking very surprised) Oh, now I think I get it. (pause) Let me know if I got this right, OK? You think you're being punished for telling and that foster care means you are in trouble. I can see why you would be mad about that. I would be mad too if they put children in foster care to punish them! Is that what you think?*

Casey: I told what happened and now they want to put me in foster care. *(spoken sternly and concretely)*

CW: *But you didn't do anything wrong by telling. (spoken gently but confidently) Telling was a brave thing to do and it was the right thing to do. Going to stay in foster care is to keep you safe to make sure no one hurts you like that anymore. (pause) Does that make sense?*

Casey: No! *(starts to cry)* I want him to get in trouble. *(pause)* HE NEVER GETS IN TROUBLE. I ALWAYS GET IN TROUBLE!

CW: *What he did was something grownups should get in trouble for doing to a child. It's against the law and that's why the caseworker wanted you to tell the police. She was not lying to you about talking to the police. You are not in trouble for telling, but things will change now in order to keep you safe from harm. (pause) Do you understand that you are not in trouble?*

Casey: Yes *(tentative and not confident)*, but I don't want to go to foster care. I wish I did not tell—then I could go home. *(appearing sad)* He should get in trouble, too. *(contradicting her understanding that she is not in trouble)*

CW: *This is a very confusing time—you're going to feel a lot of different feelings about telling. (pause) Even if it feels as though you're in trouble, I want you to know that foster care is really not meant to punish you. Foster care is to make sure you will be in a safe place until it is decided that you can be safe at home.*

Casey: Why can't I just go home? *(Casey begins sobbing and holding her head in her hands)*

CW: *I hear that you very much want to go home—but I have to tell you the truth, even if you don't want it to be true. The truth is that even if you stay in the car, the caseworker will not take you home.*

Casey: *(Softly sobbing and hiding her face, Casey says nothing, but the counselor allows a long pause to give Casey time to express her feelings.)*

CW: *This may be the hardest thing you have ever had to do. (pause) That's what makes you so brave for telling this secret—so other people can help make it stop. Children should not have to make abuse stop all by themselves. Do you know that none of this is your fault?*

Casey: *(pause)* I didn't want it to happen—I tried to make it stop because it was bad. *(pause)* What he did was a bad thing.

CW: *What he did was very, very wrong for a grownup to do to a child. Children just can't make it stop all by themselves. They need the help of some adults to make it stop and keep them safe. Right now, part of being safe is going into foster care. Do you understand that?*

Casey: *(hesitates and looks at CW)* Okay, but I don't want to stay long.

CW: *I can't tell you how long it will be—but I will try to help you get comfortable being in foster care in any way I can. (pause) Perhaps there are some special things from home that you would like to take with you or some phone numbers of your friends or teachers that I could get for you?*

Casey: Yes. *(pause)* Yes, I want my good stuff with me.

CW: *Good, I think I can help with that. I will need to write it down. Oh, I brought some juice for us to drink. I thought you might be thirsty, so I brought an apple juice and an orange juice. Would you like one?*

Casey: I'll take the apple juice.

CW: *Ummm. I need your help here. I told you when we first met that I wouldn't come any closer to the car without your permission. My arms aren't long enough to hand you the drink. Do you think it would be OK if I sat in the car with you? We could keep talking and have some juice together.*

Casey: OK.

CW: *Where would you like me to sit?*

Casey: Over here. *(pointing to the other side of the back seat)*

CW: *(gets in the car and smiles pleasantly at Casey)* Boy, I'm glad you let me come in and sit down. I really appreciate that because my legs were getting tired and numb. Are you feeling tired? *(hands the apple juice to Casey)*

Casey: Yes. *(pauses to sip her juice)* Today looked like it was going to be good. *(pause)* I got a B on a math quiz—that's good for me 'cause I mostly get Ds in everything. *(pause)* Today turned out to be the worst day of my life.

CW: *Really? (said in a surprised tone) I can see why today may be like no other day you ever had. It does seem as though it will be a really, really hard day but in the end it could turn out to be a really really good day for you. (pause) I don't know if that will make sense to you now.*

Casey: You mean . . . cause I told, don't you?

CW: *(smiling proudly at Casey) Exactly! A lot of the time it's really hard to do the right thing. The bigger the right thing we have to do, the harder it can be. (pause) I want you to know that telling what happened was the rightest, (pausing for effect) bestest, (pause) goodest, (pause) bravest, (pause) wonderfulest (pause) thing you could do!*

Casey: *(smiling proudly)* Think so?

CW: *Oh, yes. What do you think?*

Casey: I think . . . what he did was bad. He is not supposed to do . . . that. *(starting to look sad)* He just wouldn't stop. *(looks away outside the window)*

CW: *Casey, (pause) people who do that to children are wrong and almost never "just stop," even if they know it is wrong. It may not be fair that you were the one who had to tell . . . but somebody had to tell to make it stop. That's what makes you so brave. Was it hard to tell?*

Casey: Sorta. I didn't even know . . . know . . . I was going to tell. I don't think I could have . . . if I thought about it.

CW: *So how did you end up telling?*

Casey: It just kinda came out . . . when I was in guidance. *(referring to the guidance office)* Ms. Smith is so nice. It's easy to talk to her. It just came out. *(pause)* I can't believe . . . I really told.

CW: *You did the right thing by telling. (said with emphasis) Are you surprised you really told the secret?*

Casey: Yeah. I guess things will be different now.

CW: *Yes, they will. How do you think things will change?*

Casey: I . . . I'm not sure.

CW: *Let's talk about that. I don't know all the ways they will change . . . but I do know some. (pause) Hey, let's play a game. I'll name one thing I think will change, then you name one. OK?*

Casey: OK.

CW: *You will be protected from your father touching you in the wrong way.*

Casey: *(pause)* I have to go to foster care. *(sad voice)*

CW: *(pause) Going to foster care will help keep you protected from being hurt— until it is sure you will be safe. (pause) OK, that may not be a new one but I had to put the two together. Do I have to say another one?*

Casey: YES!

CW: *Humm. You will need to tell more grownups about what happened. Like the police need you to tell them about what happened.*

Casey: Do I have to talk to them now?

CW: *You will have to talk to them very soon. Probably today. Do you want me to find out if they are waiting and when you need to talk with them?*

Casey: Don't go. I don't want to know.

CW: *It's getting close to the time when we will have to get out of the car and find out.*

Casey: What if I don't get out? *(resigned and passive tone)*

CW: *Honestly, I think that would be a very poor choice to make. You really can't go home now. . . . You already know you can't live in this car. (pause) Think about it. (silly tone) How would you go to the bathroom, eat, or do fun stuff? (pause) How can I help you get ready to get out of the car and do what you need to do next?*

Casey: Can you be with me when I talk to the police?

CW: *I'm not sure, but if I can't be in the room I will be right outside the door waiting. We can talk more when you get out. Would that be OK?*

Casey: I guess.

CW: *I have an idea (sounding positive). Why don't we both get out of the car together and find out what is going to happen next? What do you think?*

Casey: OK, but I have to use the bathroom first.

CW: *No problem. We'll find the bathroom first. Then you and I will find the caseworker who drove you here and ask her lots and lots of questions about what is going to happen next. But Casey, I have one more thing to say that's really important for you to hear, OK?*

Casey: OK.

CW: *I want you to know that it is OK to disagree with something and not like some of what is going to happen. You should tell people when you feel that way. They should try to help you if they can. Not everything is going to go the way you want, but all the grownups you will talk to about what happened want to keep you safe from being hurt. But . . . but . . . but . . . are you ready? Here it comes. . . . I'm going to say it now. . . . Don't you wonder what it is I'm going to say? Why can't I just say it? Well, here it comes (pause). . . . Some of this may really stink, but none of it is your fault. Got it? (smiling)*

Casey: Right! *(smiling)*

CW: *Good. Well, let's get out of the car now. Oh, let's talk with the caseworker about the special stuff you would like to get from home, write it down, and see what can be done.*

Crisis Worker's Evaluation of Single-Session Crisis Intervention

Affect

The initial assessment of Casey's affect indicted she was experiencing shock and confusion due to the enormity of her disclosure of sexual abuse and the realization that the caseworker planned on placing her in foster care. Especially for a child, the burden of keeping the secret of sexual violation may necessitate compartmentalizing the abuse, which includes an often unconscious attempt to deny or repress the abuse in order to cope and function when the abuse is not occurring. Casey's disclosure of sexual abuse forced her to confront the emotional reality of her abuse including feelings of fear, shock, helplessness, and anger.

The crisis worker was aware that an initial disclosure of sexual abuse can temporarily compound feelings of anxiety, fear, and shame. She was aware that Casey might be having difficulty for any or all of the following reasons: (1) the perception that "telling" might get her in trouble, (2) the belief that she was at fault for the abuse, (3) the embarrassment of discussing a taboo subject, (4) the emotional intensity of putting the details of the abuse into words, (5) the fear of not knowing what was going to happen next, (6) the process of talking to a stranger, and/or (7) feelings of disloyalty or guilt related to the possibility of hurting her father.

Initially, Casey's affect could be described as blunt, stunted, bland, or numb. She was overwhelmed by the magnitude of the events that transpired in a relatively brief period of time. Her feelings of helplessness and powerlessness were amplified when she found out that she would be placed in foster care.

The crisis worker wanted Casey to understand that she recognized her anger and respected her feelings, but she also needed to begin to defuse Casey's angry resistance. The first step was for the crisis worker to present herself as a nonthreatening person who would not try to "drag her out of the car," because being in the car was providing Casey with a sense of safety, personal space, and a feeling of control.

It was important to help Casey regain a feeling of safety, personal agency, and control in a way that would not jeopardize her or lead to an escalation of the situation. The crisis worker first intervened by giving a voice to an inanimate object because Casey was displacing her anger on the seat. This element of humor and playfulness was intended to be nonthreatening. It invited Casey to respond in an atypical way that was not like talking to an adult in a position of power over her. It gave her an object through which she could project her feelings and thoughts.

Behavior

Casey's behavior clearly communicated that she (1) was displeased about going to foster care, (2) felt angry and was seeking a way to express her disagreement with what was happening to her, (3) wanted to regain a feeling of control and choice, and (4) had the strength and fortitude to take a stand against another perceived violation. It was important for the crisis worker to appreciate and respect her refusal to leave the felt safety of the car, which indicated that she wanted her voice to be heard and that she was going to express her feelings (by acting out) even if she had to reject what was expected of her and rebel against authority. These same personal qualities enabled her to survive the sexual trauma and led to her eventual disclosure of the abuse. These qualities will also serve her in healing from her trauma and coping and adapting to the subsequent changes she will face.

Casey reacted to the perceived crisis of going into foster care by putting her feelings into behavioral action by refusing to get out of the car. The crisis worker needed to assess the possibility that Casey might become a danger to herself or others. If she thought her behavior was not sending a strong enough message, she might have tried to "up the ante" and become more aggressive. The crisis worker had to assess whether Casey had the potential to harm herself and, if so, whether it would be to the degree that would necessitate hospitalization. Casey responded well to the crisis intervention and, following this session, did not seem to pose an active threat. She made no verbalizations or actions that indicated she intended to harm herself or others. Prior to this crisis session, her aggressive behavior was limited to her attempts to remain in the car and she quickly de-escalated once she was engaged and when she realized she would not be forced to leave the car.

Cognition

Casey's beliefs about why she was being placed in foster care were distorted and false. She thought the caseworker was lying to her about why she was going to the Child Protective Services office. Because childhood sexual abuse violates a child physically, emotionally, and cognitively, it is important not to assume that the child perceives reality the same way others do.

Thoughts about reality are subjective, and experiences are filtered through the lenses of past knowledge, experiences, and beliefs. Casey had a distorted perception of foster care from information her father had given her, and based her actions on this perception. Casey's father had lied to her and betrayed her in the course of her abuse and, as a result, she was more suspicious of others and doubted the veracity of what she was told.

Children Casey's age think in concrete and absolute terms. Therefore, when the caseworker told Casey that she was going to talk to the police, Casey was more apt to think that that was the only thing she was going to do, and, further, that it would get her father in trouble, but not her. In her mind, she was prepared to do that. She did not have the cognitive capacity to see the bigger picture, which would have required her to be able to predict that her disclosure would lead to a complicated series of events geared toward ensuring her safety.

When the caseworker told her that she would be going into foster care, Casey thought of it as a punishment. The single-session crisis intervention assisted Casey in understanding that foster care was not meant to be punitive, reinforced the fact that she did have to go to foster care, and focused on her need for safety and protection. The crisis worker presented this information in a manner that Casey would understand by using a child's language, being clear and honest, and not invalidating her feelings.

Development

Single-session crisis interventions with children typically do not afford the luxury of detailed information about developmental history but crisis workers can extrapolate a fair amount if they have a good knowledge base of general childhood development and an understanding of how trauma affects a child's functioning. Casey's verbalizations and behaviors were consistent for a traumatized child in her age range.

In times of trauma and crisis, children are prone to regression and decompensation in functioning. A child of Casey's chronological age may behave more like a younger child or even a toddler depending on the duration, frequency, and intensity of the trauma. In this crisis intervention, Casey behaved like a traumatized nine-year-old, in some ways acting her age and in others acting more like a younger child.

Developmentally, Casey needed to have information presented to her in a clear manner that she could understand. She was more likely to hear an adult who was empathizing with her discontent because the adult was not monopolizing the conversation or discounting her perspective. The adult must earn the right to be heard by the child through active listening and compassion. Children usually have fairly predictable and constant daily routines and function within the context of their familiar environments. Even abuse can become familiar and routine for children. Casey was struggling to find a way to comfort and soothe herself in a situation that was foreign. With no previous experience to draw upon and no previously known safe persons to aid her, Casey's intense emotions were overwhelming to her.

Ecosystem

At the time of the initial crisis session, it was evident that Casey felt she had few resources and supports available to her. Casey recognized that foster care would entail drastic changes in her environment including the loss, even if only temporarily, of many people, places, and things that were meaningful and valuable to her.

It was important for the crisis counselor to be respectful of the loss and change of environment that foster care would entail and to find ways to ease this transition, such as helping Casey to get favorite objects to take with her. Casey had created a microecosystem within the car and was identifying the car as her safe place. She needed to see that the adults outside the car wanted to help her, did not think she was bad or at fault, and could be trusted. As Casey began to perceive the helping professionals more positively, she was less resistant to leaving the safe car and facing the challenges ahead of her. When she realized that she would have support from the crisis counselor, the outside world felt less threatening to her. As she regained emotional stability she became more empowered to cope with the looming environmental changes, including being introduced into foster care.

DISCUSSION QUESTIONS

1. Compare and contrast the characteristics of childhood physical abuse and childhood sexual abuse:
   a. What are the similarities?
   b. What are the differences?
   c. What might a physically abused child be thinking and feeling when first meeting a crisis worker?

d. What might a sexually abused child be thinking and feeling when first meeting a crisis worker?

e. If a child has been both physically and sexually abused, how might the crisis worker be sensitive to both types of abuse?

2. In the process recording of the intervention with Casey, the first words she says to the crisis worker are "I want to go home and they won't take me!" As a crisis worker, how would you respond to Casey? Record exactly what you would say to her and explain why you selected that intervention.

INDIVIDUAL OR SMALL-GROUP EXERCISES

1. Compose a list of "Do's" and "Don't's" for working with abused children. Compare your list with other members of the class and decide together on the best "Do's" and "Don't's."

2. The topic of child abuse often elicits strong negative feelings. Discuss your emotional reactions to childhood physical and sexual abuse. For each reaction, identify how it might present a barrier when working with an abused child. What steps could you take to proactively reduce this potential obstacle prior to crisis work with abused children and their families?

REFERENCES

Armstrong, L. (1982). The cradle of sexual politics. In M. Kirkpatrick (Ed.), *Women's sexual experience: Explorations of the dark continent* (pp. 109–125). New York: Plenum.

Beebe, B., & Lachmann, F. M. (1988). The contribution of mother-infant mutual influence to the origins of self- and object representations. *Psychoanalytic Psychology, 5,* 305–337.

Benjamin, J. (1990). An outline in intersubjectivity: The development of cognition. *Psychoanalytic Psychology, 7,* 33–46.

Briere, J., & Runtz, M. (1988). Symptomatology associated with childhood sexual victimization in a nonclinical adult sample. *Child Abuse and Neglect, 12*(1), 51–59.

Briere, J., Smiljanich, K., & Henschel, D. (1994). Sexual fantasies, gender, and molestation history. *Child Abuse and Neglect, 18*(2), 131–137.

Chodorow, N. (1989). *Feminism and psychoanalytic theory.* New Haven, CT: Yale University Press.

Cosentino, C. E., & Collins, M. (1996). Sexual abuse of children: Prevalence, effects, and treatment. In J. A. Sechzer. & S. M. Pfafflin (Eds.), *Women and mental health* (pp. 45–65). Annals of the New York Academy of Sciences (Vol. 789). New York: New York Academy of Sciences.

Courtois, C. A. (1988). *Healing the incest wound: Adult survivors in therapy.* New York: W. W. Norton.

Davies, J. M., & Frawley, M. G. (1994). *Treating the adult survivors of childhood sexual abuse: A psychoanalytic perspective.* New York: Basic Books.

Finkelhor, D. (1981). *Sexually victimized children*. New York: Free Press.

Finkelhor, D. (1984). *Child sexual abuse: New theory and research*. New York: Free Press.

Finkelhor, D., Hotaling, G., Lewis, I. A., & Smith, C. (1990). Sexual abuse in a national survey of adult men and women: Prevalence, characteristics, and risk factors. *Child Abuse and Neglect, 14*(1), 19–28.

Gold, S. N., Hughes, D. M., & Swingle, J. M. (1996). Characteristics of childhood sexual abuse among female survivors in therapy. *Child Abuse and Neglect, 20*(4), 323–335.

Heath, V., Bean, R., & Feinauer, L. (1996). Severity of childhood sexual abuse: Symptom differences between men and women. *American Journal of Family Therapy, 24*(4), 305–314.

Helfer, M. E., Kempe, R. S., & Krugman, R. D. (Eds.). (1997). *The battered child* (5th ed.). Chicago: University of Chicago Press.

Herman, J. (1992). *Trauma and recovery*. New York: Basic Books.

Jansson, B. S. (1997). *Social policy: From theory to policy practice* (2nd ed.). Pacific Groves, CA: Brooks/Cole.

Johnsen, L. W., & Harlow, L. L. (1996). Childhood sexual abuse linked with adult substance use, victimization, and AIDS risk. *AIDS Education and Prevention, 8*(1), 44–57.

Jones, D. (1997a). Assessment of suspected child sexual abuse. In M. E. Helfer, R. S. Kempe, & R. D. Krugman (Eds.), *The battered child* (5th ed., pp. 296–312). Chicago: University of Chicago Press.

Jones, D. (1997b). Treatment of the child and the family where child abuse or neglect has occurred. In M. E. Helfer, R. S. Kempe, & R. D. Krugman (Eds.), *The battered child* (5th ed., pp. 521–542). Chicago: University of Chicago Press.

Kirschner, S., Kirschner, D. A., & Rappaport, R. L. (1993). *Working with adult incest survivors: The healing journey*. New York: Brunner/Mazel, Publishers.

Kluft, R. P. (1993). Basic principles in conducting the psychotherapy of multiple personality disorder. In R. P. Kluft & C. G. Fine (Eds.), *Clinical perspectives on multiple personality disorder* (pp. 19–50). Washington, DC: American Psychiatric Press.

Mahler, M., Pine, F., & Bergman, A. (1975). *The psychological birth of the human infant*. New York: Basic Books.

Mandell, J. G., Damon, L., Castaldo, P. C., Tauber, E. S., Monise, L., & Larsen, N. F. (1989). *Group treatment for sexually abused children*. New York: Guilford Press.

Martin, H. P. (Ed.). (1976). *The abused child: A multidisciplinary approach to developmental issues and treatment*. Cambridge, MA: Ballinger Publishing.

Mullen, T. E., Martin, J. L., Anderson, J. C., Romans, S. E., & Herbison, G. P. (1996). The long-term impact of the physical, emotional, and sexual abuse of children: A community study. *Child Abuse and Neglect, 20*(1), 7–21.

Neumann, D. A., Houskamp, B. M., Pollock, V. E., & Briere, J. (1996). The long term sequelae of childhood sexual abuse in women: A meta-analytic review. *Child Maltreatment: Journal of the American Professional Society on the Abuse of Children, 1*, 6–16.

Pearce, J. W., & Pezzot-Pearce, T. D. (1997). *Psychotherapy of abused and neglected children*. New York: Guilford Press.

Perez-Foster, R. (1997). Las mujeres: Women speak to the word of the father. In S. Schoenberg & R. Lesser (Eds.), *She foreswore her womanhood: A response to Freud's female homosexual*. New York: Routledge Press.

Putnam, F. W. (1989a). *Diagnosis and treatment of multiple personality disorder*. New York: Guilford Press.

Putnam, F. W. (1989b). Pierre Janet and modern views of dissociation. *Journal of Traumatic Stress, 2*, 413–429.

Roche, D. N., Runtz, M. G., & Hunter, M. A. (1999). Adult attachment: A mediator between child sexual abuse and later psychological adjustment. *Journal of Interpersonal Violence, 14*(2), 184–207.

Ross, C. (1989). *Multiple personality disorder: Diagnosis, clinical features and treatment.* New York: Wiley.

Runtz, M. G., & Roche, D. N. (1999). Validation of the trauma symptom inventory in a Canadian sample of university women. *Child-Maltreatment: Journal of the American Professional Society on the Abuse of Children, 4*(1), 69–80.

Russell, D. E. H. (1986). *The secret trauma: Incest in the lives of girls and women.* New York: Basic Books.

Silverman, A. B., Reinherz, H. Z., & Giaconia R. M. (1996). The long-term sequelae of child and adolescent abuse: A longitudinal community study. *Child Abuse and Neglect, 20,* 709–723.

U.S. Department of Health and Human Services, Administration on Children, Youth and Families [ACYF]. (2001). *Child maltreatment, 1999.* Washington, DC: U.S. Government Printing Office.

U.S. Department of Health and Human Services, The Administration for Children and Families, National Clearinghouse on Child Abuse and Neglect Information. (2002a, February 5 Updated). *About the federal child abuse prevention and treatment act.* Retrieved March 30, 2002, from http://www.calib.com/nccanch/pubs/factsheets/about.cfm

U.S. Department of Health and Human Services, The Administration for Children and Families, National Clearinghouse on Child Abuse and Neglect Information. (2002b, February 22 Updated). *What is child maltreatment?* Retrieved March 30, 2002, from http://www.calib.com/nccanch/pubs/factsheets/childmal.cfm

van der Kolk, B. (1999). The body keeps the score: Memory and the evolving psychobiology of post-traumatic stress. In M. Horowitz (Ed.), *Essential papers on post-traumatic stress disorder* (pp. 301–326). New York: New York University Press.

Videka-Sherman, L. (1991). Child abuse and neglect. In A. Gitterman (Ed.), *Handbook of social work practice with vulnerable populations* (pp. 345–381). New York: Columbia University Press.

Winnicott, D. W. (1953). Transitional objects and transitional phenomena: A study of the first not-me possession. *International Journal of Psychoanalysis, 34,* 89–97.

Winnicott, D. W. (1958). The capacity to be alone. *International Journal of Psychoanalysis, 39,* 416–420.

Zlotnick, C., Zakriski, A. L., Shea, M. T., & Costello, E. (1996). The long-term sequelae of sexual abuse: Support for a complex posttraumatic stress disorder. *Journal of Traumatic Stress, 9*(2), 195–205.

CHAPTER 12

School-Based Crises

LEEANN ESCHBACH

An eighth-grader at the local middle school, Amelia struggled to fit in. This was her second year at this school and most of the students had been classmates for years. It was hard to find peers that would include her. She tried out for the girls' basketball team and they made fun of her basketball shots. The science club kids joked about how much she didn't know. Other kids partied a lot and did some drinking. That didn't fit Amelia either. The popular kids ignored her and when she tried to join their group, one of the cheerleaders, Anna, started making jokes and taunting Amelia. Other kids followed Anna's lead. Amelia found herself alone at lunch and felt as though she didn't belong anywhere at the school. Previously a good student, even her schoolwork was suffering.

Anna and her group's taunting grew progressively worse. Amelia got poor grades in three English projects in a row. The "smart kids" noticed this and began telling her she wasn't smart enough for this school. Everything was wrong. Her dad had a small pistol in the back of his closet. She carried it with her to school in her backpack for three or four days. Anna and her group started making fun of Amelia's clothes, and Amelia increasingly felt alone, resentful, and alienated. On Thursday she carried her backpack to the cafeteria with her. She set her lunch tray down at Anna and her friends' table. Anna challenged her, saying, "What do you think you're doing sitting here?" Amelia took out her dad's pistol and fired it at Anna. The bullet grazed Anna's shoulder. Anna and her friends began screaming and ran out of the cafeteria. Amelia stood, still holding the pistol in her hand.

• • •

Central High School is a large comprehensive high school in an ethnically diverse and socioeconomically polarized community of 75,000. Recently, conflict escalated between students from rival groups, resulting in turf battles on school campus and an increasing amount of graffiti as both groups attempted to mark the areas they perceived they controlled.

On Tuesday night, at the community teen center, a teen from one group made lewd comments and grabbed the girlfriend of one of the leaders of a rival group. A fight subsequently broke out outside the teen center; the police stopped it but no arrests were made. The school principal was unaware of these community events and arrived at school the next morning.

• • •

Brandon immersed himself in third-grade activities at his small neighborhood school. At Highland Elementary there are two classrooms for each grade level, from kindergarten through fifth grade. Brandon's parents are thrilled with the community atmosphere at the school. In fact, the school's motto is "Highland Elementary: A Great Beginning." His mother volunteers as a library aide on Wednesdays. Many of the children in Brandon's neighborhood attend the same school, and Brandon and his friends participate in the school's basketball league and in a youth soccer league that his father helps coach.

One Sunday afternoon in October, returning home from a family trip, Brandon's family was involved in a car accident on the interstate. Brandon and his father were killed instantly. Brandon's mother was slightly injured. Early Sunday evening, Mrs. Coleman, the school counselor, saw the story on the local evening news.

• • •

Cassandra is a junior at a comprehensive high school. She has one older sister who is away at college and a younger sister, Molly, who is a sophomore at the same school. Her parents divorced approximately ten years ago, and Cassandra and Molly live with their mom. They visit Dad once a month. Dad drinks frequently, and Mom and Dad fight constantly over custody, child support, visitation arrangements, and finances.

Cassandra always felt like the "odd one" of the family who didn't fit in. Her sisters were all high achievers in school and in athletics. Cassandra had lost interest in school years ago. In eighth grade she started hanging around with an older group of friends who exposed her to alcohol and drugs. Her alcohol and substance use evolved into abuse. Cassandra started skipping school to hang out with her friends and get high. In tenth grade she was suspended and eventually ended up in a residential treatment facility. When her family came to visit, her older sister didn't know how to talk to her anymore, and even Molly was distant.

When Cassandra came home that summer she felt completely out of step. Her "group" dropped her, and her situation provided fuel for her parents' constant bickering. In eleventh grade Cassandra never caught up academically and said she didn't really care. Molly was getting straight As. Cassandra began drinking and using drugs again, and her life was abysmal—socially, academically, emotionally, and with her family. Her father set up an appointment with a psychiatrist to treat

her depression, and things seemed a little better. One day Molly re-
turned home from school and found Cassandra, who had hanged her-
self in the upstairs bathroom.

SCHOOL AS A CONTEXT FOR CRISIS

Schools serve as an important influence and context for student academic accomplishment and cognitive growth, as well as many other aspects of development: social struggles, emotional struggles, and self-identity formation. Schools are a developmental-ecological system, and school community members face unique crises as well as unique challenges in coping with those crises. Schools are critical contexts for child and adolescent development. Students spend a considerable amount of time at school, and the entire school experience has enormous potential to influence children and adolescents' lives (Bronfenbrenner, 1979).

Students and all members of the school community bring their cultural and familial values, concerns, and expectations to the school community. In many ways, schools are passive recipients of social and family problems (Astor, Pitner, Heyer, & Vargas, 2000). Societal crises such as violence, abuse, death, and gang-related activity in communities encroach and spill over into school communities.

This chapter addresses crises that have an impact on the school community. The school is an important system in the ecology of students, parents, teachers, and all members of the school community. School crises can stem from multiple sources. A crisis in the outside community has the potential to become a school crisis. A crisis affecting an individual in the school community (student, teacher, or staff member) becomes a school crisis. School crises may affect an individual, a group in the school, or the entire school community, and may occur inside the school building or outside, in the larger community.

School crises are embedded in the unique environment and context of a school as well as in the familial and cultural backgrounds of all members of the school community. There may be risk factors at schools that can increase the potential for crises such as violence among students as well as protective factors that can promote adaptive adjustment among students such as self-esteem, self-confidence, and problem-solving skills.

Pitcher and Poland (1992) conceptualized crises as important and seemingly unsolvable problems or situations that cause individuals to feel unable to cope. A hallmark of a crisis event is the severe stress reactions that negatively affect the ability to think and effectively cope. Lovre (2000) defined a school crisis as either an event, impending event, or unstable condition that "seriously impacts members of the school community; causes persons to feel distress, hardship, fear, or grief; results in temporary weakened problem-solving/coping skills or emotional insecurity; [and/or] has traumatic elements or events which may leave people vulnerable to Posttraumatic Stress Disorder or traumatic reactions" (Introduction).

As reflected in the case vignettes at the beginning of the chapter, school crises can occur either within the school setting or in the larger community outside of school. Members of the school community may bring a crisis to school, where it is identified and must be addressed. Alternatively, members of the school community may experience a crisis within the school. School crises not only affect victims and survivors but a large circle of school community members. Thus, in responding and intervening with school crises, crisis workers' clients can include students, teachers, administrators, support personnel, other school staff members, and parents. Schools must not only provide intervention for crisis situations but also prevention and long-term services for the entire school community.

Crises are rare and unexpected events, and it is daunting to anticipate and prepare for the circumstances and special challenges associated with various potential crisis events. This is true whether a crisis affects one individual or the entire school community. It is also true whether the precipitant(s) for the crisis are the result of a series of accumulating stressful situations or one devastating event. Many school-based crises begin as difficulties with one student or a seemingly isolated problem that escalate over time and eventually affect the school system or become exacerbated by the school system. From this perspective, some school-based crises are more accurately conceptualized as processes rather than events (Cornell & Sheras, 1998).

Crises occurring in a school setting generally fall into two major categories: developmental crises and situational crises (Allan & Anderson, 1986). Students often experience developmental crises while negotiating developmental tasks and transitions. Achievement of certain developmental milestones and/or changes is relatively smooth for some students; however, other students may encounter obstacles and unanticipated challenges.

Situational crises include school violence, gang-related activity, abuse, disaster, injury, and death. Typically, situational crises occur unexpectedly. Addressing situational crises in school communities is complex both because of ethical and legal considerations and because crises may cause ripple effects throughout a school community.

The School Ecosystem

Ecosystems theory emphasizes sensitivity to the interpersonal, situational, and sociocultural factors in any situation and draws attention to the transactions and interactions that occur between individuals and their environment. As an ecosystem, the school climate is unique. When a crisis occurs, the entire community reacts. The relationships between members of the school community as well as the school environment itself can provide critical buffers and essential supports for school community members in crisis. Relationships within the school system can accelerate and promote crises, or de-escalate and avert crises.

Another distinguishing characteristic of school crises is the need for both group and individual responses, in a variety of formats and school settings. Thus, a brief overview of the characteristics of a healthy school environment that can support crisis prevention and intervention is useful.

A healthy school environment promotes a sense of community through relationships, emphasizes certain pedagogical approaches, provides consistent policies (including discipline policies), fosters healthy peer relationships, and integrates developmentally appropriate social and emotional topics within the academic curriculum. Community support is a hallmark of effective schools. The level of community support for a school depends in part on the community's "social capital": the family networks, the neighborhood and religious community, and the school's integration with social service and other community agencies (McWhirter, McWhirter, McWhirter, & McWhirter, 1998). The perception of school as a personally supportive community is critical for students' positive connection and affiliation to school as well as their motivation and satisfaction (Baker, 1998). A healthy school ecosystem models collegiality and collaboration between teachers and other school staff.

Pedagogical approaches that emphasize student decision-making and problem-solving skills and self-monitoring of behavior and school progress, and that promote an attitude of shared responsibility for learning also contribute to a healthy school ecosystem. School policies, including those covering discipline, need to be consistent and clearly understood by all, and should not unintentionally alienate students who already feel isolated. Baker (1998) asserted that problem student behaviors reflect a poor fit between the performance demands of the school and students' developmental capacities. Recognizing the importance of peers on student development as well as the socializing function of the schools, a healthy school ecosystem systemically promotes positive peer interactions through student dialogue, critical thinking, mediation programs, life skills curricula, violence prevention programs, character education, and other personal and social development programs (McWhirter et al., 1998). A healthy school ecosystem fosters a sense of belonging among students as well as all members of the school community and nurtures all dimensions of student development.

An unhealthy school environment is characterized by a lack of attention to the school culture or climate as well as a failure to appropriately address the academic, personal, and social needs of school community members. An unhealthy school environment does not foster and systemically nurture connections between and among peer groups, which can breed competition among social groups with alienated and outcast students and even school staff. Students and parents do not observe collegiality and collaboration among teachers and other school staff. The lack of role modeling creates an environment in which connections among students tend to be superficial. An unhealthy school environment does not implement school routines and policies in a dependable and uniform way. The demand characteristics of the school may not fit with students' developmental capacities and enhance a broad range of critical thinking and coping skills. In summary, an unhealthy school environment misses key opportunities both for relational enhancement as well as proactive interventions addressing personal, social, academic, and cognitive development.

The Developmental Context for Crises

Students deal with crisis situations within their own unique developmental reality; thus counselors must always "take developmental considerations into account when they are trying to understand the crisis reactions of a child" (Muro & Kottman, 1995, p. 309). Students' developmental background and social milieu influences their reactions to crisis situations. To foster healthy development, all students need respect, safety from harm, freedom from stress, a caring functional family, mutually caring friendships, positive role models, relevant academic success, and positive school relationships (Blum, 1998). A student's developmental deficits can potentially exacerbate crisis situations and their own and others' reactions. Alternatively, personal traits and coping skills acquired through positive cognitive, emotional, and/or social development may enhance student coping strategies and responses to crisis events within the school community.

During middle childhood (ages six to eleven) there are many firsts in students' lives, particularly those associated with school and friends. Socialization with peers is a major concern. Developmental crises involving social relationships may be especially difficult. Cognitively, students in this age group operate concretely and are limited in their ability to reason abstractly and see diverse possibilities. They are unable to cognitively process the implications of a crisis event, as they tend to be bound to the present reality rather than future problems or outcomes of a crisis event (Muro & Kottman, 1995). "Regardless of the type of problem a child is experiencing, whether it is a normal challenge of growing up or a more serious situational problem, mental health professionals need to design interventions that are concrete in nature to engage the child in the problem-solving process. With middle-age children, simply talking about the problem is generally not very effective" (Vernon, 2000, p. 11).

During early adolescence (ages eleven to fourteen) peer relationships and peer approval are paramount. A high concern for others' opinions and fear of negative peer evaluation places early adolescents on an "emotional roller coaster" (Vernon, 2000). In crisis situations, it is often difficult for students in this age group to acknowledge and share their feelings, and they often mask underlying feelings with anger, apathy, or acting out (Vernon, 2000). These students may be oversensitive, particularly regarding relationships. Thus, feelings of grief, sadness, and loss may be overwhelming. They may have intense feelings of helplessness because of their perceived lack of power over external events (Muro & Kottman, 1995). Cognitively, these students are acquiring formal operational thinking; yet the abstract thinking process develops gradually. Given that students often regress developmentally during crises, crisis counselors must assist adolescents to look at alternatives and long-range implications, and help them verbalize their feelings.

Mid-adolescence describes students between fifteen and eighteen years of age. Peer relationships continue to be highly valued. Mid-adolescents are developing social sensitivity; thus, in crisis situations they can be attuned to others' circumstances and needs. Students in this age group are capable of insight and more able to express their emotions than younger students (Vernon & Al-Mabuk, 1995).

Mid-adolescents usually do not feel quite as vulnerable as younger students, yet a crisis situation can trigger intense feelings of vulnerability. As they develop abstract thinking, they can hypothesize and think about the future, and they are less likely to conceptualize everything in either/or terms (Vernon, 2000). During crisis situations, mid-adolescents may initially present "adult-like" reactions to a crisis. Thus, crisis counselors need to be flexible and adjust their interventions to the changing reactions of mid-adolescents. Crisis counselors need to provide opportunities for these students to share—again, and again, and again. Mid-adolescents need a safe, nonjudgmental forum to try out their logical thinking processes and alternative problem-solving possibilities in responding to a crisis situation.

Consideration of students' cognitive, social, and emotional development guides and directs developmentally appropriate crisis interventions. Variability in both maturity and development is important to consider. Although there are normal, expected age-related differences in developmental capacities, within-group differences in development are often more noteworthy than between-group differences. Thus even within a single grade or classroom, students attach their own developmentally relevant meaning to a crisis situation. Development affects students' understanding of a crisis situation, their concern for others, their emotional reactions and ability to share as well as their ability to rely on their supportive social networks. Students' development interfaces with physical, social, and community resources in their personal ecosystem to influence their response to crisis situations.

CRISES IN SCHOOL SYSTEMS

School systems are generally prepared to deal with developmental crises. Counseling professionals in schools routinely apply known developmental frameworks (e.g., cognitive, social, relational, and emotional developmental theories) when providing prevention, intervention, or remediation services to address developmental issues in the school community. School counselors implement the components of their comprehensive school counseling program in a developmentally appropriate manner. Relevant components of a comprehensive school counseling program for developmental crises include school counselors' system support activities (consultation and collaboration), guidance curriculum services (classroom guidance units and structured groups), and responsive services (individual counseling, small-group counseling, referral and consultation) (Ripley, Erford, Dahir, & Eschbach, 2003). The guidance curriculum and responsive services target students' academic, career, and personal and social needs. An ongoing comprehensive school counseling program appropriately addresses many developmental crises in school settings.

School counselors, other counseling professionals, and school staff, however, are typically less prepared to deal with sudden and unexpected situational crises. School staff may find themselves ill equipped and caught off guard for such events. Many situational crises trigger strong emotional reactions among the school staff, contributing to the complexity and difficulty of the response. Also, the school system's response to a situational crisis is often under public scrutiny. Recently, public scrutiny has resulted in criticism of school systems' responses to crises, questioning the efficacy of schools' responses both in terms of timeliness and effectiveness. Pitcher and Poland (1992) asserted one reason that school personnel are caught off guard is that school systems have not invested the necessary material resources and staff to plan and prepare for crisis events. Another reason is the ripple effect of school crises. Few, if any, institutions have as many issues to deal with during a crisis as a school. Any crisis affecting a student or anyone in the school community potentially affects the entire school community. Additionally, in responding to situational crises, mental health professionals already in the schools (e.g., school counselors, school social workers, school psychologists) must coordinate and collaborate with everyone in the school community as well as outside mental health professionals entering the school community.

Too often, school system responses to crises ignore known developmental intervention practice and reflect, instead, a chaotic "crisis mentality." Yet the developmental-ecological model of crisis intervention stresses responding to situational crises within individuals' important environments, thus it is important to mobilize the resources of the school environment. All members of the school community need developmentally appropriate opportunities for sharing. Effective and timely school system responses to crises must stem from developmental-ecological crisis intervention strategies.

Overview of Types of School Crises

Personal developmental crises Many personal developmental student crises evolve from universal developmental milestones such as school transitions or reaching puberty (Muro & Kottman, 1995). Examples of common personal developmental student crises include academic performance anxiety, not being selected for an extracurricular performance event (e.g., sports, drama, debate), physical development changes at a rate different from others in a peer group, sexuality issues, concern with personal appearance, eating disorders, teenage pregnancy, or the college admissions process. Also, Lockhart (2003) detailed several school-related situations that may trigger a crisis for students with disabilities including experiencing fear associated with a life-threatening disability, feeling awkward about addressing normal developmental tasks while being disabled, and feeling helpless.

Developmental transitions may be extremely stressful and anxiety-provoking and difficult to cope with for some students, whereas they may not be stressful at all for others. This underscores the personal and subjective nature of crises, depending on the student's interpretation of the situation (Muro & Kottman, 1995). Thus, counselors need to be flexible in their responses to developmental crises. The student's reaction can guide the counselor's response. Also, because personal developmental crises potentially affect many students, as a preventative measure school counselors can implement classroom guidance sessions addressing common concerns of various developmental groups of students.

Interpersonal or social developmental crises   Interpersonal or social developmental crises are not universal, but they do occur frequently among students. As with personal developmental crises, some students may be relatively unstressed by events in this category, and others may be extremely stressed, unable to cope, or may experience depression or anxiety. A student's family environment may precipitate a crisis for a student. For example, divorce, family dysfunction, another family member's personal crisis, or moving can each precipitate a crisis response for an individual student. The social milieu of the school environment or peer groups outside the school community may trigger a crisis for some students. For example, lack of acceptance by a desired peer group can yield feelings of alienation or loneliness, cause depression, or make a student feel like a social outcast. Further, desire for peer group acceptance often causes a preoccupation with self-image, substance abuse, sexually acting out, or engaging in other risky behaviors. Ongoing teasing and criticism can also trigger an interpersonal crisis for some students.

The discrimination and alienation commonly experienced by students in these crisis situations can be especially challenging for students with disabilities and students struggling with their sexuality. Lockhart (2003) reported that students with disabilities may be victimized because of their disability, unable to succeed in school at a level commensurate with their classmates, and worry excessively that others are talking about them. Adorno and Paris (2000) emphasized that school environmental attitudes about being gay, lesbian, or bisexual may result in feelings of isolation and/or fear. "A teen becoming aware of their same-gender sexual identity within a context of hatred, fear, shame, and secrecy with few to no resources for understanding and support, is at risk for depression and other psychosocial difficulties when hiding one's true self becomes a daily challenge" (Adorno & Paris, 2000, p. 164).

Counselors can offer small-group counseling for students negatively affected by these crises. "Many times students in crisis benefit from hearing that their experiences are similar to those of other children. They may also learn new ways of dealing with problems from other students who have encountered comparable situations" (Muro & Kottman, 1995, p. 307). Other students may need individual counseling for these crises.

Disaster events   Disasters occur when a natural or human-caused event affects large numbers of people simultaneously and suddenly. Natural disasters include forest fires and weather-related events such as earthquakes, tornados, or floods. Disasters caused by people can be unintentional, such as the recent case in which a school bus lost its brakes and crashed into a school building, killing or injuring more than twenty students, or intentional, such as the terrorist attacks of September 11, 2001.

Disasters become crises for school communities, whether the event occurs in or around the school campus, elsewhere in the local community, or outside the local community. The effects of a disaster have an impact on many members of the school community. Particularly with events occurring outside the school community, crisis response counselors may be unaware of the effects of the disaster on some students. For example, following the September 11 attacks, school counselors and other mental health professionals across the country met with students in their classrooms to discuss and process the event. They may have been unaware of students' connections to the people and places directly affected, however. Furthermore, some younger students cognitively generalized the events, expressing concern for their own and their family's future safety. In such cases, the astute crisis counselor tries to ascertain information about relationships and connections students may have to a crisis event and assesses students' developmentally situated responses.

Physical abuse and sexual abuse   Reports of both physical and sexual abuse have increased substantially in the last decade. Legal definitions of abuse vary from state to state, and uncertainty regarding the number of unreported incidents compounds the difficulty in determining the true prevalence of child abuse. In 1995, however, more than half of all child abuse reports originated with professionals affiliated with schools (as cited in Thompson & Rudolph, 2000). Thus, teachers, counselors, and school administrators play a key role in identifying and reporting child abuse.

Child abuse is a crisis that a student brings into the school community. In the school community, child abuse is identified, addressed, and then referred to professionals outside the school community. (Crisis intervention and counseling procedures for child abuse are addressed in Chapter 11.) Yet, it is important to note that child abuse precipitates a ripple effect in the school community. It is well documented in the literature that child abuse survivors struggle to succeed with both the social milieu and academic demands of the school community. Low scores on standardized tests, repeating one or more grades, classroom behavior problems, teen pregnancy, and dropping out of school are common among abused children (Kurtz, Gaudin, Wodarski, & Howing, 1993).

Student death   It is difficult to ascertain accurate statistics regarding the number of student deaths in school communities. It is appropriate to assume that all school-age children or adolescents who die are connected to a school, and that their deaths will have an impact on their school communities.

As high school graduation drew near, one high school senior discussed his upcoming commencement with a counselor:

"There are 374 students in my graduating class. Many of us have gone to school together since kindergarten . . . some of the people I've gone to school with have died. It seems as though we've lost a student from our class almost every year or every other year since elementary school. Some have been close friends. Sometimes that's harder to deal with and get through than figuring out and deciding what I'm going to do after high school."

The death of a student in a school community precipitates a bereavement crisis for the entire school. The bereavement experience for students, teachers, school administrators, and parents in the school community reflects the stages of grieving identified in Chapter 10. Reactions include denial, shock, disbelief, apparent lack of feelings, explosive emotions, somatic symptoms, and the desire to help or "do something" constructive.

Students close to the deceased may include those from the same class, those in his or her grade, those who participated in extracurricular activities with the deceased, and other students, neighborhood friends, friends of siblings, teachers, other school personnel, parents, and school administrators. When mental health professionals examine the dynamics of the school community, they may overlook some people who had close relationships with the deceased simply because they are unaware of those relationships.

Even those who did not have a close personal relationship to the deceased may be strongly affected by an accidental or unexpected death. People in the school community are likely to become acutely aware of their own mortality as well as the personal meaning they associate with death within their own developmental context.

Suicide   Suicide is the third leading cause of death among adolescents (ages fifteen to twenty-four), following unintentional injuries and homicides (National Institute of Mental Health, 2002). Because suicide is underreported, some have speculated that suicide may be the leading cause of death for adolescents, as it is difficult to ascertain motive with some accidental adolescent deaths (Studer, 2000). Specific subgroups of adolescents with very high rates of suicide include troubled adolescents, juvenile offenders, gays and lesbians, and Native Americans (National Institute of Mental Health, 2002).

A suicide attempt within a school community can also precipitate a school crisis. No annual data on attempted suicides are available; however, the National Institute of Mental Health (2002) reported an estimated eight to twenty-five attempted suicides to one completion, with a higher ratio of attempts in children, adolescents, and females. Females are three times more likely to attempt suicide than males; however, males are more likely to complete suicide.

Students who contemplate suicide often struggle with developmental adjustments or transitions that elicit feelings of depression, loss, hopelessness, helplessness, and sometimes anger. Overall, the strongest risk factors for attempted suicide in youth are depression, alcohol or other drug use, and aggressive or disruptive behavior (National Institute of Mental Health, 2002). The theme of loss is common for those contemplating suicide: parental loss through divorce or death, loss of an important relationship, loss of friends, or peer rejection. The pervasive feeling of loss may be exacerbated by substance use. The home environment for suicidal students is often dysfunctional and perceived as nonsupportive. Personal characteristics associated with suicidal ideation in children and adolescents include loneliness, impulsivity, risk-taking, low self-esteem, and faulty thinking patterns (McWhirter, Hunt, & Shepard, 2000).

Suicide was addressed at length in Chapter 5, but the school-wide impact of suicide is noteworthy. Reactions of the school community include not only typical reactions for survivors of a completed suicide such as loss, guilt, sadness, and anger, but also concern about the possibility of contagion effects.

School violence   "School violence is probably best conceptualized as a range of antisocial behaviors on school campuses, ranging from oppositionality and bullying to assaults" (Baker, 1998, p. 29). School violence includes actions between students, between students and teachers or administrators, and, even more disturbing, actions involving parents on school grounds.

Reports of young people injuring or killing their classmates and teachers contribute to the perception that schools are dangerous. In fact, some schools are violent and others are not. In 1996–1997, 57 percent of 1,234 public schools surveyed reported at least one violent incident, and 10 percent reported at least one *serious* violent crime incident (such as murder, sexual assault, suicide, physical attack with a weapon, or robbery) (Morrissey, 1998). According to the Children's Defense Fund (2002), every day in the United States, nine children or adolescents are killed by firearms, nine children or adolescents are homicide victims, and 180 children or adolescents under the age of eighteen are arrested for violent crimes, not necessarily in the school. Teachers are seriously assaulted 70,000 times each year (as cited in Morrissey, 1998).

Despite the documented violence affecting children and adolescents, evidence suggests that the number of students carrying weapons to school has declined 42 percent in recent years (U.S. Department of Education, 2001). Since 2000, there has been a continuing theme in the literature that schools are one of the safest places for children. For example, the Children's Defense Fund (2002) reported that fewer than 1 percent of students nationwide who were murdered or committed suicide during the 1998–1999 school year were at school or on their way to or from school. In 1999, students were more than twice as likely to be victims of serious violent crime while away from school than while at school, as violent youth crime peaks between 3 and 6 P.M.

Popular beliefs about violent crime among students both in and out of school continue to contribute to children's and adolescents' fears regarding their safety, erode the positive developmental contributions of the school community, and foster personal attitudes among youth that lead to violence. This persists despite continued improvements and changes in school safety.

According to studies reviewed by the National Center for Educational Statistics (2002), bullying (defined as being picked on or made to do things that a student does not want to do) is reported by females and males in equal numbers. Students in lower grades were more likely to report being bullied (about 10 percent of students in grades 6 and 7) than students in higher grades (about 5 percent of students in grades 8 and 9, and about 2 percent in grades 10 through 12). Bullying contributes to a climate of fear and intimidation in schools and erodes trust and connections among school members, and poses the danger of escalation of and retaliation among bullies and their victims.

Gang-related behavior   Many school crises involve events that take place entirely outside of school, and it may appear that school authorities can do little about them. Youth gang-related activities in the local community permeate a school community. Gang-related activities and attitudes in schools often parallel gang experiences, belief systems, and mind-sets in the community. It is not easy to gather accurate data on the number of adolescents and children affiliated with gangs and delinquent groups; however, Sandhu, Underwood, and Sandhu (2000) asserted that gang-related behavior is increasing as gang affiliation stretches from the major cities to rural areas and suburbs throughout the United States. During 1995, 28 percent of students surveyed reported that street gangs were present at their schools (National Center for Educational Statistics, 2002). Goldstein and Kodluboy (1998) emphasized that gang presence in schools occurs in all geographic locations, all socioeconomic environments, and among all ethnicities.

"A gang is a group of people that form an allegiance for a common purpose, and engage in unlawful or criminal activity" (Jackson & McBride, 1987, p. 20). One of the most frustrating characteristics of contemporary gangs is that there is little internal control over the activities of individual members, and it is difficult to predict individual gang members' behaviors (Burden, Miller, & Boozer, 1996). Parks's (1995) literature review on school-related gangs revealed that gangs operate at every level of school, including the elementary grades.

WHO PROVIDES CRISIS INTERVENTION IN SCHOOLS?

School Counselors

The primary role of school counselors is to implement a comprehensive developmental counseling program in the school (Bowers & Hatch, 2002). School counselors provide services to members of the school community in a variety of ways: classroom guidance, group counseling, individual counseling, working with peer helpers, facilitating parenting programs, collaborating on and coordinating school-wide programs, and organizing leadership and advocacy efforts (Wittmer, 2000).

School counselors often implement classroom guidance units or lessons. Allan and Anderson (1986) described a classroom guidance unit for elementary and middle school students that offers a preventive approach for crisis situations. The lessons focused on the kinds of crises that affect students, how students felt and what they thought during a crisis, and what helped them in times of crisis. Through this classroom guidance unit, students reported learning the benefits of talking about crises, that they are not alone in experiencing a crisis, and that a crisis will pass. Students learned adaptive coping skills that they could use in crisis situations.

There are three contemporary models to guide school counselors' development, implementation, and evaluation of a comprehensive school-counseling program. All three models address the role of the school counselor in preventing and responding to crisis events occurring within the school facility as well as crisis events in the outside community that affect the school system and its members.

The National Standards for School Counseling Programs (American School Counseling Association, 2002) articulate the key components of a school counseling program and describe the knowledge and skills that all students should acquire through participation in the program (Campbell & Dahir, 1997). The content focuses on personal/social, academic, and career development. Several student competencies are detailed to facilitate and encourage student development, including students' ability to identify and express their feelings, develop coping skills, and seek help with problem solving.

Myrick's (2003) developmental guidance approach is based on recognition of all students' developmental trajectory. This approach features a planned curriculum that involves all members of the school community. Understanding the school environment, understanding oneself and others, and decision making and problem solving are three of the seven essential goals identified by Myrick.

In 1996 the Education Trust (2002) proposed the Transforming School Counseling Initiative, which defined the school counselor's role as a leader and team member working with teachers, administrators, and other school personnel. This initiative emphasizes that school counselors serve the school community not only by carrying out their counseling and programming functions, but also by collaborating and coordinating joint efforts with school staff members (House & Martin, 1998).

Comprehensive school counseling programs guided by these contemporary models can facilitate student development. A comprehensive school counseling program provides a foundation for crisis intervention. Students are accustomed to meeting in classroom-size and small groups to discuss and share their personal reactions to various topics. Thus, meeting in these already established groups to share and process crisis-related information provides a familiar context for students. Also, school counselors' leadership and coordination roles combined with their developmental and counseling knowledge and skills are applicable to school-wide crisis intervention.

Teachers

Teachers are in a distinctive position, as they have more contact with students than other adults in the school community. Whether a crisis event involves violence, a personal student crisis, or students' response to an outside disaster, teachers' frontline interactions serve several key roles in both crisis prevention and crisis response.

Increasingly, teachers have to confront crisis situations directly, and sometimes independently. A crisis can erupt in a classroom, in which case the teacher is the sole provider of the initial crisis response. This situation is compounded in some schools, as many school counselors are assigned to more than one school and outside mental health professionals are also itinerant, moving from school to school. Conceivably, a crisis could occur when there were no counseling or mental health professionals in the school building.

Teacher observations of students are critical. Teachers need to be alert for warning signs that are cues to student distress. Because of their ongoing interactions with students during the school day and from day to day, teachers may notice subtle behavioral, cognitive, and emotional changes in students. Teachers have an opportunity to gather information and share their concerns (Callahan, 1998).

Further, in many middle schools teachers work in teams. School counselors are often members of these teams; yet, it is the teacher-to-teacher sharing of student behaviors and nuances that can be particularly helpful in crisis prevention. Also, teachers often supervise extracurricular activities, which provide an unstructured setting for interacting with students and identifying potential problems.

Additionally, teachers serve key roles in early intervention. In many schools, teachers are members of Student Assistance Teams or Child Study Teams. In these situations, they actively provide early intervention services for students struggling with academic, personal, or social difficulties, or for students who lack coping and/or problem-solving skills.

The richest resource teachers have to offer in crisis prevention and intervention is the knowledge they have about their students and their connections with students. Because students and teachers spend so much time together in the school setting, many teachers serve as positive role models or significant adults in students' lives.

The implications of these key teacher roles are clear. First, school counselors and mental health professionals in the school community need to foster good relationships with teachers that emphasize frequent and effective sharing. Second, professional preparation and in-service training for teachers in crisis prevention, crisis response and intervention, and developmentally appropriate communication or basic counseling skills with students is critical. Although teachers should be aware of their limitations as counselors and understand the counseling referral process, teachers who have developed competencies in crisis work are capable of effectively providing single-session crisis interventions and serving on crisis response teams.

School Psychologists

School psychologists typically work in teams with school counselors, teachers, parents, and other mental health professionals "to ensure that every child learns in a safe, healthy and supportive environment" (National Association of School Psychologists, 2003). Core services that school psychologists provide include consultation, assessment, intervention, and education. Many school districts assign a school psychologist to several schools in the district; thus the psychologists may not have a strong relationship to a school community when there is a crisis situation. Also, in many school districts the focus of school psychologists' assessment and intervention efforts is on students' needs to effectively cope and succeed in the school environment. Given legislative and state department of education demands for special student populations, this tends to be a major, time-consuming portion of their work.

Cornell and Sheras (1998), however, asserted that school psychologists are best trained to provide two important crisis responses. First, their training and knowledge in organizing and decision making regarding meaningful, timely, and psychologically appropriate interventions is valuable to all members of a school community affected by a crisis. Second, school psychologists may be uniquely positioned within a school community to understand and appropriately respond to the needs of school administrators and/or teachers.

School psychologists can provide significant insights and knowledge of anticipated crisis dynamics and victim/survivor responses. Further, because school psychologists routinely engage in program evaluation. they can organize evaluations of the crisis response efforts and highlight strengths and effective actions and recommend improvements in the school's response capabilities.

School Social Workers

School social workers facilitate the social, psychological, and educational adjustment of students. School social workers are charged with enhancing the educational and human potential of students and their families as well as promoting sound public policies to meet student needs. School social workers not only provide individual services to students but also coordinate services between schools, families, community organizations, and the court system. In Astor and colleagues' (2000) large survey of school social workers, respondents raised multiple concerns related to their school districts' management of crisis situations. Identified concerns included poor funding, district-level policy restraints, and extremely large case loads that did not permit school social workers to adequately attend to student and family needs.

School districts vary greatly in the way they use school social workers. Some school districts rely on school social workers for primary individual and group intervention with students. In other school districts, school social workers provide services to identified students' families, particularly with those families whose members are involved with multiple social agencies (e.g., child welfare, drug and alcohol, juvenile probation). They may function as coordinators or case managers who strive to develop coordinated and integrated systems of services for students and families. In other school districts, the position of school social worker does not exist. If there are school social workers on the school staff, their knowledge and skill backgrounds are extremely useful in planning, implementing, and evaluating crisis response services in a school community. School social workers are able to conceptualize systemic crisis response services. They have a keen understanding of and ability to interact with other social service agencies and community organizations.

Other Mental Health Professionals

Increasingly, community social service and mental health agencies provide direct services to their school-age clientele within a school building. Some schools designate specific counseling space for mental health professionals to provide individual and group counseling. Other mental health professional services include therapeutic staff support in classrooms and case management and coordination. Whatever the role or presence of outside mental health professionals in a school community, they are valuable resource persons and potential crisis service providers in schools because of their skill, knowledge, and training.

THE DYNAMICS AND IMPACT OF CRISES IN SCHOOLS

The discussion about the school ecosystem earlier in this chapter emphasized the uniqueness of schools as a context for crisis events. School system crises are distinctive in terms of the dynamics as well as the impact of the crisis event. Crises occurring either on or off a school campus become crisis events in a school's ecosystem. Both the experience of someone in a crisis situation and the short- and long-term influence of a crisis are moderated by the school environment and change the school climate. Because school-based crises affect more than one person, crisis workers need to be prepared to provide intervention and counseling to the entire school community.

Appropriate response is critical to prevent further harm and additional stress. The culture and history of a school community must guide the response to school-related crisis events. Environmental conditions and the social functioning of school community members help define a school culture. School culture includes school routines, policies, and roles of school community members as well as interpersonal relationships, support resources, and school community members' reliance on others to assist with problems and crises.

This section examines the dynamics and impact of four school crises: student death, suicide, violence in schools, and youth gang-related behavior. In a school setting it is relevant to explore the dynamics and impact of a crisis event not only among those directly involved, but also among others in the school community. This section also includes a brief overview of prevention and intervention approaches.

Student Death

An unexpected student death in a school community affects everyone, as the loss is experienced by and permeates the entire interpersonal system of a school (Thompson, 1995). When students, teachers, and other school staff learn about a student's death, they may experience the loss in a very personal way in a very public setting, the school building.

Mental health professionals working in the school community are confronted with a number of serious issues following such a loss. Some of the initial tasks they need to tackle include verifying what actually happened, informing the school community, helping students and teachers cope with the death, working directly with concerned parents, protecting the privacy of the family, and communicating with the media, if necessary.

The way members of the school community receive information about unexpected deaths influences emotional responses. Teachers should be notified first, preferably in small groups meeting either in the school counseling office or another private location in the school. It is important to share information with students in a supportive atmosphere. Having two adults (preferably a teacher and either a school counselor or crisis worker) share the information with each class-room-size group facilitates identifying students who may be struggling and who may need immediate individual attention. It is best to contact those closely connected to the deceased and inform them individually or in small groups. A delay in informing the school community provides the opportunity for rumors to spread, which can quickly precipitate another crisis.

The reactions of survivors, students, teachers, and other school staff who learn of an unexpected death are likely to be diverse and complex. Besides sadness, typical reactions to unanticipated death include denial, anger, blaming, guilt, fear, intellectualization, persistent thoughts of the accident, and/or hostility. Individuals may deny the importance of their relationship with the deceased or deny the reality of the unexpected death. Anger or hostility may center on blaming the deceased student for "unsafe behavior," or may be directed toward those assumed to be at fault. Because a young person's death is untimely, survivors often attempt to find someone or something to blame in order to reduce the dissonance the death creates.

Student reactions   Children and adolescents often feel invulnerable and believe that they, their friends, and their favorite adults will live forever. Death and loss seem like strangers in the hustle and bustle of school life. When death does intrude, particularly the death of a significant person in students' lives, the bereavement and grief process becomes one of the most important influences in their subsequent emotional development (Worden, 1996).

There are many reasons grounded in developmental theory why the loss of a close friend may create difficulties for students. Erikson (1963) theorized that a major task of late childhood and early adolescence is identity formation. One of the ways students define themselves is through their interpersonal relationships with peers. Students increasingly see themselves as members of a peer culture. "Thus, the loss of a peer can upset identity formation which may already be unstable" (O'Brien, Goodenow, & Espin, 1991, p. 431). The degree of disruption for students may depend, in part, on the closeness of the student to the deceased peer.

A student's developmental conceptualization of his or her peer's death also influences the impact of the crisis. For example, younger students with middle childhood cognitive development think egocentrically and concretely. Although they will grieve the loss of a friend, their primary concern may be that something similar could happen to them. Adolescents, by contrast, have developed greater social sensitivity and may focus more on surviving family members as well as their own emotional responses.

School counseling professionals must support a variety of reactions, reflecting different developmental levels and a wide range of feelings. Students need to know details about the circumstances of the death. Students interviewed by

O'Brien et al. (1991) said that hearing about the death of a significant person in their life in an impersonal way increased the difficulty of discussing the loss later.

Students often feel alone in their grief and may be unable to recognize the resources and potential support others can provide, but their recovery is facilitated when they have a chance to share with others who are also experiencing the loss. Some students need additional time to internalize the information, but all students can benefit from the opportunity to reminisce about their deceased friend and talk about the loss. Some students are forthcoming in expressing their feelings, raising questions and talking about the loss of their peer, whereas others are more reserved. It is common for students to share disbelief, positive and negative feelings, strong emotional reactions, and questions about details surrounding the circumstances of the death.

Students' cognitive and emotional grief reactions reflect their developmental levels. It is noteworthy that what students say may not mirror what they have internalized; that is, they may say one thing but their internal cognitive and emotional meanings may not be consistent with their verbalizations. Also, there is fluctuation and instability in both cognitive and emotional reactions to the crisis of death.

Students interviewed by O'Brien and colleagues (1991) stressed the importance of speaking about the death of their friend. They reported that a year after their peer's death, although they still felt the need to talk about the loss, there were few people they could speak with about their feelings and reactions. It remained difficult yet important to talk. "I think that all my peers could say was 'I'm sorry,' but it just didn't cut it when someone close dies. Basically, no one would sit down and ask me about it; people just didn't know how" (p. 436).

In reacting to an unexpected death, students' normal coping mechanisms may break down. Students may have pervasive feelings of anxiety, confusion, or failure. After the memorial service and the initial shock have passed, students are confronted with returning to their normal school routine and activities in their daily life. Students may feel guilty for going on with life and having fun. Later, it is not uncommon for students to withdraw socially, display problem behaviors (both in the classroom and at home), have emotional outbursts, regress in their emotional or cognitive development, or manifest physical symptoms (Thompson, 1995).

Recovery from grief ebbs and flows. Students may experience a short span of sadness, unable to endure their painful feelings for long stretches of time. They may express their grief in short, intense emotional outpourings, followed by periods during which they seem to be no longer affected by the loss (Grollman, 1995; Winter, 2000).

Academically, teachers should not expect peak performance from students following a peer's death. Students may be unable to concentrate and may act out in class. Arena, Hermann, and Hoffman (1984) reported that teachers struggled with students' difficult behavior following the death of a classmate, as students were more restless, talkative, and distracted than usual. Younger children, developmentally unable to verbalize their feelings, frequently act out their upset feelings.

After-school activities or active classroom assignments can be an outlet for some of their excess physical energy.

If students cannot reach some resolution of the grief they may become vulnerable to further developmental crises and emotional disorders. Potential for such vulnerability is typically assessed through clusters of warning signs. Although these markers may be expected in initial grief, if they persist over time, children and adolescents may be struggling with more complicated grief responses. Physical signs of continuing difficulty include altered eating and/or sleeping habits or chronic complaints of physical ailments. Emotional warning signs include overwhelming and persistent anxiety, dependency, absence of all grief, resistance to forming new attachments, and/or a desire to die. Behavioral cues include uncharacteristic behaviors, unwarranted hostility or anger toward peers, alienation, regression, continued overachievement or underachievement, and substance use/abuse. Persistent inability to concentrate and distorted or confused thinking are cognitive signs that may also indicate poor adjustment to the loss. These warning signs may signal that a student is not healing and that he or she could benefit from additional support (Lovre, 2000; Winter, 2000).

Teachers and school staff reactions   Teachers should also be given the opportunity to express their own grief. Teachers may expect themselves to be strong, but this is an unfortunate and unhealthy self-imposed mandate. When counselors or administrators share information about an unexpected death with teachers, it is also important to provide them a safe setting to discuss their own needs. Arena and colleagues (1984) identified three needs of teachers: (1) Specific information so that they can respond to the questions and concerns of students and parents. All teachers need the same details about the crisis so the information they share is consistent. (2) The opportunity to express their own grief. This may mean relieving teachers of their classroom responsibilities for a short period of time if they need to be alone or to interact with peers or support professionals to deal with their own personal responses. (3) Prior training and specific guidelines through previous in-service professional development meetings to handle the diverse developmental reactions and experiences of students. All adults in the school community need to be encouraged to take care of themselves—to get adequate sleep; eat regularly; and share with peers, school counselors, mental health professionals, and other crisis workers.

Following school or religious memorial services, teachers confront a number of issues surrounding their students' recovery. How soon should they attempt to return to normal classroom routines? When can they expect students to return to prior levels of academic functioning? What should they do with the deceased student's desk? How often should the death be discussed in the class? Parents may also approach teachers with a variety of concerns. Teachers need to be educated to anticipate and address changes in the classroom behavior of students.

In summary, all school community members have their own developmentally anchored cognitive, social, and emotional responses to the crisis of student death. Individual grief reactions are also influenced by familial and cultural values and beliefs and the responses of support networks. Reactions may range from immobilization to eagerness to return to the normal school routine. The school system must be prepared to respond to the losses precipitated by the unexpected death of a student for a considerable length of time.

Suicide

As described, there are many more suicide attempts than completions among children and adolescents, and some experts believe that suicidal ideation and suicide attempts and completion among youth are much higher than statistics indicate (Studer, 2000). Thus, suicide prevention needs to be a major concern for school personnel. Student suicides differ from other school-based crises because of the self-initiated behavior, the complex underlying motivations, and the various cultural values and interpretations associated with suicide.

Indicators of potential suicide There are numerous characteristics associated with children's and adolescents' suicide attempts. Although it is beyond the scope of this chapter to address suicide prevention, this section provides a brief overview of suicide indicators within the context of the ABCDE model as they impact the dynamics of suicide in the school system.

Affect

A vast majority of suicidal students have affective disorders, primarily depressive disorders. Not all depressed children and adolescents consider suicide, but depression is an important indicator of suicidal ideation, as is hopelessness (Negron, Piacentini, Graae, Davies, & Shaffer, 1997) reported a high level of hopelessness prior to a suicide. "Compared with nonsuicidal peers, ideators reported significantly more overall emotional and behavior problems as well as lower self-esteem, which contributed to suicidal gestures by age eighteen" (Studer, 2000, p. 271).

Behavior

Three behavior patterns are correlated with student suicide. First, students who have difficulty in coping with the academic challenges of school, poor problem-solving skills, and negative peer group involvement are at risk of suicide (Wagner, Cole, & Schwartzman, 1995). This pattern of behavior can lead to social isolation and, for some, to suicidal behaviors. A second pattern of behavior is frequently exhibited by academically gifted students who approach academics with perfectionist standards and have had minimal experience with failure. These students may experience a crisis when their accomplishments do not measure up to their expectations or their perceptions of significant others' expectations (Snyder, 2000). Third, substance-abusing behaviors are frequently present in the lives of suicidal students (Studer, 2000).

Cognition

Overall, suicidal children and adolescents do not manage stress or negative life events well. Many children and adolescents contemplating suicide possess poor coping skills, often based on inaccurate or distorted thinking and resultant problem-solving deficits (Wagner et al., 1995). For instance, an individual may perceive a particular stressor (e.g., switching to a new school, breaking up with a boyfriend, caught cheating on a college entrance exam) as more than he or she can handle and concludes "there is no way out." Studer (2000) noted that "suicide attempters, in comparison with depressed adolescents, have a cognitive style that attaches more negativity and paranoia to a situation" (p. 271).

Development

Those who contemplate suicide tend to believe that their particular developmental problems, issues, and concerns are unique. These high-risk students, who are confronting developmental problems, often lack experience in implementing problem-solving strategies. Their problem-solving difficulties multiply when one negative event is compounded by another negative event. This becomes catastrophic in these students' frames of reference.

This is compounded for certain special-needs youth who are thus at a high risk for suicide. Adorno and Paris (2000) reported that gay and lesbian students are two to three times more likely to attempt or commit suicide than their heterosexual peers. Identity formation is a primary developmental task of adolescents, which can be overwhelming for adolescents struggling with their sexual identity. Gay and lesbian students often face ostracism and struggle with multiple negative peer group issues. McWhirter and colleagues (1998) linked suicide attempts with significant developmental events such as "coming out."

Ecosystem

The transactions between students and their environments are critical to consider when assessing suicide risk. Several researchers have documented a link between family discord and suicide (Henry, Stephenson, Hanson, & Hargett, 1993; Reinherz, Giaconia, Silverman, Friedman, Bilge, Frost, & Cohen, 1995). Some children and adolescents withdraw and isolate themselves from support systems when confronted with disrupted or conflicted family life and parental and family changes. Physically removing oneself from daily stressors by running away from home is another characteristic of children and adolescents who become suicidal, particularly younger adolescents (Studer, 2000). Knowing someone who has attempted or committed suicide is also an important risk factor. Loss within one's environment is a common theme associated with suicidal youth. External life-changing events are often beyond students' control and leave them feeling helpless.

Contagion or cluster suicides   Contagion or cluster suicides occur when more than one suicide attempt or completion happens in similar surroundings—in a peer group, school community, or geographic community. There is some evidence for increased contagion suicide among student populations; thus, the possibility of a compounding suicide event is critical to address. Kirk (1993) paralleled contagion to the infectious disease concept: when an infection is introduced into a vulnerable group of individuals, the probability of infection spontaneously increases. Although some have asserted that it is difficult to prove that one suicide attempt or completion directly causes another, Kirk maintained that there is too much evidence of suicide clustering to dismiss the contagion phenomenon, particularly in school settings. It is critical for crisis workers to be aware of the possibility of contagion or clustering in planning and implementing school-wide postvention.

Key elements hypothesized to increase contagion effects in a school include sensationalizing the suicide, portrayal of teen suicide in the media, and failure to address the suicide at developmentally appropriate levels for students. A suicide must not be glorified or made heroic or others who feel hopeless may consider it as a solution that receives a great deal of attention. For this reason schools should not hold or endorse commemorative memorial services or rituals as might happen following other types of deaths.

It is inappropriate for the media to sensationalize the reporting of a student suicide. Also, Kirk (1993) claimed that there was an increase in suicides following certain television programs and movies depicting suicide in the lives of troubled adolescents. Suicide needs to be discussed carefully within students' developmental context. A common, but inaccurate, myth is that talking about suicide in a classroom makes students more likely to try to kill themselves. In fact, when students are confronted with a peer's death by suicide, they need to talk about it and receive assistance in trying to make sense of a senseless act.

The counselor can portray the student who committed suicide as an individual with problems who did not find an avenue to effectively deal with his or her problems. This should be done without abusing the victim's character (Brock, Sandoval, & Lewis, 1996). Many people have suicidal thoughts, but this does not mean that they are strange. Persistent suicidal ideation is a signal to utilize resources within one's support system. The counselor can portray suicide as a permanent solution to a temporary problem for which help is available (Brock et al., 1996).

Group work to address impact   Bereavement support groups are often recommended to help students cope with loss following the suicide of a friend. Siblings or other family members should receive individual counseling rather than participating in a group with the deceased's peers. Student participation in a school-based bereavement support group needs to be voluntary. The best strategy for identifying potential group members is to contact friends of the deceased and students struggling with the suicide. It is important to acknowledge but not glorify the suicide, and to support survivors in their grief. What needs to be recognized is the individual loss for group members.

Structured group sessions can help student group members with the grief process. Students need to accept the reality of the loss, work through the pain of their loss, adjust to the school environment without the deceased, and move on with life and continue with developmentally appropriate school, extracurricular, and community activities (Hoff, 2002).

Themes to discuss in a group setting to help survivors cope with the impact of a suicide include (1) Identification of clues and signs prior to the suicide that make it more understandable from the deceased's point of view. Group members should also examine the faulty logic or style of thinking that led to suicide as a solution. (2) Recognition of the positive traits of the deceased and positive aspects of student group members' relationships with the deceased. Group members need time to reflect on their relationships with the deceased and their own personal loss. (3) Identification of viable alternatives to suicide. (4) Addressing "survivor guilt" so group members can acknowledge that they are not responsible for their peer's decision. (5) Follow-up that includes appropriate referrals, recognizing that those affected by a suicide may experience problems years after the suicide occurs (Hoff, 2002).

Impact on survivors   Bereaved family members blame themselves more for suicide than any other form of death or loss (Thompson & Range, 1992). In addition to the death itself and all the emotions associated with the loss of a loved one, survivors also confront social stigma, guilt, responsibility, unfinished business, perceived rejection, a search for meaning, and even anger (Rando, 1983; Studer, 2000). Survivors may "feel the pain" of their deceased loved one, ruminate over memories and thoughts of what they should have done, and be haunted by their search for clues.

Reactions are even more complicated when the survivor is a child or adolescent. The individual who committed suicide may be a sister, brother, cousin, or even a parent. The child's or adolescent's cognitive, social, and emotional developmental capacity to make sense of the suicide also influences his or her ability to cope and understand what occurred. Children or adolescents must return to a public life in school, often unsure about how to handle the truth of their loss with others. Student survivors of a family member's suicide usually need ongoing crisis counseling, as illustrated in the case example at the end of this chapter.

Violence in Schools

Juvenile violence, particularly in school settings, has become an issue of growing concern across the nation. School violence reflects a complex set of social problems and has quite different social dynamics than violence among adults (Astor et al., 2000). Many educational professionals feel that school violence is a classic example of outside crises spilling over into the school environment. Pietrzak, Petersen, and Speaker (1998) cited societal changes, the breakdown of family relationships, violent role models in the media, and media-modeled violence as contributors to school violence. Dupper and Meyer-Adams (2002) attributed many incidents of school violence to the escalation of and victim reaction to low-level violent peer behaviors such as bullying, sexual harassment, and victimization based on sexual orientation.

Violence on a school campus tends to occur in common or public areas. Pietrzak and colleagues (1998) surveyed elementary and middle school personnel about school violence. Nearly one-third of the respondents reported that violent incidents occurred in hallways, cafeterias, classrooms, and buses. Incidents also occurred in the offices of administrators and counselors, at athletic events and extracurricular activities, and in gymnasiums and restrooms.

Researchers have attempted to analyze and identify indicators of potentially violent students. A broad spectrum of social, emotional, and behavioral factors contribute to a perpetrator's actions. Potentially violent students are not always those students who act out in an aggressive manner. For example, Hunter (1999) described a violent student at the bottom of the social ladder who had been the brunt of jokes and taunting for years. The case example of Amelia, described at the beginning of this chapter, also reflects this dynamic. Hazler and Carney (2000) examined the developmental nature of peer-on-peer abuse and how such abuse plays a role in the escalation of violence against self and others. They described a downward spiral for some students as they move from victim to aggressor.

Another important risk factor for violence is substance abuse, especially when accompanied by serious emotional disturbance, which significantly increases the risk of violent behavior (Cornell & Sheras, 1998; Pietrzak et al., 1998). School personnel have perceived lack of parental monitoring, poor parental supervision, and a dysfunctional family structure as correlates of student violence (Pietrzak et al., 1998). These same researchers identified below average academic performance and overall low self-concept among students who resorted to violent behaviors in the school community. School personnel must be vigilant in identifying and responding proactively to troubled and at-risk students.

Media sources have reported on several instances of school violence in which some students apparently knew in advance what was planned but did not tell anyone. Rettig (1999) suggested that school communities provide a means for students to share information and seek help for themselves or others. It is essential that school staff create an environment in which students can communicate their fears in a way that maintains confidentiality, respect, and safety. A large percentage of school violence perpetrators are middle school and elementary school students (Pietrzak et al., 1998), and middle school students often experience intense peer pressure against "telling on someone" (Rettig, 1999). There is some indication that this is changing, but, clearly, school communities must work hard to keep open communication within the school environment.

An incident of school violence can sweep through an entire school community and create a climate of fear. A school violence incident not only affects the students involved in the altercations but also affects witnesses, observers, and virtually everyone in the school community (Astor et al., 2000).

Youth Gang-Related Behavior

Reasons for gang affiliation   Children and adolescents are attracted to gangs and engage in gang-related behaviors for a variety of social, self-image, and cultural affiliation reasons. From a developmental standpoint, gang affiliation meets students' need for socialization, peer acceptance, and an opportunity to demonstrate caring for other members in their group.

Group membership appeals to students' need for connection, which is so prominent in their social development. Youths seek and find kinship, alliance, support, companionship, protection, and peer relations in gangs (Molidor, 1996; Soriano, Soriano, & Jimenez, 1994). Too often, parents and families of students connected to gangs do not provide a sense of belonging, structure, and stability. Also, these students are not connected to the school community. Instead, they form their own subculture in the school community as well as the larger community outside of the school. Childhood physical and sexual abuse are also common themes in the family experience of student gang members (Benda & Corwyn, 2002). Attachment to family and connection to the school community are important protective factors against gang affiliation (Franke, 2000).

Young people mistakenly perceive the prestige, status, and power associated with gang involvement as an antidote for low self-esteem, self-image, and feelings of academic or social failure. They view gang members as dynamic, exciting, and engaging in purposeful behaviors. Gang members may even serve as role models in some community neighborhoods served by schools. Gangs offer a sense of strength in numbers as well as a distorted perception of individual identity (Burden et al., 1996). Young people who have experienced many blows to their dignity through abuse, rejection, and neglect may try to regain it by asserting themselves in gang-related behaviors. The gang subculture has its own special rules for living, as members value several "honor-related" qualities (Sandhu et al., 2000).

There are various levels of involvement in gangs, from affiliation for the sake of protection or sense of belonging to leadership roles. Most gang members perceive that the benefits from gang membership (e.g., friendship, sense of belonging, protection) outweigh the negatives, especially because only a minority of young gang members actually get involved in hard-core gang activities such as violent crime and large-scale drug sales.

Gangs offer a sense of community and an important cultural affiliation for dealing with community-wide problems such as racism, oppression, discrimination, and marginality. Ethnicity is a factor in youth gangs because gangs usually form from existing friendship or acquaintance patterns. The common traits among a peer group of children or adolescents that set them apart from the rest of the community are frequently ethnic identification and racial pride.

Consequences of gang involvement   Despite the benefits gang members perceive in gang affiliation, research suggests gang involvement threatens students' physical well-being and safety, and has deleterious effects on their personal and social development. Students involved in gangs have also been found to experience increased psychological distress (Macmillan, 2001). Shafii and Shafii (2001) identified comorbid depression and suicidal ideation and suicide attempts among youth gang members. The social life and social networks of children and adolescents connected to gangs is constricted. Students may prematurely foreclose on developmentally appropriate social activities and voluntarily exclude themselves from positive social interaction.

Youth affiliated with gangs tend to compromise their school experience. They do not value and may sabotage academic achievements (Macmillan, 2001; Weist & Cooley-Quille, 2001). Students involved with gangs tend to have continuous problems with school behaviors, and often fail to engage in developmentally appropriate goal setting, including setting career-related goals.

School gang activities include drug use and sales, graffiti to indicate "owned" territory, roaming hallways, class disruptions, assaults (especially on female students), and possession of weapons (Arthur & Erickson, 1992). Levels of violence exhibited by gangs often increase as gang members compete for territory and drugs. Parks (1995) found that at the elementary school level a form of gang activity revolved around providing "protection" from threats or assaults and giving "permission" to enter or leave the school or pass through a common area of the school.

There are also adverse consequences of gang presence and gang-related behaviors in a school community for non-involved students. For example, Slovak and Singer (2001) reported that third through eighth graders exposed to gun violence displayed more anger, dissociation, and posttraumatic stress. Several researchers have also noted aggression, depression, and symptoms of Posttraumatic Stress Disorder in children and adolescents witnessing gang-related violence (Fehon, Grilo, & Lipschitz, 2001; Scarpa, 2001; Slovak & Singer, 2001). McGee and Baker (2002) noted different effects for male and female students (ages twelve to eighteen). Female victims frequently had depressive symptoms, whereas male victims had poor self-images, engaged in avoidance behavior, or subsequently engaged in violence. Finally, Purnell (1999) identified a cluster of classroom behaviors among students who had reported a high incidence of witnessing or being victims of gang violence. These classroom behaviors included hypervigilance, difficulty concentrating, problems with memory, emotional distance, and difficulty meeting goals.

Proactive interventions   Adults in the school community must become proficient at identifying signs of gang involvement and countering its damaging effects.

Signs of gang involvement include gang clothing, graffiti, and suspicious behavior. Such behavior includes reports that a student is not returning home at night; increased substance abuse; abrupt changes in behavior, personality, and values; newly acquired and unexplained "wealth," often shared with peers; requests to borrow money; and/or hanging out with others who share a dress code that applies only to a few (wearing a particular color, style, or item of clothing, or another symbol of identification) (Burden et al., 1996).

The school community can foster an environment that promotes the school experience as an alternative to gang involvement. Several trends in school districts, however, contribute to a school building ecosystem conducive to gang formation and development:

1. *Failure to address school building transitions.* When the elementary, middle, and high schools in a school district are programmatically distinct and not integrated, students may get "lost in the shuffle." Transitions are an important element of all developmental pathways, particularly with academic and social development.

2. *Consolidation of small neighborhood schools* into budget-saving, large community-wide comprehensive schools. This is a growing trend intended to maximize school district resources. An important consequence of this trend is that it makes it more difficult for students to get involved in school life and extracurricular activities. Transportation difficulties and limited opportunities for joining a team or club lead to lack of student involvement in extracurricular activities. This contributes to students feeling excluded and viewing themselves as outsiders. Marginalized students have fewer opportunities to connect with the school community. (Goldstein & Kodluboy, 1998).

3. *Uneven and unequal communication* between school administrators and students. Often, the "good students" seem to have the ear of the administration. Marginalized students have limited experience in sharing their "voices" with adults in the school community and perceive minimal opportunities to communicate with school staff about positive events. Thus, marginalized students stay marginalized.

4. *School safety* is often considered an issue of physical well-being. School safety also involves a sense of psychological well-being (Brock et al., 1996) and connection to the school community.

5. Lack of attention to *changing school populations* and increasing racial and ethnic diversity among students. An unwillingness to modify school policies and procedures, established extracurricular activities, and school-wide activities because "this is the way we've always done it" can alienate culturally diverse students. A culturally relevant academic curriculum and a constellation of diverse extracurricular activities are essential in contemporary schools. All students need to be integrated into the school community and to be able to find a connection and an outlet for involvement (Feshbach & Feshbach, 1998; Goldstein & Kodluboy, 1998).

6. *Limited parental involvement* in the school community. Parent organizations fail to thrive in some schools because attendance and participation is minimal. Parent education in understanding, monitoring, and curtailing violent behavior is critical, and parent involvement is a key in gang reduction programs. When parents perceive a school community as a welcome environment, students do too.

7. *Lack of attention to reentry programs* for suspended students. Students returning to school may feel like outcasts in their home school. Innovative programming is essential to reintegrate suspended students into the school community and facilitate a connection to the school system. Structured, planned, and frequent positive adult contacts as well as culturally and developmentally appropriate role models are essential.

8. Conceptualizing a school's purpose in *isolation from community organizations*. Successful school communities are connected to community organizations, including religious groups and community programs. When adults in the school community interact with the community, the nature and frequency of gang incidents is clarified. Further, when school leaders connect with community groups there are proactive opportunities to address gang-related behaviors.

CRISIS INTERVENTION

The ability of students as well as other school community members to understand and process the meaning of a crisis event, to develop strategies to sort out their feelings, and to maintain control over everyday life experiences ultimately depends on their coping skills, the assistance they obtain, and the resources provided to them through a timely and organized crisis response plan. Collective efforts involving many school personnel as well as social service and community agency representatives are necessary. A well-developed and regularly reviewed crisis response plan for a school system is essential for appropriately dealing with crises in a school community. Crisis intervention strategies must include initial single-session interventions as well as guidelines for ongoing crisis counseling. A crisis response plan must provide details about how the school community will respond to a crisis, including who will provide the initial crisis intervention services and how they will be coordinated. Although beyond the scope of this chapter, a plan also needs to articulate how the safety of school community members will be assured.

School Crisis Response Plan

A comprehensive crisis response plan is a priority for all school districts. Development of a crisis response plan takes a considerable amount of planning and commitment by the school staff. Although school crisis plans have common dimensions, each school community is unique and has its own peculiarities in regard to physical facilities, staffing characteristics, student population, and extended community; thus, each school's plan must be individualized.

Crisis response planning committee   Development of a school crisis plan requires a team of individuals who represent a cross section of school district personnel, community social services, and agencies that would need to respond to a crisis in any facility within a school district. This group can generate school district-wide crisis response policies and procedures. A second, building-specific crisis response team can focus on plans for a specific school community or building. Committee members need to be familiar with the school facility and the characteristics of its constituents, including developmental needs, family supports, and the social/cultural milieu of the community served by the school. Coordination between the two groups is essential. A school building crisis response team can build upon and expand district-wide policies and procedures, identifying realistic implementation strategies for its school building and school community.

Components of the crisis response plan   School-wide needs assessment clarifies the specific types of potential crises that must be addressed in the crisis response plan and identifies school staff training needs. The needs assessment process also generates school community acceptance of the crisis response plan. The crisis response plan should address a variety of potential crises in the school and include a caveat acknowledging that many crisis situations cannot be anticipated. A schedule for annual school-wide staff training on the specifics of the plan is important. All school personnel need to know essential details of the crisis response plan, including what is going to happen, who is responsible for specific components of the plan, and the anticipated timing for crisis response interventions.

The crisis response plan should clearly articulate interventions that can easily be implemented during the initial phase (the first twenty-four hours) of the crisis, the first three days, and the first week following the crisis (American School Counseling Association, 2002). During the initial phase the crisis response team needs to assess how many students and which students are affected, what level of response will be required, how to inform the school community, how to provide group and individual services, how to communicate with parents, and which services are needed (e.g., immediate crisis intervention, safe room discussion groups, and classroom intervention with trained personnel).

Thompson (1995) and Lovre (2000) suggested creating a special crisis resource kit that summarizes the crisis response plan. This kit can be a box (e.g., toolbox), bag, file, or packet that provides necessary information and resources: a school map with locations of school phones, designated meeting rooms and care centers, keys to all doors of the school, name tags for crisis team members, an updated master schedule of classes, a list of students enrolled in the school, telephone numbers of mental health counselors in the community, home and work numbers of parents in parent networks, names and contact information for local clergy, and emergency numbers for all faculty and staff. This resource should be accessible by all team members so it can be utilized during the initial response to the crisis. The crisis resource kit could even include activity sheets for elementary school students, a general brochure about crisis situations for distribution to parents, and sample letters and/or news releases, which could be adapted for a specific crisis.

Development of and implementation plans for a "safe room" are recommended components of the crisis response plan (Lovre, 2000). The safe room is a place set aside for students who are struggling with the consequences of the crisis. The safe room is for all students, including students directly affected by the crisis and students for whom this crisis is a trigger. "Providing a safe room facilitates a return to normalcy in the classroom. When those students who are not ready to return to academics have an alternate place to be, the teacher can return to academics more easily" (Lovre, 2000, p. A-4).

Crisis response team   The crisis response team consists of school counselors, school psychologists, school social workers, administrators, selected teachers, and possibly a mental health counseling professional from an outside agency with a specialization in children and/or adolescent issues. The team participates in crisis intervention training, meets regularly to maintain its team identity, and schedules opportunities to practice responses using table-top exercises. "In combination, these individuals have strong clinical skills, knowledge of how school buildings function, experience with crisis intervention and education in systems thinking" (Sorensen, 1989, p. 426). Crisis response team members must be committed to professional development training in crisis intervention, willing to give time beyond the school day when necessary, and approved by an immediate supervisor for release time in the event of a crisis (Perea & Morrison, 1997).

Assigning team members specific roles when the plan is formulated facilitates their acquiring specific professional development training relevant to their duties. It also clarifies team members' duties during the crisis response. There are several specific roles team members must be prepared to assume:

1. The *crisis response coordinator* is typically a school administrator with decision-making capabilities and good communication links within and outside the school system. The crisis response coordinator is in charge of managing and evaluating the crisis response plan.
2. The *crisis intervention coordinator* may be a school counselor, school psychologist, or other mental health professional who works primarily in the school building. This individual needs to be confident about delegating responsibilities and capable of coordinating a number of activities and people under stressful conditions (Brock et al., 1996). The crisis intervention coordinator is responsible for implementation of the crisis response plan.
3. The *media liaison* is the individual who will communicate with the media, providing press releases if necessary. Lovre (2000) emphasized the concept of management of the media, balancing their need to know with protecting the privacy of school community members.

4. The *security liaison* implements safety procedures and maintains the safety and location of students (Brock et al., 1996). This may involve moving large groups or the entire school community to a safe location. The security liaison coordinates releasing students from the school building appropriately.

5. The *parent liaison*'s sole responsibility is interacting with parents. Parents need information and support so they can remain calm and patient as the school community initiates its crisis response plan. During a crisis, parents often want to remove their child from the school facility. If this need is acknowledged, parents are more willing to be patient as crisis response protocol is followed. Some parents may need crisis support services. Others may want to help, and may, in fact, be of great help in the school. Lovre (2000) noted: "No untrained people should be working directly with impacted students in a crisis response effort. There are, however, many support roles carefully chosen parents might fulfill" (p. A-2).

6. *Crisis counselors* provide direct services to those affected by the crisis. It is advantageous to utilize school employees such as school counselors and selected teachers who have strong rapport with students, in this role. This will enhance students' favorable response to crisis workers' interventions. It is a good idea to have more than one crisis response team member trained in each role. Then, if the primary crisis response team member assigned to a specific role is directly involved in the crisis, another team member can assume that role.

Mobilization of the crisis response team   Upon initial notification of the crisis, the crisis response team is activated. Team members can come together in a pre-arranged school office. The two objectives for this initial meeting are assessing the impact the crisis will have on the school and planning an appropriate intervention. There are several considerations in assessing the impact of the crisis on the school community: the intensity and nature of the crisis, the school community's history, whether the school community has faced a similar crisis and, if so, how recently, the degree of exposure by staff and students, the emotional needs of students and staff, identification of the high-risk population, parental involvement and contact, the popularity of the victim(s), resources currently available, and timing (Sorensen, 1989). It is helpful to try to anticipate anything else that could happen. The crisis response team must quickly review and clarify the specific roles and responsibilities members will have in responding to the crisis.

The crisis response team needs to quickly, thoroughly, and accurately assess the specific and overall needs of everyone in the school community and develop an intervention plan specific to those needs. Most crisis intervention plans include strategies for communicating news of the crisis to the school community; a combination of classroom, group, and individual interventions; and optional methods for working with parents and others. The team must be prepared to adjust and revise the crisis response plan, as no two crises are identical (Center for Safe Schools, 2002).

Communicating with the school community   A designated response team member should always immediately notify teachers and close friends of a crisis victim or victims. It is also helpful to have procedures in place for communicating relevant information to the entire school community. Minimizing the rumors that invariably start in a crisis is critical to calming fears and anxieties that can quickly incite a school community. A previously prepared packet of handouts that includes tips on how to talk with students and parents as well as suggested classroom activities could be distributed to teachers (Perea & Morrison, 1997).

Communication among team members/support for team members   In any crisis situation, and particularly in large-scale disasters, crisis response team members have needs too. Team members need time for their own emotional processing of the crisis event. It is helpful to include some mechanism in response system protocols that provides crisis team members some "time out" and an opportunity for team members to support each other.

For the first week following a major school crisis, the crisis response team should hold a morning planning session, with all team members present. The crisis response coordinator can use that opportunity to provide information, review responsibilities, and facilitate a discussion to plan the next interventions (Brock et al., 1996). At the end of each day, there should be a summary of actions, an examination of weaknesses and strengths, and a review of referred students, staff, and parents. The end-of-the-day activities can be handled by the crisis response coordinator or in a crisis response team-debriefing meeting. Plans can then be made for the next day.

Team member debriefing and follow-up   As a crisis subsides, crisis team members need to be able to process their individual experiences and to integrate the experience into their lives. Members need to objectively discuss the team's response and evaluate the process. The crisis response coordinator often collaborates in an overall evaluation and the preparation of a written report, including a description of the crisis event, interventions conducted, and recommendations for changes in the future. A debriefing provides the opportunity to both emotionally vent and critically evaluate and is an important learning opportunity; the team can summarize suggestions for improvement or refinements in the crisis response plan. Debriefing provides valuable feedback on training and targets components of the crisis response plan and protocol for modification. The follow-up report can also be used to justify budget allocations.

SINGLE-SESSION CRISIS INTERVENTION

This section presents a single-session group crisis intervention with homeroom students whose classmate died in an automobile accident. The intervention refers to the third case vignette at the beginning of this chapter. The steps of single-session crisis intervention are integrated with the classroom group approach frequently used in schools.

After adults in the school community (teachers and other school staff) have been informed of a student's death, the deceased student's close friends and classmates should be told either individually or in small groups. Crisis workers can gather close friends and other students involved in activities with the deceased student (e.g., athletic teams and school clubs) in small groups to communicate relevant information and process immediate reactions. Depending on the family relationships in the community and developmental needs of these closely connected students, it may also be appropriate to contact the parents of these individuals. Students whose families are close to the deceased students' family may also need to be contacted individually. Each of these individual or small group sessions are single-session crisis interventions.

It is also useful to consider initiating individual single-session crisis interventions with students who are known to be at risk due to other factors. Crisis response team members can consult with teachers and school counselors for assistance in identifying students currently experiencing psychological difficulties or known to have recently experienced a death or similar accident in their family, extended family, or community network.

Finally, news about the death should be shared with the remaining students in the school building through classroom meetings.

Single-Session, Classroom-Based Crisis Intervention

Several authors stress utilizing a classroom meeting approach to share the crisis-related information and initially assess students' level of functioning (Brock, 1998; Pitcher & Poland, 1992). This allows students to react to the crisis within their own familiar, supportive environment, and also gives them access to the school support system. Existing connections among classmates facilitate group sharing and support (Brock, 1998). The classroom meeting described here is a single-session crisis intervention in a group format. Ideally, the school counselor or crisis response team member and the classroom teacher meet with each classroom to communicate the news of the unexpected death. At least one adult leading the classroom meeting should be already familiar to the students (Brock, 1998). The two adults function as the classroom meeting facilitators. Having two facilitators for each classroom meeting allows one to present the information and the other to observe students and note which students are having severe reactions, requiring further individual or small-group counseling interventions.

The classroom meeting approach is contraindicated with certain classrooms or environmental situations. For example, if a class has a history of being unsympathetic, insensitive, or conflict-ridden, it would be prudent to consider intervening with smaller numbers of students. Also, if crisis workers know in advance that some class members may be deeply affected by news of the death whereas others are not, a classroom meeting is not recommended (Johnson, 1993).

The first classroom meeting should be held with the deceased student's class and followed by meetings with other classrooms at that grade level. Subsequent classroom meetings can then address students in the grade levels above and below. This sequence can be viewed as a series of concentric circles moving outward from the deceased's classroom until all classes in the school are contacted. In each classroom the students' cognitive and emotional development levels are the primary considerations in planning what to say (Winter, 2000). As crisis workers move to different grade levels, they must make adjustments in content and focus in order to be developmentally appropriate. What are the students able to understand, to internalize, to make sense of? Do they have a "real" sense of time and lasting loss? The answers to these questions help the team determine what constitutes meaningful support for each group of students.

Step 1:
Support and empathically join with the students.

The first step must always be to introduce the crisis workers, especially if students do not know them. The second step is to explain the purpose of the meeting (Brock, 1998). It is useful for the crisis workers/group facilitators to share their own concerns for the students and for the deceased student and his or her family. The facilitators' personal sharing at the beginning of the meeting demonstrates both empathy and authenticity as well as modeling for student sharing. This helps lessen some of the students' anxiety and encourages them to express their thoughts and feelings.

All interactions with students in crisis must be responsive to the cognitive, emotional, and language capacities of the student(s). Honest information about the facts and relevant details must be appropriate to students' developmental capacities. Facts may be difficult to understand; thus, facilitators may need to repeat them—sometimes several times during the course of the classroom meeting. For early or mid-adolescents, a well-written newspaper article about the accident can be helpful in clarifying what happened. With younger students this would be inappropriate; younger students would require simpler descriptions. The initial goal is to make certain students have a reality-based understanding of the crisis (Brock, 1998). Students need the opportunity to ask questions about how their peer died, and it is essential to answer those questions directly without using euphemisms.

Step 2:
Intervene immediately to create safety, stabilize the situation, and handle students' immediate needs.

An important component of any intervention in a school crisis is to ensure that students are, in fact, safe, physically and emotionally, and that their environment is stabilized. In some circumstances, students need to be reassured about their own safety. Younger students may generalize knowledge of a peer's death by expressing concern that something similar will happen to them or someone they know. When a student's death has occurred on the school grounds, there may still be considerable chaos with police, emergency personnel, students being dismissed early, and other nonroutine activities. It is important to stabilize the environment within the school system by emphasizing continued school structure—maintaining the normal school routine as much as possible and announcing any adjustments to the school schedule as soon as possible.

A second component of this step is to help students attain short-term control of themselves emotionally. A common reaction to crises is for students to experience high levels of emotionality and anxiety. Crisis workers can help students de-escalate by empathizing with their feelings while simultaneously helping them to understand that they are in control of themselves, their thoughts, and their emotions.

The third component of this step is to handle the immediate needs of students. Each student's grieving process is unique (Schuurman & Lindholm, 2002). Students reacting to a crisis situation often begin verbalizing immediate concerns and decisions to be made. Allowing students to address immediate issues gives them a sense of power and control over themselves and the situation. It also opens the door for students to deal with the aspects of the crisis that are most personally distressing.

At this time one of the facilitators can meet individually with students who are having a particularly difficult time coping and perhaps give them the opportunity to leave the classroom and get individual help. A safe room is particularly helpful for these students. The facilitators must be attentive to each individual student and to the class as a whole.

Step 3:
Explore and assess the dimensions of the crisis and the students' reactions to the crisis.

Crisis workers can encourage students to talk extensively about their reactions and concerns about what has happened and to express their thoughts and feelings. Comprehending students' reactions requires understanding each student's developmentally based meaning of the death. As students begin to talk, crisis workers can listen and observe them in order to develop an understanding of both individual and group responses. Listening and observing focuses on five discrete areas: affect, behavior, cognition, development, and the students' ecological context.

Affect

The facilitators can emphasize that it is normal and therapeutic for students to express their feelings, share memories, and even cry together. Gender, culture, and social/emotional development have an impact on affective expressiveness. For example, early adolescents may work hard to mask feelings, and younger children may be uncertain how to label affective responses. Lovre (2002) underscored the importance of adults modeling feelings and the willingness to express them. Students reveal their emotions in a variety of ways; thus, facilitators need to be sensitive to both verbal and nonverbal clues, aiming to identify the range and intensity of feelings in a classroom-size group during this phase of initial student reaction. Sometimes facilitators can demonstrate this by stating the obvious: *"I can see that you are sad."* It is important for facilitators to verbally identify and validate student feelings.

Students who were not close friends of the deceased can also have intense emotional reactions. The student's death can serve as a trigger for them. Or they might express guilt regarding their overwhelming feelings, which they feel are inappropriate. "I shouldn't feel so sad. I hardly knew him/her." Normalization of thoughts and feelings is the appropriate intervention with these students.

Behavior

A classroom-size group of students will probably display a wide range of behaviors, from talking about the death to avoiding it by making inappropriate comments or jokes, to seeming immobility. Facilitators can convey the fact that this is expected behavior, and that it is all right. The classroom meeting can also provide opportunities for students to process the event either verbally or more actively (e.g., talking, drawing pictures, listening to stories, listening to others talk) (Lovre, 2002).

Cognition

Facilitators can begin to determine how students perceive and interpret the significance of a peer's death by listening carefully to the types of questions they ask. The reality of the loss sinks in at different rates for different children. Because of denial, a common initial response to crisis, facilitators need to repeat the details of the event until students actually grasp it (Brock, 1998). Lovre (2002) suggests that instead of deciding yourself what you can do to help students, find out from the students by using probes such as *"Help me understand how this is for you"* or *"What do you wish adults understood about this?"* Probes such as these may draw students out and provide insight regarding their ways of thinking. Students' perceptions and interpretations of bereavement crises are embedded in their own and their families' belief systems and self-perceptions, and depend on their individual cognitive development. It can also be helpful for facilitators to share information about grief, for example, that pain eases over time as we talk about it and cry and that it does not last forever.

Development

Learning of a peer's death precipitates a crisis for many students, as the emotional reaction derails previously acquired coping and problem-solving skills. It also accentuates feelings of loss. Because peer connections are crucial to young people's development and how they identify themselves, a student's relationship with the deceased may have been a vital component of how the student sees him- or herself. Crisis workers can help normalize sometimes overwhelming responses by anticipating students' developmentally situated reactions (Brock, 1998). Terr (1992) suggested that in a classroom-based crisis intervention, facilitators share with students what they know to be developmentally common reactions, and ask students to raise their hands if any of them have experienced any of the named reactions. Facilitators can then ask students for examples, make summarizing comments about the examples identified, and discuss reactions that students can anticipate in the future.

Facilitators can also reassure students that what they are feeling, thinking, and questioning is normal for kids their age who have to face a peer's death. Again, reassurances must reflect an understanding of what students at different levels of cognitive and social-emotional development need. For example, young students may have a strong need for reassurance. With any age group, reassurances must be honest and must not promise things that cannot be controlled (Lovre, 2002).

Ecosystem

It is important to be attentive to students' social, family, and cultural backgrounds, as they all influence the meanings students attribute to the crisis event. For example, depending on their own family interactions, students may be concerned with how the deceased student's family is doing. Also, crisis counselors need to be sensitive to diverse family and cultural belief systems that may convey different messages regarding the meaning of death.

O'Brien and colleagues (1991) found that students used religious beliefs for support and as an explanation for death. Although crisis counselors in a public school may not feel comfortable addressing specific aspects of students' various religions, they cannot ignore religious constructs, which are important aspects of some students' ecosystems. It would certainly be inappropriate, however, for group facilitators to assume a particular religious stance.

As noted, the school itself is an important component of students' personal ecosystems. The school-based peer group is central to students' social and personal world. Thus, when crisis occurs, students need to come together in groups with their peers. As Lovre (2002) stated, there are social components to grieving and it is best to share with others who knew the friend who died. "It is comforting to share memories and put words to our sadness with others who nod in recognition and shared memory" (p. 10). Most individuals grieve in the environment of the loss. When a student peer dies, children and adolescents may not be able to go home and process the loss with parents who didn't know the deceased in the way fellow students did (Lovre, 2000).

Step 4:
Identify and examine alternative actions and develop options.

During this stage of the classroom meeting the primary goal is to identify possible solutions to students' immediate needs. Crisis counselors can be more directive during this step and students should be as actively involved as possible. Encouraging independent thinking reinforces that students are effectively problem solving (Brock, 1998). Students can learn that no matter how difficult circumstances are, there are things they can do to improve their situation (Brock, 1998). Group facilitators can engage students in a discussion of what they could do together or individually to cope with the news. Often, the strategies students generate involve "doing something" such as writing cards and letters to the family of the deceased student. Students in Perea and Morrison's (1997) crisis intervention wrote sentiments on paper sheets in the school dining hall that they later shared at a memorial service. Another group of students suggested a moment of silence in the deceased student's memory.

Step 5:
Help students mobilize personal and social resources and connect with other community resources, as needed.

Facilitators may need to prepare students for discussing their peer's death at home. It may surprise some crisis workers to realize that some students have fears about disclosing this type of news to their families. Students may be concerned that their family members will not comprehend the significance of the death or their friendship with the deceased student. Students may also worry that such news would be too troubling or disconcerting to a family member, or they may fear that they will start to tell the story and have strong emotional reactions that they are uncomfortable expressing.

Helping students identify their own supports and resources is always helpful. There may be resources they can draw on to help them accomplish the actions they identified. For example, they may have resources that could assist with fund raising or help write a letter to the editor about drunk driving.

Further, crisis workers should initiate individual counseling services for those students who have been most directly affected or are most distressed by the death. Efforts to help individuals with such needs include identifying and contacting follow-up services. Such efforts might include making a follow-up appointment with a professional in the school community or with a community mental health professional.

Step 6:
Anticipate the future and arrange follow-up contact.

Students need to engage in activities that will help bring a sense of closure to the crisis. During this step, group facilitators can also answer any remaining questions (Brock, 1998).

It is important to remember that all cultures have rituals. Funerals and memorial services are culture-specific and provide a means of saying good-bye. If students will be attending a funeral, individually or as a group, it is helpful to give them as much information as possible about it. Students need to be prepared for attending a funeral (Lovre, 2000), especially if many students are attending. They need to have some ideas about what to expect and know how to behave appropriately.

Experience has shown that a school-based memorial event is often very helpful to the entire school community, unless the death was caused by suicide. School-based memorial events can help the school community return to normal. "It provides a time for students to make amends by saying positive things about the friend who has died and marks a time when the formal period of grief is over. We acknowledge that individuals will go on grieving for some time, but having a memorial event provides a helpful turning point" (Lovre, 2002, p. 11). School-based memorial events provide an opportunity for needed closure.

Crisis workers could discuss the possibility of a school-based memorial event with students as part of ending the initial crisis intervention discussion. It is important to help students understand what to expect with a school-based memorial event, and to provide information regarding possible emotional responses and where and whom to contact for help. Crisis workers should convey the message that holding a school-based memorial event does not assume that individuals are over their grief.

It is also helpful to let students know that going in and out of grief is normal, and experiencing grief intermittently allows breaks for fun and reprieve. It is not unusual for students to begin to engage in normal activities again and then start feeling very sad again.

Although crises bring pain and sadness, crisis counselors can also lead students to become more compassionate and giving. Crises present opportunities for personal and relational growth, and interventions in crisis situations should always assume that as an ultimate goal.

Other Contacts Following a Classroom-Based Single-Session Intervention

Parent meeting   Depending on the community networks in a school community and the needs of students, a parent meeting may be helpful. The type of crisis determines the best timing for this meeting. For example, after a student death a meeting can be held after the initial crisis response and prior to funeral services and a school-based memorial event. Typically, disaster and school violence crises have an impact on the school facility, the school environment, and the safety of members of the school community. Some school community members are directly affected and others indirectly. In these cases, a parent meeting should be held earlier in the crisis response process. Also, when there is a potential for inaccurate information or rumors to spread, it is important to share accurate information immediately with parents and other interested adults in the community.

Key agenda items are to provide information as needed, discuss aspects of the situation that may affect other students' experience, and review developmental considerations (Lovre, 2000; Winter, 2000). For some crisis events, it is necessary to share short-term changes in school routine and outline mechanisms and strategies to ensure safety of the school community. Also, it is useful to share warning signs that will let parents know whether their children are starting to develop symptoms worthy of referral. This can be done via a slide presentation or with handouts on tips for talking with different children and adolescents about death and the grief process. Crisis workers can also distribute referral information with appropriate phone numbers.

Support for the principal   As the leader of the school, the principal is responsible for taking charge and helping the school community resolve the crisis and return to the normal school routine. Handling an intense emotional crisis such as a student death, however, may not be comfortable or familiar territory for the principal. As the primary representative of the school, it is often the principal who makes the official contact with the deceased student's parents. School counselors or mental health professionals can help principals with this task.

Armstrong (1997) provides several suggestions for preparing for contact with bereaved parents. First, it is useful to identify some stories and/or memories of the student that the principal can share with the parents. Consulting with teachers can be helpful as they are likely to have many memories and stories to share. It is very important to talk about the child when meeting and talking with his or her parents. "Death of a child makes loved ones desperately hungry for details of his or her life. They crave new insights into this unique person who was with them for only a short time, and they realize the deceased can no longer provide any clues . . . discovering how many people a child touched in a brief lifetime can be both humbling and comforting" (Armstrong, 1997, p. 35). Crisis workers can also reassure the principal or the school community's liaison with the bereaved family that it is acceptable to share their own tears and emotions.

ONGOING CRISIS COUNSELING

For individuals who continue to experience adverse reactions and difficulties coping with a crisis event, ongoing crisis counseling may be useful. In a school setting the counselor and student can meet for multiple sessions; the length of the counseling process depends on the specific needs of the student.

Most frequently, the school counselor becomes aware of a student's need for crisis counseling either through ongoing contact, a self-referral, or a teacher referral. Depending on the time constraints for counseling and the competencies of the school counselor, either the school counselor, a mental health professional working in the school building, or a counseling professional outside the school system can provide ongoing crisis counseling.

The purpose of crisis counseling is to assist the student in achieving affect stability, making appropriate behavioral adjustments, achieving cognitive mastery through meaning making and reframing, accomplishing developmentally appropriate tasks, and establishing and maintaining healthy relationships and social connections in his or her ecosystem. All counseling strategies are aimed at assisting the student to make the personal and interpersonal changes necessitated by the crisis. Through an empowering counseling relationship, the student becomes a fully participating partner in the counseling process in terms of problem definition, the pace and tempo of counseling, and termination of the crisis counseling process.

One of the case vignettes at the beginning of the chapter introduced the case of Cassandra, a junior in high school who committed suicide by hanging herself. In the following section, crisis counseling with Cassandra's younger sister, Molly, is used intermittently to illustrate the components of ongoing crisis counseling.

CASE EXAMPLE: MOLLY

Ongoing Crisis Counseling

Cassandra's family consisted of divorced parents and two sisters. One sister was older and lived away from home. The other sister, Molly, was two years younger, lived at home, and attended the same school. Cassandra committed suicide at her home after school while her mother was working and Molly was at basketball practice. Molly found her sister. The suicide happened in early November.

In February, Molly joined the school's theater program. This was a new venture for her, but Cassandra participated in this program the year before. The theater teacher observed that Molly seemed to connect with the other theater students in only a very limited way and often seemed disengaged, sitting by herself in the prop room. After a while, it was clear to the theater teacher that Molly was still having difficulty coping. The teacher contacted the school counselor.

The counseling sessions began in March, approximately four months after Cassandra's death. The school counselor (SC) initiated the first counseling session.

SC: *Hi, Molly. It's good to see you.*

Molly: Hi, Mrs. A.

SC: *How's everything going?*

Molly: OK, I guess. What did you want to meet with me about?

SC: *Well, I know this year has been a rocky road for you and I thought it would be a good idea for us just to check in with each other and see how things are going.*

Molly: I guess you're right. It hasn't been that great.

SC: *First, tell me how school and basketball are going.*

Molly: School is OK. I mean, I'm still getting good grades and my classes aren't that difficult and I have lots of time at home to do the work. It's kind of hard to concentrate and I find myself just spacing out. It takes me a lot longer to do homework than it used to. Coming to this high school from middle school was easier than I thought. Now, basketball . . . that's another story. I quit basketball after that game in November.

SC: *Oh, I'm sorry to hear that. I know basketball was important to you.*

Molly: I just couldn't do it, after . . . you know. . . . *(voice softens and trails off)*

SC: *I am still sad sometimes about Cassandra's death. Sometimes I still get caught up thinking about her.*

Molly: You do? I do too, and everything is just so different, it doesn't feel as though there's any place that fits.

Establishing a Supportive Relationship and Beginning to Assess Needs

The school counselor began the counseling session by focusing on relationship building with Molly. Because of the size of the student body, the counselor had fairly superficial relationships with a number of students. She realized that she would need to establish a trusting and supportive relationship with Molly. Molly needed to be reassured regarding the safety of the counseling process before she would be ready to discuss her intensely personal emotions and distress. The school counselor's expression of her own concerns and sadness communicated that it was OK to talk about Cassandra, and that Molly is not alone in her feelings.

This paves the way for Molly to share several stories about what has been happening since Cassandra's death, many of which focus on others rather than her own grief process. The school counselor's role during this phase of counseling is to reflect feelings and summarize events. As Molly feels heard, understood, accepted, and supported, she feels safer and is able to focus more on her personal reactions.

Molly: I just feel so alone at home; you know, I'm the only one at home, except for mom. My sister at college calls home a lot. Mostly she talks to mom and I know mom is crying about Cassandra, and when she gets off the phone I don't want to bother her with my problems, so I don't say anything. I feel bad for mom, but there's nothing I can do.

SC: *Your mom talks about the loss of Cassandra with your sister, and you feel kind of left out of it. So, whom do you talk to about it?*

Molly: Lately, not too many people. My friends just really don't know what to say. So, they don't say much. We don't even talk about as much "regular" stuff as we used to. My sister says we have to help Mom. Dad is useless, as usual. After my sister went to college, Cassandra and I would go to Dad's together. Now, I go by myself, and sometimes he even works late. I'm alone there, which is really hard.

SC: *It might help to talk about Cassandra and sort out where everything is for you. Would you like to do that with me?*

Molly: Yeah, I think I need to know that someone has time and room left inside to talk with me about where I'm at.

SC: *OK, good. I'm concerned you feel so alone after Cassandra's death. We probably need to sort out what ground we need to cover and what is most troubling to you now. We could meet weekly for several weeks. There's a little over two months until the end of the school year.*

Molly: When would we meet? You know, I missed a couple of weeks of school last semester, and I've got to do well in everything this semester. Also, there's school play practice.

SC: *What if we meet during your study hall on Tuesdays? Would that work for you?*

Molly: Yes.

The school counselor lays out the time frame for counseling (we have up to the end of the school year), joins with Molly in goal setting, and provides support. Molly begins to allow herself to share her emotions; the counselor responds to communicate to Molly that she is heard, understood, accepted, and supported.

Affect stability:
Help Molly to express and process memories and emotions related to Cassandra's death.

Molly: I don't feel as if I have anyone to talk to, and sometimes it feels as though no one cares what I'm feeling.

SC: *I'm really concerned that you feel as if you're coping with this all alone, and it's hard to find support in either your family or friends.*

Molly: It's not really easy *(begins to tear)*. Sometimes, I think she's just gone away for a while, like she did when she went to the treatment program last year.

SC: *Tell me about you and Cassandra.*

The school counselor begins with the problem statement offered by the student and encourages Molly to reminisce about time spent with Cassandra. Molly reveals several experiences she shared with Cassandra during the year before her death. Themes recurring in this discussion include "I should have done more," "I should have protected her," "Because of our close ages, it was just the two of us." This was intensely emotional for Molly, and the school counselor stayed with her, emotionally supporting her and helping her stay with her feelings. Even after this focus diminishes, the counselor realizes that Molly still needs to talk about and process her memories and feelings, and that this will continue to be a counseling focus. As they have been talking, the counselor at times has guided the conversation, and at other times has responded to Molly's conversation. She has been listening for the purpose of ongoing assessment and to understand the various areas of Molly's life that continue to be adversely affected in the aftermath of Cassandra's suicide. Several important developmental and grief themes have emerged thus far, and the counselor will come back to them at a later time, as she wants Molly to determine the pace of the counseling process. Molly is having difficulty concentrating on her homework; she quit and withdrew from an important activity, basketball; she feels slightly alienated from her friends and is experiencing a loss of peer support; she is also missing some connection with her family members. During later sessions, the counselor explores these and other dimensions of her psychosocial functioning including behavioral adjustments and coping strategies, cognitive mastery, developmental mastery, and the health of Molly's ecosystem.

SC: *Molly, since you gave up basketball, have you gotten involved in any other activities?*

Molly: Well, I'm in the school play this spring. I've never done that before, but Cassandra once did. You know, we always called her the "drama queen."

SC: *The school play is a lot of work. I'm impressed.*

Molly: Yeah, it's hard to get my homework done, but at least I don't have to go home after school and be alone until Mom gets home. Cassandra would have loved to be in this play, and I'm trying to do it for her. It's the least I can do.

SC: *Drama is a great activity, but I want you to be in drama because it's right for you, not just Cassandra.*

Molly: It is hard because the drama kids are so different; I can see why Cassandra could more fit in with them. I don't know if I fit in with them or not. Also, that might be part of the reason why I'm missing out on my friends. They're in the gym after school shooting hoops and I'm over in the theater. Then, I have to rush home in order to get all my homework done. That's got to be perfect, you know. So, I really have to stick with my homework when my sister calls in the evening.

SC: *So, you miss basketball with your friends.*

Molly: Yeah, kind of. But it would just be too much. Too hard. Mostly, it's just awkward silence with them, and that makes me feel like crying.

SC: *So you're missing just being comfortable with your friends and it sounds as though you're missing out on some opportunities with your family, too.*

Molly: Maybe I am.

SC: *Molly, you've always done very well in school. I'm wondering if it is somehow more important to get good grades this semester than in the past. None of us has to be perfect.*

Molly: I know. I don't think I am, but dad says now I'm the only one left to go to college. I really have to do well so I can go to a good college and major in something really important.

Behavioral adjustments:
Help Molly to make and sustain necessary behavioral changes.

The school counselor helped Molly formulate strategies to eliminate negative or maladaptive behaviors and to develop or strengthen effective and constructive patterns of behavior. Maladaptive behaviors often center on either avoidance or overemphasis of typical developmental activities; for example, either steering clear of important extracurricular activities or academic pursuits, or imposing extremely high standards of performance. In Molly's case it was both, as she had stopped basketball and reduced her social interactions with family and friends. She had also become overly goal-oriented to the point where it was crowding out her ability to have a normal and developmentally appropriate balance in her life. Adaptive behaviors encompass the typical developmental activities appropriate for students of this age group.

As the focus turned to behavioral change, the counselor's approach became more active, directive, and behaviorally focused. Yet, she also continued to communicate empathy as Molly struggled with problem solving, decision making, and increased self-reliance.

Cognitive mastery:
Help Molly to examine and reformulate beliefs, expectations, and personal meanings threatened by the suicide.

Molly also needed to reappraise some of her beliefs and conclusions, choose developmentally appropriate activities, and establish goals that fit her lifestyle, not Cassandra's. To a certain extent, Molly has been attempting to live both Cassandra's life and her own life. There are some clear avenues that the counselor can encourage Molly to pursue. The counselor worked on increasing adaptive behaviors, clarifying her cognitions, and strengthening her ecosystem as Molly continued to engage in more developmentally appropriate activities, such as the play, finding time for fun with friends, and even playing basketball again once in a while. As is true of most ongoing crisis counseling, these goals and counseling processes are interwoven.

SC: *Molly, how are things going for you today?*

Molly: Much better. Performances for the play are this weekend, and I'll be glad to be done with that. I think I've learned I can't really be involved with the drama group. I just don't fit in and now I know I don't have to. Also, I'm just too self-conscious to be on a stage dressed up in some outfit in front of people. I can be in front of people, but it's better to be showing them something I'm good at. . . .

SC: *Like basketball.*

Molly: Yeah.

SC: *I've been looking through the brochures I get for summer programs, and I saw one for a girl's basketball camp that looks pretty interesting at the local university.*

Molly: You did? Does it cost a lot?

SC: *I don't really recall, but I think it's fairly reasonable. I can give you a brochure if you like.*

Molly: That would be great because I'm going to see my dad this weekend and I could ask him if he could pay for it. Also, I could talk to some of my friends about going with me. That would give us something fun and not serious to do together. I think that's OK, don't you?

SC: *Yes, I do.*

Molly: I hope I could make it. I haven't been playing basketball since last fall, before . . . you know . . .

SC: *It is natural to think that playing basketball, an activity you were doing when Cassandra died, will remind you of that tragic time.*

Molly: How will I ever be able to go out on to the court again and not think about it?

SC: *What could you do to make approaching an activity you used to enjoy, like basketball, easier and maybe even enjoyable again?*

Molly: My first reaction is to say I should take it in small steps.

SC: *That's a good idea.*

Molly: Well, a small step might be just playing around after school.

SC: *Whom would you want to do that with?*

Molly: Elise—I was always just a bit better than she was, but I'm afraid she's probably gotten better during this past season.

SC: *I don't know about that—I remember watching you at games last year, and you seemed pretty sure of yourself. You were pretty good at hitting some shots from far away.*

Molly: I used to be. Maybe playing with Elise will give me confidence again. I used to be pretty good.

SC: *Molly, playing basketball is about you. It used to be part of who you were as a high school student. Maybe it will be again. It was an important way you grew in self-confidence.*

Molly: Maybe it will be again.

SC: *It sounds as though you're ready to try and see.*

Molly: Yeah.

Developmental mastery:
Help Molly to examine the impact of Cassandra's death on her stage-of-life needs and to make plans for her ongoing developmental mastery.

Molly and the school counselor also explored how Cassandra's death altered her view of the world and her place in it. Reestablishing meaningful peer and sibling relationships and talking about components of Molly's religious beliefs also became a focus. Counseling subgoals that emerged included developing greater self-reliance in order to pursue normal developmental tasks. For example, as she continued the process of thinking about her own identity, Molly needed to set realistic goals relevant to academic endeavors, reconnect with peers, get involved in an appropriate array of social activities, clarify her role in significant relationships, and identify important aspects of emotional sharing.

Molly: Guess what? In the last two weeks, Elise and I have gone to the park and played basketball together a few times.

SC: *That's great, Molly. It sounds as though you feel good about yourself for doing that.*

Molly: You know, in some ways, I kind of do . . . even though I procrastinated doing my homework in order to do it.

SC: *How are the other areas of your life going outside of school?*

Molly: OK.

SC: *I've been concerned about the time you're spending alone at home in the evenings. What has that been like for you?*

Molly: You know what? I'm almost embarrassed to say this. I've been reading a book on personal reflections for teens that the youth minister at our church gave me.

SC: *I bet that's helping to clarify some of your own personal meanings about your sister.*

Molly: Yeah, I feel pretty certain that I was the best little sister I could be. I did what I could. Once I even went over to her friends and told them: "Be kind to Cassandra. She's my sister."

SC: *Good for you. I'm so glad you're examining and reworking some of your beliefs. It is work, isn't it?*

Molly: Yes it is, but sometimes I do feel better.

SC: *Have you talked to anyone about what you're reading?*

Molly: No, you're the first person.

SC: *Do you feel it would be helpful to talk about the parts of the book that are most helpful?*

Molly: I suppose I could talk to the youth minister. You know I was thinking about joining the youth group he runs at church. Praying about this does help. Is it weird to say that?

SC: *Not at all. I'm glad you're at a place where you can do that. I'm proud of the steps you're taking to stay true to your beliefs and who you are as a person.*

Molly: You know, there is something else I keep thinking about. I think part of what goes on with me is that I'm still a little embarrassed around kids at school. With my friends it's not that bad because I know they know the whole story. What do other kids at the school know? What happened at school after Cassandra died? What was the rest of the school told and what did the school do?

Molly's need at this time is to find out what everyone else knows and how the school dealt with her sister's death. The school counselor shares that the suicide was briefly discussed in classrooms. The school counselor shares an outline of the information that was shared with students in the school, emphasizing that consistent information was shared in each class and that students were offered the opportunity to meet in smaller groups with the school counselor. The school counselor shared the information with Molly to reassure her about "what everyone else knew."

Another area that is important to explore at this stage is Molly's perception of herself in relation to her school and academic performance. Molly imposed perfectionist standards of performance on herself academically. She was trying to perform for two people, herself and Cassandra. This is important to address. She also wants her parents to view her in a positive light and to "earn" attention from them that she may have lacked as her parents processed their own grief. It would be important to readdress this issue later with the developmental issue of post-high school planning. The choice of a college, a college major, and even the college experience need to reflect Molly's aspirations, strengths, and core beliefs. Developmentally, this could be another stage when Molly strives to perform for both her sister and herself.

Ecosystem healthy and intact: Help Molly to make changes in her personal support system in order to reestablish connections and community.

In some ways, this issue was the crux of the crisis and thus a part of ongoing work with Molly in that Molly needed to adjust to an environment in which her deceased sibling was missing. Her personal/familial ecosystem was shattered by her sister's suicide.

For any similarly situated individual student, subgoals during this step of crisis counseling would include "ground to be recovered" as well as "new ground to be broken." Old coping strategies, such as seeking support from certain individuals, may no longer be effective. The student may need to be assertive in asking for support from his or her family, peer network, and/or other significant adults. Often family members may be dealing with their own grief issues. Peers of a student coping with a suicide in the family may be afraid to broach the subject; thus, the student may need to initiate a discussion of the deceased or concerns related to personal coping. Similarly, significant adults in the student's life may be unsure of the student's needs and the best way to offer connection and support.

The final aspect of this step of crisis counseling involves cementing changes and thinking about the future. The student will have implemented some immediate solutions and engaged in concrete actions that brought about needed changes. In the case of Molly, the school counselor communicated her continued availability as well as reiterating the importance of Molly continuing to use her natural support system.

SCHOOL-CRISIS WEB SITES

American Counseling Association. This professional organization offers a variety of resources for school-related crises. Its link on resources addresses many issues in school-related crises. http://www.counselor.org

American School Counseling Association. This professional organization provides a variety of resources for school-related crises. http://www.schoolcounselor.org

The Counselor's Classroom. This column presents a monthly feature-length article on school-based issues. A majority of the 2002 issues addressed crises and traumatic responses for students. This column is maintained by the Guidance Channel. http://www.guidancechannel.org

Crisis Management Institute. This organization provides services and materials on crisis responses in schools, peaceable schools, and school violence prevention. http://www.cmionline.org

International Critical Incident Stress Foundation, Inc. (ICISF). This nonprofit foundation provides training and support services for a variety of professionals responding to crisis situations. http://www.icisf.org

The National Alliance for Safe Schools (NASS). This is a nonprofit organization offering training, school security assessments, and technical assistance. http://www.safeschools.org

National Association for School Psychologists. This professional organization has a section of its web site devoted to the National Emergency Assistance Team (NEAT), which helps schools, families, and communities cope with crisis. http://www.nasponline.org/NEAT

National Center for Children Exposed to Violence. This is a national resource center for information about the effects of violence on children and the initiatives designed to address the problem. http://www.nccev.org

The National Education Association. This professional organization has a section of its web site titled "Crisis Communications Guide and Toolkit." http://www.nea.org/crisis

The National Organization for Victim Assistance (NOVA). NOVA is a private, nonprofit membership organization of individuals committed to the recognition and implementation of victim's rights. http://www.try-nova.org

National Resource Center for Safe Schools (NRCSS). This national organization's web site offers articles on a variety of school-crisis situations as well as several documents on strategies to assess the potential for specific crises and intervention strategies. http://www.safetyzone.org

State Department of Education. The web sites of many state departments of education have extensive resources on crisis response planning and developing a crisis response team.

Students Against Violence Everywhere (SAVE). SAVE is a student-run organization providing alternatives to violence. http://www.nationalsave.org

DISCUSSION QUESTIONS

1. Review the case studies presented in this chapter and compile a list of characteristics of each type of crisis. What generalizations can you formulate for each of the crises described in the case studies?

2. What can a counseling professional do to foster good relationships among school staff and other members of the school community?

3. What can a school counselor do to promote a healthy school environment?

4. What prevention activities would you include in a comprehensive school counseling program?

5. Outline a training session for crisis response team members.

6. What supplies and materials would you include in a "safe room" in a school? What different materials would you supply for elementary schools, middle schools, and high schools? What reading materials would you make available?

7. How would you conduct a single-session crisis intervention differently with students in different grade levels? How do your intervention ideas reflect students' developmental levels?

8. Family, culture and societal experiences are important components of a student's ecosystem. What strategies would you use to uncover these experiences for students in a school community? How would you specifically address these issues and incorporate them into your crisis interventions?

9. Think about your community or a school you are familiar with. What unique components of the ecosystem of the school and school community members are important to recognize during a crisis intervention?

ATTITUDE/AWARENESS ACTIVITY

Square Activity and Loss

Start with four pieces of paper.

Identify four personal material possessions that you care about. Tear one piece of paper into four squares and write one material possession on each square. Then identify four nonmaterial possessions. Tear a second piece of paper into four squares and write one nonmaterial possession on each square. Repeat this process with relationships and personal beliefs.

Place all sixteen squares facedown in front of you. Pick up one square at random, wad it up, and throw it on the floor. Then have the student to your left and the student to your right each select one square and throw it on the floor.

In a brief class discussion, students can share their concerns about what they may have lost. What items do you hope you did not lose? What are your fears?

After the discussion, the instructor will walk around and randomly take none, one, two, or three of the remaining squares from each student. This demonstrates the randomness of crisis, as some students have several squares removed and some have none.

After the instructor has finished taking away squares, turn over your remaining squares. After determining what you have lost, you now have the opportunity to bargain. This illustrates Kubler-Ross's (1969) stage of bargaining. For example, if you lost a key relationship, what would you give up to get it back?

Discussion questions:
- What do your sixteen squares reveal about your values?
- How do these losses affect your life?
- Which loss is most difficult to comprehend and makes it most difficult to plan moving forward?
- What did you learn about the bargaining process of grieving?
- What was it like to experience the randomness, unpredictability, and unfairness of losses associated with the impact of a crisis event?
- How did it feel when the instructor unexpectedly took additional squares?
- As a crisis worker meets with a client, which losses experienced in this exercise are you aware of? Which ones are you unaware of? How does this awareness affect your intervention?

Source: Adapted from Dougherty, L. (1998). Unpublished Lackawanna County Red Cross HIV/AIDS Training Materials.

SKILL EXERCISE

Crisis Cards

Prior to conducting this activity, class instructors prepare a set of crisis cards, with a brief crisis vignette described on each card. Prepare approximately two to five more cards than there are students in the class.

Fan the deck out in front of students, with the crisis vignettes facedown. Each student selects one card from the deck, simulating the randomness of crisis events. Students may fill in extra details of the crisis event that are not included in the brief vignettes.

Reflection. Individually or in groups of two, ask students to reflect on the following questions:

1. What are your feelings about this crisis, and which components of the crisis event affect your feelings?
2. What are your needs as you face this crisis?
3. What aspect of the crisis situation would you want to change if you could? How would you want to change it?

Trading. After this initial reflection, offer students the opportunity to trade crises. Note the discussion and criteria for the trades. Students may even select one of the remaining cards in the deck. Note: Sometimes when students select a new crisis it can be worse than the one they had before.

Intervention. Students take turns reading their crisis out loud. Other class members act as crisis workers and discuss intervention strategies. Organize the discussion around (1) filling in any extra background details (the student holding the card can make these decisions), (2) preparing for intervention, (3) single-session crisis intervention, and (4) crisis counseling.

Processing. The processing component of the discussion focuses on the experience from the perspective of the person experiencing the crisis as well as the crisis workers. Sample questions: What were the cognitions, feelings, and anticipated behaviors of the person experiencing the crisis event? What were your concerns as a crisis worker as you contemplated this crisis intervention? How would you vary the single-session crisis intervention as well as the crisis counseling model for this crisis?

Sample crisis vignettes

- You are a teacher in a school. A parent storms into the school, interrupts your class, and threatens you.
- A tornado destroys the housing development you live in. You have not seen many of your neighbors since it happened, but your parents thought it best for you to just come to school anyway today.
- You are a fourteen-year-old student who stops by the office before school with a crumpled piece of paper. "This is my new address." You were placed in foster care yesterday afternoon because of sexual abuse.
- • You are a fifteen-year-old student and you casually make an appointment to see the school counselor during your study hall. As you begin talking, you start crying and, with probes from the counselor, disclose that you are pregnant.
- You are a football team coach. After the big game of the season, many fans come out onto the field and begin fighting with the opposing team.
- You are a middle school student. A group of students who hang together all the time and even wear the same kind of clothes control the hallway where you have to pass to get from your second- to third-period class.
- You are a high school student with a 98 average. After school you find out you did not get a part in the spring school play. You walk home and find rejection letters from three colleges you applied to. You feel hopeless and helpless, as there is nothing to look forward to in the future.
- Your friend attempted suicide last week by cutting her wrists in the bathroom. You and your other friends have heard no news about how she is doing. You make a pact and go into the bathroom after lunch. You break the mirrors in your make-up compact to cut your wrists.
- Your parents recently divorced, and they don't communicate with each other. Custody arrangements require you to change schools to a school on the other side of town.
- Your father came home drunk last night and was displeased with something. He hit you a few times. You wore clothes with long sleeves (even though it is warm outside) to try to cover it up. Your best friend sees you get off the bus and walks you to the school counselor's office.

Source: Barber, G. (2002). Unpublished classroom materials for Crisis Intervention course.

REFERENCES

Adorno, G., & Paris, P. (2000). Counseling gay and lesbian students. In J. Wittmer (Ed.). *Managing your school counseling program: K–12 developmental strategies* (pp. 161–172). Minneapolis, MN: Educational Media Corporation.

Allan, J., & Anderson, E. (1986). Children and crises: A classroom-guidance approach. *Elementary School Guidance and Counseling, 21,* 143–149.

American School Counseling Association. (2002). *Position statements.* Retrieved June 2, 2002, from http://www.schoolcounselor.org

Arena, C., Hermann, J., & Hoffman, T. (1984). Helping children deal with the death of a classmate: A crisis intervention model. *Elementary School Guidance and Counseling, 19*(2) 107–115.

Armstrong, C. (1997). What to say to bereaved parents. *Principal, 76*(3), 34–36.

Arthur, R., & Erickson, E. (1992). *Gangs and schools.* Holmes Beach, FL: Learning Publications.

Astor, R. A., Pitner, R. O., Heyer, H. A., & Vargas, L. A. (2000). The most violent event at school: A ripple in the pond. *Children and Schools, 22,* 199–217.

Baker, J. A. (1998). Are we missing the forest for the trees? Considering the social context of school crisis. *Journal of School Psychology, 36,* 29–44.

Benda, B. B., & Corwyn, R. F. (2002). The effect of abuse in childhood and in adolescence on violence among adolescents. *Youth and Society, 33,* 339–365.

Blum, D. J. (1998). *The school counselor's book of lists.* West Nyack, NY: The Center for Applied Research in Education.

Bowers, J. C., & Hatch, P. A. (2002). *The national model for school counseling programs* (draft). Retrieved October 5, 2002, from http://www.schoolcounselor.org

Brock, S. E. (1998). Helping classrooms cope with traumatic events. *Professional School Counseling, 2*(2), 110–116.

Brock, S. E., Sandoval, J., & Lewis, S. (1996). *Preparing for crises in the schools.* Brandon, VT: Clinical Psychology Publishing.

Bronfenbrenner, U. (1979). *The ecology of human development.* Cambridge, MA: Harvard University Press.

Burden, C. A., Miller, K. E., & Boozer, A. E. (1996). Tough enough: Gang membership. In D. Capuzzi & D. R. Gross (Eds.), *Youth at risk: A prevention resource for counselors, teachers, and parents* (2nd ed., pp. 283–306). Alexandria, VA: American Counseling Association.

Callahan, C. J. (1998). Crisis intervention model for teachers. *Journal of Instructional Psychology, 25,* 226–234.

Campbell, C., & Dahir, C. (1997). *Sharing the vision: The national standards for school counseling programs.* Alexandria, VA: American School Counselor Association.

Center for Safe Schools. (2002). *Facts and figures.* Retrieved June 1, 2002, from http://www.safetyzone.org

Children's Defense Fund. (2002). *For all U.S. children: Everyday in America.* Retrieved June 15, 2002, from http://www.childrensdefense.org/everyday.htm

Cornell, D. G., & Sheras, P. L. (1998). Common errors in school crisis response: Learning from our mistakes. *Psychology in Schools, 35,* 297–307.

Dupper, D. R., & Meyer-Adams, N. (2002). Low-level violence: A neglected aspect of school culture. *Urban Education, 37,* 350–364.

Education Trust. (2002). *The National Initiative for Transforming School Counseling.* Retrieved October 9, 2002, from http://www.edtrust.org.main/main/school-counseling

Erikson, E. H. (1963). *Childhood and society*. New York: W. W. Norton.

Fehon, D. W., Grilo, C. M., & Lipschitz, D. S. (2001). Correlates of community violence exposure in hospitalized adolescents. *Comprehensive Psychiatry, 42,* 283–290.

Feshbach, N. D., & Feshbach, S. (1998). Aggression in the schools: Toward reducing ethnic conflict and enhancing ethnic understanding. In *Violence against children in the family and the community* (pp. 269–286). Washington, DC: American Psychological Association.

Franke, T. M. (2000). The role of attachment as a protective factor in adolescent violent behavior. *Adolescent and Family Health, 1*(1), 40–51.

Goldstein, A. P., & Kodluboy, D. W. (1998). *Gangs in schools: Signs, symbols, and solutions*. Champaign, IL: Research Press.

Grollman, E. A. (Ed.). (1995). *Bereaved children and teens: A support guide for parents and professionals*. Boston: Beacon Press.

Hazler, R. J., & Carney, J. V. (2000). When victims turn aggressors: Factors in the development of deadly school violence. *Professional School Counseling, 4*(2), 105–112.

Henry, C. S., Stephenson, A. L., Hanson, M. F., & Hargett, W. (1993). Adolescent suicide and families: An ecological approach. *Adolescence, 28,* 291–308.

Hoff, S. (2002). *Adolescent suicide assessment and intervention*. Workshop presented at the Pennsylvania Counseling Association Conference, October, 2002, Harrisburg, PA.

House, R. M., & Martin, P. J. (1998). Advocating for better futures for all students: A new vision for school counselors. *Education, 119,* 284–291.

Hunter, D. (1999, March 2) There are deeper reasons why kids bring weapons to school. *The Knoxville News-Sentinel,* p. A7.

Jackson, R., & McBride, D. (1987). *Understanding street gangs*. Sacramento, CA: Custom Publishing.

Johnson, K. (1993). *School crisis management: Team training guide*. Alameda, CA: Hunter House.

Kirk, W. (1993). *Adolescent suicide: A school-based approach to assessment and intervention*. Champaign, IL: Research Press.

Kubler-Ross, E. (1969). *On death and dying*. New York: Macmillan.

Kurtz P. D., Gaudin, J. M., Wodarski, J. S., & Howing, P. T. (1993). Maltreatment and the school-aged child: School performance consequences. *Child Abuse and Neglect, 17,* 581–589.

Lockhart, E. J. (2003). Students with disabilities. In B. Erford (Ed.), *Transforming the school counseling profession* (pp. 357–409). Upper Saddle River, NJ: Pearson Education, Inc.

Lovre, C. (2000). *The crisis response manual* (2nd ed.). Salem, OR: Crisis Management Institute.

Lovre, C. (2002, May–June). Helping students grieve a friend's death. *ASCA School Counselor,* 10–11.

Macmillan, R. (2001). Violence and the life course: The consequences of victimization for personal and social development. *Annual Review of Sociology, 27,* 1–22.

McGee, Z. T., & Baker, S. R. (2002). Impact of violence on problem behavior among adolescents: Risk factors among an urban sample. *Journal of Contemporary Criminal Justice, 18*(1), 74–93.

McWhirter, E. H., Hunt, M., & Shepard, R. (2000). Counseling children and adolescents at risk. In A. Vernon (Ed.), *Counseling children and adolescents* (2nd ed., pp. 259–298). Denver, CO: Love Publishing Company.

McWhirter, J. J., McWhirter, B. T., McWhirter, A. M., & McWhirter, E. H. (1998). *At-risk youth: A comprehensive response* (2nd ed.). Pacific Grove, CA: Brooks/Cole.

Molidor, C. E. (1996). Female gang members: A profile of aggression and victimization. *Social Work, 41,* 251–257.

Moore, M. M., & Freeman, S. J. (1995). Counseling survivors of suicide: Implications for group postvention. *Journal for Specialists in Group Work, 20*(1), 40–47.

Morrissey, M. (1998). Mitigating school violence requires a system-wide effort. *Counseling Today, 40,* 36–37. Alexandria, VA: American Counseling Association.

Muro, J. J., & Kottman, T. (1995). *Guidance and counseling in the elementary and middle schools: A practical approach.* Dubuque, IA: Brown and Benchmark Publishers.

Myrick, R. D. (2003). *Developmental guidance and counseling: A practical approach.* Minneapolis, MN: Educational Media Corporation.

National Association of School Psychologists. (2003). *What is a school psychologist?* Retrieved June 2, 2002, from http://www.nasponline.org/about_nasp/whatisa.html

National Center for Educational Statistics. (2002). *Indicators of school crime and safety, 1998* (No. 98251). Washington, DC: Author.

National Institute of Mental Health. (2002). *Suicide facts.* Retrieved October 8, 2002, from http://www.nimh.gov/research/suicidefact

Negron, R., Piacentini, J., Graae, F., Davies, M., & Shaffer, D. (1997). Microanalysis of adolescent suicide attempters and ideators during the acute suicidal episode. *Journal of American Academy of Child and Adolescent Psychiatry, 36,* 1512–1519.

O'Brien, J. M., Goodenow, C., & Espin, O. (1991). Adolescents' reactions to the death of a peer. *Adolescence, 26,* 431–440.

Parks, C. (1995). Gang behavior in the schools: Reality or myth? *Educational Psychology Review, 7*(1), 41–68.

Perea, R. D., & Morrison, S. (1997). Preparing for a crisis. *Educational Leadership, 55*(2), 42–44.

Pietrzak, D., Petersen, G. J., & Speaker, K. M. (1998). Perceptions of school violence by elementary and middle school personnel. *Professional School Counseling, 1*(4), 23–29.

Pitcher, G. D., & Poland, S. (1992). *Crisis intervention in the schools.* New York: Guilford Press.

Purnell, L. A. (1999). Youth violence and post-traumatic stress disorder: Assessment, implications, and promising school-based strategies. In C. W. Branch (Ed.), *Adolescent gangs: Old issues, new approaches* (pp. 115–127). New York: Brunner-Mazel.

Rando, T. A. (1983). An investigation of grief and adaptation in parents whose children died from cancer. *Journal of Pediatric Psychology, 8*(1), 3–20.

Reinherz, H. Z., Giaconia, R. M., Silverman, A. B., Friedman, A., Bilge, P., Frost, A. K., & Cohen, E. (1995). Early psychosocial risks for adolescent suicidal ideation and attempts. *Journal of American Academy of Child and Adolescent Psychiatry, 34,* 599–611.

Rettig, M. A. (1999). Seven steps to schoolwide safety. *Principal, 79*(1), 10–13.

Ripley, V., Erford, B., Dahir, C., & Eschbach, L. (2003). Planning and implementing a twenty-first century comprehensive developmental school counseling program. In B. Erford (Ed.), *Transforming the school counseling profession* (pp. 63–119). Upper Saddle River, NJ: Pearson Education.

Sandhu, D. S., Underwood, J. R., & Sandhu, V. S. (2000). Psychocultural profiles of violent students: Prevention and intervention strategies. In D. S. Sandhu & C. B. Aspy (Eds.), *Violence in American schools: A practical guide for counselors* (pp. 21–42). Alexandria, VA: American Counseling Association.

Scarpa, A. (2001). Community violence exposure in a young adult sample: Lifetime prevalence and socioemotional effects. *Journal of Interpersonal Violence, 16*(1), 36–53.

Schuurman, D., & Lindholm, A. B. (2002). Teens and grief. *The Prevention Researchers, 9,* 1–3.

Shafii, M., & Shafii, S. L. (2001). Diagnostic assessment, management, and treatment of children and adolescents with potential for school violence. In M. Shafii & S. L. Shafii (Eds.), *School violence: Assessment, management, prevention* (pp. 87–116). Washington, DC: American Psychiatric Association.

Slovak, K., & Singer, M. (2001). Gun violence exposure and trauma among rural youth. *Violence and Victims, 16,* 389–400.

Snyder, B. (2000). School counselors and special needs students. In J. Wittmer (Ed.), *Managing your school counseling program: K–12 developmental strategies* (pp. 172–180). Minneapolis, MN: Educational Media Corporation.

Sorensen, J. R. (1989). Responding to student or teacher death: Preplanning crisis intervention. *Journal of Counseling and Development, 67,* 426–427.

Soriano, M., Soriano, F., & Jimenez, E. (1994). School violence among culturally diverse populations: Sociocultural and institutional considerations. *School Psychology Review, 23,* 216–235.

Studer, J. R. (2000). Adolescent suicide: Aggression turned inward. In D. S. Sandhu & C. B. Aspy (Eds.), *Violence in American schools: A practical guide for counselors* (pp. 269–284). Alexandria, VA: American Counseling Association.

Terr, L. C. (1992). Mini-marathon groups: Psychological "first aid" following disasters. *Bulletin of the Menninger Clinic, 56*(1), 76–86.

Thompson, C. L., & Rudolph, L. B. (2000). *Counseling children* (5th ed.). Belmont, CA: Wadsworth/Thompson Learning.

Thompson, K. E., & Range, L. M. (1992). Bereavement following suicide and other deaths: Why support attempts fail. *Omega: Journal of Death and Dying, 26*(1), 61–70.

Thompson, R. A. (1995). Being prepared for suicide or student death in schools: Strategies to restore equilibrium. *Journal of Mental Health Counseling, 17,* 264–277.

U.S. Department of Education. (2001). Fiscal year 2001 program performance reports: Safe and drug-free schools program—state grants program and national programs. Retrieved from http://www.ed.gov/about/reports/annual/2001report/edlite-283.html

Vernon, A. (2000). Counseling children and adolescents: Developmental considerations. In A. Vernon (Ed.), *Counseling children and adolescents* (2nd ed., pp. 1–30). Denver, CO: Love Publishing Co.

Vernon, A., & Al-Mabuk, R. (1995). *What growing up is all about: A parents' guide to child and adolescent development.* Champaign, IL: Research Press.

Wagner, B. M., Cole, R. E., & Schwartzman, P. (1995). Psychosocial correlates of suicide attempts among junior and senior high school youth. *Suicide and Life-Threatening Behavior, 25,* 358–372.

Weist, M. D., & Cooley-Quille, M. (2001). Advancing efforts to address youth violence involvement. *Journal of Community Psychology, 30*(2), 147–151.

Winter, E. (2000). School bereavement. *Educational Leadership, 57*(6), 80–85.

Wittmer, J. (2000). Implementing a comprehensive developmental school counseling program. In J. Wittmer (Ed.), *Managing your school counseling program: K–12 developmental strategies* (pp. 14–34). Minneapolis, MN: Educational Media Corporation.

Worden, J. (1996). *Children and grief.* New York: Guilford Press.

CHAPTER 13

Crisis Intervention and Disaster Trauma

BARBARA G. COLLINS

Disaster can strike anyone at any time, quickly and without warning. Each year multiple disasters occur in the United States and throughout the world, and each year millions of individuals face disasters' devastating consequences. Disasters can take many forms, from natural disasters like floods, hurricanes, tornadoes, and earthquakes, to accidents like hazardous chemical spills or radioactive contamination, to intentional disasters like political attacks or terrorism. Whether natural, accidental, or intentionally created, they affect not only individuals but entire communities. The effects of disasters often extend well beyond the immediate incident, as recovery and reconstruction of homes, businesses, and community infrastructures can continue for months and, in some cases, years. The biopsychosocial impact on individuals, especially those directly confronted with great personal loss, horror, and destruction, is also frequently long lasting.

According to the Federal Emergency Management Agency (FEMA), an independent federal agency reporting directly to the president, a major disaster is defined as "any natural catastrophe, or regardless of cause, any fire, flood, or explosion that causes damage of sufficient severity and magnitude to warrant assistance supplementing state, local, and disaster relief organization efforts to alleviate damage, loss, hardship, or suffering" (FEMA, 1995, p. 1). Created in 1979, FEMA is the only federal agency responsible for providing both individual assistance (e.g., disaster housing, low-interest loans, crisis counseling) and public assistance (e.g., debris removal, emergency provision of public services) to states and locales where disaster has overwhelmed the local and state governmental capacity to respond effectively.

In 2001, there were forty-five major disaster declarations in the United States that resulted in FEMA involvement, the majority of which were natural disasters including severe storms and flooding in the South and Midwest and tropical storm Allison, which affected five states. Also included were the terrorist attacks against the Pentagon and the World Trade Center in New York City (FEMA, 2002). In each case, the request for FEMA involvement was made to save lives and protect public health, as these large-scale disasters posed community-wide environmental concerns, destroyed water supplies, transportation systems, and waste management systems, and in some instances resulted in levels of injuries and deaths that overwhelmed the capacities of local hospitals and morgues.

The cost to individuals who were directly affected by these large-scale disasters was high—in loss of resources (e.g., employment, homes) as well as physically, relationally, and psychologically. Victims were injured physically, overwhelmed psychically, and had material resources decimated. Although most individuals recover emotionally following disasters, without lasting psychological impairment, "peritraumatic stress symptoms"—those stress reactions that occur during and in the immediate aftermath of a firsthand traumatic disaster experience—are ubiquitous.

Although exposure to disaster creates extreme losses and challenges, most individuals evidence amazing resilience. And, perhaps even more impressive, many individuals "exhibit heroic altruism, generativity, and existential shifts in appreciation of their survival" (Abueg, Woods, & Watson, 2000, p. 244). This was nowhere more evident than in the actions of the hundreds to thousands of New York police officers, firefighters, and citizens who responded heroically and altruistically in the aftermath of the September 11 attacks.

IMPACT ON SURVIVORS

Two general points are important in considering the impact of disasters on survivors. First is the recognition that each survivor's disaster is unique. Individuals may face relatively similar objective circumstances such as terrifyingly close encounters with injury and/or death, or relocation and rebuilding in the wake of a flood or fire. Each survivor's personal, familial, and cultural history, gender, age, socioeconomic status, psychological/relational resources, community practices, and resources, however, affect his or her reactions. Directly influencing individual responses are additional factors such as prior traumatic experiences or particularly stressful experiences immediately following the disaster.

This latter issue is specifically important in considering the effect of disasters on rescue and emergency personnel. Rescue workers may be directly involved in the immediate disaster situation and have ongoing traumatizing experiences as they provide assistance to other survivors and/or engage in various recovery efforts. One young police officer interviewed by the author described being at the World Trade Center as the buildings collapsed. Two days later, when on patrol several blocks from the site, he stumbled over a charred boot that still contained a foot. He then spent a week on duty sifting through debris that slowly passed on a long conveyer belt; his job was to search for body parts or personal effects that might assist in identifying bodies. The smell of death and the sights and sounds of destruction surrounded him daily. For individuals like this young police officer, the disaster was prolonged with repeated potentially traumatizing exposure.

The second point, related to the above example, is that prolonged or repeated traumas and those that have "high levels of powerful impact with low levels of predictability and controllability" (Meichenbaum, 1994) can produce longer-lasting symptoms. Technological disasters like toxic waste or radioactive contamination, for example, may produce ongoing, intermittent symptoms of anger, bitterness, and alienation as individuals cope with continuing fears and uncertainty regarding future health effects (Green, Lindy, & Grace, 1994).

Phases of Response

Several researchers have identified changing responses that occur over time as people struggle to cope in the aftermath of a disaster. During the *emergency or acute phase,* which includes the days and weeks immediately following the disaster, individuals tend to be highly aroused physically and emotionally, preoccupied with thoughts about their experience, and tend to openly discuss their anxieties and feelings with others (Pennebaker & Harber, 1993). A common pattern of posttraumatic stress response includes emotional effects (e.g., anger, despair, guilt, grief, helplessness, loss of pleasure), cognitive effects (e.g., impaired concentration and decision making, confusion, intrusive thoughts and memories, worry), physical effects (e.g., fatigue, insomnia, hyperarousal, headaches, gastrointestinal problems, decreased libido), and interpersonal effects (e.g., alienation, social withdrawal, relationship conflict, school or work impairment) (Young, Ford, Ruzek, Friedman, & Gusman, 1998).

Researchers specifically examining the pathogenesis of PTSD have noted that survivors frequently report intrusive thoughts and memories, including nightmares, and that survivors exhibit a high incidence of acute stress disorder symptoms in the first several months following exposure to disasters (Aguilera & Planchon, 1995; McFarlane, 1995; Wood, Bootzin, Rosenhan, Nolen-Hoeksema, & Jourden, 1992). For example, researchers found that 53 percent of high-exposure victims of an airplane crash exhibited symptoms that met the criteria for PTSD four to six weeks later (Smith, North, McCool, & Shea, 1990), and even minimally exposed college students who lived in the vicinity of the Loma Prieta earthquake in California were much more likely to have nightmares, particularly with earthquake content, than were an unaffected control group of college students (Wood et al., 1992).

More extreme peritraumatic stress symptoms that have been noted in both children and adults include dissociation, flashbacks, panic episodes, depression, and anxiety. Those who experience more extreme initial stress reactions have been found to be at greater risk for ongoing psychological disorders including PTSD, major depression, and substance abuse (Abueg et al., 2000; Vernberg & Vogel, 1993; Young et al., 1998). Meichenbaum (1994) contended that those who respond in a more dissociative fashion, appearing inappropriately calm, composed, and unfazed, might be at greatest risk for developing posttraumatic problems like anxiety and flashbacks at a later time.

The *inhibition or avoidance phase* appears to emerge as people stop talking about the disaster and their responses but continue to have thoughts and dreams about it. Pennebaker and Harber (1993), who interviewed survivors of the Loma Prieta earthquake, found that as weeks passed survivors' significant others were no longer receptive to hearing about the earthquake. As survivors curtailed their expression of memories and emotions, however, relational conflicts and increased nightmares and health problems emerged. Shalev (1992), who studied injured survivors of a terrorist attack, found that the avoidance symptoms of PTSD including feelings of numbness and social withdrawal, tended to develop later than intrusive symptoms—perhaps, he suggested, as a strategy for coping with the unsettling memories.

Pennebaker and Harber (1993) found that after about six weeks an *adaptation phase* emerged and, for most individuals, troubling symptoms gradually decreased and ultimately ended. Most other researchers have found adaptation to emerge less rapidly, particularly for individuals most directly affected by a disaster. A time period of six to eighteen months may be a more realistic estimate of the time necessary for full recovery from moderate stress reactions for most people. Green and Solomon (1995) proposed a time line of adjustment, with time demarcations of zero to three months, three to eighteen months, and longer than eighteen months.

Young et al. (1998) identified three phases of disaster mental health response. The first phase focuses on the initial delivery of emergency crisis intervention services immediately following the disaster. In the second phase, postimpact services focus on facilitating psychological and interpersonal stabilization and last from the day after the disaster until the eighth to twelfth week following onset. And, finally, a restoration phase usually begins around the eighth to twelfth week after onset of the disaster and generally coincides with the implementation of long-term FEMA recovery programs.

Building on the anecdotal observations of crisis workers, particularly those who have worked with survivors of natural disasters, Raphael (1986, 2000) posed an alternative model as a heuristic for envisioning the pattern or phases of adjustment. The first phase, referred to as the *heroic phase,* emerges during the hours and first few days following a disaster. During this time of high physiological arousal, energy, and behavioral activity, individuals are involved in rescuing and helping one another and providing shelter and emergency assistance. This is followed by the *honeymoon phase,* which lasts from three days to three weeks, during which time there is frequently a considerable amount of media and official attention. Individuals and communities are reassured that their homes and communities will be restored and rebuilt quickly, leading to a sense of optimism and hopefulness. As the media disappear, crisis support and rescue resources dwindle, and the reality of what has been lost and the enormity of the task of rebuilding become more apparent, however, *disillusionment* sets in. During this phase, which generally lasts from three to six months after the disaster, individuals struggle to overcome bureaucratic red tape and feelings of hopelessness and abandonment. In some instances, posttraumatic stress symptoms reemerge as the stressors become overwhelming. Gradually, individuals reach a point of *restabilization.* By this time most of the initial processes of seeking assistance are completed, and rebuilding and reconstruction of homes and lives has begun to bring results. Although there are exceptions, within six months to two years most persons regain their prior equilibrium (Green & Lindy, 1994; Green & Solomon, 1995).

What all typologies of postdisaster response indicate is that in the early days, weeks, and, perhaps, months following direct disaster exposure, most people suffer high levels of distress, and many experience symptoms that meet the diagnostic criteria of acute stress disorder. What is also apparent is that for the majority of these individuals there is a gradual lessening of symptoms, although for some, symptoms are exacerbated as the stressors of rebuilding and confronting personal and material losses continue. As previously noted, however, although common aspects of coping and the expected time line for adjustment have been identified, the impact that a disaster has on any one individual is unique and depends on a number of variables. Several authors have suggested that the individualized impact of a disaster is influenced by three broad factors: (1) characteristics of the disaster, (2) characteristics of the postdisaster response and environment, and (3) characteristics of the individual and group (predisaster characteristics) (Freedy, Kilpatrick, & Resnick, 1992; Meichenbaum, 1994).

Characteristics of the Disaster

Type of disaster   Although any disaster experience can include close encounters with death, devastating personal and material losses, and exposure to horrific images of pain and suffering, some types of disasters have been found to be particularly traumatizing. *Technological disasters,* particularly toxic contamination, pose a particular psychological risk. Often, toxic contamination disasters may not have a clear beginning and ending. Individuals may be told that their homes and communities are contaminated, when the event that caused the contamination is removed and invisible. Survivors of toxic contamination disaster are thus at risk of ongoing stress as they contend with an unseen, unpredictable, and uncontrollable enemy, and must depend on the word of authorities to tell them when (and if) they are safe. Often they also have to confront the reality of specific health problems and ongoing fears and suspicions regarding the cause of their physical maladies (Baum & Fleming, 1993; Green et al., 1994).

Green et al. (1994) proposed a specific syndrome to describe the symptoms of individuals who have been exposed to radioactive contamination; although the symptoms are similar to PTSD, the traumatic precipitant is future-oriented and ongoing rather than an event that occurred in the past. They found that survivors of a radioactive leak in Fernald, Ohio could not escape their ongoing obsessive fears and ruminations regarding the contamination in their homes and community. They were alienated and distrustful of authorities and experienced ongoing unrelenting concerns about their presumed physical deterioration.

Intentionally caused disasters have also been associated with increased traumatization and resultant psychological difficulties (Ursano, Fullerton, Kao, & Bhartiya, 1995). Disasters that involve political or criminal intent may result in more intense emotional responses including rage, depression, and anxiety, and individuals may have difficulty comprehending or attributing meaning to what occurred (Aguilera & Planchon, 1995). Events like the bombing of the Murrah Federal Office Building in Oklahoma City or the destruction of the World Trade Center in New York City may be particularly likely to cause relatively quick onset of post-traumatic stress symptoms, particularly when there are continued fears of another attack, as was the case in New York.

Degree of exposure to mass destruction or death   A second characteristic of disasters with direct implications for the extent of traumatic impact is the severity of exposure. Young et al. (1998) reviewed the research literature and found that the degree of exposure of individuals and families as well as neighborhoods or communities were predictive of individual psychological impairment, although community exposure was less a factor in predicting negative outcomes than was individual exposure. Meichenbaum's (1994) review of the literature concluded that the "dose" of the disaster, or the magnitude of the stressor, is directly related to development of PTSD.

Variables related to exposure include the speed of onset, the amount of destruction and loss of life, and the magnitude, intensity, and duration of impact (Ursano et al., 1995; Vogel & Vernberg, 1993). A two-year follow-up study with the survivors of a flood disaster caused by a dam break found that the presence of continuing and severe depression was directly related to witnessing death, experiencing personal injury, and sustaining extensive material losses (Green et al., 1990).

Additional disaster characteristics   Several other factors characterizing the disaster itself have been found to influence postdisaster impact: specifically, the scope of community impact and perceived control over future impact. The latter issue was mentioned in the discussion of toxic contamination. When there is a high potential for recurrence or little sense of control over future impact (as with the effects of radiation), there is an increased likelihood of continuing psychological impairment, as individuals are likely to be more isolated in their suffering and there is no point at which they can inventory their losses, mourn, and return to normal life.

The scope of community impact is somewhat paradoxical because, on one hand, a significant amount of property destruction and a significant number of injuries and deaths increases the potential of trauma. Community-wide disasters can lead to breakdowns in social codes for behavior, activities, communication, transportation, and community appearance, resulting in disillusionment, loss of normal routines, and diminished appreciation of community physical character and beauty. At the same time, the fact that community members have shared both the experience of the disaster and its burdens means that they may be more readily able to share feelings and memories with one another, facilitating healthy ventilation and mourning. Community members may band together, sharing resources, and providing each other social support. Steinglass and Gerrity (1990) found that disaster survivors who lived in communities in which the disaster was defined in community terms, and where individuals felt that they were part of a community, were less likely to experience PTSD than survivors of community disasters where this community identity was not present.

Finally, in addition to the above factors, adverse outcomes for survivors have been correlated with direct injury to self or family members, direct life threat, extensive loss of property, relocation or displacement, separation from family, and the experience of panic or horror during the disaster experience (Young et al., 1998). Each of these factors is thus important to assess when attempting to identify those individuals most at risk and therefore most in need of more intensive intervention.

Subjective perceptions of the disaster experience   As noted in Chapter 1, it is not just objective circumstances that define a crisis, but also an individual's perception of the event and interpretations of its meanings. This caveat is fundamental in understanding the impact of a disaster, regardless of other objective characteristics of the disaster. Meichenbaum (1994) suggested that in considering the subjective, individual meaning of a disaster, disaster crisis workers consider the following questions: Did the survivor view the disaster as completely unexpected and sudden? Did the survivor perceive it as a threat to life survival? Did the survivor believe someone or something to be at fault? Does the survivor see him- or herself as behaving in a way that resulted in others being hurt or killed? Does the survivor perceive an absence of social support, believing that there is no one to turn to for help? An affirmative response to any of these questions suggests an increased risk of an unfavorable psychological outcome.

Characteristics of the Recovery Environment

A number of issues already discussed also relate to understanding the role of the environment in facilitating recovery. For example, in discussing Pennebaker and Harber's (1993) study with survivors of the Loma Prieta earthquake in California, it was noted that when people were discouraged from expressing their feelings and thoughts to others, increased health and social problems ensued. Similarly, in the study examining community impact (Steinglass & Gerrity, 1990), it was noted that identification with community appeared to be correlated with lower levels of PTSD symptomatology among community members in the aftermath of a community-wide disaster. Both cases point to the importance of the postdisaster environment as a factor influencing recovery.

McFarlane (1995) contended that the postdisaster environment may, in some cases, be an even more significant factor than memories of the event itself in influencing ongoing levels of distress and the maintenance of posttraumatic stress symptoms. Further, the acute stress of the disaster experience frequently exacerbates other chronic stressors including marital stress, financial stress, and ecological stress (Young et al., 1998). The result is increased relational and psychological distress that becomes inseparable from the disaster response. For example, a couple that was experiencing financial pressures and marital discord prior to the disaster may find that the disaster further hurts them financially, and that they cannot process their acute disaster stress responses within the relationship because of lack of trust and already fragile bonds. It is the interplay of these multiple forces that ultimately determines ongoing impact.

Psychosocial resources   Several writers have documented the potential decimation of resources with a disaster and the negative effect of resource loss on physical, psychological, and interpersonal/familial functioning (Freedy et al., 1992; Hobfoll, 1989; Hobfoll & Lilly, 1993). Hobfoll and Lilly (1993) suggested that disasters can imperil both individual and community resources. According to their "conservation of resources" model, resource loss can occur in a number of areas, including loss of *objects* (e.g., homes, cars, roads, public buildings), *conditions* (e.g., loss of employment, health, social and community relationships), personal and community *characteristics* (e.g., self-esteem, sense of meaning and purpose, sense of community, community pride), and *energies* (e.g., money, food, time, credit, fuel reserves, government financing).

Social support   Considerable research suggests that psychosocial resources are extremely influential factors affecting responses in the aftermath of disasters, both in affording individuals protection against negative psychological outcomes and, alternatively, in precipitating negative outcomes (NCPTSD, 2002b). Three factors have been found to positively affect postdisaster coping and survival: *social embeddedness* (size and closeness of survivor's social network), *received social support* (actual help that is provided to individuals), and *perceived social support* (survivor's belief that he or she is cared for and that help is or will be available). These sources of social support are also vulnerable in the aftermath of disasters, however, as individual family members may be killed or injured, other members of individuals' support networks may be overwhelmed, relocated, or unavailable, and community-wide devastation may result in changes in social routines and activities. Accumulated data has documented that attenuation of social support is a primary factor contributing to declines in individual psychological functioning (Edwards, 1998; Solomon & Smith, 1994; Vernberg, La Greca, Silverman, & Prinstein, 1996). This fact argues for the importance of postdisaster interventions that promote and sustain natural helping networks. Resource mobilization can also assure the provision of timely and accessible emotional, informational, and concrete assistance to survivors and their families.

Characteristics of the Individual

There are a number of individual characteristics that also influence how a survivor processes and resolves a disaster including demographic characteristics (e.g., age, gender, culture and ethnicity, socioeconomic status), prior mental health and a history of positive coping skills and resources, prior exposure to traumatic events, and an individual's social position (e.g., geographically isolated, on the "margins" of community).

Demographic characteristics Numerous studies have shown that girls and women have a greater risk of negative postdisaster outcomes than boys and men. One review of the literature found that in 93 percent of studies reviewed (42 of 45), females were more adversely affected than males, with the strongest negative effect being a 2:1 likelihood of developing PTSD. Women in more traditional cultures appeared to be the most vulnerable to negative psychosocial effects, particularly in the context of severe exposure. This greater negative impact is probably related to a number of gender-based factors including greater caregiving demands and less social support (e.g., single parents).

Children as a vulnerable group The effects of age are not entirely consistent from study to study; however, it does appear that children are a high-risk group. One large review of the empirical literature examined 130 distinct samples of individuals who had experienced a total of more than 80 different disasters, 60 percent of which were in the United States (NCPTSD, 2002c). School-aged youth were the most likely group across samples to evidence severe impairment, defined as having symptoms that met the criteria for a *DSM*. Sixty-two percent of the school-age survivors studied suffered severe impairment, compared to 39 percent of the adult survivors.

Children respond to disaster trauma in a number of different ways. Like adults, children have intrusive memories, reexperience traumatic events, and experience increased physiological arousal as well as emotional numbing and behavioral avoidance. Children's most severe negative reactions appear to be associated with (1) higher levels of exposure to life threat, witnessing the death or injury of others, and/or hearing screams and calls for help; (2) closer proximity to the disaster; (3) previous experience of trauma; and (4) poor parental response or psychopathology (NCPTSD, 2002e). Children's responses are also mediated by their developmental age and maturity, their relationships with parents and siblings, their gender, and their learned coping capacities. Parental distress, particularly parental psychopathology, and family disruption are the factors most predictive of children's distress (NCPTSD, 2002d; Young et al., 1998).

Typical responses of children are developmentally determined (Monahon, 1997; NCPTSD, 2002e; Pynoos & Nader, 1993). Very young children (ages one to six) have the greatest difficulty comprehending what has occurred and identifying and verbalizing their feelings and thoughts. Young children's responses are thus likely to be physiological and behavioral. Young children may have stomachaches or headaches, and may be fussy, clinging, needy, and may cry frequently. Alternatively, young children may appear passive, lack their usual responsiveness, and/or may display regressive symptoms such as bedwetting or loss of speech. Some young children have nightmares and other sleep disturbances and are fearful of separation from their caregivers.

School-age children (ages six to eleven) may show some of the same physiological and behavioral responses; however, they are also likely to be emotionally and cognitively responsive to their developmentally based confusion and misunderstandings of what has occurred (e.g., magical thinking, self-centered explanations, high attunement to parent's responses). School-age children are more likely to engage in repetitious retelling and acting out of the trauma, may feel responsible or guilty for things that occurred, and may be preoccupied with fears about their own and their family's safety. They may not want to go to school and may be less able to concentrate at school and/or may become more aggressive and angry. They also may experience noticeable changes in behavior, mood, and personality (Monahon, 1997; NCPTSD, 2002e; Pynoos & Nader, 1993).

Adolescents (ages twelve to eighteen) may also display some of the same physiological and behavioral responses including somatic complaints, nightmares, sleep and eating disturbances, and generalized anxiety and depression. Adolescents, however, are also more likely to engage in acting-out behaviors that are potentially reckless and self-injurious such as sexual acting-out, engaging in risk-taking/life-defying games, or abusing drugs or alcohol. They may also display abrupt changes in attitudes and social relationships, and declines in school attachment and performance. Adolescents may also be more likely to wish for revenge and engage in action-oriented responses, particularly if the disaster was caused intentionally, as in a terrorist attack (Monahon, 1997; NCPTSD, 2002e; Pynoos & Nader, 1993).

Older adults The effects of older age on responses to disaster are also somewhat inconsistent. Some empirical research indicates that middle-aged adults are the most adversely affected adult population. These studies suggest that middle-aged adults' greater risk for adverse psychological outcomes reflects the greater stress, responsibilities, and burdens they faced prior to the disaster, which are compounded in the aftermath of extensive resource loss (NCPTSD, 2002d).

Young et al. (1998) suggested that older adults (over age sixty-five) should be considered a "special" or "at risk" population because their postdisaster stress reactions may be complicated by age-related developmental vulnerabilities. For example, older adults may already be experiencing increased stress as the result of health changes, role changes, and the deaths of parents, friends and/or partners. Further, the trauma and losses associated with a disaster may lead to increased levels of hopelessness and futility among older adults because they may lose family keepsakes (e.g., photographs, memorabilia) and homes, which simultaneously destroys their connections to their history and family identity. And unlike younger family members, older adults face the possibility that they will not live long enough to rebuild what they have lost.

Older adults may also have already experienced a deterioration of functioning that negatively affects their ability to cope in the aftermath of a disaster. For example, an older person's senses (e.g., hearing, vision) may be less acute. Older adults may be taking multiple medications (e.g., blood pressure medication, thyroid medication, insulin, pain medication). They may have arthritis or other chronic illnesses and/or suffer from impaired mobility. Some may have memory disorders. Because of multiple impairments, older adults may be more susceptible to victimization by con artists and other criminals, less able to navigate the bureaucratic processes of applying for and receiving aid, and physically, cognitively, and emotionally less able to deal with the compounded, multiple losses they face (Young et al., 1998).

Culture, ethnicity, socioeconomic status   According to a National Center for Post-Traumatic Stress Disorder (2002d) review of the empirical literature, in five studies that considered ethnicity among adults, minority groups suffered greater negative effects following disasters than majority cultural groups. It was suggested that the disproportionate risk of psychological impairment stemmed from a greater likelihood of exposure to more severe aspects of a disaster (e.g., living in trailers or more crowded and less well-constructed homes that were more susceptible to destruction) as well as from cultural attitudes that may have prevented minority group members from seeking help. Some studies have documented that being a member of an American minority group places individuals at higher risk for developing postdisaster psychological distress than being a member of a majority group (Abueg & Chun, 1996; Kulka, Schlenger, Fairbank, Jordan, Hough, Marmar, & Weiss, 1991).

Abueg et al. (2000) asserted that culture's impact extends well beyond differential symptom expression, as culture also affects notions about trauma and some cultures view the general Western psychiatric notion of mental health sequelae with suspicion. They suggested, for instance, that avoidance and psychological numbing, identified as one criterion in diagnosing PTSD, may be indistinguishable from culturally specific patterns of emotional inhibition and lack of expression. They also cautioned, however, that in such cultural settings attention must be paid "to the degree to which victims have a voice in their cultural system," and they suggested that interventions should be "aimed at squarely addressing how to empower victims in those settings" (p. 263).

Lower socioeconomic status (SES) was similarly related to more negative outcomes. In 91 percent of the studies reviewed by Norris for the National Center for Post-Traumatic Stress Disorder (2002d), lower SES was correlated with significantly higher levels of postdisaster psychological distress. The increased risk for negative outcomes is likely the result of compounding stressors including greater exposure to severe aspects of the disaster (as with ethnic minorities), and fewer resources to replace or repair the more often substantial material losses. Poverty is also a likely contributor to the increased likelihood of severe impairment following disasters that occur in developing countries, where death tolls often measure in the thousands, and fewer services and resources are available to provide aid in the aftermath of disaster.

Prior mental health and previous trauma exposure   Of all the factors that can influence psychological outcomes following a disaster, predisaster mental health conditions are almost always the best predictor of postdisaster conditions. Individuals with prior psychiatric histories are much more likely to develop disaster-specific PTSD and to be diagnosed with other postdisaster mental health disorders (e.g., generalized anxiety disorder, major depression) than are those without prior mental health problems. Individuals with persistent mental illness who live in the community may experience deterioration or exacerbation of symptoms or even complete decompensation as a result of the increased stress and trauma associated with a disaster. In such instances an immediate referral to intensive community mental health providers is essential and, in some cases, psychiatric hospitalization may be necessary (Meichenbaum, 1994; NCPTSD, 2002d; Young et al., 1998).

Similarly, survivors with prior trauma experiences have been found to be at higher risk of postdisaster psychosocial impairment (Bland, O'Leary, Farinaro, & Trevisan, 1996; Hiley-Young, 1992; Hodgkinson & Shepherd, 1994). Individuals who have successfully adjusted to a prior traumatic experience may find that exposure to disaster trauma reactivates problems associated with the original trauma, including intrusive thoughts and memories.

Hiley-Young (1992) differentiated between two types of trauma reactivation. In *uncomplicated reactivation,* individuals who previously recovered from trauma symptoms experience a reemergence of their traumatic symptoms in response to exposure to the present disaster. Symptoms may include increased arousal and emotionality, sensory sensitivity, and intrusive memories and nightmares. In *complicated reactivation,* an individual who is still experiencing residual PTSD from a prior trauma experiences an exacerbation of symptoms upon exposure to the current disaster. In complicated cases, the individual experiences increased sensitivity and arousal to a range of stimuli not necessarily directly related to either trauma. Such individuals may also exhibit more serious impairments in identity (e.g., dissociation) and interpersonal skills.

CRISIS INTERVENTION WITH DISASTER SURVIVORS

The nature of the crisis intervention services provided in the aftermath of a disaster differs depending on the phase in which they are provided. The type of services provided is also affected by where they are delivered and to whom they are provided. In general, interventions can be envisioned as occurring during three phases: the *emergency phase* immediately after the disaster occurs; the *early postimpact phase,* which includes the days and weeks after the disaster occurs; and the *restoration phase,* which generally begins in the eighth to twelfth week after the disaster and often coincides with the implementation of long-term recovery programs. Crisis intervention services may be delivered at "ground zero" directly where the disaster occurred or at off-site areas where survivors congregate, including shelters, morgues, first-aid stations, schools or neighborhood community centers, or Red Cross service centers. People receiving assistance may include child and adult survivors, surviving family members, emergency personnel, and/or other community helpers (Young et al., 1998).

Crisis intervention services provided in the aftermath of disasters have commonly been referred to as "disaster mental health" services (DMH). Common wisdom, however, suggests *not* referring to "mental health services" when speaking with survivors, as it may interfere with their comfort in receiving assistance. Recent American Red Cross training sessions have identified those who provide services as *crisis responders.* We use the terms *crisis counseling* and *disaster mental health services* interchangeably, in all cases referring to the range of supportive, psychoeducational, and therapeutic interventions provided by human service professionals to survivors or to other crisis responders (e.g., emergency workers, police officers, firefighters, construction workers) in the aftermath of a large-scale disaster.

During the immediate impact phase, most "first on the scene" crisis workers are likely to be affiliated with local police, fire, or medical emergency personnel, or local mental health or other human service professionals with immediate access to the site of the disaster. This might include school counselors, psychologists, and social workers, human service agency personnel, hospital social workers, and, possibly, local American Red Cross disaster mental health providers.

The American Red Cross (ARC) established a formal disaster mental health service in 1989 and, since that time, has developed "Statements of Understanding" with a variety of professional organizations (e.g., the American Counseling Association, the American Psychological Association, the National Association of Social Workers, the National Association of Marriage and Family Counselors) for the purpose of enhancing the recruitment and deployment of professionals trained to provide disaster mental health services. One important goal of these alliances is to ensure that services are coordinated and delivered through identified administrative bodies such as FEMA or ARC. Red Cross service centers are usually fully established and staffed early during the postimpact phase, whereas FEMA-sponsored crisis counseling services often do not begin until much later.

Despite efforts to enhance and coordinate the deployment of crisis assistance in the aftermath of a disaster, there is usually some bureaucratic confusion in the early days following a large-scale disaster when the goals and priorities of different agencies may conflict. For instance police, firefighters and emergency medical personnel have distinct jobs to perform, large urban police departments and fire departments may have their own mental health experts, and local and state mental health agencies may view the provision of crisis intervention services as their responsibility. In large-scale disasters when there is a presidential declaration of disaster, FEMA establishes a local Disaster Field Office with representation from public health services, state mental health services, and the American Red Cross and assumes responsibility for the overall coordination of all emergency services.

Defusing and Debriefing

The terms *defusing* and *debriefing* currently refer to a variety of interventions hypothesized to reduce the likelihood of psychological impairment following exposure to traumatic incidents including disasters. Mitchell (1983) first used the terms *defusing* and *critical incident stress debriefing* (CISD) to describe specific components of a multicomponent crisis intervention system, *critical incident stress management* (CISM), developed to prepare and support emergency medical personnel and other first responders including rescue and disaster personnel, military personnel, and mental health care professionals.

The components of CISM include preincident preparedness training, demobilization and informational briefings, defusing, individual psychological support,

CISD, family crisis intervention and support, and follow-up and referral mechanisms for further assessment and/or treatment, as needed. CISM and its components, defusing and debriefing, rest on the hypothesis that through structured group communication individuals can be assisted to recall their traumatic experiences, share memories and emotions, and express fears, concerns, and regrets leading to an enhanced ability to understand and accept what they have witnessed or experienced (Everly & Mitchell, 1997).

Defusing—in essence, a shortened version of debriefing—ranges (depending on the model) from a three-phase to six-phase structured small group discussion or one-on-one intervention provided within hours of the event. Whether in a group format or individual intervention, the purpose of defusing is to provide an opportunity for survivors to disclose their experiences and obtain some relief of symptoms.

CISD refers to a structured group discussion with survivors in the days or weeks following exposure. The ideal intervention includes seven phases: (1) introduction and guidelines; (2) fact phase; (3) thought phase; (4) reaction/emotional processing phase; (5) symptom phase; (6) education phase; and (7) reentry/information and referral phase. According to this model, after participants are prepared, the crisis worker leads them through a process of recalling the facts of what occurred and the thoughts they had as the event unfolded. This cognitive recall is conceptualized as preparatory to the reaction/affective phase during which the crisis worker asks participants to speak about the most emotionally troubling and difficult aspects of the event. Discussion of symptoms begins to move participants back into a more cognitive realm, and debriefings end with information sharing both about symptoms, symptom relief strategies, and referrals (Mitchell & Everly, 2002; Young, 1998).

As noted, CISD was originally intended to assist first responders who had been briefed prior to their mission and were then debriefed afterward. Since their development, however, many helping professionals advocate defusing and debriefing strategies for a much wider range of situations, and CISD is currently utilized as the standard of care for responding to survivors of both natural and manmade disasters.

We have devoted considerable attention to these intervention strategies because they have been the dominant approach to intervention following large-scale disasters. We do not advocate the adoption of debriefing strategies as a primary intervention with survivors, however, as there is a growing body of literature cautioning against their routine use. Recent research suggests that psychologically oriented group debriefings of survivors may *not* assist recovery, and, on the contrary, may actually *exacerbate* individuals' traumatic stress (NCPTSD, 2002a; National Institute of Mental Health, 2002).

At a recent workshop convened by the National Institute of Mental Health (NIMH, 2002), fifty-eight disaster mental health experts from six countries met to review the current research on early psychological interventions following exposure to mass violence and to identify what works, what doesn't work, and what knowledge is needed to determine best practices. Workshop attendees also addressed questions related to the timing of interventions, assessment and screening, and the expertise and training necessary for providing early intervention services. One of the most important and controversial recommendations to come out of this workshop was the recommendation that the term *debriefing* be used only to describe operational debriefings conducted by organizations and provided to staff responders. *Operational debriefing* was defined as routine individual or group review of the factual details of an event for the purposes of identifying what actually happened, improving future missions, and increasing the ability of individuals to return to duty.

The report issued by the attendees concluded that current research does not support the one-time "recital of events and expression of emotions evoked by a traumatic event" (as advocated in some forms of psychological debriefing), as it has not been found to reduce the likelihood of developing trauma-related disorders and some survivors "may be put at heightened risk for adverse outcomes as a result of such early interventions" (NIMH, 2002, p. 8). Similar cautions have also been issued by the National Center for Post-Traumatic Stress Disorder (2002a): "While operational debriefing, which involves clarifying events and providing education about normal responses and coping mechanisms, is nearly always helpful, care must be taken before delivering more emotionally focused interventions. . . . Available evidence shows that it may in some instances increase traumatic stress or possibly complicate recovery" (p. 4).

What do these research-based cautions suggest about intervention in the aftermath of a large-scale disaster? First, it appears that the heightened arousal survivors may experience in the early posttrauma period that is associated with long-term trauma disorder is not easy to identify in individuals in one group intervention. Second, the one-time verbalization of emotionally traumatic material may increase rather than decrease arousal because habituation to emotional and physiological distress cannot occur during such a brief intervention. Rather, intervention strategies that emphasize individual and family psychological first aid, and that foster resilience, facilitate natural support networks, and provide outreach and information are preferred (and empirically supported) intervention responses. Further, triage, the process by which crisis workers evaluate and respond to victims according to the immediacy of their treatment needs, is essential. Such an approach permits more individualized mental health responses while still attending to the important role of outreach and information dissemination.

SINGLE-SESSION CRISIS INTERVENTION

Early crisis intervention must be an integrated component of comprehensive disaster relief/disaster management plans. It must be provided in a manner that fully reflects the survivor's hierarchy of needs, with survival, safety, and security clearly primary. Therefore, initial mental health interventions must focus on protecting survivors from further harm—physical as well as psychological harm. This means reducing survivors' exposure to traumatic experiences and helping them connect with loved ones and with individuals who will be able to provide support, information, and needed resources. First contacts with survivors frequently occur in chaotic circumstances, as when assistance is provided at the site of the disaster, in mass shelters, or in hospitals and morgues.

Single-session interventions may occur during the emergency phase (the immediate period after disaster strikes) and/or during the early postimpact phase. Although crisis responders are advised to expect that most individuals will recover normally following exposure to disasters, research also suggests that in some types of disasters, particularly exposure to mass violence, large numbers of individuals experience significant psychiatric disturbances. One study of individuals directly exposed to the Oklahoma City bomb blast found that nearly half of them had a diagnosable trauma-related disorder (North, Nixon, Shariat, Mallonee, McMillen, & Spitznagel, 1999). Researchers have also documented, however, that despite experiencing significant distress, most individuals do not voluntarily seek mental health services. Given these paradoxical findings, crisis interventionists must recognize the barriers to help seeking and provide outreach to individuals identified as at risk.

The following discussion of single-session intervention draws heavily on the recommendations for disaster mental health services developed by Young and colleagues (1998) for the National Center for PTSD and on the recommendations in the report produced by the workshop on psychological intervention following exposure to mass violence (NIMH, 2002). It is important to reiterate that in highly chaotic or volatile situations the single-session model is rarely applied in a linear fashion. Thus in a disaster setting, particularly during the impact phase, the crisis worker must be able to assess the situation, connect with the survivor or survivors, and begin to de-escalate and create safety—and do it all simultaneously. In many instances single-session interventions are provided to families or small groups.

Step 1:
Supportively and empathically join with survivor(s).

Initial contacts with survivors of disasters must help them connect with human caring. Individuals who have experienced large-scale disasters, particularly those involving traumatic loss of life, have been temporarily disconnected from their known world of human experience, safety, and relationships. However brief the interaction one has with a survivor, supportive, compassionate, and caring relational connection will be reparative. When an individual is in acute distress, a crisis worker's simple presence may assist the individual to manage fears and sorrow.

Young et al. (1998) suggested a pragmatic range of initial activities: "Protect, direct, connect, triage." When mental health professionals enter a disaster site in the immediate impact period, their first responsibility is often to identify "natural helpers" who have begun to provide care and to sensitively relieve them of that responsibility. Creating a shelter or safe haven where both survivors and natural helpers can be protected from further exposure to traumatic stimuli is helpful, as is providing gentle but firm direction to individuals who may be stunned or in shock.

During the early postimpact phase, crisis intervention providers frequently move to shelters and other sites where many survivors are gathered. Crisis workers should begin by observing the setting and the people who are congregated, quickly assessing the environmental stresses and resources. First contact with survivors can be facilitated by efforts to provide practical assistance such as serving food or water. For example, *"Can I get you something to make you more comfortable?"* or *"Have you been waiting long?"* It is essential to avoid comments that survivors may perceive to be trivializing. Statements or questions that might seem appropriate in other circumstances are often not appropriate in the aftermath of a disaster when the answer to such questions is apparent. For instance, survivors would find it naïve, condescending, or trivializing if a crisis worker asked them how they were feeling, tried to cheer them up, or compared their loss or suffering to others'.

When survivors initiate contact, crisis workers can begin to establish relational contact by listening carefully and responding to whatever concerns or questions they identify. When the crisis worker initiates contact, he or she can ask questions such as, *"How are you managing?"* or *"May I help you in some way?"* to facilitate connection and further the conversation gradually, allowing the crisis worker to assess the individual's current functioning and/or needs.

Step 2:
Intervene to create safety, stabilize the situation, and handle the survivor's immediate needs.

As we have noted, during the impact phase of a disaster protecting survivors from further physical danger and further exposure to traumatic stimuli is often the first responsibility for crisis interventionists who are among first responders. Crisis interventionists can firmly and gently move ambulatory survivors away from potentially dangerous areas and away from other more seriously injured individuals. This protection and direction is particularly helpful for children; it is important to prevent children from experiencing further harm, either through continuing exposure to physically dangerous circumstances and/or through repeated exposure to psychologically traumatizing images and the sounds of others' anguish.

Assessment of individual needs is ongoing from first contact, and triage—identifying individuals who are experiencing the most intense psychological/emotional responses—is essential so that crisis workers can provide further care to those who need it. Indicators of severe stress reactions like panic and/or grief include being immobilized or engaging in erratic behavior, trembling, extreme agitation, loud screaming, and/or wailing. Crisis workers can provide some relief by quickly establishing an empathic connection and validating the survivor's experience while simultaneously providing calm, firm direction. Individuals in acute distress may need someone to remain with them, and crisis workers can consult with a physician or other medical personnel regarding medication to promote short-term stability.

During the early postimpact phase, efforts continue to stabilize and de-escalate those in acute crisis. Crisis interventionists also continue to assist survivors by helping them handle immediate needs. These needs range from physical survival needs (shelter, food, clothing, medical problems), to reconnecting with loved ones, to obtaining accurate information and identifying resources for additional information and/or support, and managing grief and acute traumatic stress reactions.

Step 3:
Explore and assess the dimensions of the crisis and the survivor's reaction to the crisis, encouraging ventilation.

As crisis interventionists begin to make contact with survivors and meet their immediate needs, they are simultaneously engaged in assessment. Young et al. (1998) suggested a format that utilizes informal socializing as the vehicle for beginning relational connection and assessments. Crisis worker can gradually assist individuals who are able and willing to discuss their current issues and needs to speak more directly about their exposure during the disaster's impact and their current emotional state.

Single-session interventions are not intended to provide in-depth therapeutic exploration of the meanings of the disaster experience or its emotional impact. Rather, the purpose is to enable individuals to obtain greater control over themselves and their situations, and to prevent the development of posttraumatic symptomatology. All assessment and intervention begins with sensitivity to the person's developmental needs. Children have special needs, many adults have significant social role responsibilities as spouses and parents that directly affect their needs and concerns, and older people may suffer from declining physical abilities, may have handicapping medical conditions, and/or have suffered previous losses.

Because level of exposure is a clear risk factor, it is useful to gradually shift the focus of a conversation with a survivor from the immediate situation to one that facilitates assessment of exposure to life threat and other traumatic stimuli. Crisis interventionists can begin with questions like *"Where were you when it happened?," "What do you remember seeing, smelling, and hearing?," "Where were other people?,"* and/or *"What did you do first?"* Such open questions encourage the individual to speak about his or her experience, but in a concrete and factual manner. The crisis interventionist can then build on these facts to facilitate the survivor's expression of his or her thoughts, for example, *"What were your first thoughts?"* or *"Is there anything that you keep thinking about?"* As survivors describe their experiences and their thoughts, crisis workers can respond empathically, validating their emotions and responding in ways that depathologize their reactions. Probes that help survivors describe how they've been feeling since the disaster happened can also be useful at this juncture. In this manner, crisis interventionists intervene to both promote ventilation and assess.

A primary purpose of assessment is to determine which individuals are most at risk of significant psychological difficulty in order to provide the necessary immediate intervention and to identify those in need of follow-up crisis services. Individuals who did not have high levels of exposure to traumatic events (e.g., witnessing massive loss of life, exposure to horrifying sights or sounds, being terrified about harm or loss of one's own life) are usually considered to be at relatively *low risk*. Survivors who appear to be able to appropriately express grief and loss, and who describe only low to moderate levels of normal stress responses including anxiety, depression, arousal, and reexperiencing would also be considered low risk. Individuals at *moderate risk* were probably directly exposed to massive deaths and/or horrific injury, and may be experiencing higher levels of emotional distress. The *highest risk* category includes survivors who had direct traumatic exposure, who may also have experienced the deaths of people close to them, and are frequently either exhibiting intense emotions of panic, anxiety, and/or grief, or are numb, hopeless, avoidant, and/or possibly dissociative. Continuing intervention and the timing of that intervention should reflect the survivor's level of risk. Whereas crisis workers can usually assist those at low risk with educational/informational group interventions, they should see those at higher risk in individual or family single-session interventions, and provide follow-up care. Those in the highest risk category should receive intensive interventions aimed specifically at treating acute stress disorder symptoms (Abueg et al., 2000).

Previously described cautions about psychological debriefings are equally applicable to defusing protocols, particularly those advocated for use with groups of survivors. Therefore, initial group interventions should be primarily informational, with more extensive discussion of individual survivors' experiences handled in one-on-one or family interventions. In all interventions, crisis workers must carefully monitor individual responses and avoid contributing to a heightened sense of vulnerability and/or anxiety, particularly for those individuals who may already be at greatest risk.

Assessment must also consider survivors' concrete needs and the characteristics of the recovery environment. Individuals who have survived floods, hurricanes, or fires may have lost their homes, automobiles, and other possessions. Communities may be devastated. Most individuals are unaware of what kinds of assistance may be available to assist them or how to obtain access to that help.

Step 4:
Identify and examine alternative actions and develop options.

The impact of disasters on individuals, families, and communities is frequently so far-reaching that the list of immediate needs is long. Correspondingly, the resources to assist survivors may be limited. Individuals may have experienced the death of family members and/or friends, or loved ones may be missing. Homes and possessions may have been damaged or destroyed. Survivors may be emotionally traumatized. The concrete problems of finding housing, seeking medical tests and/or treatment, and pursuing property and/or medical insurance claims may overwhelm survivors' coping capacities.

Given the enormity of many survivors' needs, crisis workers can help them take a step toward regaining control by providing assistance in prioritizing concerns, examining options, and choosing discrete steps to take. Issues requiring immediate attention must be identified. Because the nature of a disaster determines the types of needs that arise, crisis workers must be sensitive to a range of possible scenarios. For instance, some disasters (e.g., the attacks in Oklahoma City, New York City, and Washington, DC) are traumatic events that cause great injury and loss of life. Many survivors may nonetheless still have families and homes to which they can return. (One year after the attack on the World Trade Center in New York, however, many people in the area surrounding the Twin Towers were still unable to return to their homes because of collateral damage to their buildings, and police and firefighters were exposed to continuing trauma throughout the long period of rescue, cleanup, and recovery of bodies.) In other disasters, like hurricanes and floods, there may routinely be continued exposure to severe conditions and stressors (e.g., decimation of homes and surrounding community, environmental destruction, cleanup and rebuilding) that continues for months or years.

Immediate needs can be conceptualized on a continuum, with personal coping needs at one end of the spectrum and concrete practical needs at the other. In both cases, in single-session interventions, consideration of alternatives and options focuses on "what comes next." Asking survivors about their personal coping responses and needs can lead to an exploration of immediate concerns as well as potential coping strategies. It can also give crisis workers an opportunity to provide educational information that will help survivors recognize potential problems, improve coping, and take care of themselves. For example:

- *"After what you and your family have been through, and given what you all still face, it's going to be really important to identify some ways to get some relief and perhaps some help along the way. Let's talk about some ways that you can take care of yourself over the next days and weeks."*
- *"The kind of stress you and your family have been under makes everyone vulnerable. Let's try to think of some ways you may be able to help your children cope."*
- *"What you have been through and still face is pretty overwhelming. As you think about getting through the next couple of days physically and emotionally, what are the things that you believe can help you?"*

The goal is for individuals to utilize active coping strategies, to identify and utilize their natural support systems, and to identify formal sources of support should they be necessary. Helpful questions to guide this exploration of alternatives also include:

- *"What has helped you get through this so far?"*
- *"Whom do you usually turn to/talk to when you're having difficulty?"*
- *"It's unlikely that anything quite like this has happened to you before, but when you have had really stressful times in the past, what has helped you get through?"*

In the course of this exploration, crisis workers can educate survivors about the importance of taking care of themselves and managing stress; can encourage the ongoing expression of fears, anxieties, and other trauma-evoked emotions; and can help survivors identify sources of strength and resilience in themselves, their families, and their support systems.

It is equally important to explore alternatives and options in relation to immediate concrete needs. Crisis workers can initiate an exploration of those immediate needs and alternatives for addressing them. For example:

- *"It sounds as though you're about to be allowed to return to your neighborhood. Have you considered the possibility that someone might accompany you to your home?"*
- *"From what you've been told, it sounds as though you will be unable to stay in the building where you were living. What options have you considered for where to go when you leave the shelter?"*
- *"It sounds as if just thinking about all that needs to be done is pretty overwhelming. Maybe we could try and prioritize the steps so at least you'd have an idea about where to start."*

Exploration of alternatives is a primary tool for helping the survivor switch from survival mode to problem solving. It is important to remember the utility of compartmentalizing as a strategy for enhancing coping. When there are many interrelated needs, the ability to identify discrete issues often leads to a sense of positive movement and increased sense of self-efficacy. And, as previously discussed, survivors' perceived control and self-efficacy are strongly and positively related to positive mental health outcomes (NCPTSD, 2002b). Furthermore, as survivors successfully take the identified actions, they are likely to achieve greater stability. Thus, for example, it will be much easier emotionally and physically for an older woman who lived alone to go to survey the damage to her house if she is accompanied by a stable and caring family member or friend.

Step 5:
Help the survivor mobilize personal and social resources and connect with other community resources, as needed.

Resource deterioration, the extent to which a survivor loses material and social resources, is an important factor contributing to psychological distress following disasters. Survivors who believe that they are cared for and that help is available to assist them fare better and experience fewer negative psychological sequelae (NCPTSD, 2002b; Vernberg et al., 1996). Therefore, interventions that help survivors connect with sources of concrete assistance and social support are critical.

As crisis workers explore survivor responses to the disaster experience and engage in the process of problem solving by identifying immediate needs and alternatives, they also begin to identify potential personal, social, and concrete supports and resources that they can enlist to assist survivors to go forward. These potential resources include survivors' predisaster psychological strengths, their social embeddedness, and their material resources.

Social embeddedness—the size, closeness, and involvement of an individual's social support network—can be a paradox. Social embeddedness is characteristically related to positive mental health, and the active involvement of a survivor's social support network in the aftermath of a disaster provides protection against negative mental health outcomes. Survivors' natural social support systems, however, are also vulnerable to the impact of a disaster: many individuals who would normally be supportive may themselves be directly affected by the disaster; neighbors and other community members may be forced to relocate; and community-wide devastation often results in the cancellation of social activities, school activities, and other activities. Attending to the social needs of disaster victims is therefore particularly helpful in protecting survivors from adverse outcomes (NCPTSD, 2002b).

Crisis workers can assist survivors to identify their natural support systems and reinforce the importance of utilizing them. "Naturally occurring social resources are particularly vital for disaster victims. Professionals and outsiders are important sources of assistance when the level of need is high, but they must not and cannot supplant natural helping networks" (NCPTSD, 2002b, p. 3). Crisis workers can encourage survivors to maintain routine social activities and can educate them about the difficulties individuals in their personal support systems may be experiencing. Crisis workers can encourage the development of community support groups. Relief organizations sometimes organize such groups to disseminate information. These groups, if they continue to meet, can provide survivors with ongoing emotional support, concrete assistance, and the opportunity to share information about resources.

It is also helpful to produce a handout that provides contact information for formal community resources such as mental health and other social services as well as specific disaster relief information. The provision of early financial and emotional support can both concretely meet needs and contribute to the perception of support availability, which, as previously noted, is a factor positively correlated with recovery. Norris and Kaniasty (1997) found that racial or ethnic minorities and those of lower socioeconomic status often receive less assistance than other survivors even when they experience similar losses and have a similar need for resources. Further, because families of lower socioeconomic status often had fewer resources before the disaster, they are more vulnerable in the face of a disaster. Crisis workers can provide information to members of these vulnerable groups about gaining access to resources and provide assistance in applying and obtaining aid. In addition, crisis workers can advocate for the equitable distribution of assistance to the most needy individuals and families.

Step 6:
Anticipate the future and arrange follow-up contact.

Although crisis workers provide information to survivors throughout the process of single-session crisis counseling, a final goal is always to ensure that individuals have information that prepares them for what may occur in the days, weeks, and, perhaps, months to follow. Disaster survivors always benefit from knowledge about the potential onset of a variety of posttraumatic symptoms including recurring memories and nightmares about the event and some degree of emotional distress. For low-risk survivors, anticipation of negative symptoms can normalize their responses and facilitate their ability to express their feelings and accept support to aid coping. Crisis workers can also inform survivors about the likelihood of recurring symptoms during times that remind them of the disaster (e.g., anniversaries, memorial services, return to the site). For moderate- and high-risk survivors, education about the nature of Acute Stress Disorder and PTSD and the identification of resources that can provide specialized assistance enhance the likelihood that survivors will seek and receive these continuing services.

Follow-up crisis counseling should always be offered to individuals who are at risk for developing difficulties. According to the NIMH (2002) work group on best practices, at-risk individuals include (1) those who have acute stress disorder or other clinically significant symptoms, (2) those who are bereaved, (3) those who have required medical or surgical care, and (4) those survivors whose exposure to the disaster was intense and/or of long duration (p. 9). Workshop participants observed that survivors who have not experienced clinically significant symptoms after approximately two months do not routinely need follow-up, although it should be provided, if requested.

Even during large-group informational debriefings, crisis workers can identify individuals who appear to have strong emotional responses and attempt to provide both immediate follow-up and ongoing follow-up care, if indicated. One benefit of having two facilitators in a postdisaster group is to allow one facilitator to attend to the educational agenda and the other to focus on individual responses. As the case study at the end of the chapter illustrates, a facilitator can approach individuals who appear to be having a particularly difficult time and provide them the opportunity to further process their immediate reactions as well as offer follow-up counseling. Follow-up counseling can either be with the group leader or another identified crisis counselor skilled in providing intervention to trauma survivors.

According to American Red Cross guidelines for referral, crisis responders should refer a survivor for follow-up crisis counseling whenever a survivor demonstrates any of the following: an inability to care for personal needs or to perform everyday functions, an inability to make simple decisions, preoccupation with a particular idea, pressured speech or other psychotic symptoms, excessive avoidance of emotion and withdrawal from interpersonal contact, suicidal or homicidal talk or gestures, frequent flashbacks and/or nightmares, dissociation, developmental regression, and/or abuse of alcohol or drugs (Young et al., 1998).

ONGOING CRISIS COUNSELING WITH DISASTER SURVIVORS

Ongoing crisis counseling following disasters, as with most crises, is provided to individuals and families who are still experiencing difficulty after the immediate postimpact period. Some individuals accept offers of follow-up by a crisis worker who provided crisis services during the impact or early postimpact phase. Other individuals recognize at a later time that they are experiencing continuing or renewed distress in the aftermath of the disaster and seek assistance. Follow-up services can also be initiated by crisis service provider outreach.

Routine Follow-up Services

Ideally, crisis workers should provide all survivors with follow-up information "to help normalize common reactions to trauma, improve coping, enhance self-care, facilitate recognition of significant problems, and increase knowledge of and access to services" (NCPTSD, 2002a, p. 6). More intensive follow-up meetings with subgroups of survivors, with specific families, and/or with individuals who were initially identified at highest risk for onset of PTSD may enhance the likelihood that these individuals will seek ongoing crisis counseling services. Clearly, survivor readiness affects whether a survivor accepts outreach efforts but efforts at follow-up can provide the opportunity for rescreening and repeated referrals even if individuals are still not ready to face the emotional aspects of the trauma.

Outreach follow-up services can also be timed to coincide with events that may be retraumatizing such as anniversary and/or memorial events or criminal trials for perpetrators whose violent actions precipitated the disaster.

In some instances, survivors who present for ongoing crisis counseling suffer from complex PTSD or are highly dissociative, frequently as the result of experiencing previous unresolved traumas prior to the disaster trauma. In such cases, crisis workers must take extreme care in assessment and before engaging in interventions aimed at eliciting trauma memories. Unless the crisis counselor has specific training and competence in providing interventions that include recall of traumatic memories, he or she should refer the survivor to an individual with the requisite expertise.

Assessment of individuals who seek ongoing crisis counseling must be holistic and responsive to biopsychosocial needs. In addition to the potential negative impact on affective, behavioral, cognitive, developmental, and ecological functioning, trauma survivors often experience significant physiological manifestations of acute stress including high arousal, heart palpitations, and headaches. Most theories of PTSD posit an important relationship between physiological and psychological functioning. Thus, crisis workers may need to consult with physicians or other medical providers in order to evaluate for possible psychopharmacological intervention as well.

Importantly, not every survivor who requests follow-up crisis counseling is suffering from ASD or PTSD. For some individuals, the disaster trauma triggers problematic personal or interpersonal responses that seem more urgent to confront after the trauma. For example:

Renee is a thirty-four-year-old married woman who was seen several months after her escape from a chemical explosion in a building where she was employed. Although crisis counseling was offered at the time, she chose not to participate. She stated that what precipitated her seeking help was her dissatisfaction with what she described as her husband's "shallow" reactions to what she went through and the impact it had on her. She described a marriage that had long ago "lost its passion" and that had become even less satisfactory since the explosion. She described questioning her lifestyle and her beliefs, and felt driven to engage her life more fully. She felt that the event had had an enormous impact on her, yet it seemed invisible and inconsequential to her husband. Although the crisis counselor examined and worked with her continuing anxieties and dysphoria, the overarching focus of her crisis counseling centered on understanding the way the experience had changed her and reevaluating her relationship with her husband in terms of those changes.

For some, the feelings of fear, vulnerability, guilt, or shame may resonate with long-standing personal or familial concerns. For others, the disaster may reactivate unresolved prior losses or traumas. And some individuals may indeed experience acute symptoms of posttraumatic stress and/or a combination of the above.

Assessment Instruments

After crisis counselors have established the general parameters of the needs for which the survivor is seeking ongoing counseling, screening measures can help pinpoint the nature of the specific stressors and assess the types and levels of distressing symptoms. For the first purpose, Young et al. (1998) recommended the use of their *Personal Experiences in Disaster Survey (PEDS),* an instrument for adult respondents consisting of a series of questions regarding the types of physical injury sustained or observed in others, the dangers faced, and the extent of personal and/or material losses. It also contains a number of questions designed to elicit details about the types of resultant crises (e.g., relational, spiritual) and about the types and degree of social supportiveness experienced. Young et al. also recommended the use of a PTSD measure (*PCL;* Weathers, Litz, Huska, & Keane, 1995) to specifically assess levels of PTSD symptomatology. There are also a number of screening measures for children that can provide specific information relative to hurricane-related trauma (*HURTE;* Vernberg et al., 1996) and PTSD (*CAPS-CA;* Nader, 1996).

Establishing an Empowering Relationship

As is true of survivors of any traumatic event, individuals who have survived disaster traumas often begin the counseling relationship relatively alienated and guarded. In some instances, the postdisaster experience may have disrupted a survivor's normal social supports. In other instances, survivors may feel shame and/or guilt over something they did or failed to do that they believe resulted in further harm to others. Or survivors may have been exposed to scenes or events that were emotionally overwhelming and may feel that they cannot convey their experience to someone who was not there.

Despite, and at times because of, these challenges, it is essential that crisis workers establish a helping alliance. Empathic recognition of these barriers coupled with attention to current needs can create the necessary context for the disaster survivor and crisis counselor to gradually establish a trusting relationship.

The initial focus of all postdisaster crisis counseling is on crisis management and stabilization (Young et al., 1998). Thus, establishing the helping relationship occurs concurrently with assessment (of symptoms, stressors, coping, and personal and social resources) and beginning interventions to provide the immediate relief of symptoms. Individualized education about the types of stress reactions and/or symptoms a survivor is experiencing can also have a significant impact on reducing initial resistance and establishing the credibility of the helper. Information gained through initial assessment processes (a clinical interview and/or the use of screening measures) allows the crisis counselor to provide information that is specific to the survivor's experience and needs, as opposed to the more generic information most often provided in group outreach efforts.

Ongoing Crisis Counseling Goals and Processes

The following sections examine the goals and processes of crisis counseling, attending to issues of assessment and intervention with disaster survivors.

Affect stability:
Help survivors to express and process memories and emotions related to the disaster.

The affective dimensions of survivor responses cannot be separated from the cognitions that underlie them. Thus interventions to help survivors attain greater emotional stability include those directly focused on evoking emotions and those focused on evoking thoughts and images of the trauma experience.

Interventions that target emotions assist survivors to identify and work through the range of emotions they may be experiencing. Because easily recognized emotions such as anger or sadness may be dominant, survivors may not recognize other emotions that they are experiencing. For example, fear may be masked by anger, shame, or guilt, and/or grief may be masked by sadness (Young et al., 1998).

The crisis worker's goal is to bring to the foreground those emotions that may be discounted, hidden, and out of conscious awareness so that the survivor can acknowledge them, express them, and gradually work through them. The process of working through emotions includes ventilation in the safe confines of an empathic relationship and identifying the thoughts and beliefs that trigger the emotions. In this manner, for example, the crisis worker can help the survivor link feelings of hopelessness, powerlessness, and separateness to the precipitating cognitions, which he or she can also attempt to change.

Crisis workers also target survivors' emotions indirectly as they assist them to recall their narrative disaster record—the images and memories of the disaster experience. Processing memories often begins with the survivor's conscious recollection of the factual chain of events. As crisis workers guide survivors through the remembering process, they help them connect their emotional and physiological reactions to their factual account. The process of remembering with attention to the physical and emotional aspects of the experience is intended to gradually desensitize survivors to those images and attendant reactions so they are more able to tolerate them without high levels of arousal distress. Unlike mass debriefings in the immediate postimpact phase of a disaster, this individualized focus on processing memories and emotions is preceded by the crisis counselor's attention to the survivor's capacity to handle this process and by ongoing assessment of and responsiveness to attendant difficulties.

Behavioral adjustments:
Help survivors to make and sustain behavioral changes conducive to personal and social functioning.

Disaster survivors, like survivors of any crisis or trauma, must be able to return to patterns of eating, sleeping, working, and playing that are healthy and satisfying. They may need to continue efforts to rebuild homes or to move and relocate. They may need to follow through with ongoing medical and/or rehabilitative care for themselves or family members. Or they may need to find ways to cope with the demands and challenges of a family constellation changed by loss of a family member. For example:

Sarah and her husband, David, were traveling in Israel when a suicide bomber detonated a bomb in the market adjacent to where they were having lunch at an outdoor café. The explosion knocked both of them to the ground, and David was struck in the head by flying debris. He was one of twenty-one people who died from the attack.

Sarah and David had two young children who were at home in the United States with Sarah's widowed mother. In addition to dealing with her own responses to the disaster trauma and the grief of losing her husband, Sarah also had to resolve insurance problems, assume the management of David's fledgling small business, and be a single parent to her sons. She was physically exhausted, had lost twenty pounds, and had not slept for more than five hours a night since David died four months ago, in part because she didn't want to dream. Apart from handling the paperwork necessary for the funeral and insurance claims, she has been unable to begin to sort through David's papers and/or personal belongings.

Clearly, Sarah faces many challenges in the aftermath of this traumatic disaster. One focus for crisis counseling must be assisting her to engage in behaviors that will contribute to her well-being so that she is capable of fulfilling the many demands she faces. Beginning work with Sarah must focus on improving her eating and sleeping patterns or she will eventually collapse from sheer physical exhaustion and/or ill health. She also will need assistance in gradually approaching the specific tasks of sorting through David's personal effects. Some of the behavioral challenges she faces intersect with issues she must address regarding her relationships with others, the business, and her need for assistance. Her developmental stage in life and the accompanying roles she occupies and tasks she faces also affect and, in many ways, define her emotional and behavioral challenges.

All crisis counseling must emphasize the development and/or enhancement of positive behavioral coping strategies. This may include encouraging survivors to verbalize their needs and concerns and/or to reach out to other survivors. As noted, disasters frequently affect many individuals and, indeed, whole communities at the same time. Crisis workers can encourage survivors to work with other community members to establish mechanisms for ongoing mutual emotional support and to combine efforts to garner the resources necessary for family and community rebuilding and recovery. Teaching and practicing positive coping strategies such as systematic relaxation or breathing strategies to better manage anxieties or fears are also useful. Meichenbaum (1994) suggested that behavioral strategies for emotional soothing, use of social supports, and direct-action problem solving are all positive coping behaviors that can be developed and/or enhanced.

Crisis workers can also encourage children to develop positive coping skills including expressing their concerns and engaging in constructive activities. Participating in commemorative rituals, letter writing, and assuming developmentally appropriate responsibilities within the home can all contribute to children's renewed sense of personal control and power. Crisis workers can assist parents to assess their children's behavior and to develop "rules and limits, incentives and logical consequences, and activities that instill an atmosphere of empathy and encouragement to assist their children with fear and anxieties or with impulsive or aggressive behavior problems" (Young et al., 1998, p. 86).

Behavioral interventions may also entail addressing comorbid drug and alcohol issues. Previously undetected substance abuse may come to the fore, or drug and alcohol abuse may have become a maladaptive coping strategy in the aftermath of a disaster. Crisis workers should always assess survivors' drug and alcohol use, identifying active abuse or dependence behaviors and targeting them for change.

Finally, assessment of potential lethality must be an initial and ongoing focus, with interventions targeted to level of assessed risk. Crisis workers must identify both cognitive and behavioral indicators of risk and intervene to eliminate potentially lethal behavior.

Cognitive mastery:
Help survivors to examine and reframe their core beliefs, expectations, and personal meanings threatened by the disaster.

The sheer magnitude of a disaster experience and the multitude of losses experienced suggest that they frequently shatter survivors' beliefs about personal control and safety. They may also call into question survivors' spiritual beliefs, appraisals of life's fairness, views of other people's character and trustworthiness, or ideas regarding independence and dependence. The cognitive impact of a disaster experience and the subsequent changes in personal beliefs and meanings are different for all survivors. Thus one individual may emerge from a disaster experience with a renewed appreciation of other people's generosity and caring or of his or her own strength and determination. Another individual may harbor the conviction that God is punishing him or her by meting out unbearable unhappiness and suffering.

For crisis counselors engaged in ongoing crisis counseling, the primary question is whether individuals' cognitions are realistic and are contributing to their adaptation and ongoing mastery of their lives in the aftermath of the disaster experience. And ultimately, how can crisis counselors help individual survivors ascribe meaning to their experiences that contributes to that healthy adaptation?

Because personal safety is always a major concern, identification of beliefs or thoughts that contribute to or prolong emotional and/or physiological difficulties must be an initial focus of counseling attention. For example, beliefs that interfere with help-seeking or expression of needs, or self-deprecating thoughts that result in isolation can be targeted through cognitive restructuring/reframing techniques. Consider the following example:

Margaret is a seventy-four-year-old widow who believed she should not complain and bother her children (i.e., express her needs for assistance) because it would take them away from the many challenges they were facing in the aftermath of the hurricane that badly damaged both of their homes. The crisis counselor helped her see how her insistence on being a martyr was actually distracting her family from attending to their other needs because they were concerned about her. The counselor also helped her realize that she was not a burden. The counselor helped her identify her role as a pillar of family solidarity and continuity, and recognize her ability to be a source of help rather than merely her children's responsibility.

Abueg et al. (2000) noted that guilt is often pervasive in the aftermath of traumatic disasters. They suggested that crisis counselors explore questions related to survivors' perceptions regarding whether they did or did not do enough, whether they made a devastating mistake, or whether they were somehow responsible for a negative outcome. Meichenbaum (1994) also suggested that counselors assess individual survivors' perceptions of their personal responsibility. For example, he suggested that crisis counselors attend to any indications that the individual perceives him- or herself in a role that "resulted in injury or death to others because of what he/she did or failed to do" or that he/she offered assistance that "proved to be unhelpful . . . futile . . . or even made things worse" (p. 506). These concerns may be particularly relevant for rescue personnel and other first responders. In each case, intervention must focus on correcting distortions and creating realistic appraisals of personal control.

Cognitive interventions often include teaching survivors to connect their troubling reactions and symptoms to the unique trauma they experienced. A useful first step is often asking the survivor to tell the story of the disaster so the crisis worker can identify the most troubling aspects of it and the thoughts that the survivor has about his or her experiences. The crisis worker can specifically address the thoughts that are connected to the survivor's current psychological and interpersonal distress for the dual purpose of producing clearer recollection and correcting cognitive distortions or thoughts underlying irrational fears.

Repeated reviewing of memories with attention to their cognitive, sensory, and emotional aspects gradually contributes to the survivor's ability to tolerate those memories with less arousal and distress. As Young et al. (1998) noted, "If, after several sessions, the client experiences a sense of relief from having reviewed the trauma in tolerable 'doses,' the sense of fear, helplessness, and horror gradually shift to a healthy blend of feeling sad and acceptance of having been changed by the trauma" (p. 81).

A troubling issue for both adult and child survivors of disasters is how to feel secure and safe again. Thus it can also be quite useful to help individuals realistically establish whether they are in continued danger and determine specific steps they can take to increase their belief in their safety. Ultimately, survivors benefit from the development of increased hope about the future.

Family interventions are particularly effective in that they can assist family members to develop a shared narrative of the disaster experience and what Figley (1988) called a "family healing theory." In the course of developing this narrative, parents and children remember together, weaving their shared experience into a common story that identifies both the most troubling and the most hopeful aspects of their experience. This process of working together to articulate what happened and to envision surviving and coping in the future can contribute to family openness about the disaster experience and strengthen family unity in survival efforts (Abueg et al., 2000; Figley, 1988; Young et al., 1998).

On a final note, crisis counselors are most helpful to survivors when they facilitate the survivors' ability to discuss any and all views of themselves, others, and the universe that may have changed as the result of the disaster. Individuals are *changed* when they have survived a traumatic event like a disaster, but their losses, pain, and dislocation do not need to compromise survivors' futures. Indeed, considerable research has documented "salutogenic" effects on cognitions following traumatic incidents, including positive changes in perceptions of self, perceptions of relationships with others, and beliefs and perceptions about the value of life (Stuhlmiller & Dunning, 2000).

<u>D</u>evelopmental mastery:
Help survivors to examine the impact of the disaster on their stage-of-life needs/tasks and to make the adjustments necessary to attain ongoing developmental mastery.

Assessment and intervention that encompass a developmental perspective target those developmental tasks that may be interfered with as the result of a crisis event. Assessment and intervention also must consider the individual's developmental capacities as they affect the individual's ability to comprehend, cope, and adapt.

We have considered the impact of development each time we have discussed age-related issues. Developmental issues have also been present in each case example we have discussed. For example, Sarah's stage of life and its accompanying demands and tasks clearly affected the types of challenges she faced. She and her husband had just started their family, and he had just started his business. They were relatively vulnerable financially, and her family lost its primary wage earner. They had just acquired a sizable mortgage. Sarah's father was deceased and her mother was getting older, although she was still a great support to Sarah. Sarah's children experienced the death of their father at ages two and four. Their young ages directly affected both their ability to comprehend what happened and the numerous ways their lives would be changed by his absence.

Similarly, the hurricane affected Margaret in developmentally specific ways. She had already experienced the loss of her husband. She was alone except for her adult children, and they, too, were dealing with the impact of the hurricane in terms of their own stage-of-life tasks and responsibilities. Margaret was clearly at risk for adverse effects. She was still grieving the death of her husband and had recently had a hysterectomy. Although she had recovered quickly and her prognosis was excellent, the entire process had been stressful and frightening. Her initial appraisal of herself as a burden and as useless furthered her feelings of hopelessness.

In each of these cases, consideration of the developmental impact was essential to comprehending the ways in which the disaster affected each individual. Similarly, intervention must then focus on assisting individuals to continue to master their developmentally situated life tasks.

Intervention with older adults   Because of the greater vulnerability associated with older adults' adaptation in the aftermath of a disaster, developmentally sensitive intervention is particularly essential. In part, this means being attuned to the increased insecurity, physical vulnerability, and isolation that they may experience, as well as prior losses they may have suffered. Crisis counselors can best assist older adults if they recognize their need for security, stability, and reconnection. It is important to assist older adults to reaffirm their attachments and relationships so that they continue to experience themselves as connected to a family, group, or community (Young et al., 1998).

Family interventions that include multiple generations are particularly helpful in that older adults are more likely to be receptive to assistance in the context of the family. Also, family relationships may suffer from the stress and strain of confronting so many external demands. Interventions that build and sustain family connection and unity are useful for all family members, but they serve the additional function of emphasizing older adults' continued importance as extended family members. Quickly assisting older adults to reestablish their routines and a stable living environment are also critical so they can maintain developmental continuity.

Children and adolescents We have previously described children as a vulnerable group, and we have given some examples of ways to intervene with parents and families to assist them in meeting their children's needs. Because parental distress and family environment are strongly predictive of children's distress, interventions to assist parents and families as a whole are most often the intervention of choice.

Children may be susceptible to severe reactions to disaster particularly when there has been severe exposure. For example, in one study of survivors' reactions two years after a dam collapsed, causing severe flooding and destruction, 37 percent of children directly involved were found to have a probable PTSD diagnosis (Green, Korol, Grace, Vary, Leonard, & Gleser, 1991). Young et al. (1998) suggested that crisis counselors talk with parents to assess the degree of traumatic exposure experienced by their children. For example, counselors can ask parents the following questions: *Where was your child when the disaster struck? What did your child witness? Do you know what your child saw/heard/felt?* Young et al. also suggested that counselors question parents about their children's behavior and problems since the disaster, including eating, sleeping, physical problems, behavioral problems, nightmares, or disaster reenactments in play (p. 99).

Specific interventions to assist children must be developmentally and contextually appropriate and may take place within schools or in formal counseling groups, and may involve individual or family counseling. In general, intervention focuses on activities or discussions that encourage children to express their experiences and concerns, promote positive coping and problem solving skills, and strengthen supportive relationships, including those with family members and classmates. Specific activities counselors can employ with children range from drawing and storytelling to the modified use of exposure techniques to treat a child's PTSD (Meichenbaum, 1994; Young et al., 1998).

E̲cosystem healthy and intact:
Help survivors to examine and make healthy changes in their personal ecosystem.

A disaster, by definition, involves widespread destruction that affects many individuals simultaneously. In the immediate aftermath of disasters, survivors are often gathered in shelters and family assistance centers. Ongoing recovery frequently requires community members to work together to garner resources and assistance from state and federal agencies. Grieving and commemorating losses and heroes is also often a process of coming together.

To the extent that individuals experience a sense of community and relational embeddedness, they benefit. As we have noted, research has documented that when disaster survivors live in communities in which the disaster is defined in community terms and individuals experience themselves as part of the community, personal and resource recovery are aided (Steinglass & Gerrity, 1990).

As Raphael (1986, 2000) noted, however, there comes a time after every disaster when the media go home and the outside world's attention turns to other matters. At this time most individuals and communities are left to deal with the disaster's impact alone. Raphael described this as a period of disillusionment, when individuals struggle with bureaucratic red tape and feelings of hopelessness and abandonment. For some individuals, PTSD symptoms reemerge or become more acute. Family relationships may suffer as the emotional and physical stressors take their toll.

What this research reiterates is the importance of assisting disaster survivors to connect with others and to remain connected. Family connections, connections to friends, and connection to community groups all serve as protective psychosocial resources. Vulnerable groups like children and the elderly are particularly at risk if they do not have this protective web of relationship safety, but all survivors benefit from it.

Those engaged in providing ongoing crisis counseling to disaster survivors must be particularly attentive to the presence or absence of a variety of social supports, and should work to enhance relational and community connections throughout involvement. This entails identifying obstacles and assisting individuals to reach out both to previous members of their social support networks and to form new contacts and alliances with other survivors.

Crisis counselors must also be aware of how systems that allocate community resources may marginalize or underserve certain individuals, families, or groups as they go through the processes of recovery and rebuilding. Many individuals continue to need financial assistance and other concrete assistance for months and years after a disaster. Crisis counselors' familiarity with standard sources of assistance prepares them to educate and advocate for individual families when necessary.

CASE EXAMPLE: WORLD TRADE CENTER DISASTER

By JoAnn Packer, Psy.D.

The terrorist attacks of September 11, 2001, created the need to provide crisis intervention services to large numbers of people in diverse circumstances. Varying modes of service delivery were employed in an effort to respond to the thousands of individuals directly and indirectly affected by these events. I was engaged as a consultant to a crisis intervention organization utilized by employee assistance programs and corporate human resource departments to respond to trauma in the workplace. This organization and many others provided interventions in the days following the September 11 attacks on the World Trade Center during a time when the infrastructure of New York City life was severely changed. It is impossible to describe the degree to which normal life was changed during the days immediately following September 11th. Air travel was halted and the absence of the usual jet noise was very noticeable. Fighter planes flew overhead frequently, which was both reassuring and frightening in its implications. Bridge and truck traffic was disrupted. The air in the city was acrid and sirens wailed continuously. I was repeatedly struck by the sight of perfectly groomed people with briefcases wandering around in a state of shock. People were startled by the most minute stimuli and a very high level of emotional arousal was the norm.

Security precautions were apparent, with police and military personnel continuously patrolling the streets. The degree of tension was palpable and many people expected another attack. A friend described hearing screams after a sudden thunderclap, as people assumed another attack had begun. It was in this context that consultants were brought in to aid various groups of people in beginning the recovery process, in part so they would be able to return to functioning at work.

Our interventions were intended to provide psychological first aid, to assess needs, and to provide information, education, and referrals. Two crisis counselors provided all interventions to relatively large groups; one crisis counselor provided interventions to smaller groups. We worked collaboratively to intervene and assess individual responses to the extent that we could within the large group format.

The first group comprised about fifty individuals who worked for a company that had offices in the World Trade Center: support staff, secretaries, paralegals, and librarians. Some of them had also worked for the same company at the World Trade Center at the time of the 1993 bombing.

Many of these individuals were already in their offices at the time the first plane crashed into the neighboring tower. A manager who had experienced the 1993 bombing insisted that all employees evacuate the building despite announcements by authorities that personnel should remain in their offices. All individuals who evacuated from the company offices survived. Many then walked for hours to their homes in the New York boroughs in a state of shock. Most of these survivors were in the debris storm created by the collapse of the towers and at the time of the crisis intervention meeting still had lacerations, respiratory problems, and glass shards in their hair. A few employees had been on the Staten Island ferry en route to work and had witnessed the planes crashing into the buildings, the ensuing fire, and people jumping from upper floors.

The format we employed was as follows. The group gathered in a large meeting room in the firm's temporary headquarters in midtown Manhattan, several blocks from the World Trade Center site. My colleague and I were introduced and explained that we were consultants who were invited to help and were not employees of the company. We emphasized this fact in order to help people feel free to express whatever they needed to without worrying that their comments would be shared with company managers. We spoke briefly about ourselves, talking about our own experiences and reactions to the attacks, in a warm, open, and nonclinical manner. Sharing our experiences showed group members that some of our reactions were similar to theirs and allowed them to remain in a receptive mode rather than immediately having to speak themselves.

The group appeared to gradually relax and feel more at ease as we talked about our own responses and suggested that most people probably felt at least some of the same things that we were describing. Heads nodded and comments were offered in response. After this early joining with the survivors, my colleague and I shared the task of providing information about the nature of the trauma response including its physical, emotional and spiritual components, while monitoring the group for signs of individuals in obvious distress. During our talk some people relaxed and became more visibly comfortable, whereas others were clearly having a very difficult time coping. The more distressed individuals were often crying softly, did not make eye contact, were holding themselves, and were frequently rocking back and forth and/or visibly shaking. One of us went to each individual who was noticeably upset, made brief contact, and offered to talk one-on-one. Several people accepted the offer of individual time and we followed through with each of them after the large group meeting.

This ongoing assessment began when we entered the room and continued until the meeting ended. With such a large group, people were of different ages, had different degrees of attachment to the company and the building in which they had worked, had varying levels of premorbid functioning, and different types of outside support. These factors influenced their immediate adaptation to their disaster experience. It was essential that we pay continuous attention to signs of severe individual responses requiring more intensive intervention.

For example, while my colleague was talking to the group I noticed a middle-aged woman sitting apart from the others and crying. I made eye contact with her and, when she seemed receptive, went to her, placed my hand lightly on her arm, and asked if she would like some time to talk after the presentation. She nodded and thanked me, saying she felt alone and overwhelmed. Later, during our conversation she described being new to the firm, recently divorced, having just completed treatment for breast cancer, and said that she had been given a significant amount of complex work to be ready for the company in a few days time. I commented that she was already dealing with major life issues even before the building was attacked. She opened up further and spoke about a vision of moving to a farm and being able to watch cows outside her windows. She felt torn by the need to earn money and felt she owed it to the company to stay on, although she did not really want to. I suggested that traumatic events such as the one she had just experienced can help people readjust their priorities and that it was good and healthy for her to gradually reassess her needs and wants. She calmed considerably, and by the end of our conversation had a clearer sense of what she was going to do in the immediate future as well as a sense of freedom, knowing that she could continue to reconsider her options. She also felt more able to manage her emotional responses.

An older woman in the group was also in a great deal of distress, crying despondently. When I approached, she clung to my arm but was unable to stop crying. I held her hand and told her I would sit with her. She began to talk about the terrible guilt she felt over having survived both the 1993 bombing and this one without a scratch, whereas so many younger people had died. She struggled to find reasons and meaning for her survival. I shared with her that those were questions that greater minds than mine had grappled with, but that I understood how she was struggling to make sense of tragedies that were so senseless. She talked about the importance of faith in her life, and I suggested that at some point talking to her pastor might help her in her efforts to find a way to comprehend what had happened. After our presentation, my colleague and I spent time circulating around the room, talking briefly with some people and more extensively with others. On several occasions, coworkers brought someone they were concerned about to one of us to facilitate a connection.

These sessions were quite helpful in identifying who might be in need of immediate follow-up care in the community and allowed us to explore with the individual how best to reach out for assistance. One of the most gratifying aspects of working with this group of people, all of whom experienced a frightening and devastating traumatic event, was observing the grace with which they responded to one another and the resilience they showed in coping with what had happened to them. They were able to laugh at appropriate times in our conversations, and we pointed out to them that their laughter was a sign of health, not callousness. We attempted to impart hope about their ability to recover from this trauma, and it was this message that seemed to resonate most deeply with people. Many individuals came to us as they were leaving and thanked us warmly, saying that they had a better understanding of their physical and emotional reactions and were less upset by them. Delineating the nature of the trauma response allowed these survivors to understand their reactions as normal and expected responses to a horrifying and aberrant situation. They no longer needed to fear that they were crazy or that they would never regain their usual functioning.

The second group of people I worked with were employees at a public relations firm whose offices were in a skyscraper two blocks north of the World Trade Center. These people had watched for hours from the vantage point in their offices as the attacks occurred, as people jumped from the upper floors, and as the towers collapsed. They were told not to leave their building so as not to interfere with the evacuation of the attack site and therefore they watched the events unfold as firsthand observers. This was a smaller group than the first, about a dozen people, and we gathered in a small conference room around a table. A manager directed employees to the conference room, where I greeted each one and introduced myself as each person arrived. I explained to the group, as I had with the first group, that I was a volunteer consultant brought in to help them and that I had no ties to the company. I outlined the format of our meeting and explained that I would speak about the nature of the trauma response and the recovery process. I invited people to ask questions and to make comments at any time while I was speaking, and said I would welcome the interruption because it would give me a chance to collect my thoughts. With this small group I wanted to create a cozier, more informal setting than was possible with the larger group of employees.

Indeed, this group quickly evidenced a small group process dynamic, owing to its size and to the fact that it comprised many creative artistic individuals. Some people in this group expressed surprise that they were as deeply affected as they were, saying they had "only watched" the events rather than being directly involved in them. Several people described a physical reaction, also described by people on the ferry, of shaking so violently that they were "afraid they would shake apart."

I explained that research has documented that witnessing violent death and catastrophe while feeling helpless is highly traumatizing. This began to dispel the notion that their feelings were somehow invalid and allowed them to acknowledge and accept their feelings as a step in moving on. This group differed from the first in that the survivors from the World Trade Center workgroup had been in imminent danger of dying. For this group, their experience of the trauma was watching violence and destruction unfold while worrying that another round of attacks might target their building.

Many in this group had difficulty returning to their workplace, and several had begun to question whether the type of work they did had merit. One woman angrily threw a doll into a corner, saying that it seemed "beyond stupid" to be absorbed in marketing a toy when their city had just experienced such a devastating attack. We talked about the fact that, for many people, what was usual and acceptable last week might very well look different in light of the events of September 11.

Another theme that emerged in this group was the issue of ongoing safety and security. A number of people stated that they no longer felt safe at work or in the city and that their fear was a source of much anger and confusion. I explained that we all function in normal circumstances with a healthy amount of denial of danger and threat, which helps us get out of bed each morning. For many people, seeing their city under attack tore away that protective shield of denial and left them suddenly feeling uncomfortably vulnerable.

Before the group session began, I was informed that one man in the group had been "ranting" about vigilante justice and about the need for everyone to be armed at home. During the group meeting he brought up these issues with intense affect. I let him speak while monitoring the group for signs that others were becoming too distressed by his talk. I had an obligation to assess his mental state, with attention to homicidal ideation and the possible need for emergency psychiatric care, and a concomitant responsibility to protect the group from becoming further traumatized. I explored whether this man had felt this vulnerable at other times in his life, and how he had handled himself in those situations. He spoke about more familiar aspects of city life. He explained that his neighborhood bordered a dangerous area, which made him aware of keeping doors and windows locked at home. He spoke of his difficulty in protecting his children from danger in the course of their lives. As we examined these aspects of his life, his coworkers began to share similar concerns and to empathize with his intense feelings of vulnerability and helplessness since the attacks. We talked about the illusion of safety under which most of us operate in normal circumstances, and also discussed how this intense awareness of danger might fade.

One of the most meaningful moments for me from this period of time in NYC occurred when this man looked at me at the end of our group meeting and said, "You've been so helpful to us, but tell me, how are you doing?" His humanity in expressing his concern for me underscored the fact that reactions to trauma, even violent and devastating events like this one, may only temporarily cloud the basic health, caring, and decency of individuals.

A third group of individuals I worked with were employees of another company whose offices had been in one of the buildings destroyed in the attacks. At the time of the intervention they were sharing corporate space on a temporary basis in lower midtown Manhattan. This group comprised about forty people who were seated in a large room around three conference tables. As with the first group, the format utilized with this group consisted of a short talk outlining the major features of the trauma response and stages in the recovery process, followed by one-on-one meetings. This group was also invited to ask questions and share comments and experiences at any time during my presentation. Perhaps due to the fact that this group convened a week after the attack occurred, these survivors already appeared less in shock than the previous groups had been.

Although these individuals continued to experience respiratory problems, they did not emphasize their physical discomfort as much as members of the first group had. Their lacerations, mostly on their hands, faces and scalps, were healing well. I was able to use their physical healing to remind and reassure people that their psyches had a similar innate healing mechanism. This group had moved beyond the initial stage of shock and disbelief, and group members were becoming aware that some aspects of themselves and their lives would be forever changed.

A young woman spoke privately to me after the presentation, saying that she was sad that her fiancé, who was not directly affected by the attack, could not seem to appreciate its impact on her. His response that she was "fine and lucky" and "should stop thinking about what had happened" left her feeling disconnected from him and wondering whether she should remain in the relationship We discussed the various defense mechanisms people employ to help themselves cope with life events, and I suggested that she explore with him what he thought and felt when he learned about the attack. My goal was to help her preserve her relationship, at least for the time being, as it appeared that she was inclined to precipitously leave it in hurt and anger. My concern was that to create more losses at a time when she was just beginning to recover from this psychological trauma would have complicated her recovery. I urged her not to make a decision about the relationship at this time, and we discussed the value of her continuing with counseling, both to assist in her continuing recovery from the trauma experience and in exploring her relationship in more depth. At the time I had no way of knowing whether her relationship had always been turbulent or even whether leaving a relationship in a reactive angry way was a pattern in this young woman's life. What was apparent was that these issues were outside the realm of single-session crisis intervention and that she could benefit from ongoing crisis counseling.

Another individual in this group, a man of about forty-five years old, spoke movingly to the group about his pain upon hearing that his son, a teenager with a dark olive complexion, was afraid to leave the house for fear of being mistaken for an Islamic militant. This man struggled with how to protect his son as well as teach him lessons in tolerance when he himself was overwhelmed by his own responses. I suggested that his son's immediate safety needed to be a priority and validated his concerns about the city's potential for vigilante justice. The group offered empathic advice to this man, who cried when giving voice to his pain and confusion. He shared that as an American he suffered because of what had occurred, yet his fears for his son's physical and emotional safety made him feel like an outsider.

This group of survivors, even more than the group from several days earlier, was grappling with cognitive issues that were at times deeply dissonant and painful for them to confront. Many expressed surprise that a traumatic event challenged them not only emotionally but mentally and spiritually as well. Some people spoke about a changed sense of the world and their place in it. Some spoke of feelings of hate and intolerance that they were ashamed of. Others struggled with their notions of God and feared that their spiritual base was threatened and not available to comfort or guide them. It occurred to me at various times when working with this group that they needed not only a crisis counselor but a theologian and philosopher, as well. I attempted to convey to the group that in the face of so great a tragedy the feeling that one's innermost beliefs were in question was normal. We discussed the fact that people are necessarily shaken and changed by experiences such as the one they survived, but that many individuals emerge from their struggle to adapt feeling tested and stronger as a result.

Although each group was unique, as were the individual survivors, the goals of crisis intervention in each instance were to assist individuals to achieve greater control over their trauma responses and to provide them with the education and referral information that would assist them both then and in the future. In order to accomplish those goals, I needed to establish a relational connection so that group members perceived me as someone they could trust and speak with openly. Individuals needed an opportunity to speak about what they had experienced, and I needed the opportunity to assess their crisis reactions in order to identify those individuals most in need of individual attention and/or follow-up. I provided information that could begin to normalize their common reactions. In group settings, the process of thinking about "next steps" in coping and decision making occurred synergistically as individuals responded not only to me but to each other. Each intervention ended with information that would help survivors anticipate their future reactions and encourage them to utilize other community resources.

Individuals and groups differed in the dominant focus of their concerns. For some individuals, like the young police officer discussed at the beginning of the chapter, a dominant focus was ongoing peritraumatic responses experienced in the form of nightmares and waking intrusive images, smells, and sounds. For others, like the last group of survivors described, the efforts centered around finding meaning in the disaster. And for still others, like the woman who struggled with her desire to move to a farm, the disaster raised issues regarding major life choices.

As is true in any single-session crisis intervention, only a limited amount could be accomplished, the boundaries determined by time. It is my belief that, although constrained by time and scope, these interventions were helpful to the survivors, and many described their enhanced sense of calm and understanding. I left New York knowing that I had witnessed both the devastation caused by evildoers and the strength, resilience, and humanity of the many survivors.

DISCUSSION QUESTIONS

1. Invite a representative from a local branch of the Red Cross to speak in class about the role of the Red Cross in disasters and about Red Cross training programs for disaster mental health volunteers. Prior to the visit, have class members prepare questions for the representative to address.

2. This chapter made the point that ethnic minorities and those of lower socioeconomic status often suffer greater losses as the result of natural disasters. Further, these same groups also appear to receive less assistance than other survivors even when experiencing similar losses. Discuss reasons why this may be the case and what can be done to correct this unfair burden.

EXERCISES

1. A number of assessment instruments were recommended for determining both the nature of specific stressors experienced and the types of symptoms survivors may be experiencing. Divide the class into groups and ask each group to acquire a copy of one recommended assessment instrument. Have each group present its instrument and information about how to use it to the rest of class.

2. There are numerous natural disasters in the United States every year. Prior to class, obtain a list of the previous year's FEMA-declared disasters (available from http://www.fema.gov/library). Divide the class into groups and have each group select one disaster from the list. Then instruct each group to research that disaster to determine the extent of personal and community losses suffered and the types of assistance that were provided. Groups can then present their findings to class. Visual images are particularly helpful in presentations of this type, and can be obtained from popular news journals such as *Newsweek* or *Time)* and from TV news footage.

REFERENCES

Abueg, F. R., & Chun, K. (1996). Traumatization stress among Asians and Asian-Americans. In A. J. Marsella, M. J. Friedman, E. Gerrity, & R. M. Scurfield (Eds.), *Ethnocultural aspects of post-traumatic stress disorders*. Washington, DC: American Psychological Association.

Abueg, F. R., Woods, G. W., & Watson, D. S. (2000). Disaster trauma. In F. M. Dattilio & A. Freeman (Eds.), *Cognitive-behavioral strategies in crisis intervention* (2nd ed., pp. 243–272). New York: Guilford Press.

Aguilera, D. M., & Planchon, L. A. (1995). The American Psychological Association—California Psychological Association Disaster Response Project: Lessons from the past, guidelines for the future. *Professional Psychology: Research and Practice, 26*, 550–557.

Baum, A., & Fleming, R. (1993). Implications of psychological research in stress and technological accidents. *American Psychologist, 48*, 665–672.

Bland, S., O'Leary, E., Farinaro, E., & Trevisan, M. (1996). Long-term psychological effects of natural disasters. *Psychosomatic Medicine, 58*, 18–24.

Edwards, M. L. (1998). An interdisciplinary perspective on disasters and stress: The promise of an ecological framework. *Sociological Forum, 13*, 115–132.

Everly, G. S., & Mitchell, J. (1997). *Critical incident stress management, CISM, a new era and standard of care in crisis intervention*. Ellicott City, MD: Chevron.

FEMA. (1995, November). Publication 299 (4).

FEMA. (2002). *2001 disaster activity*. Retrieved July 19, 2002, from http://www.fema.gov/library

Figley, C. (1988). A five-phase treatment of post-traumatic stress disorder in families. *Journal of Traumatic Stress, 1*, 127–139.

Freedy, J. R., Kilpatrick, D. G., & Resnick, H. S. (1992). Natural disasters and mental health: Theory, assessment, and intervention. *Journal of Social Behavior and Personality, 7*, 1–55.

Green, B. L., & Lindy, J. D. (1994). Post-traumatic stress disorder in victims of disasters. *Psychiatric Clinics of North America, 17*, 301–309.

Green, B. L., Lindy, J. D., & Grace, M. C. (1994). Psychological effects of toxic contamination. In R. Ursano (Ed.), *Trauma and disaster* (pp. 154–176). New York: Cambridge University Press.

Green, B., Korol, M., Grace, M., Vary, M., Leonard, A., & Gleser, G. (1991). Children and disaster: Age, gender, and parental effects on PTSD symptoms. *Journal of the American Academy of Child and Adolescent Psychiatry, 30*, 945–951.

Green, B., Lindy, J., Grace, M., Gleser, G., Leonard, A., Korol, M., et al. (1990). Buffalo Creek survivors in the second decade: Stability of stress symptoms. *American Journal of Orthopsychiatry, 60*, 43–54.

Green, B. L., & Solomon, S. (1995). The mental health impact of natural and technological disasters. In J. Freedy & S. Hobfoll (Eds.), *Traumatic stress: From theory to practice* (pp. 163–180). New York: Plenum.

Hiley-Young, G. (1992). Trauma reactivation assessment and treatment: Integrative case examples. *Journal of Traumatic Stress, 5*(4), 545–555.

Hobfoll, S. (1989). Conservation of resources: A new attempt at conceptualizing stress. *American Psychologist, 44*, 513–524.

Hobfoll, S., & Lilly, R. (1993). Resource conservation as a strategy for community psychology. *Journal of Community Psychology, 21*, 128–148.

Hodgkinson, P., & Shepherd, M. (1994). The impact of disaster support work. *Journal of Traumatic Stress, 7,* 587–600.

Kulka, R. A., Schlenger, W. E., Fairbank, J. A., Jordan, B. K., Hough, R. L., Marmar, C. R., & Weiss, D. S. (1991). Assessment of posttraumatic stress disorder in the community: Prospects and pitfalls from recent studies of Vietnam veterans. *Psychological Assessment, 3,* 547–560.

McFarlane, A. C. (1995). The severity of the trauma: What is its role in posttraumatic stress disorder? In R. J. Kleber, C. R. Figley, & B. P. R. Gersons (Eds.), *Beyond trauma: Cultural and societal dynamics.* New York: Plenum.

Meichenbaum, D. (1994). *A clinical handbook/practical therapist manual for assessing and treating adults with post-traumatic stress disorder (PTSD).* Waterloo, Ontario, Canada: Institute Press.

Mitchell, J. T. (1983). When disaster strikes . . . The critical incident stress debriefing process. *Journal of Emergency Medical Services, 8*(1), 36–39.

Mitchell, J. T., & Everly, G. S. (2000). Critical incident stress management and critical incident stress debriefings: Evolutions, effects and outcomes. In B. Raphael & J. P. Wilson (Eds.), *Psychological debriefing: Theory, practice and evidence* (pp. 71–90). New York: Cambridge University Press.

Monahon, C. (1997). *Children and trauma: A guide for parents and professionals.* San Francisco: Jossey-Bass.

Nader, R. (1996). Assessing trauma in children. In J. Wilson & T. McKeane (Eds.), *Assessing psychological trauma and PTSD* (pp. 291–348). New York: Guilford Press.

National Center for Post-Traumatic Stress Disorder. (2002a). *Mental health intervention for disasters.* Retrieved July 21, 2002, from www.ncptsd.org/facts/disasters

National Center for Post-Traumatic Stress Disorder. (2002b). *Psychosocial resources in the aftermath of natural and human-caused disasters: A review of the empirical literature, with implications for intervention.* Retrieved July 21, 2002, from www.ncptsd.org/facts/disasters

National Center for Post-Traumatic Stress Disorder. (2002c). *The range, magnitude, and duration of effects of natural and human-caused disasters: A review of the empirical literature.* Retrieved July 21, 2002, from www.ncptsd.org/facts/disasters

National Center for Post-Traumatic Stress Disorder. (2002d). *Risk factors for adverse outcomes in natural and human-caused disasters: A review of the empirical literature.* Retrieved July 21, 2002, from www.ncptsd.org/facts/disasters

National Center for Post-Traumatic Stress Disorder. (2002e). *Terrorist attacks and children.* Retrieved July 21, 2002, from www.ncptsd.org/facts/disasters

National Institute of Mental Health. (2002). *Mental health and mass violence: Evidence-based early psychological intervention for victims/survivors of mass violence. A workshop to reach consensus on best practices.* NIH Publication No. 02-5138, Washington, DC: U.S. Government Printing Office.

Norris, F. H., & Kaniasty, K. (1997). Received and perceived social support in times of stress: A test of the social support deterioration deterrence model. *Journal of Personality and Social Psychology, 7,* 498–511.

North, C., Nixon, S., Shariat, S., Mallonee, S., McMillen, J., & Spitznagel, E. (1999). Psychiatric disorders among survivors of the Oklahoma City bombing. *Journal of the American Medical Association, 282,* 755–762.

Pennebaker, J. W., & Harber, K. D. (1993). A social stage model of collective coping: The Loma Prieta earthquake and the Persian Gulf War. *Journal of Social Issues, 49,* 125–146.

Pynoos, R., & Nader, K. (1993). Issues in the treatment of posttraumatic stress in children and adolescents. In J. P. Wilson & B. Raphael (Eds.), *International handbook of traumatic stress syndrome* (pp. 535–549). New York: Plenum.

Raphael, B. (1986). *When disaster strikes: A handbook for the caring professions.* London: Hutchinson.

Raphael, B. (2000). *Disaster mental health response handbook: An educational resource for mental health professionals involved in disaster management.* New South Wales, Australia: New South Wales Institute of Psychiatry.

Shalev, A. Y. (1992). Posttraumatic stress disorder among injured survivors of a terrorist attack: Predictive value of early intrusion and avoidance symptoms. *Journal of Nervous and Mental Disease, 180*(8), 505–509.

Smith, E. M., North, C. S., McCool, R. E., & Shea, J. M. (1990). Acute postdisaster psychiatric disorders: Identification of persons at risk. *American Journal of Psychiatry, 147,* 202–206.

Solomon, S. D., & Smith, E. M. (1994). Social support and perceived control as moderators of responses to dioxin and flood exposure. In R. Ursano, B. McCaughey, & C. Fullerton (Eds.), *Trauma and disaster.* New York: Cambridge University Press.

Steinglass, P., & Gerrity, E. (1990). Natural disaster and post-traumatic stress disorder: Short-term versus long-term recovery in two disaster-affected communities. *Journal of Applied Social Psychology, 20,* 1746–1765.

Stuhlmiller, C., & Dunning, C. (2000). In J. Violanti, D. Paton, & C. Dunning (Eds.), *Posttraumatic stress intervention* (pp. 10–42). Springfield, IL: Charles C. Thomas Publisher, LTD.

Ursano, R., Fullerton, C., Kao, T., & Bhartiya, V. (1995). Longitudinal assessment of posttraumatic stress disorder and depression after exposure to traumatic death. *Journal of Nervous and Mental Disease, 183,* 36–42.

Vernberg, E. M., La Greca, A., Silverman, W., & Prinstein M. (1996). Prediction of posttraumatic stress symptoms in children after Hurricane Andrew. *Journal of Abnormal Psychology, 105,* 237–248.

Vernberg, E. M., & Vogel, J. M. (1993). Interventions with children after disasters. *Journal of Clinical Child Psychology, 22,* 485–498

Vogel, J. M., & Vernberg, E. M. (1993). Children's psychological responses to disasters. *Journal of Clinical Child Psychology, 22,* 464–484.

Weathers, F. W., Litz, B. T., Huska, J. A., & Keane, T. M. (1995). *PCL-C.* Portland: Oregon Health Sciences University.

Wood, J. M., Bootzin, R. R., Rosenhan, D., Nolen-Hoeksema, S., & Jourden, F. (1992). Effects of the 1989 San Francisco earthquake on frequency and content of nightmares. *Journal of Abnormal Psychology, 101*(2), 219–224.

Young, B. H. (1998). Initial debriefing protocol. In B. H. Young, J. D. Ford, J. I. Ruzek, M. J. Friedman, & R. D. Gusman, *Disaster mental health services: A guidebook for clinicians and administrators.* Menlo Park, CA: National Center for PTSD.

Young, B. H., Ford, J. D., Ruzek, J. I., Friedman, M. J., & Gusman, F. D. (1998). *Disaster mental health services: A guidebook for clinicians and administrators.* Menlo Park, CA: National Center for PTSD.

CHAPTER 14

Helping the Helpers: Avoiding Burnout, Compassion Fatigue, and Secondary Traumatic Stress

In the preceding thirteen chapters we have examined various types of crises that individuals face and what crisis counselors can do to assist them to cope and ultimately survive. Given the intensity inherent in responding to persons in the immediate aftermath of a crisis and the corresponding emotional demands of being attuned to individuals confronting what are often overwhelming losses, it is essential that crisis workers also attend to their own psychological well-being.

Some authors have suggested that even exposure to and intensive study of stories of trauma and violence in the classroom can be stressful to students. These authors thus recommend anticipating and addressing the emotional consequences in order to facilitate self-care (O'Halloran & O'Halloran, 2001). This has been our experience as well, particularly for students who have their own trauma histories. For example, one of the authors' female students tried twice unsuccessfully to complete a class on crisis intervention with sexual assault and domestic violence. She eventually completed the course, but only after seeing a crisis counselor to resolve her own sexual assault history.

Numerous authors have recognized and addressed the personal psychological toll that working with death and destruction takes on police, emergency workers, and firefighters (Mitchell, 1985; Mitchell & Bray, 1989; Raphael & Wilson, 1994). A corresponding effect has been identified in the experiences of counselors, social workers, psychologists, and other human service personnel working in crisis settings with individuals who have been traumatized, victimized, or have experienced significant losses. Whether called burnout, compassion fatigue, secondary trauma, or vicarious traumatization, the primary concern has been to name and describe the emotional strains of working in high-stress, sometimes seemingly hopeless situations, with people in great emotional turmoil (Corey, Corey, & Callanan, 1988; Figley, 1995; Maslach, 1982; McCann & Pearlman, 1990; Pines, 1983; Saakvitne & Pearlman, 1996).

Inherent in these concepts, sometimes used interchangeably, are two fairly distinct ways of responding to the emotional stress of working with high-risk people in difficult circumstances. The first type of response was described by Wilson and Lindy

(1994), who suggested that some helpers respond to emotional stress by gradually becoming exhausted, disengaging, and withdrawing from emotional and empathic connections. The second type of response is overidentification, or empathic enmeshment, with trauma clients. The first type of response is most frequently associated with burnout and compassion fatigue; the second type of response is more closely aligned with secondary trauma or vicarious traumatization, although aspects of compassion fatigue are also endemic to the numbing aspects of vicarious traumatization. In this chapter we examine burnout and secondary traumatic stress. Our overriding goal is primary prevention. Crisis workers must be aware of the emotional and professional risks of working with crisis clients in order to prevent negative personal outcomes. A secondary aim, perhaps best conceptualized as secondary prevention, is to teach crisis workers to recognize signs of burnout and secondary traumatic stress so that they can take the actions necessary to heal. Some authors have suggested that although there are actions that helpers and the agencies that employ them can take to decrease the vulnerability of crisis workers to vicarious traumatization, the "occupational hazard" that comes with "knowing, caring, and facing the reality of trauma" is unavoidable (Saakvitne & Pearlman, 1996, p. 25).

BURNOUT

Maslach (1982) defined burnout as "a syndrome of emotional exhaustion, depersonalization, and reduced personal accomplishment" that emerges in helping professionals in response to the "chronic emotional strain" of working with people who are troubled or having problems (p. 3). Individuals who are experiencing burnout may no longer have the emotional energy necessary to use in the interest and care of others. They are emotionally fatigued and drained. Although they continue to work with clients, they do so without energy or enthusiasm.

Depersonalization in this domain refers to the tendency to be less personal or authentic and caring in relation to others. Helping professionals who are experiencing burnout are unlikely to genuinely and authentically connect to a client's emotional pain and sorrows, and instead seem detached, callous, and uncaring. Burnout also manifests itself as a sense of reduced adequacy and accomplishment. Individuals may feel unappreciated, unimportant, and powerless, yet at the same time may paradoxically feel unreasonably responsible for client successes or failures. Crisis workers may lose their idealism and feel victimized by clients, colleagues, and the system. Young professionals, who are at high risk for burnout, find their excitement and enthusiasm turn to discouragement and dread. Many simply turn off emotionally and go through the motions of performing their jobs (Cormier & Hackney, 1993; Hagen, 1999; Maslach, 1982).

Clearly, burnout is destructive for helpers and clients alike. Helpers lose a sense of vitality and connection to their work. Clients sense the helper's detachment and callousness, and are deprived of a therapeutic relationship grounded in empathy and trust necessary to meet their needs. The helper who experiences burnout is an impaired professional. Understanding the reasons for burnout may help individuals avoid it.

CASE EXAMPLE: MARCUS

Marcus has been employed as a mental health caseworker in an intake unit at a community mental health center for more than five years. The intake unit serves as the sole mental health crisis response for the full range of crises from relationship conflicts, to psychiatric emergencies, to suicide attempts. Over the last few years, Marcus has begun to use sick time more frequently, especially on Mondays and Fridays. His fellow workers in the unit are well trained and manage to cover for him when he is not there, but there is growing tension over the amount of extra intervention they need to provide in his absence. His colleagues have also begun to notice that when they go out for drinks after work, he drinks to excess and, inevitably, at the end of the evening they are trying to take his keys away before he drives off. There are no indications of any accidents or DUI charges. When Marcus is actually working at the unit, staff members note that he responds to clients in a perfunctory manner and rushes clients through crisis appointments—to the extent that his colleagues have had to follow up with an increasing number of clients who were unsure how to proceed once they left his office. Marcus has also begun to mimic clients and talk disparagingly about families of low socioeconomic status and their inability to function in the real world. University student interns have complained to faculty supervisors about not only the lack of supervision when working with Marcus but also his constant negative attitude toward clients. In addition, Marcus has begun to flirt with university interns and has asked other staff members to cover for him when he was unavailable to answer his wife's telephone calls at work.

When Marcus fails to appear for his weekly group clinical supervision, his supervisor manages to arrange an appointment for the following morning. Marcus arrives to the appointment fifteen minutes late.

Marcus: Sorry, Janet. I don't know what happened this morning. The time just got away from me. Have you ever had one of those mornings?

Janet: *Yeah, I've had mornings like that. Pretty hard to get started on those days.*

Marcus: Thanks for understanding. What did you want to see me about? I want to make sure that I get back to the unit in case they need me.

Janet: *I'll make sure you get back soon, but I want to spend some time with you right now. Actually, I've wanted to talk personally with you for quite a while. It just seems as though there's always so much going on around here that I don't get the time.*

Marcus: Yeah, we've been busy all right. Full moon's coming.

Janet: *I guess so . . . but I've had a difficult time tracking you down.*

Marcus: Janet, I've been a good employee for five years. I'm not sure where you're going with this conversation.

Janet: *Marcus, I'm worried about you, that's all. You used to be the one at the end of the year who had the most sick leave left over, and now you've been* *using it as soon as you earn it. In fact, you've been cutting into the sick time you saved up for emergencies.*

Marcus: Geez, Janet, I didn't know you were watching me so closely but I can assure you I'm fine. Just had a physical. I'm fine. Should I have the union shop steward sit in on this conversation?

Janet: *No, Marcus. I just want to talk. I'm pleased to hear that you're OK, Marcus, but my concern for you goes beyond that. It seems as though something has changed in you. You're not the same guy who couldn't wait to come to work and didn't want to leave at the end of the day. You started that master's program in counseling and you bagged it after one semester. That was a couple of years ago and it seems as though something has changed for you and it's not in a positive direction.*

Marcus: Nobody stays the same, Janet. You know that. Haven't you used sick time for a mental health day along the way yourself?

Janet: *Marcus, I'm not here to compare you and me. It goes beyond that anyway. Something tells me you don't care about your job the way you used to, and that bothers me. You always were one of the best, and I haven't seen that Marcus for a long time.*

Marcus: This is pretty heavy, Janet. Did you get some bad press on me or something?

Janet: *As a matter of fact, I have been getting some feedback that concerns me.*

Marcus: I thought colleagues were supposed to come to each other if they had problems with a fellow worker. Who complained about me? Ray?

Janet: *No, it wasn't any of your colleagues. You know they care about you a great deal and would probably help you through anything.*

Marcus: Who is it, then?

Janet: *Well, Marcus, the things I've been hearing come from clients who have seen you for emergencies and also from student interns from the past couple of semesters. It's not easy for people who don't have any power to complain so I take it seriously when I get feedback.*

Marcus: You're going to take the word of some nutcases who talked to you about me and a couple of students who don't know jack about crisis work?

Janet: *Marcus . . . that type of response does not sound like the same professional I have worked with for the past five years. You were one of those students who interned here and stayed on. You know I valued your perspective then, and I still do. I've never heard you refer to our clients as "nutcases." I get a little upset when I hear one of our best talking in those terms.*

Marcus: All right, Janet, touché. I'm pissed.

Janet: *You're pissed.*

Marcus: Damn right. You bust your ass for this agency and these clients for years and nothing ever changes. You still get shit on at the end of the day. These people don't want to change. This agency can't afford to have people change. I should have gone into business like my folks told me. This work sucks. I need a life and it's not this one.

Janet: *Can we slow this down a little bit? I feel as though we're on different tracks going in the opposite direction and I'm not getting my point across.*

Marcus: I'm sorry, Janet. I haven't wanted to be here for a long time and I guess you stepped in it. I'm trapped and I don't know how to get out of it. I did love being here and sometimes I still do, but it's rare. I just get so sick of hearing people's shit that I don't want to hear any more. I know they're good people but I just don't know what to do sometimes. I just don't know how to help them and it seems as if no matter what we do, the same shit keeps on happening over and over again for these families, their kids, themselves. I'm not sure that what we do really makes a dent in the problems in these people's lives.

Janet: *Their problems certainly are complex and it does seem sometimes that the harder we work, the more work there is. But I guess I remember that optimistic crisis worker and all the people he has helped through the years. Something changed a couple of years ago and I'm wondering if you know what it was?*

Marcus: Well, I know when things really started to go downhill, if that's what you mean.

Janet: *When was it, Marcus?*

Marcus: I'm not sure I want to talk about it right now, but it was when we committed the Dixon kids' father and when he got out of the psych unit, he killed their mother and the kids before shooting himself. That's when things started to change for me.

Janet: *That is one of my saddest moments here, too, Marcus. You were the petitioner on that one, weren't you?*

Marcus: Yeah, I met the mother at the ER after he had threatened to kill her and the kids. He was convinced that she was a witch and that the kids were Satan's children. They were just normal kids, and she actually loved him. It was so sad. They actually loved him, and he got out and went right to the house and killed them. The involuntary commitment, the inpatient stay, the psychiatrists, the medication . . . nothing stopped him. I felt as though what we did didn't help a bit.

Janet: *How did it change you?*

Marcus: I was sad. I was pissed at everyone. I was pissed at myself . . . and I haven't gotten over it. I gave up on school because all the education in the world wasn't going to stop that type of crap from happening. Nothing. I haven't felt the same since. Everything seems out of control to me and the only time I feel better is when I drink, but even that doesn't help me sleep.

Janet: *Why didn't you bring this up in the supervision group?*

Marcus: I couldn't. I didn't want everyone to think I couldn't handle it. They've always given me the most difficult cases because I was good at it . . . I was good at it. *(begins to tear up)*

Janet: *Marcus, you are good at it but you lost the thread somewhere in the mix. I think we have to help you find it again. In fact, I think we owe it to you. The agency and your colleagues owe it to you.*

Marcus: How is that going to happen?

Janet: *Well, for one thing . . . I think you might benefit from talking with someone outside of here because my sense is that if your work has been affected, then other parts of your life may need looking at, too. I think you need some distance from the agency to do that—someone from the EAP, for example, or someone completely separate. I guess the second thing I'd like you to do is to begin to talk about what you've been feeling to the supervision group. I think you may be surprised how helpful your colleagues might be. I think then we go from there and plan out the future further down the road. I want to provide you with as much support as possible, and I especially want to keep you working for the agency. We need you.*

Reasons for Burnout

There are a number of factors that contribute to burnout including individual characteristics, characteristics of the helping relationship, the work environment, and broader societal stressors (Hagen, 1999).

Individual characteristics   Maslach (1982) concluded that risk factors for burnout include being a young professional with high ideals and aspirations, lacking self-confidence, needing others' appreciation and approval, and lacking an understanding and acceptance of self-limitations. It may seem contradictory that a young person's excitement and idealistic enthusiasm to make a difference or to create a more just world could ultimately contribute to burnout, but in some instances, this is the case. Difficulty arises when one cannot reconcile his or her lofty ideals with the reality of slow change and, at times, minimal progress. When idealistic helpers find that they cannot easily solve clients' problems and that social changes occur incrementally and only with significant compromise of desired goals, they are apt to experience disillusionment. This outcome is even more likely if the individual is impatient and uncompromising.

Other individual characteristics that contribute to an increased risk of burnout include a high need for recognition, approval, and affection. Individuals who depend on recognition of their work in order to feel good about themselves find that these needs are unrealistic when working in the helping professions. It is unreasonable and unethical to expect clients to fulfill those personal needs, as the helper's role is to serve clients' needs, not his or her own. And, unfortunately, it is likely that in the highly demanding and stressful environment of most social agencies, little time will be spent on nurturing the needs of agency staff.

Last, the nature of the individual crisis worker's own support system is an important factor in considering the risk of burnout. When one's relationships are stressed or conflicted, or when individuals are relationally overextended or over-involved, the risk of work stress and eventual burnout increases (Koeske & Kelly, 1995; Koeske & Koeske, 1989).

The helping relationship   The nature of the helping relationship has often been identified as the crux of burnout. The stress of constantly working with people with intractable problems over a long period of time can be a major contribution to burnout. Also, it is within the helping relationship that the symptoms of burnout are manifested as the helper's feelings toward the client become hardened and/or uncaring (Maslach, 1982; Pines, 1983; Pines, Aronson, & Kafry, 1981). What is it about the helping relationship that creates vulnerability for burnout?

One precipitant is the constant demand to serve the needs of other people with little attention to one's own needs. Unless crisis counselors are taking good care of their own needs, the constant giving to others in need may lead to emotional emptiness.

Similarly, helping relationships can be stressful or frustrating. For example, crisis workers who serve victims of political torture, domestic violence, or sexual assault may find themselves drained by exposure to a constant barrage of brutality and violence. Crisis workers who work with abused children may be reminded too often of their own powerlessness within a legal system that often places greater emphasis on family preservation than child safety. Crisis workers who work with addicted individuals or other involuntary clients may find it difficult to constantly engage with clients who are unappreciative and may be angry with them.

And last, the problems presented by clients may sometimes resonate with personal problems in the crisis counselor's own life. When crisis counselors share life experiences with their clients, unresolved emotions may be triggered. They may overidentify with clients and find it difficult to maintain their professional objectivity. They may even find that they cannot escape their clients' problems, which become enmeshed with thoughts and emotions regarding their own problems (Koeske & Kelly, 1995). Having survived similar crises may lead to enhanced counselor sensitivity and awareness of survivor needs. If crisis counselors have not adequately resolved their own issues, however, overidentification may lead to reduced capacity for objectivity, to the lowering of appropriate boundaries, and to burnout.

The work environment   A number of factors have also been identified within the work environment that may contribute to burnout. One factor relates directly to the crisis worker's position, which, particularly in large public bureaucratic organizations like child welfare or community mental health agencies, often includes large caseloads and little individual autonomy or power (Arches, 1991; Maslach, 1982; Maslach & Leiter, 1997). In identifying causes of burnout, Corey and Corey (1998) listed three issues that directly relate to the work role: not having opportunities to take initiative, having unrealistic demands placed on one's time and energy, and being in a personally and professionally difficult role with little supervision or continuing education.

A second factor pertains to relationships with coworkers, supervisors, and administrators. Organizations that are impersonal, competitive, or conflicted are unlikely to provide the support, encouragement and attention to staff needs that prepare crisis workers for the difficult work they must perform. Positive relationships with coworkers and the availability of supervisor support and direction result in decreased burnout among workers (Corey & Corey, 1998; Himle, Jayaratne, & Thyness, 1991; Poulin & Walter, 1993).

Societal factors   Some crisis workers experience constant, critical public scrutiny of their job performance. This seems particularly true for those who work in child welfare agencies, where every decision made and action taken is open to criticism. This may also be true for crisis counselors who work in rape crisis or domestic violence crisis settings. Criticism emerges in response to controversies related to societal ambivalence about these victims and the veracity of victims' reports.

Meichenbaum (1994) identified the danger that individuals who work with trauma survivors, particularly sexual abuse survivors, face because of the public's fear that crisis counselors may suggest abuse to their clients and thus create false accusations of sexual abuse. He points out that such insinuations can be particularly stressful because workers may actually face litigation alleging that they have contributed to false reports.

In some situations crisis workers are publicly perceived as heroes, as was the case following the September 11 attacks on the World Trade Center and the Pentagon. The sense of doing something that is recognized personally and publicly as meaningful can be a major contributor to crisis and rescue workers' own emotional survival. In many other situations, however, including large-scale natural disasters like fires and floods, crisis workers often toil in harsh and difficult circumstances with scant recognition or praise.

Preventing and Countering Burnout

The first step crisis workers can take to avoid burnout is to inventory the factors in their own situation that place them at risk. A second step is to assess themselves for emotional, cognitive, or physical signs indicating vulnerability to burnout. If one identifies factors in one's situation that may contribute to burnout (as there are for most crisis workers), and especially if there is evidence to suggest that one is already vulnerable, it is important to initiate preventive action. Prescribed steps can assist crisis counselors to avoid burnout and/or deal with it effectively.

Perhaps the most fundamental strategy to avoid burnout is to develop self-awareness: awareness of one's strengths and competencies as well as of one's needs and limitations. Crisis workers who are self-aware can set realistic expectations of themselves and not assume responsibility for clients' decisions. They know when it is necessary to say "no" to unrelenting or inappropriate demands, identify when they need help or support, and recognize the importance of taking care of themselves. They also recognize subjective emotional responses to clients and seek supervisory assistance in processing and addressing their reactions.

TABLE 14.1
SIGNS OF BURNOUT

- Do you no longer care about your clients and their struggles as much as you once did?
- Do you feel emotionally empty or drained most of the time?
- Do you dread going to work or miss work regularly?
- Do you feel powerless to really help your clients change?
- Do you feel unappreciated for all your hard work?
- Have you lost your idealistic belief that you can make a difference?
- Do you feel as though you just go through the motions of doing your job?

If you answered YES to any of these questions, what can you do?

- Acknowledge that you are in trouble.
- Take a personal inventory of ways you can improve self-care (e.g., healthy eating, sleeping, exercising, relaxing, leaving work at work).
- Set realistic expectations for yourself regarding what your responsibility is and what belongs to others.
- Identify specific needs for ongoing education and training and seek out continuing education opportunities.
- Seek out and make good use of supervision.
- Work to maintain positive relationships with colleagues and supervisors.
- Advocate for proactive agency attention to preventing burnout (e.g., provide consistent, empowering supervision, provide continuing education opportunities).
- Reexamine your commitment to empowering intervention with clients.

Second, crisis workers can develop essential personal and professional resources. This includes acquiring the knowledge and skill to perform their jobs competently. Feeling competent in a professional role can be a major contributor to feelings of job satisfaction, and feeling good about one's job can be a prime antidote to burnout (Corey & Corey, 1998; Harrison, 1983). Corey and Corey (1998) identified the loss of intellectual curiosity and interest in new ideas and developments as part of the experience of burnout. They also contended that an organizational cause of burnout among workers was the lack of opportunity for supervision, continuing education, and other forms of ongoing training. It follows that one way to avoid burnout is to initiate and make good use of supervisory sessions and to engage in professional development. The fact that state licensing and certification boards expect credentialed professionals to complete a requisite number of continuing education hours provides additional encouragement and incentive.

A third important way to avoid burnout is to take care of oneself. This includes eating and sleeping adequately, exercising, relaxing, engaging in soothing activities like listening to music or getting a massage, and most important, leaving your work at work (Meichenbaum, 1994). Taking care of oneself also includes ensuring that one has mutually caring and supportive relationships with family, friends, and colleagues. Supportive relationships with colleagues provide opportunities to share the frustrations, quandaries, joys, and satisfaction of working in crisis situations with others who share those experiences. Colleagues can function as a sounding board as well as provide technical assistance and support. Hagen (1999) noted that "Energy invested in developing relationships with colleagues is repaid many times over through access to their expertise and support" (p. 506). Maintaining rewarding relationships with family and friends is equally important. Having a fulfilling personal life outside of work is one of the primary ways one guards against work taking over one's life (Maslach, 1982).

Last, an important way to avoid burnout is *not* to restrict one's work to crisis counseling. Balancing crisis and noncrisis counseling and victim and nonvictim caseloads gives one a break from the unrelenting tragedy of crisis and victimization. Having variety in one's work can also counteract the boredom or disillusionment that may come from a constant barrage of similar problems and needs.

SECONDARY TRAUMATIC STRESS AND VICARIOUS TRAUMATIZATION

The concepts of secondary traumatic stress and vicarious traumatization have been developed to describe the emotional, cognitive, and physiological changes that may occur in those who are secondarily exposed to stories and experiences of trauma survivors. They involve the transfer of trauma symptoms from those who were directly traumatized to those who have extended and close emotional contact with them (McCann & Pearlman, 1990; Pearlman & Saakvitne, 1995). Our primary concern in this text is the effect of these changes on crisis workers and counselors who treat trauma survivors. As previously noted, compassion fatigue is a related concept that more narrowly describes the physical and psychological exhaustion that may result from extensive professional work in intensely emotional and stressful situations and high empathic connections with individual suffering. Compassion fatigue has been identified as a risk for police officers and a variety of helping professionals and volunteers who work in situations that demand high levels of empathy and compassion (Figley, 1995, 1999; Rainer, 2000).

Working with trauma survivors, either in the immediate aftermath of traumatic crisis or in longer-term crisis counseling, involves exposure to disturbing images of human suffering. In some cases, one directly observes mutilation, physical and emotional injury, or death and destruction, as is the case with emergency personnel and crisis workers who are responding at the site of a natural disaster or a violent human-caused disaster. When providing services in the aftermath of an individual trauma or large-scale disaster, the crisis worker hears in-depth stories and witnesses the emotional impact of those traumatic experiences. Trauma touches the life of the crisis worker and potentially leaves its emotional scars.

Raphael and Wilson (1994) reviewed the literature examining prolonged stress responses among rescue workers and analyzed the major themes in rescue work that appeared to contribute to a high incidence of stress reactions. Among the themes identified were the force and destruction involved, the confrontation with massive and gruesome death, feelings of hopelessness, a sense of the "helplessness of humanity," feelings of both anger and grief, survivor guilt, and discomfort and confusion about being a voyeur or an onlooker who watches others in deep personal pain and suffering.

Although some of these themes are more descriptive of the rescue worker's environment and experience than they are of most crisis workers' experiences, there are also many commonalities. Although many crisis workers are not in the field at the site of a disaster, those who work with trauma survivors are exposed to graphic details of abuse and human cruelty. They also may experience difficult and stressful relationship experiences in working with victims who engage in a variety of self-destructive and acting-out behaviors (Gamble, Pearlman, Lucca, & Allen, 1994). Trauma survivors may mutilate themselves, experience repeated suicidal thoughts and wishes, deliberately put themselves in risky situations, or regularly engage in dangerous games with their health. A client of one of the authors who was an insulin-dependent diabetic would deliberately eat disallowed foods when she was depressed, putting herself at high risk for insulin shock. In a study of shelter workers in a domestic violence program, 65 percent reported the following events as highly stressful: witnessing the damage from battering and then seeing battered women return to their homes even though future abuse was likely, feeling intense anger at perpetrators of domestic violence, and "dealing with the overwhelming pain and horror of domestic violence" (Brown & O'Brien, 1998).

Larson (2000) suggested that those who constantly work with death and grieving clients may experience a form of disenfranchised grief. Hospice workers and workers who provide crisis intervention in medical settings empathically experience survivor grief as well as their own grief because individuals they have assisted and companioned through the process of dying eventually do die. What Larson means by disenfranchised grief is that crisis workers may have few opportunities to work through their own grief process. Crisis counselors who work with death and grieving survivors may censor the expression of their own emotions, believing that it is unprofessional to experience such grief, or they may be discouraged by peers, family, and friends from expressing and processing their feelings. This diminished opportunity to express grief may lead to burnout, personal distress, and compassion fatigue.

Signs of Secondary Traumatic Stress and Vicarious Traumatization

As a result of secondary exposure to traumatic experiences, some crisis counselors and therapists have reported developing symptoms similar to PTSD. Research also documents, however, that not everyone involved in such work experiences this negative sequelae. Some individuals report positive effects from working with traumatized individuals (Brown & O'Brien, 1998; Foa & Rothbaum, 1998; White, 2001). The task is to understand which conditions may place individual crisis workers at risk of developing either compassion fatigue or secondary traumatic stress responses and to identify factors that appear to insulate individuals from that negative outcome. Before addressing those questions, it is useful to elaborate on our description of secondary traumatic stress/vicarious traumatization in order to develop a clearer picture of the negative impact it can have on crisis workers.

Saakvitne and Pearlman (1996) described vicarious traumatization as the "transformation of the therapist's or helper's inner experiences as a result of empathic engagement with survivor clients and their trauma material" (p. 25). They further explained this transformation as changes in the helper's "frame of reference" (e.g., their underlying sense of identity, worldview, and spirituality), their "self capacities" (e.g., affect tolerance, sense of self as "viable" and deserving love, continuing capacity to be in connection with others), their "ego resources" (e.g., self-awareness skills, interpersonal and self-protective skills), their "psychological needs and cognitive schemas" (e.g., beliefs about safety, trust, self control, intimacy), and their "memory and perceptions" (e.g., sequential narrative memories that include the appropriate visual, affective, and sensory components).

Following this outline, signs of vicarious traumatization would be expected in the same areas. For example, a crisis counselor who works with cancer patients might find himself no longer caring about his client's lives and emotions (disconnected from his identity as a caring person), or a crisis counselor who works in a rape crisis center might find that she is increasingly distrustful of and angry at men (disrupted fundamental beliefs about a just world with basically good people in it). Additionally, a crisis counselor might find that she constantly feels vulnerable to breaking down and crying, or that she is making poor decisions regarding boundaries and setting limits with her clients.

Some crisis workers experience intrusive imagery, nightmares, obsessive thinking, and emotional flooding. Saakvitne and Pearlman (1996) described one individual who had very close contact with children who had been abused. He described feeling "triggered" when he was with his granddaughter at a playground and saw a man pushing a little girl on a swing. "I couldn't get it out of my head that he was untrustworthy and would harm her later. I had been so immersed . . . I had lost all perspective. I kept having intrusive imagery . . . I had to look away to get them out of my head" (p. 39). One of the authors of this text began having nightmares of a client's sexual abuse.

Schechter (1998) suggested that crisis workers' own emotional responses are a reaction to the responses of the victims they are counseling. For example, when a victim's response is fear (of getting hurt again, of being killed), a crisis worker's response may also be one of fear—fear of getting involved, fear of getting hurt, and fear that what happened to the victim could happen to him or her. When a victim's is emotionally overwhelmed (by the lack of options and resources, by feelings of terror and rage and helplessness, or by the drastic changes that need to be made), the crisis counselor may feel overwhelmed by the same issues. A crisis counselor may also feel overwhelmed by having heard so many similar stories and knowing from experience that a victim is not safe. Schechter (1998) described similar countertransference responses to denial, discouragement, anger, guilt, trust, depression, and ambivalence. On a positive note, a skilled and self-aware crisis counselor can also use such personal reactions therapeutically as tools for increased understanding.

Risk Factors

As with burnout, the interplay of multiple factors contributes to the likelihood of developing secondary traumatic stress responses including characteristics of the individual and aspects of the work and the work environment.

Individual factors

Prior trauma history   A crisis counselor's own experience of trauma is the most frequently identified individual factor that may contribute to an increased risk of experiencing secondary trauma responses (Brady, Guy, Poelstra, & Brokaw, 1999). When one has a personal trauma history, a client's stories and emotional pain may reawaken one's memories and emotions (Figley, 1995; McCann & Pearlman, 1990; Pearlman & Saakvitne, 1995). Secondarily, as the result of his or her own trauma history, a crisis counselor may be "particularly sensitive to certain transferences" (Saakvitne & Pearlman, 1996, p. 44) including the trauma survivor's idealization of the crisis counselor as someone who can make him or her feel safe. As van der Kolk (1996) observed, "Patients' fragility and vulnerability is reflected in therapists' attempts to be perfect and in control. It is a tremendous strain on therapists to maintain an honest appraisal of their own capacities while tolerating their patients' intense need for rescue . . ." (pp. 553–554).

Additionally, traumatized individuals, especially those who were abused as children, have routinely experienced extreme boundary violations. As a result, they may attempt to engage with counselors in overly familiar, perhaps even flirtatious or sexual, ways. They may desperately seek a relationship that is not bound by professional limits. Counselors who have not worked through personal trauma issues may have a more difficult time recognizing and resisting the idealization, boundary violations, and dependency expectations of clients. They may overidentify with and/or enable overly dependent relationships to develop and continue. Although these issues can affect crisis counselors who do not have their own trauma histories, an unexamined or unresolved prior trauma experience can increase the risk.

Researchers who have tested this hypothesis have reached contradictory conclusions. Some empirical data have supported the contention that crisis counselors with a history of trauma also had higher levels of traumatic symptoms than those without such a history (Follette, Polusny, & Milbeck, 1994; Pearlman &

MacIan, 1995). Other studies have not supported that conclusion, however, find-ing, instead, that crisis counselors with a history of victimization/trauma were not more likely to have experienced vicarious trauma (Schauben & Frazier, 1995). The nature of a crisis counselor's prior traumas (childhood sexual abuse versus adult sexual assault) may explain some of this variation.

Age, education, and experience   Demographic characteristics such as age, level of education, and number of years working as a crisis counselor have also been identified as factors likely to affect one's susceptibility to experiencing secondary trauma. The general assertion is that younger counselors with less education and fewer years of experience are more susceptible to traumatic stress as the result of having less time to develop the personal and professional knowledge, compe-tence, and coping strategies that may serve to protect the older, more educated, and experienced crisis counselor (Saakvitne & Pearlman, 1996). Empirical find-ings, again, are mixed. For example, Neumann and Gamble (1995) found that being a less experienced crisis counselor increased the risk for secondary trauma. Landry (2001), who investigated secondary traumatic stress disorder in the thera-pists involved in the aftermath of the Oklahoma City bombing, however, found that more years of counseling experience had no significant effect on lowering risk for secondary traumatic stress.

Coping strategies   Every crisis counselor develops ways of coping with the stresses inherent in working with crises and trauma. It is clear, however, that some ways of coping are better than others. Certainly, some negative ways of coping are as unhealthy for crisis counselors as they are for our clients. For example, using drugs or alcohol to numb oneself or to feel able to relax is, in the long run, too costly a strategy. Similarly, it is self-defeating to isolate oneself from people and situations that require intimacy and connection because one is too emotionally overwhelmed or physically exhausted.

Some researchers have investigated whether there is a direct relationship be-tween "style of coping" and reported secondary stress reactions. Truman (1997) explored this issue with a sample of fifty-seven trauma counselors who worked with survivors of crime-related, war-related, or natural disaster trauma. Her data suggested that those who engaged in either "escape-avoidance" coping or "posi-tive appraisal" coping had a significantly elevated risk of experiencing secondary stress when compared to those with other styles of coping. Anderson (2000) ex-amined how Child Protective Services investigators, the individuals who have first contact with children identified for suspected abuse or neglect, coped with job stress and assessed a hypothesized relationship between coping strategies and "levels of emotional exhaustion," "depersonalization," and a "sense of reduced personal accomplishment." CPS workers who relied on "disengaged/avoidant" strategies were more likely to score high on "emotional exhaustion." She con-cluded that the problem-focused strategies many crisis workers learn are not use-ful for coping with the intense emotional aspects of their work.

What these studies suggest is that individuals who work in highly emotional sit-uations cannot escape, reappraise, or avoid directly coping with the emotional aspect of their work. Problem-focused coping and positive appraisal coping may offer a respite. These approaches, however, are insufficient in situations that are intensely emotional unless individuals also employ strategies that allow them to express their emotions and receive emotional support.

Professional behaviors   Another individual factor that may contribute to the risk of vicarious traumatization is the failure to take advantage of opportunities to grow professionally. This area obviously intersects with work environment issues because the work setting must ensure the availability of such opportunities. Individuals who are reluctant to utilize supervision or consultation, however, or who fail to seek and take advantage of continuing education rob themselves of an important opportunity to gain knowledge and skills that might contribute to a sense of competence and satisfaction. They also deprive themselves of the opportunity to gain emotional and technical support from supervisors or consultants (Saakvitne & Pearlman, 1996). With fewer professional resources to draw upon, crisis counselors are less able to recognize potential stresses or problems in helping relationships (e.g., transference/countertransference, boundary violations, overdependency, and reduced effectiveness). Both contribute to a loss of hopefulness and increased anxiety and/or fatigue.

Aspects of the work and the work environment   The sine qua non of compassion fatigue and secondary traumatic stress responses is the nature of the work and the nature of the clients' problems crisis counselors engage with (Figley, 1995; Leon, Altholz, & Dziegielewski, 1999; McCann & Pearlman, 1990; Saakvitne & Pearlman, 1996). For crisis counselors who work in emergency settings, contacts with trauma survivors are brief. However, the enormity of survivors' needs, the intensity of emotional impact, and the survivors' experience of powerlessness exert a tremendous pressure on crisis counselors to make a difference. Further, although the contact may be brief, the exposure to injury, destruction, death, and detailed accounts and images of traumatic experiences may be longer lasting. The empathic sharing of clients' emotional, physical, and spiritual pain cannot help but touch those who allow themselves to care and help. As Saakvitne and Pearlman (1996) observed, "We connect, we care, and then our clients are gone; we do not know the rest of their healing process" (p. 42).

Crisis counselors who work with trauma victims through the healing process have the opportunity to share their journeys toward becoming survivors, which can provide a sense of closure and hopefulness for the counselors. They also intimately share the experience, however, including the protracted pain and difficulty inherent in the journey. And they must bear witness as victims struggle with the awful reality they have experienced and may continue to experience in remembering.

The individuals seen by crisis workers engaged in both brief and long-term counseling interventions often continue to face dangers (e.g., abused children, battered women, some rape victims). They may have limited personal or material resources and multiple problems and may engage in or be at risk for a variety of self-destructive behaviors. Their despair, the "poignancy and intensity of their suffering, and the not infrequent histories of multiple abuses adds to the traumatic and stressful potential for those who seek to give aid" (Saakvitne & Pearlman, 1996, pp. 43–44).

Yet, as previously noted, although every caring and compassionate crisis worker is emotionally affected by these conditions, not all suffer ill consequences, and some report feeling both gratification and fulfillment. A primary factor that may make the difference is the work environment. Maslach and Leiter (1997) contended that it is a myth that characteristics of individuals or the type of work individuals do cause burnout, emotional fatigue, and job stress. Rather, they suggested that blame lies squarely on the shoulders of the organizations that employ crisis workers. The presence of impaired workers is a sign of dysfunction within an organization. Maslach and Leiter asserted that although the nature of the work may be emotionally difficult, organizational health is what determines how counselors fare. This may be a generalization, not based specifically on trauma work, but their general point about the importance of the work environment is well supported.

As Saakvitne and Pearlman (1996) stated, organizations that "provide no respite for staff," "require staff to have unrealistically high caseloads," "fail to provide enough qualified supervisors," and fail to recognize and attend to crisis workers' needs create a context for increased worker stress and diminished resilience and positive coping (p. 43).

Prevention and Healing

The recognition of factors that may place individual crisis counselors at risk for experiencing secondary traumatic stress and/or compassion fatigue points toward steps that can be taken to prevent this outcome. There are also some positive actions and attitudes than can contribute to one's personal and professional well-being.

Once again, both prevention and healing begin with an honest appraisal and identification of the ways an individual crisis counselor may be at risk due to either individual characteristics or work-related factors. Honestly assessing one's own personal and professional functioning in order to identify early warning signs of vulnerability is essential. When self-assessment reveals signs of looming difficulty, crisis counselors must take action. Even if risk factors are not identified, however, every crisis counselor can contribute to his or her ongoing wellness by attending regularly to personal and professional needs for self-care and support and by creating and sustaining balance and meaning in their lives.

Self-care and support   Because the crux of secondary traumatic stress for crisis workers is vicariously experiencing others' suffering and despair, often in highly charged, emotional situations, taking care of oneself is fundamental. Self-care begins with decreasing stress and nurturing oneself. This can include daily rituals that allow one to unwind and relax such as taking a walk, sitting under a tree, gardening, meditating, or reading a story with a child. Other positive strategies include balancing one's responses to the needs of family members and friends, attending to one's needs for solitude or quiet, and maintaining supportive relationships. Research has demonstrated the relationship between using social support as a coping strategy and fewer trauma symptoms (Schauben & Frazier, 1995). Getting sufficient rest, eating healthfully, and getting regular exercise are equally important.

Self-care also necessitates planning time away from work and being inaccessible to the demands of work (e.g., being on call or expected to keep up with e-mail). Planning and taking vacations and spending time with friends and family who are not helping professionals can also decrease the likelihood of being consumed by work.

Meichenbaum (1994) suggested that crisis counselors bring "signs of life and hope" such as plants, pictures of nature, and pictures of children into their homes and offices. Images that remind one of beauty, joy, and hopefulness can be a helpful antidote to the stress of trauma work.

Creating personal meaning   Some theorists have suggested that a cornerstone of vicarious traumatization is a "transformation of meaning" wherein crisis counselors' dominant beliefs about self, identity, the world, humanity, and spirituality change in a negative way. It is important to note here that empirical data supporting this assertion is limited and some studies examining aspects of this hypothesis have not affirmed it. For instance, Brady et al. (1999) conducted a national survey with 1,000 female therapists to assess hypotheses related to vicarious traumatization. One hypothesis focused on the impact of trauma work on respondents' reported spiritual well-being. The researchers concluded that respondents' "underlying assumptions and worldview were undisturbed" and, further, that those who did more work with trauma survivors actually reported a "more spiritually satisfying life" than those who did less work with them.

Despite this conclusion, these researchers emphasized the importance of counselors who engage in trauma work pursuing activities that promote their spiritual well-being (Brady et al., 1999). Other experts have similarly identified the importance of adopting a "philosophical or religious outlook" (Meichenbaum, 1994). Saakvitne and Pearlman (1996) asserted that the strategies most successful in "transforming" vicarious traumatization are those that "infuse meaning into our lives" (p. 73). Because the experience of trauma, directly or indirectly, often creates cynicism and loss of meaning, strategies that challenge negative beliefs, build community, and infuse one's life with meaning may be most helpful in countering that outcome. For some crisis counselors, simply recognizing the meaningfulness of the work may promote resilience.

Professional behavior   Professional behavior and organizational health are symbiotically related. Because many professional strategies known to contribute to counselor well-being depend on organizational climate and supports, most of those are addressed in the next section.

Schechter (1998) examined counselors' transference responses when working with battered women. She also identified specific actions that crisis counselors could take when they found themselves mired in fear, guilt, or ambivalence. Two of her suggestions are particularly germane. First, she urged counselors not to discount their fears, as they are frequently based in reality. Instead, she urged counselors to both talk out their fears and establish realistic safety procedures. When there are real dangers, it is not paranoid to feel afraid. Second, rather than being afraid of or trying to deny anger, she suggested that crisis counselors acknowledge it and use it, directing it into agency and political advocacy and change. She also advocated the importance of humor.

Organizational health   As noted earlier, some researchers and other authors have concluded that the organizational climate in which counselors work is the most important factor influencing their well-being. Brady et al. (1999), in concluding remarks in their study of vicarious traumatization with female psychotherapists, urged organizations and agencies whose staff members provide services to trauma survivors to "take responsibility for reducing the likelihood of vicarious traumatization in the workplace" (p. 390).

Factors in the organizational setting that contribute to crisis counselors' well-being include supportive consultation teams or staff meetings. In addition to individual supervision, clinical team meetings can serve multiple purposes including support, consultation, instruction, feedback, camaraderie, and humor. Talbot, Manton, and Dunn (1992) suggested that one component of clinical staff meetings should be routine debriefings in which counselors discuss (within the confidential confines of supervision) specific cases, including what they are seeing and hearing and how they are responding personally to the traumatic material clients present. Taking the time to address the feelings and concerns counselors have in response to their crisis work is a primary means of preventing the exacerbation of secondary stress responses. A related strategy is to provide continuing education to staff. Education should focus both on increasing knowledge and competence in working with traumatized clients and increasing knowledge about compassion fatigue and secondary traumatic stress as potential effects of working with trauma.

A second organizational issue concerns safety. Organizations that serve trauma clients must ensure that their work environment is physically and emotionally safe, respectful, and comfortable (Brady et al., 1999; Brown & O'Brien, 1998; Saakvitne & Pearlman, 1996). This includes having prearranged, specific safety mechanisms and plans in place in those settings where services are provided to individuals for whom continuing violence may be a problem (e.g., battered women shelters, child welfare offices, and some mental health crisis centers).

Social support is one of the variables with the greatest influence on whether individuals are able to cope adaptively with crises. This is true for victims of trauma or other crises as well as for those who serve them, empathically sharing their experience. Organizations must ensure that their counselors have specific social and professional supports and an overall supportive climate within which to work.

ON A POSITIVE NOTE: COMPASSION SATISFACTION AND WORK FULFILLMENT

This chapter focuses the reader's attention on the potential personal and professional difficulties inherent in working with crisis survivors. The dangers of burnout, compassion fatigue, and secondary traumatic stress are real. Those who work in crisis environments must attend to their own well-being, and the organizations and agencies that employ them must accept the responsibility to create work environments that nurture and support their staff.

That said, we could not end this text without identifying the very positive and fulfilling aspects of providing crisis intervention services to people in need. The truth is that most individuals who work in this capacity do not suffer debilitating outcomes and do not experience loss of meaning or the capacity to care. On the contrary, many express appreciation for having the opportunity to engage in such powerful and meaningful work.

Empirical studies that have examined burnout, compassion fatigue, and secondary traumatic stress have documented some negative symptoms in the lives of professionals serving as emergency responders and crisis counselors. The same studies, however, have also noted that although individuals who treat trauma survivors may be at higher risk of developing PTSD-like symptoms (e.g., intrusive imagery), *for most individuals those symptoms were mild, and long-term negative effects on beliefs and meaning structures were rare.* Studies support the fact that although prolonged exposure to clients' trauma is associated with counselors' distressful symptoms, most counselors seem to be able to cope with their experiences in a healthy way (Minnen & Keijsers, 2000).

Perhaps more important, some evidence exists that those who work with trauma survivors experience positive effects. For example, as noted earlier, one study found that those who treated trauma survivors reported a more "existentially and spiritually satisfying life" than did those who did not (Brady et al., 1999). These researchers compared their findings to the findings from a study of Holocaust survivors, who also showed higher levels of spiritual belief than those who were not Holocaust survivors. Trauma, whether experienced directly or indirectly, appears to challenge systems of meaning and spiritual faith. For many, however, the outcome of such an existential crisis is not alienation but a strengthening of their sense of meaning.

Although we reviewed literature that suggested that idealism and enthusiasm may backfire for some individuals, causing them to experience burnout, the other side of this issue is that individuals who take a job because they regard the work as important and worthwhile are likely to experience feelings of job satisfaction and accomplishment. Studies of shelter workers in battered women's programs (Brown & O'Brien, 1998) and hospice workers (White, 2001) have documented that although there is potential for secondary trauma and burnout, when the work environment is supportive and individuals have the opportunity to engage in tasks that they view as worthwhile, they are fulfilled in their work. White (2001) found that social workers reported that the most satisfying aspect of their work with dying patients was their perception of hospice as a calling and their ability to facilitate a peaceful death for patients and their families. This study found that "compassion satisfaction," which was universally reported by the respondents, appeared to be an antidote to secondary traumatic stress.

Research previously reviewed similarly suggested that strong emotional responses to clients' crises may lead to compassion fatigue. Studies have also documented, however, that some crisis counselors view those emotional responses as an important part of their work and their effectiveness. Thus, rather than being conceptualized within a "vicarious trauma framework," those intense emotional reactions may also serve as resources for crisis counselors working with crisis survivors (Wasco & Campbell, 2002).

Finally, those of us who enter the professional world of crisis counseling and work with traumatized individuals do so because of a commitment to a greater end. We believe in the human capacity for good, for relationship, for change, and for growth. As Foa and Rothbaum (1998) noted, our work is similar to that of hospital and other medical personnel caring for medical trauma survivors. It is hard for compassionate people to see pain and loss and not feel upset and sometimes emotionally exhausted or even devastated. We must keep this in mind, however:

> Even in the worst atrocities, there are opportunities for the resilience of the human spirit to shine through. These experiences may be perceived as "gifts" that are only available to those of us who are working "in the trenches." Seeing an assault victim who accepts what has happened to her with dignity and self-respect, and who sometimes even finds a positive message in it, is an example of such an uplifting experience. Working with a terminally ill cancer patient who is leaving behind a legacy of love and integrity and is dying with such dignity as to make us marvel that such people exist is another example of such a gift. We truly gain an understanding of what people are capable of, both good and bad, and we are doing something that not everyone can do. (Foa & Rothbaum, 1998, p. 175)

The authors and contributors to this text share this observation. As a group we have worked extensively with crises and trauma. We have worked in the fields of cancer care, rape, domestic violence, and hospice. We have provided crisis services to individual victims of rape and battery, torture, and natural and human-caused disasters. In that work we have experienced the need for attention to our own needs and personal and professional self-care. Above all, however, we have found our work with people surviving crises and trauma to be some of the most meaningful work we have experienced in our professional lives.

We end this text with a personal reflection by Dr. Grace Telesco, a twenty-year veteran in the New York City Police Department. On September 11, 2001, she was asked to coordinate the crisis intervention response to the families of the victims of the attacks on the World Trade Center. Under her leadership, over 5,000 families were provided crisis intervention and related services through the family assistance center at Pier 94.

In the following section, Telesco describes the effects of that experience—on herself and on the hundreds of city workers and volunteers she supervised during the days and weeks following one of the worst single disasters the United States has ever endured.

A CAREGIVER'S REFLECTION ON SEPTEMBER 11, by Grace Telesco

A Sea of Human Suffering

In the immediate hours following the September 11th attacks in New York City a temporary family assistance center was set up near the city morgue, later moved to the armory on Lexington Avenue in Manhattan, and ultimately moved to Pier 84, where crisis intervention and other support services were offered to the families of the victims. The agency responsible for the safety, security, and coordination of service delivery was the New York City Police Department's Community Affairs Section. As a police lieutenant with a doctorate in social work and extensive background in crisis intervention, I coordinated the interagency mental health response along with a team of officers chosen for their expertise in crisis intervention. This work lasted from the hours immediately following the attacks until early December 2001.

The response began for us on September 11 at approximately 1:30 P.M. at the city morgue where the police mental health team was involved in assisting hundreds of families with the preparation of the "missing persons report." That first day's response seemed to never end and, in a surreal way, became the next day and the next day and the next day. For the longest time, even months later, it never stopped being September 12, the day after, for us. Those first few days following the attacks, prior to the arrival of the Red Cross, clinicians volunteered their services by offering support and assisting in crisis intervention for the families who came to the morgue en masse. Families were also assisted in negotiating a traumatic and chaotic bureaucratic process.

In the first few weeks, service providers observed the various crisis reactions of individuals ranging from denial, shock, and disbelief to desperation, frustration, and ultimately anger. A classification of "premourning" was probably the most fitting during this time. As time moved on and no word came of more survivors, despair and grief became more evident as people began to move into deeper stages of mourning.

Individual shock, anger, disbelief, denial, and grief were expressed in the words of many languages and in the tears, gestures, and body postures that crossed the barrier that language can sometimes be to effective communication. A sea of humanity, displayed in the photos held in the hands of thousands representing the missing and the dead symbolized the severity of this enormous tragedy. On a cognitive level, the crisis workers and service providers knew that this was an enormous task before them and one that would require a unique and eclectic response.

On an emotional and spiritual level, there is no training to prepare the practitioner for such an assignment. The sea of human pain coupled with the magnitude of the death toll and the severity of the disaster created an atmosphere of despair that was overwhelming.

In the days and weeks following the attacks, various agencies and organizations became part of a unique support team. This team consisted of law enforcement, medical personnel, mental health practitioners, spiritual care providers, pet therapy professionals, and family survivors from Oklahoma City who lost loved ones in the Murrah Federal Building bombing. The Community Assistance Unit from the mayor's office and the New York Police Department's Community Affairs Section coordinated the delivery of services. The services included assisting family members in the preparation of the missing persons report, DNA sampling, release of patient and deceased lists, distribution of death certificates and memorial urns, and escorting families to Ground Zero. The eventual impact this would have on the workers would not be realized until months after the work had been completed.

McCann and Pearlman (1990) described how providers' own cognitive assumptions and beliefs about safety and power can be disrupted in the face of client trauma. This indescribable trauma triggered an array of emotions in crisis intervention professionals. From clinician to police officer, feelings of grief, loss, fear, and the questioning of one's own mortality were evident (Dick, 1996).

Many families refused to let go of the notion that their loved one would be rescued while others hoped to find them wandering disoriented in lower Manhattan. Still others believed that their friend, mother, lover, partner, son, or daughter, whose "missing person" photo they carried with them, was unconscious and unidentified in a hospital. One woman was screaming in rage that she wanted to go and dig her baby brother out of the rubble. Questions abounded.

"How current is this hospital list?" "If she was disoriented, she wouldn't be able to spell her name correctly—can I check again for a different spelling?" "Is this list really all-inclusive?" "Is this deceased list as of this morning?" "I have his photo and dental records. Should I give it to you?" "She was wearing a red shirt that morning and she has a wristwatch engraved with her initials." "How do I fill out this nine-page form?" Unsure of how to respond, crisis workers would answer, "I'm sorry, it doesn't look as though his name is here." Those fourteen-hour days were filled with tears, unanswered questions, shock, denial, disbelief, thousands of photos, toothbrushes, dental records, and extraordinary hope that a missing relative was not dead and might be "the unconscious one in the hospital."

As the days and weeks went on and the term "rescue effort" was gently changed to "recovery," with very few bodies being recovered and no one being rescued alive, families turned from premourning to mourning. Comfort rooms were set up at the center, where we could offer support privately and provide crisis intervention. Spiritual care providers also gave support to those who often turn to faith in times of grief.

Most of all, people wanted their questions answered and neither the police nor the mental health practitioners could offer a resolution. In many cases, those in crisis screamed in frustration, and active listening was the only appropriate intervention. Family members cried in fear of the worst and crisis workers listened with quiet support and empathic connection. Those of us who were aware that people's worst fears had been realized, gently and compassionately broke the news to one person at a time.

The volume of clients, some of whom continued to come back daily to check lists despite the fact that the lists remained unchanged, slowly began to wear on the crisis workers. For those of us in leadership positions, the juggling of territorial jurisdiction, authority, and political objectives became the quintessential bureaucratic nightmare.

Challenging aspects of the work also centered on issues of organizational development. Initially, there was no plan of action, and the resultant lack of designated leadership created confusion over authority. Unclear roles and responsibilities led to frustration and stress for crisis workers, who were already at risk for vicarious trauma. Ordinarily, the Red Cross maintains jurisdiction over the initial mental health response at disaster sites and will thus take the lead; however, the City Department of Mental Health also assumed jurisdiction because of their responsibility for the mental health of the New York City community. This jurisdictional struggle, the enormity of the crisis, and the looming fear of another terrorist attack created an ad-hoc mental health response that put my police community affairs mental health team at the center of the coordination.

The emotional energy necessary to balance the needs of the clients with the political objectives of each of the agencies involved was often more frustrating and painful than the actual work itself. Many of us had become "overprotective" of the families and felt it was our responsibility to shield them from the political and bureaucratic processes.

"Take Care of My People"

Figley (1995) and others describe compassion fatigue as a deleterious effect of helping others in trauma. Others define the psychological effect on workers who offer assistance to those in trauma and grief as vicarious traumatization or vicarious bereavement (McCann & Pearlman, 1990; Rando, 1997; Saakvitne & Pearlman, 1996). I believe that one of the most important factors that contributes to compassion fatigue is found in the empathic response itself. In order to intervene effectively, it is necessary to make a genuinely empathic connection with the individual in need. Figley (1995) maintained that the interpersonal competence of the caregiver is one characteristic of compassion fatigue. In letting suffering individuals into the inner depths of one's self, and by feeling their pain as your own, you create a connection that is at the very center of effective intervention. I listened to some of the cops who worked at the pier say, "I can't let them in, because once I do that I'm finished. I don't want to know their story because it will hurt too much."

On September 22 the mayor's office asked my police mental health team to lead an ongoing collaborative effort to escort families by ferry to the sacred place of ground zero in order for them to view the site and see the place where their loved ones were last alive. In addition to the ground zero visit, families were to be escorted to a memorial site nearby, where they could pay tribute to their loved ones by leaving flowers, cards, and bears donated by Oklahoma City families. There was no plan to follow and little direction given yet the police mental health team, with the guidance of Jeannie Straussman, C.S.W., from the State Office of Mental Health, and Ken Thompson and Diane Leonard, Oklahoma City family survivors, put together an initiative that would prove to make the difference in the lives of thousands of mourners. The support team would consist of community affairs officers assigned to the mental health team, Red Cross mental health practitioners, spiritual care providers including Coast Guard chaplains, paramedics, New York state troopers, the New Jersey Special Operations group, city mental health practitioners, pet therapy dogs, and family survivors from Oklahoma City.

Our plan was to make three trips a day, taking fifty people by ferry to the World Financial Center and walk them reverently and gently to the burial place of their loved ones, known to the world as Ground Zero. The mission was to provide emotional, spiritual, and physical support to families as they witnessed the incomprehensible destruction and said their good-byes. Family members' safety was of grave concern to us, particularly in light of the heightened alert and the possibility of another attack, so law enforcement professionals from all over the tri-state area provided additional security. Because the integrity and dignity of the process was critical to me, I established a policy prohibiting the photographing of families.

The grieving process is a personal one, and mourning rituals in most cultures and religious faiths are particularly private events, created and developed individually. Because of the vast numbers of people who died, however, grieving families were forced into a situation in which their mourning became a matter of public view. The nonsectarian ritual that was created for them was simultaneously conducted with hundreds of strangers. These families from various races, ethnicities, and cultures, who were strangers to each other before the trip, ultimately shared a ritual that bonded them as a group. It would not bring closure, but hopefully it would help them begin their process of recovery.

We could not be fully aware of the effect this work would have on us until many months later. One of the factors that I believe contributed to compassion fatigue for many police crisis workers was the fact that they "went the distance." Most mental health volunteers, whether they were sponsored by the Red Cross or by the city's Department of Mental Health, were limited to one ferry trip per day, twice a week.

Out of necessity, however, our officers were assigned to a minimum of two trips per day for two months. Lacking empirical evidence to support limiting the number of trips to moderate deleterious effects of vicarious grief for the providers, we can only report anecdotally on the effect on the officers who were consistently involved in the intervention.

Despite efforts to prevent vicarious traumatization and compassion fatigue by conducting regular debriefings with these officers, negative psychological outcomes have been observed. At a recent follow-up with officers who were directly involved with families at the pier, conducted six months after September 11, symptoms of posttraumatic stress, depression, vicarious trauma, and compassion fatigue were clearly evident. These officers were vessels within which thousands of people deposited their grief, and they were full. Very few of us know how the families we assisted are currently functioning. For most of us, our memory is of their despair.

During formal and informal debriefing sessions, officers talked about the importance of the work. For most of us it was a ministry. We were answering a call to serve and take care of the families of thousands who had died. We saw ourselves as serving the many victims by trying to take care of their loved ones. We had to let the stories in and care for these families as if they were our own. As a result, some of us "crossed the line." We psychologically adopted those families and for that interpersonal competence, as Figley (1995) labeled it, we now pay the price with remnants of grief that remain in us.

Moderating Outcomes of Compassion Fatigue

As the leader of the mental health team, in addition to the responsibility I felt to the thousands of families, I was continually concerned about the team members. I worried that the officers were taking in too much, working too hard, staying too long, taking too many trips each day, and not taking enough time off. I limited the number of trips per day to two and insisted that officers take off at least once a week. I convinced my chief to prohibit officers from working seven days straight and, although they grumbled because they wanted to be there, it was beneficial to their psychological well-being in the end.

In attempting to moderate the deleterious effects of the work and prevent vicarious traumatization and compassion fatigue, I conducted daily check-in sessions with my officers. Each morning at 7:00 A.M., we would gather in what we called "the circle of trust" and share our fears, frustrations, sadness, nightmares, despair, and sometimes, humorous stories of the prior day's events. Utilizing an indigenous spirituality version of the "talking stick," we would pass an Oklahoma City bear around the circle and officers would share their feelings when the bear made its way to their lap.

Some officers described dreaming of hundreds of people waiting to view hospital lists in their living rooms, spilling over into their bathrooms and hallways. Other officers cried as they shared their personal grief and loss relative to the incident. Still others talked about the effects of witnessing the horrific devastation of Ground Zero. Because they trusted each other, their team leader, and the process, they felt safe enough to freely share their feelings. We conducted these "circles of trust" daily for three months until our work at the pier was completed. On the day of our last ferry trip to Ground Zero, the "family" that had become known as the mental health team and, to some, the "boat people," had an informal termination session at an Italian restaurant where we shared food and emotions and ceremoniously marked the end of our "ministry."

Concerned that there would be ongoing negative effects, I arranged a follow-up retreat for the officers who had been assigned to the mental health team to be conducted by an outside clinician from Safe Horizon. In a beautiful and peaceful setting, far from the devastation of Ground Zero and the pain of Pier 84, we assembled for a day of healing and emotional recovery. A six-month follow-up retreat was also conducted to "check in" once again. Many shared that they could not sleep, were feeling sad, had a hard time getting the pain out of their psyche, and that the suffering of the families was still with them. It was amazing how easily these feelings could be stirred up. Six months later, it was still very close to the surface.

No Pain, No Gain

In the worst of times, it is through pain that we see the greatness in humanity and in the capacity of humans to do good work (Foa & Rothbaum, 1998). It is in this light that officers shared how proud they were to do such important work. Some officers described it as the best work of their careers and as the "most painful, yet most fulfilling." It was difficult to leave it behind and go back to routine assignments. All else seemed meaningless by comparison. The families were not the only ones who benefited from our work. We also received a tremendous, once-in-a-lifetime gift that would forever change each of us—as individuals and as mental health service providers.

When caregivers reflect on the importance of a particular crisis intervention, particularly a traumatic crisis, you realize that effective intervention does not come cheaply. The emotional exhaustion that is its aftermath can be the cost of good caring (Figley, 1995; Kinzel & Nanson, 2000; Saakvitne & Pearlman, 1996). This idea was a recurring theme at the six-month follow-up discussion with the police mental health team. Officer after officer shared how they believed they had accomplished an incredible feat in holding the families of thousands of souls in their arms, and what a privilege it was to have been able to serve them. To a person, we would not have wanted to be anywhere else. And believing we made a difference enabled us to begin to restore our sense of meaning and personal control.

Self-Care Plan

As anniversaries of September 11 approach, there are several ways we can take care of ourselves and "transform the pain of vicarious traumatization" (Saakvitne & Pearlman, 1996). Following are some of the suggestions that were made at the six-month anniversary retreat for the officers of the mental health team that seem to relieve and lessen the symptoms of compassion fatigue and vicarious traumatization:

• Avoid the "physician, heal thyself" syndrome.

As mental health practitioners and clinicians, we sometimes avoid seeking help and believe that we know what is best for ourselves. The intensity of intervening with those in crisis or trauma can take its toll, however, and professional help to deal with personal responses can be helpful.

- Sleep deprivation is dangerous.

For those of us who were engaged with the crisis work of September 11 or for those engaged in any other work involving victims of a traumatic incident, sleep may be difficult. Knowing that this is normal and to be expected is not enough. Your body, mind, and spirit require sleep. You may need a sleep aid or other medication. Some herbal teas may help as well as meditation exercises, but you may need a prescription drug to help you get a good night's sleep while you talk out your feelings with a professional clinician.

- Identify your personal issues.

Critical incidents can stir up personal feelings of loss, grief, depression, and anxiety. It is important to recognize that your own issues may be triggered and thus you need to also identify and utilize the personal coping strategies that normally work for you as they relate to those issues and losses.

- Ritualize the work.

To remember the work in its detail is important to healing. Preparing a scrapbook or journal that documents and ritualizes the work may help to put some sense of closure on the incident so that the healing can begin. For some, the ritual of going to the river or ocean and letting the "pain and suffering" go seems to be helpful.

- Find some distance.

It is important to leave the work behind. Let go of helping for a bit and acknowledge that others will be OK and will get along without you. Realize that "they need to do for themselves and now you need to do for you." To continue to feel responsible for clients, coworkers, and "the work" can become destructive. Even just to leave it for a while and then come back to it later may be emotionally and spiritually beneficial.

- Relax.

Meditate, exercise, pray, play, take a vacation, go to the beach, or visit the ocean.

Whatever it is that gives you comfort in a positive and constructive way is what you need right now. Alcohol, substance indulgence, and poor nutrition, despite the false feeling of pleasure and comfort they can provide, are destructive and should be avoided. Engage your personal "tried and true" coping skills.

- You are not alone.

It is important to remind yourself that what you are feeling is a consequence of excellence and that other crisis workers are feeling the same effects of a job well done. Now is the time for you to engage in therapeutic exercises of self-care.

Conclusion

As the nation, the cities affected directly and indirectly, and the families of the victims begin to heal and move on in their recovery process, so too must we, the caregivers, begin our healing. First we must give ourselves permission to feel and then to enter into the journey of healing. Failing to do this makes the tragedy of these events and traumatic incidents like it that much more disastrous. We then become victims rather than survivors who are healthy and whole caregivers.

SMALL-GROUP OR CLASS DISCUSSION QUESTIONS

1. How would you know if you were experiencing burnout or compassion fatigue? How would you respond?

2. If you were working in a setting where you routinely worked with people in crisis (e.g., a rape crisis or battered women's program or a hospital emergency room), how would you take care of yourself on a day-to-day basis? If you were a supervisor or manager, how would you ensure a psychologically safe environment for your staff?

3. Foa and Rothbaum (1998) regard their experiences in working with trauma survivors as "gifts" that are only available to those who work in the trenches. What do they mean by this? Can you give examples of how such difficult professional work might be considered a gift?

REFERENCES

Anderson, D. G. (2000). Coping strategies and burnout among veteran child protection workers. *Child Abuse and Neglect, 24,* 839–848.

Arches, J. (1991). Social structure, burnout, and job satisfaction. *Social Work, 36,* 202–206.

Brady, J. L., Guy, J. D., Poelstra, P. L., & Brokaw, B. F. (1999). Vicarious traumatization, spirituality, and the treatment of sexual abuse survivors: A national survey of women psychotherapists. *Professional Psychology: Research and Practice, 30,* 386–393.

Brown, C., & O'Brien, K. M. (1998). Understanding stress and burnout in shelter workers. *Professional Psychology: Research and Practice, 29,* 383–385.

Corey, G., & Corey, M. S. (1998). *Becoming a helper* (3rd ed.). Pacific Grove, CA: Brooks/Cole.

Corey, G., Corey, M. S., & Callanan, P. (1988). *Issues and ethics in the helping professions.* Pacific Grove, CA: Brooks/Cole.

Cormier, L. S., & Hackney, H. (1993). *The professional counselor: A process guide to helping.* Boston: Allyn & Bacon.

Dick, L. C. (1996). Impact on law enforcement and EMS personnel. In K. Doka (Ed.), *Living with grief after sudden loss: Suicide, homicide, accident, heart attack, stroke* (pp. 173–184). Washington, DC: Hospice Foundation of America.

Everly, G. S., Boyle, S. H., & Lating, J. M. (1999). The effectiveness of psychological debriefing with vicarious trauma: A meta-analysis. *Stress Medicine, 15,* 229–233.

Figley, C. R. (1995). Compassion fatigue as secondary traumatic stress disorder: An overview. In C. R. Figley (Ed.), *Compassion fatigue: Coping with secondary traumatic stress disorder in those who treat the traumatized* (pp. 1–20). New York: Brunner/Mazel.

Figley, C. R. (1999). Police compassion fatigue: Theory, research, assessment, treatment, and prevention. In J. M Violanti & D. Paton (Eds.), *Police trauma: Psychological aftermath of civilian combat* (pp. 37–53). Springfield, IL: Charles C. Thomas, Publisher.

Foa, E. B., & Rothbaum, B. O. (1998). *Treating the trauma of rape: Cognitive-behavioral therapy for PTSD.* New York: Guilford Press.

Follette, V. M., Polusny, M. M., & Milbeck, K. (1994). Mental health and law enforcement professionals: Trauma history, psychological symptoms, and impact of providing services to child sexual abuse survivors. *Professional Psychology: Research and Practice, 25,* 275–282.

Gamble, S. J., Pearlman, L. A., Lucca, A. M., & Allen, G. J. (1994, October). *Differential therapist stressors in psychotherapy with trauma vs. non-trauma clients.* Paper presented at the New England Psychological Association Conference, Hamden, CT.

Hagen, J. L. (1999). Burnout: An occupational hazard for social workers. In B. R. Compton & B. Galaway, *Social work processes* (6th ed., pp. 501–508). Pacific Grove, CA: Brooks/Cole.

Harrison, W. D. (1983). A social competence model of burnout. In B. A. Farber (Ed.), *Stress and burnout in the human service professions* (pp. 29–39). New York: Pergamon.

Himle, D. P., Jayaratne, S., & Thyness, P. (1991). Buffering effects of four social support types on burnout among social workers. *Social Work Research and Abstracts, 27*(1), 22–27.

Kinzel, A., & Nanson, J. (2000). Education and debriefing: Strategies for preventing crisis in crisis-line volunteers. *Crisis, 21*(3), 126–134.

Koeske, G. F., & Kelly, T. (1995). The impact of over-involvement on burnout and job satisfaction. *American Journal of Orthopsychiatry, 65,* 282–292.

Koeske, G. F., & Koeske, R. D. (1989). Workload and burnout: Can social support and perceived accomplishment help? *Social Work, 34,* 243–248.

Landry, L. (2001). *Secondary traumatic stress disorder in the therapists from the Oklahoma City bombing.* Dissertation Abstracts International, Section B: Sciences and Engineering, 61(7–8), 3849.

Larson, D. G. (2000). Anticipatory mourning: Challenges for professional and volunteer caregivers. In T. A. Rando (Ed.), *Clinical dimensions of anticipatory mourning: Theory and practice in working with the dying, their loved ones, and their caregivers* (pp. 379–395). Champaign, IL: Research Press.

Leon, A. M., Altholz, J. A. S., & Dziegielewski, S. F. (1999). Compassion fatigue: Considerations for working with the elderly. *Journal of Erotological Social Work, 32*(1), 43–62.

Maslach, C. (1982). *Burnout: The cost of caring.* Englewood Cliffs, NJ: Prentice-Hall.

Maslach, C., & Leiter, M. P. (1997). *The truth about burnout: How organizations cause personal stress and what to do about it.* San Francisco: Jossey-Bass.

McCann, I. L., & Pearlman, L. A. (1990). Vicarious traumatization: A framework for understanding the psychological effects of working with victims. *Journal of Traumatic Stress, 3*(1), 131–149.

Meichenbaum, D. (1994). *A clinical handbook/practical therapist manual for assessing and treating adults with post-traumatic stress disorder.* Waterloo, Ontario, Canada: Institute Press.

Minnen, A. V., & Keijsers, G. P. J. (2000). A controlled study into the (cognitive) effects of exposure treatment on trauma therapists. *Journal of Behavior Therapy and Experimental Psychiatry, 31*(3–4), 189–200.

Mitchell, J. T. (1985). Healing the helper. In NIMH (Ed.), *Role stressors and supports for emergency workers.* Washington, DC: NIMH.

Mitchell, J. T., & Bray, G. P. (1989). *Emergency services stress.* Englewood Cliffs, NJ: Prentice-Hall.

Neumann, D. A., & Gamble, S. J. (1995). Vicarious traumatization in the new trauma therapist. *Psychotherapy, 32,* 341–347.

O'Halloran, S., & O'Halloran, T. (2001). Secondary traumatic stress in the classroom: Ameliorating stress in graduate students. *Teaching of Psychology, 28*(2), 92–96.

Pearlman, L. A., & MacIan, P. S. (1995). Vicarious traumatization: An empirical study of the effects of trauma work on trauma therapists. *Professional Psychology: Research and Practice, 26,* 558–565.

Pearlman, L. A., & Saakvitne, K. W. (1995). *Trauma and the therapist: Countertransference and vicarious traumatization in psychotherapy with incest survivors.* New York: W. W. Norton.

Pines, A. (1983). On burnout and the buffering effects of social supports. In B. A. Farber (Ed.), *Stress and burnout in the human service professions* (pp. 158–160). New York: Pergamon.

Pines, A., Aronson, E., & Kafry, D. (1981). *Burnout: From tedium to personal growth.* New York: Free Press.

Poulin, J. E., & Walter, C. A. (1993). Social workers' burnout: A longitudinal study. *Social Work Research and Abstracts, 29*(4), 5–11.

Rainer, J. P. (2000). Compassion fatigue: When caregiving begins to hurt. In L. Vandecreek & T. L. Jackson (Eds.), *Innovations in clinical practice: A source book,* Vol. 18 (pp. 441–453). Sarasota, FL: Professional Resource Exchange.

Rando, T. (1997). Vicarious bereavement. In S. Strack (Ed.), *Death and the quest for meaning: Essays in honor of Herman Feifel* (pp. 257–274). Newark: Jason Aronson.

Raphael, B., & Wilson, J. P. (1994). When disaster strikes: Managing emotional reactions in rescue workers. In J. P. Wilson & J. D. Lindy (Eds.), *Countertransference in the treatment of PTSD* (pp. 333–350). New York: Guilford Press.

Saakvitne, K. W., & Pearlman, L. A. (1996). *Transforming the pain: A workbook on vicarious traumatization.* New York: W. W. Norton.

Schauben, L. J.,& Frazier, P. A. (1995). Vicarious trauma: The effects on female counselors of working with sexual violence survivors. *Psychology of Women Quarterly, 19,* 49–64.

Schechter, S. (1998). *Responses as guides to action: Working with victims of domestic violence.* Albany: New York State Office for the Prevention of Domestic Violence.

Talbot, A., Manton, M., & Dunn, P. J. (1992). Debriefing the debriefers: An intervention strategy to assist psychologists after a crisis. *Journal of Traumatic Stress, 5,* 45–62.

Truman, B. M. (1997). *Secondary traumatization, counselor's trauma history, and styles of coping.* Dissertation Abstracts International: Section B: The Sciences and Engineering, 57(9-B), 5935.

Van der Kolk, B. A., McFarlane, A. C., & Weisaeth, L. (Eds.), *Traumatic stress: The effects of overwhelming experience on mind, body and society*. New York: Guilford Press.

Wasco, S. M., & Campbell, R. (2002). Emotional reactions of rape victim advocates: A multiple case study of anger and fear. *Psychology of Women Quarterly, 26*(2), 120–130.

White, S. D. (2001). *A microethnography of secondary traumatic stress in hospice culture.* Dissertation Abstracts International: Section A: Humanities and Social Sciences, 62(5-A), 1945.

Wilson, J. P., & Lindy, J. D. (1994). *Countertransference in the treatment of PTSD*. New York: Guilford Press.

Acknowledgments

Table, "Blocher's Life Stages and Developmental Tasks," from D. H. Blocher, *Counseling: A Developmental Approach,* Fourth Edition. Copyright © 2000 by John Wiley & Sons, Inc. This material is used by permission of John Wiley & Sons, Inc.

"Rape Poem," by Marge Piercy, from *Circles on the Water* by Marge Piercy. Copyright © 1982 by Marge Piercy. Used by permission of Alfred A. Knopf, a division of Random House, Inc.

"Alcoholic's Anonymous Twelve-Steps." The Twelve Steps are reprinted and adapted with permission of Alcoholics Anonymous World Services, Inc. (A.A.W.S.) Permission to reprint and adapt the Twelve Steps does not mean that A.A.W.S. has reviewed or approved the contents of this publication, or that A.A.W.S. necessarily agrees with the views expressed herein. A.A. is a program of recovery from alcoholism only-use of the Twelve Steps in connection with programs and activities which are patterned after A.A., but which address other problems, or in any other non-A.A. context, does not imply otherwise.

"A Humanist Alternative to A.A.'s Twelve Steps: A Human-Centered Approach to Conquering Alcoholism," from *The Humanist*, Vol. 47, 5. Reprinted by permission of the B. F. Skinner Foundation.

G. Unterberger, "Twelve Steps for Women Alcoholics." Copyright © 1989 Christian Century Foundation. Reprinted with permission from the December 6, 1989 issue of *The Christian Century*.

Name Index

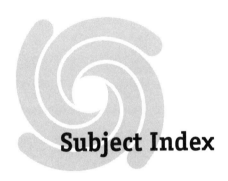

Subject Index